# ESSENTIALS OF
# ANORECTAL SURGERY

# ESSENTIALS OF ANORECTAL SURGERY

## STANLEY M. GOLDBERG, M.D., F.A.C.S.

*Clinical Professor and Director*
*Division of Colon and Rectal Surgery*
*Department of Surgery*
*University of Minnesota*
*Minneapolis, Minnesota*

## PHILIP H. GORDON, M.D., F.R.C.S. (C), F.A.C.S.

*Assistant Professor of Surgery (McGill University)*
*Associate Surgeon (Colon and Rectal), Jewish General Hospital*
*Montreal, Quebec, Canada*

## SANTHAT NIVATVONGS, M.D., F.A.C.S.

*Assistant Professor*
*Division of Colon and Rectal Surgery*
*Department of Surgery*
*University of Minnesota*
*Minneapolis, Minnesota*

### *Illustrated by*

### MARTIN E. FINCH, M.A.

*Director and Assistant Professor*
*Biomedical Graphic Communications, and*
*Assistant Professor*
*Division of Surgical Sciences*
*Department of Surgery*
*University of Minnesota*
*Minneapolis, Minnesota*

**J. B. LIPPINCOTT COMPANY**     **Philadelphia and Toronto**

3 5 6 4 2

**Library of Congress Cataloging in Publication Data**

Goldberg, Stanley M
  Essentials of anorectal surgery.

  Includes index.
  1. Anus—Surgery.  2. Rectum—Surgery.  I. Gordon,
Philip H., joint author.  II. Nivatvongs, Santhat,
joint author.  III. Title.  IV. Title: Anorectal
surgery.
RD544.G63        617′.555        79-24994
ISBN 0-397-50417-9

The authors and publisher have exerted every effort to ensure that drug selection
and dosage set forth in this text are in accord with current recommendations and
practice at the time of publication. However, in view of ongoing research,
changes in government regulations, and the constant flow of information relating
to drug therapy and drug reactions, the reader is urged to check the package insert for each drug for any change in indications and dosage and for added warn-
ings and precautions. This is particularly important when the recommended agent
is a new or infrequently employed drug.

# *Dedication*

The authors would like to dedicate this book to their wives
and their children
Luella, Ellen, Fredric, and Martha Goldberg;
Rosalie, Laurel, and Elliot Gordon;
and Wantana, Marisa, and Nitara Nivatvongs
from whom we stole the precious
hours and energy to write this book.

# *With the Collaboration of*

**Gregory W. Brabbee,** M.D.
Clinical Instructor of Surgery
Columbia College of Physicians and Surgeons
Junior Assistant Attending
Roosevelt Hospital,
New York, New York
(Chapter 26, Strictures of the Anorectum)

**John G. Buls,** MB., BS., FRACS
Senior Lecturer and Assistant Surgeon
University of Melbourne at St. Vincent's Hospital
Melbourne, Australia
(Chapter 6, Hemorrhoids)
(Chapter 11, Inflammatory Conditions of the Anorectum)
(Chapter 12, Sexually Transmitted Diseases of the Anorectum)

**William R. Johnson,** FRACS, FRCS
Lecturer, Department of Surgery
Monash University
Surgeon, Alfred Hospital
Melbourne, Australia
(Chapter 15, Benign Neoplasms of the Rectum)
(Chapter 16, Malignant Neoplasms of the Rectum)
(Chapter 17, Retrorectal Tumors)

**Philip Juno,** MB., BS., FFARACS
Assistant Professor of Anesthesia
University of Minnesota
Hennepin County Medical Center
Minneapolis, Minnesota
(Chapter 5, Principles of Anesthetic Management in Anorectal Surgery)

**Frederic D. Nemer,** M.D.
Clinical Instructor
Division of Colon and Rectal Surgery
University of Minnesota
Minneapolis, Minnesota
(Chapter 4, Pre- and Postoperative Management of Anorectal Wounds)
(Chapter 23, Injuries to the Anus and Rectum)
(Chapter 24, Complications in Anorectal Surgery—Their Prevention and Treatment)

**John D. Nicholson,** M.D.
Clinical Instructor
Department of Surgery
State University of New York
Upstate Medical Center
Syracuse, New York
(Chapter 10, Perianal Dermatology)
(Chapter 22, Anal Incontinence)

**Steven E. Olchowski,** M.D.
Clinical Instructor
Department of Surgery
Wayne State University
Detroit, Michigan
(Chapter 9, Pilonidal Sinus)

**David A. Rothenberger,** M.D.
Clinical Instructor
Division of Colon and Rectal Surgery
Department of Surgery
University of Minnesota
Minneapolis, Minnesota
(Chapter 25, Rectovaginal Fistula)

# Foreword:
## The History of Anorectal Surgery

### PART I

The history of the development of surgical treatment of diseases of the large intestine is long, interesting and, in some respects, very romantic. The abolition of barber surgeons as practitioners of surgery is directly related to the successful operation which cured Louis XIV of his fistula-in-ano and led to the teaching of surgery as a part of the medical school curriculum. In the post-Civil War period in the United States anorectal diseases were treated mostly by itinerant quacks and charlatans. This circumstance compelled the members of the medical profession to give more attention to these maladies and led to the specialty of proctology with its subsequent expansion to colon and rectal surgery. Operation on the anorectum antedated intra-abdominal colonic surgery by many centuries.

The first known treatise completely devoted to anorectal diseases is the Chester Beatty Medical Papyrus written about 1250 B.C. and translated in 1947. This treatise describes forty-one treatments for diseases of the anorectum. That specialists in anorectal diseases were present in ancient Egypt is attested to by the discovery of markers on graves of ancient Egyptian physicians, on one of which is inscribed ''Shepherd of the Anus'' and on another ''Guardian of the Anus.''

The writings of Hippocrates on hemorrhoids and fistula, circa 400 B.C., of Albucasis of Egypt on fistula, circa A.D. 1000, and of John Arderne of England on hemorrhoids, fistula, and clysters, circa A.D. 1367, testify to the surgical procedures in vogue in ancient days. The thought of using a red-hot iron, without benefit of anesthesia, to burn off protruding hemorrhoids is a shuddering thought in the 20th century. It was, however, an accepted method of treatment for Hippocrates. In the Hippocratic era fistulas were treated by the application of extracts of herbs and barks and by caustics applied to the interior of the fistulous track. Occasionally a seton was applied which was tightened daily until the tract was cut through.

The foundation upon which the present principles of good anorectal surgery was built was the *Treatise on Fistula, Hemorrhoids and Clysters* written by John Arderne of England in 1367 (Fig. 1). He stated that before any

# Early English Text Society.

### Original Series, 139.

# Treatises

### of

# Fistula in Ano

### Haemorrhoids, and Clysters

BY

## JOHN ARDERNE,

FROM

AN EARLY FIFTEENTH-CENTURY MANUSCRIPT TRANSLATION.

EDITED,

WITH INTRODUCTION, NOTES, ETC.,

BY

## D'ARCY POWER, F.R.C.S. ENG.

SURGEON TO, AND LECTURER ON SURGERY AT, ST. BARTHOLOMEW'S HOSPITAL.

PUBLISHED FOR THE EARLY ENGLISH TEXT SOCIETY

BY KEGAN PAUL, TRENCH, TRÜBNER & CO., LTD.,

DRYDEN HOUSE, 43 GERRARD STREET, SOHO, LONDON, W.

AND BY HENRY FROWDE, OXFORD UNIVERSITY PRESS,

AMEN CORNER, E.C., AND IN NEW YORK.

1910.

*Price Fifteen Shillings.*

FIGURE **1**

operation on the anorectum is undertaken, the surgeon should explore the anorectum with his finger to be sure that no hard masses are present. In the event that a mass is found, a cancer is probably present and surgery should not be performed because the case is incurable. Arderne's treatise was written before the advent of the printing press. His writings were read by few physicians and the treatment of anorectal diseases by physicians fell into disrepute.

The operation which cured Louis XIV of his fistula-in-ano in 1686 was the turning point not only for anorectal surgery but for surgery in general. That operation was of monumental historical importance for the following reasons. First, it established once and for all the necessity of laying open the fistula tract and the overlying sphincter muscle to cure a fistula. Second, prior to this operation, the monarch's physician, Philip, at the king's direction, conducted a full year of clinical trials on all methods known for the treatment of fistula. Only when it was determined that a fistulotomy was the only method which could cure a fistula did the king submit to surgery. This was the first recorded clinical research project supported by public funds. Third, by the official decree in 1715 of Louis XV, the grandson of Louis XIV, barber surgeons were forbidden to practice surgery and medical schools in France were ordered to include the teaching of anatomy and surgery in their curricula. Thus did surgeons gain their rightful place in the medical profession. The Royal Society of Surgeons in France came into existence in 1731, followed by the Royal College of Surgeons in England in 1800.

In 1765 Percivall Pott of St. Bartholomew's Hospital in London published his *Treatise on Fistula-in-Ano*. Pott refused to believe that such fistulas had their origin within the anorectum and felt that most anorectal abscesses were not fistulous and could never become fistulous without "the most supine neglect on the part of the patient or the most ignorant mismanagement on the part of the physician." He did, however, feel that all large anorectal abscesses could be cured by cutting the main wall of the abscess or the track with one clean cut into the lumen of the bowel and letting the wound granulate. He denied that this was a fistula operation but rather the proper treatment of an anorectal abscess. However, other surgeons, namely Cheselden of London and LeDran and De la Faye of Paris, did not agree with Pott and followed the principles handed down by Arderne.

The great advance in the treatment of anorectal disorders occurred with the opening of St. Mark's Hospital in London in 1835. Frederick Salmon was the founding father of that institution and served as its chief surgeon until 1859 when he was succeeded by James Lane and Peter Gouilland. The first name of the hospital was The Infirmary for the Relief of the Poor Afflicted with Fistula and Other Diseases of the Rectum. In his address on the occasion of the opening of the Hospital, Salmon referred to anorectal diseases as diseases "of which it may with truth be said that there are none more afflicting or distressing to bear, or which are productive of more serious consequences; whilst it may be doubtful whether there may be any branch of medical knowledge for the acquisition of which less facility has hitherto been afforded." Over the years an illustrious group of dedicated surgeons and pathologists have served St. Mark's Hospital with distinction and have made it the Mecca where surgeons learn the latest and best means of treating surgical diseases of the colon and anorectum.

The first published paper by Frederick Salmon was entitled "On the Causes, Symptoms and Morbid Anatomy of Simple and Malignant Stricture of the Rectum." This appeared in *The Lancet* in 1831.

In 1882, William Allingham, one of the early surgeons at St. Mark's Hospital, published the first comprehensive text on surgical diseases of the anorectum (Fig. 2). In it he gives the description of Salmon's operation for internal hemorrhoids. This is the first published description of the ligature and excision method for the removal of hemorrhoids. In 1903, in Volume I of the *British Medical Journal,* A. B. Mitchell of London published a paper on the clamp and ligature method, which was a modification of Salmon's technique. Mitchell's technique is still in use today, while Milligan and Morgan's

FISTULA, HEMORRHOIDS, PAINFUL ULCER,

STRICTURE, PROLAPSUS,

AND OTHER

# DISEASES OF THE RECTUM

THEIR

DIAGNOSIS AND TREATMENT.

BY

WILLIAM ALLINGHAM, M.D.,

FELLOW OF THE ROYAL COLLEGE OF SURGEONS OF ENGLAND; SURGEON TO ST. MARK'S HOSPITAL FOR
FISTULA AND OTHER DISEASES OF THE RECTUM, ETC.

FOURTH REVISED AND ENLARGED EDITION.
WITH ILLUSTRATIONS.

PHILADELPHIA:
P. BLAKISTON, SON & CO.,
1012 WALNUT STREET.
1882.

FIGURE **2**

modification of the ligature and excision technique described in 1937 enjoys great popularity.

## PART II

The story of the development of anorectal surgery in the United States is equally fascinating. Until 1878 there were no trained anorectal surgeons in the United States. The treatment of most anorectal diseases fell to the lot of the itinerant quacks and charlatans whose main method of therapy was the injection of sclerosing solutions into hemorrhoids. Doctor Mitchell of Clinton, Illinois, originated this form of treatment in the United States in 1871. He had gone to Europe to learn the technique and to acquire the formula of the sclerosing solutions which were being used in Ireland and Germany. Upon his return to Clinton he kept his formula secret, sold geographic franchises to other charlatans and sold his secret solutions at great profit. This disgraceful practice irked the ethical members of the medical profession and had the good effect of compelling their interest in learning more about anorectal diseases. Thus it was that Dr. Joseph W. Matthews of Louisville, Kentucky, journeyed to London to spend a year in training at St. Mark's Hospital and returned to Louisville as America's first proctologist. Dr. Matthews struck out against the charlatans and their methods. He began to teach the principles of anorectal surgery and, in 1899, became one of the founders and the first president of the American Proctologic Society. Because of his dedication and leadership in his chosen field, Matthews became known as ''The Father of Proctology'' in the United States.

In 1837, Dr. George Macartney Bushe, who was affiliated with Rutgers Medical School, published a *Treatise on the Malformation, Injuries, and Diseases of the Rectum and Anus* that received international recognition. This book is known as the first American book on proctology.

At about the time of Matthews's return to Louisville in 1878, Edmund Andrews and E. W. Andrews, professors of surgery in the Chicago Medical College, published the first popular textbook on rectal and anal surgery in the United States (Fig. 3). It contains a description of the secret methods of the itinerants. Considering the era in which it was written, it was an excellent dissertation on anorectal diseases.

In 1931 W. A. Fansler of Minneapolis introduced a new method (which he chose to call the anatomic dissection technique) for the surgical removal of hemorrhoids. He did not close the entire wound, but preferred to leave the distal centimeter or so open for drainage. In use at the University of Minnesota hospitals since its inception, and refined by Ferguson and Heaton who in 1959 described it as the ''closed hemorrhoidectomy,'' this technique is the one presented in this text. Because of its meticulous method of removing pathological tissue, controlling bleeding, and closing wounds, this operation has rightfully taken its place among modern advances in surgical techniques.

By the early part of this century the United States had developed many illustrious general surgeons and surgical teachers: J. B. Murphy, John B. Deaver, William S. Halsted, Charles and William Mayo, Frank Lahey, George W. Crile, Sr., and O. H. Wangensteen, to name a few. Many names could be added to the list. All of these men had a great interest in surgical diseases of the gastrointestinal tract; however, none of them had a major interest in anorectal surgery. In due time, men such as L. A. Buie, Sr., at the Mayo Clinic, Tom Jones at the Cleveland Clinic, Harry E. Bacon at Temple University, Neil Swinton at the Lahey Clinic, and Patrick H. Hanley at the Ochsner Clinic became the alter egos of the chiefs of surgery in their respective institutions in performing surgery of the anorectum. These men and others worked diligently to improve the quality of anorectal surgery in the United States and to establish training programs in colon and rectal surgery for future generations of surgeons.

Until the establishment of the American Board of Proctology in 1949, later to become the American Board of Colon and Rectal Surgery, most anorectal surgeons were self-taught, either by limiting their practices or by joining established anorectal surgeons. Many of these men became very expert in the field of anorectal surgery, but few had acquired the basic training in

# RECTAL AND ANAL SURGERY,

WITH

A DESCRIPTION OF THE SECRET METHODS
OF THE ITINERANTS.

BY

EDMUND ANDREWS, M.D., LL.D.,

PROFESSOR OF CLINICAL SURGERY IN THE CHICAGO MEDICAL COLLEGE,
SENIOR SURGEON TO MERCY HOSPITAL,

AND

E. WYLLYS ANDREWS, A.M., M.D.,

ADJUNCT PROFESSOR OF CLINICAL SURGERY IN THE CHICAGO MEDICAL
COLLEGE, SURGEON TO MERCY HOSPITAL.

WITH ORIGINAL ILLUSTRATIONS.

CHICAGO:
W. T. KEENER,
96 WASHINGTON ST.
1888.

FIGURE 3

general surgery so necessary for working within the abdomen. Today applicants for the Board of Colon and Rectal Surgery are qualified and/or board certified in general surgery and have completed a formal residency training program in colon and rectal surgery or an approved preceptorship program in this field.

Surgical residents in training programs which do not have qualified colon and rectal surgeons on their staffs find that their teaching in anorectal surgery is markedly deficient. In many institutions anorectal surgery is still regarded as minor surgery which can be delegated to the junior resident staff. Such errors of allowing surgery to be performed by inexperienced operators, if perpetuated, can only yield results which leave much to be desired. Only when trained and experienced colorectal surgeons are on the teaching staffs of surgical training programs can we expect an improvement in the quality of the surgery being performed.

Postgraduate courses in this specialty as a part of Continuing Medical Education Programs are now very popular, and, without question, this will result in better care for patients with anorectal surgical problems.

The American Board of Colon and Rectal Surgery has served this specialty well in setting high standards of practice and in accrediting only those training programs which measure up to the standards set by the Board. The task of conducting the work of the American Board is indeed an arduous one requiring many hours of hard work by the secretary and other members of the Board. The rewards of these efforts are great, however, when measured by the quality of the work performed by Board certified surgeons compared to those whose training has not qualified them for certification. The progress which has been made in medicine and surgery in general during the past century is well reflected in the quality of anorectal surgery being performed today compared to a century ago. Much of this improvement can be attributed to the work of the American Board of Colon and Rectal Surgery.

William C. Bernstein, M.D.
Emeritus Clinical Professor
Colon and Rectal Surgery
University of Minnesota
Minneapolis, Minnesota

# *Preface*

Most textbooks of surgery have a chapter or a subchapter on anorectal diseases and describe selected topics so briefly that the information provided is barely adequate for clinical application. With this in mind, we set out to write a practical book for the busy practicing surgeon, who can extract information from it in the shortest possible time and with the least possible effort. To help achieve this goal, we felt it beneficial to include over 300 illustrations. At the conclusion of our work on the book, we realized that many of its sections were longer than initially planned, but we believe, nevertheless, that this will be helpful to the reader who is interested in a fuller accounting of a given problem.

The subjects covered in *Essentials of Anorectal Surgery* are not exhaustive. The topics were selected to cover the majority of the day-to-day problems in practice. Emphasis was placed on the fundamentals of the diseases, explaining etiology and pathogenesis when applicable so that the rationale of the proposed treatment would be better understood. In addition to this "why" and "what," the reader will ascertain "how" and "when" to institute therapy. We thus believe that this book will prove useful not only to surgeons but as well to medical students and physicians interested in this field.

Stanley M. Goldberg
Philip H. Gordon
Santhat Nivatvongs

# Acknowledgments

We asked Dr. William C. Bernstein to write the Foreword to this book, for which we gratefully thank him. More important, we would like to acknowledge his keen interest in us as individuals, for he has been, in great part, directly responsible for our training.

His dedication to and foresight in the specialty have been extraordinary. Throughout his career, he has been an inspiration, promoting enthusiasm for the specialty. Early on, he recognized the need for training programs associated with major teaching centers and was the driving force in establishing a residency program in a university setting (University of Minnesota). Long before it was considered fashionable and eventually became mandatory, he recognized the need for postgraduate continuing medical education and expanded the course in the principles of colon and rectal surgery which has been continued annually to the present day. He is responsible for the training of many fine colon and rectal surgeons who are currently practicing and teaching the specialty. He has contributed numerous scientific papers to the colon and rectal literature. Consequently, we the authors would like to salute Dr. Bernstein, a special pioneer who has tirelessly dedicated himself to the betterment of the quality of care of the unfortunate patient afflicted with a colon or anorectal disorder.

Many individuals contributed to the preparation of this text and the authors would like to acknowledge their assistance with deep gratitude.

Certain chapters were written in collaboration with various colleagues. They include Drs. Gregory W. Brabbee, John G. Buls, William R. Johnson, Philip Juno, Frederic D. Nemer, John D. Nicholson, Steven E. Olchowski, and David A. Rothenberger. Their contributions are separately acknowledged in what follows.

Any textbook requires an enormous amount of secretarial support and we feel quite fortunate in having had the aid of a group of very competent people. For typing of the manuscript our thanks go to Rosalind Michaels, Judy Kern, Nancy Tomlinson, and Marsha Spon. For supervising the typing and organizing the manuscripts as well as for her faithful prodding and encouragement, particular thanks go to Joyce Hustleby.

The illustrations were drawn by Martin E. Finch, M. A. His talented work has converted many words into pictures, and for his outstanding effort we would like to thank him.

We would like to thank the staff of J. B. Lippincott, especially Stuart Freeman, Editor-in-Chief, and Lisa Biello, Associate Editor, for their patience and their confidence in us during the preparation of the text.

# Contents

# 1

# Anatomy of Rectum and Anal Canal

## RECTUM

The rectum is arbitrarily described as beginning at the level of the S3 vertebra, descending along the curvature of the sacrum and coccyx, and ending at the upper aspect of the pelvic diaphragm. There it abruptly turns downward and backward, passes through the levator ani muscles, and becomes the anal canal. It measures 12 to 15 cm. in length. In its short course, the rectum describes three lateral curves: the upper and lower are convex to the right and the middle is convex to the left. At their inner aspect these in-foldings are recognized as the valves of Houston. Their clinical values are that they must be negotiated during successful proctosigmoidoscopic examination, and, more important, they are an excellent location for a rectal biopsy because the inward protrusion makes an easy target. They do not contain all the layers of the bowel wall and, therefore, biopsy here carries a minimal risk of perforation. The middle fold is the internal landmark corresponding to the anterior peritoneal reflection. Consequently, extra caution must be exercised in removing polyps above this level. Due to the curves, when the rectum has been completely straightened, as in performing a low anterior resection, one may gain 5 cm. in length; hence, a lesion initially appearing at 7 cm. from the anal verge may actually be located 12 cm. from it, after complete mobilization (Fig. 1-1).

The transition from the sigmoid colon to the rectum is a gradual one. It is characterized by the taeniae coli spreading out from three distinct bands to a uniformly distributed layer of longitudinal, smooth muscle, which is thicker on the front and back than on its side, thus accounting for the lateral flexures. The rectum lacks a mesentery, sacculations, and appendices epiploicae.[24]

### Peritoneal Relations

For descriptive purposes, the rectum is divided into upper, middle and lower thirds. The upper third is covered by peritoneum anteriorly and laterally, the middle third is covered anteriorly only, and the lower third is devoid of peritoneum. The peritoneal reflection shows considerable individual and sexual variation. In men it is usually 7.0 to 9.0 cm. from the anal verge, while in women it is 5.0 to 7.5 cm. above the anal verge. The middle valve of Houston roughly corresponds to the anterior peritoneal reflection. The posterior peritoneal reflection is usually 12 to 15 cm. from the anal verge (Fig. 1-2).

### Fascial Attachments

The posterior part of the rectum is devoid of peritoneum but it is covered with a thin layer of pelvic fascia called the fascia propria. On each side of the rectum below the peritoneum there is a condensation of fascia, known as the lateral ligaments or lateral stalks, which connects the rectum to the parietal pelvic fascia. These require ligation during excision or mobilization of the rectum. The sacrum and coccyx are covered with a strong fascia, which is part of the parietal pelvic fascia, and is referred to as the presacral fascia. It covers the middle sacral vessels. At approximately the

*1*

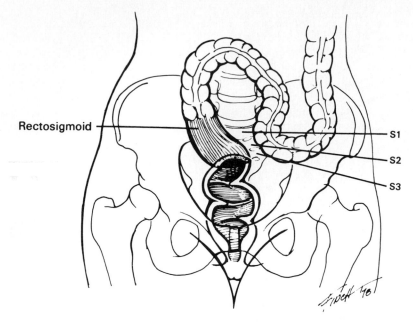

Rectosigmoid ——————— S1

——— S2

——— S3

FIGURE **1-1.** *The curves of the rectum.*

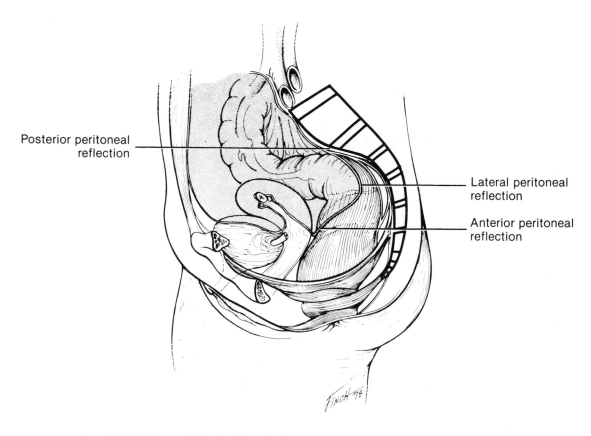

Posterior peritoneal
reflection ————————

———— Lateral peritoneal
reflection

———— Anterior peritoneal
reflection

FIGURE **1-2.** *Peritoneal relationship of the rectum.* (*Modified from Netter, F.: Ciba. Found. Symp. 3:57, 1969).*

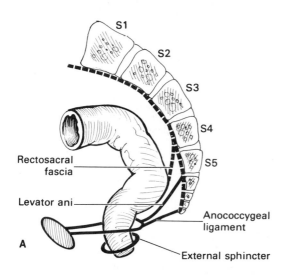
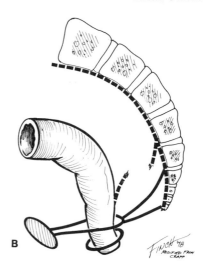

**FIGURE 1-3.** (*A*) *Rectosacral fascia.* (*B*) *Division of the rectosacral fascia for full mobilization of the rectum.* (*Modified from Crapp, A., et al.: Surg. Gynecol. Obstet., 138:252, 1974*).

level of the fourth sacral segment there is a strong avascular fascia, which runs forward and downward, and attaches to the fascia propria at the anorectal junction. This is referred to as the rectosacral fascia or Waldeyer's fascia (Fig. 1-3A).[8] It is necessary to sharply divide this fascia for full mobilization of the rectum (Fig. 1-3B). The posterior space below the rectosacral fascia is the supralevator or infrarectal space (Fig. 1-10). Anteriorly, the extraperitoneal portion of the rectum is covered with a visceral pelvic fascia known as Denonvillier's fascia. This fascia extends from the peritoneal reflection to the uro-genital diaphragm, and becomes continuous with the front of the lateral ligaments. It separates the rectum from the prostate and seminal vesicles or vagina.

## ANAL CANAL

The anal canal is the terminal portion of the intestinal tract. It begins at the anorectal junction, is 3 to 4 cm. in length, and terminates at the anal verge. It is surrounded by strong muscles, and due to the tonic contraction of these muscles it is completely collapsed and represents an antero-posterior slit (Fig. 1-4).

The musculature of the anorectal region may be regarded as two tubes, one surrounding the other.[19] The inner tube, being visceral, is smooth muscle and innervated by the autonomic nervous system while the outer, funnel-shaped tube is skeletal muscle and has somatic innervation. This short segment of the intestinal tract is of paramount importance because it is essential to the mechanism of continence and is prone to many diseases.

### Lining

The lining of the anal canal consists of epithelium of different types at different levels (Fig. 1-5). At approximately the mid point of the anal canal there is an undulating demarcation referred to as the dentate line. This line is approximately 2 cm. from the anal verge. Because the rectum narrows into the anal canal the tissue above the dentate line takes on a pleated appearance. These longitudinal folds, of which there are six to 14, are known as the columns of Morgagni. Between adjacent columns, at the lower end, there is a small pocket or crypt. These crypts are of surgical significance in that foreign material may lodge in them, obstructing the ducts of the anal glands, which results in sepsis. The mucosa of the upper anal canal is lined by columnar epithelium. Below the dentate line, the anal canal is lined with a squamous epithelium. The change, however, is not abrupt. For a distance of 6 to 12 mm. above the dentate line there is a gradual transition where columnar, transi-

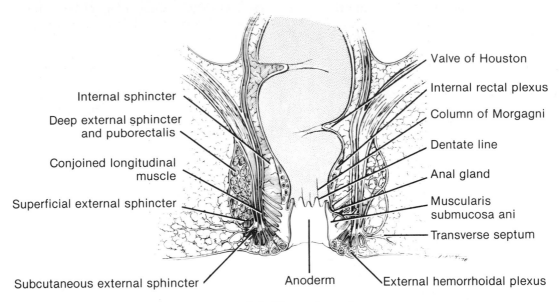

Internal sphincter

Deep external sphincter and puborectalis

Conjoined longitudinal muscle

Superficial external sphincter

Subcutaneous external sphincter

Valve of Houston

Internal rectal plexus

Column of Morgagni

Dentate line

Anal gland

Muscularis submucosa ani

Transverse septum

Anoderm

External hemorrhoidal plexus

FIGURE **1-4.** *The anal canal.*

tional or squamous epithelium may be found.[15,17] This area has been referred to as the cloacogenic zone and is important when neoplasms which arise here are considered.

A color change in the epithelium is also noted. The rectal mucosa is pink, whereas, the area just above the dentate line is deep purple or plum color, due to the subjacent internal hemorrhoidal plexus. Subepithelial tissue is loosely attached to and readily distensible from the internal hemorrhoidal plexus. Subepithelial tissue at the anal margin, which contains the external hemorrhoidal plexus, forms a lining which adheres firmly to the underlying tissue. At the level of the valves, the lining is anchored by what Parks called the mucosal suspensory ligament.[19a] The perianal space is limited, above by this ligament, and below by the

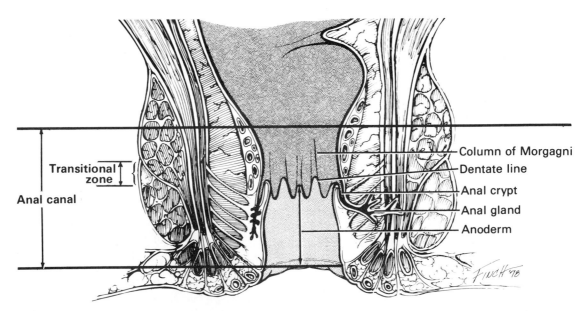

Transitional zone

Anal canal

Column of Morgagni

Dentate line

Anal crypt

Anal gland

Anoderm

FIGURE **1-5.** *The lining of the anal canal.*

attachments of the longitudinal muscle to the skin of the anal verge. The area below the dentate line is not true skin since it is devoid of accessory skin structures (*i.e.*, hair and sebaceous and sweat glands). This pale, delicate, smooth, thin, and shiny stretched tissue is referred to as anoderm, and runs for approximately 1.5 cm below the dentate line. At the anal verge the lining becomes thicker, pigmented, acquires hair follicles and glands, and other histologic features of normal skin.[17] In the circumanal area there is also a well marked ring of apocrine glands which may be the source of the clinical condition called hidradenitis suppurativa. Proximal to the dentate line, the epithelium is supplied by the autonomic nervous system, while distally the lining is richly innervated by the somatic nervous system.[10]

### Anal Intramuscular Glands

There is a variable number of intramuscular glands (4–10) in a normal anal canal. Each is lined by stratified columnar epithelium and has a direct opening into an anal crypt.[17] Occasionally two glands open into the same crypt, while half the crypts have no gland communication. These glands were first described by Chiari in 1878.[6] The importance of their role in the pathogenesis of fistulous abscess was presented by Parks in 1961.[19] These tubular structures enter the submucosa, two thirds of them entering the internal sphincter and half of these crossing into the intersphincteric plane. They do not penetrate the external sphincter. Their general direction is outward and downward. They may also be the site of origin of an adenocarcinoma.[9]

## MUSCLES

### Internal Sphincter

The downward continuation of the circular, smooth muscle of the rectum becomes thick and rounded at its lower end and is referred to as the internal sphincter. Its lowest portion is just above the lowest portion of the external sphincter and is 1.0 to 1.5 cm. below the dentate line (Fig. 1-4).

### Conjoined Longitudinal Muscle

At the level of the anorectal ring, the longitudinal muscle coat of the rectum is joined by fibers of the levator ani and puborectalis muscles. The conjoined longitudinal muscle so formed, descends between the internal and external anal sphincters (Fig. 1-4).[23] Many of these fibers traverse the lower portion of the external sphincter to gain insertion in the perianal skin, and are referred to as the corrugator cutis ani.[14] Fine and Lawes described a longitudinal layer of muscle lying on the inner aspect of the internal sphincter and named it the muscularus submucosae ani.[11] These fibers may arise from the conjoined longitudinal muscle. Some fibers which traverse the internal sphincter, and become inserted just below the anal valves, have been referred to as the mucosal suspensory ligament.[19] Some fibers may traverse the external sphincter to form the transverse septum of the ischiorectal fossa (Fig. 1-4). It has been suggested that the role of the conjoined longitudinal muscle is to affix the anal canal and to evert the anus during defecation.[21]

### Voluntary Muscle

*External Sphincter.* This elliptical cylinder of skeletal muscle which surrounds the anal canal was originally described as consisting of three distinct divisions: the subcutaneous, superficial, and deep portions.[16] This account was shown to be invalid by Goligher who demonstrated that a sheet of muscle runs continuously upward with the puborectalis and levator ani muscle.[13] The lowest portion of this muscle occupies a position below, and slightly lateral to, the internal sphincter. A palpable groove at this level has been referred to as the intersphincteric groove. The lowest part (subcutaneous fibers) is traversed by the conjoined longitudinal muscle with some fibers gaining attachment to the skin. The next portion (superficial) is attached to the coccyx by a posterior extension of muscle fibers, which combine with connective tissue, forming the anococcygeal ligament. Above this level the deep portion of the external sphincter is devoid of a posterior attachment and proximally becomes continuous with the puborectalis. Anteriorly, the higher fibers of the external sphincter are inserted into the perineal body where some merge and are continuous with the transverse perineal muscles. The external sphincter is supplied by the inferior rectal nerve and a perineal branch of the fourth sacral nerve.

Recently, Shafik has suggested that the anal sphincter mechanism consists of three

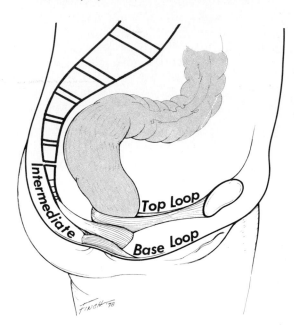

FIGURE **1-6.** *The external anal sphincter.*

U-shaped loops (Fig. 1-6).[23] The top loop, comprised of the deep portion of the external sphincter fused with the puborectalis, is postulated to function as one muscle. It arises from the lower part of the pubic symphysis and loops around the upper part of the anal canal with a downward inclination. The intermediate loop, directed horizontally, roughly corresponding to the superficial external sphincter, surrounds the anal canal, and is attached via the anococcygeal ligament to the coccyx. The base loop corresponds to the subcutaneous portion of the external sphincter. Its fibers pass from the lowest portion of the anal canal, directed anteriorly and downward, and attach to the perianal skin. Shafik believes that during voluntary contraction the three loops contract in different directions. The top and base loops, innervated by the inferior rectal nerve, will bring the posterior anal wall anteriorly; whereas, the intermediate loop, supplied by the fourth sacral nerve, pulls the anal canal posteriorly. Thus each loop is a separate sphincter and complements the others to help maintain continence.

*Levator ani muscles.* The levator ani muscle is a broad, thin muscle which forms the greater part of the floor of the pelvic cavity, and is innervated by the fourth sacral nerve. This muscle has traditionally been considered to consist of three muscles: the iliococcygeus, pubococcygeus and puborectalis.[12] More recent work, by Oh and Kark, and Shafik, suggests that it consists only of the iliococcygeus and pubococcygeus, and that the puborectalis is part of the deep portion of the external sphincter since the two are fused and have the same nerve supply (Fig. 1-7).[18,22]

THE ILIOCOCCYGEUS arises from the ischial spine and posterior part of the obturator fascia, passes downward, backward, and medially, and becomes inserted on the last two segments of the sacrum and the anococcygeal raphe.

THE PUBOCOCCYGEUS arises from the anterior half of the obturator fascia and back of the pubis. Its fibers are directed backward, downward and medially where they decussate with fibers of the opposite side.[22] This line of decussation is called the anococcygeal raphe (Fig. 1-7). Some fibers, which lie more posteriorly, are attached directly to the tip of the coccyx and last segment of the sacrum. This muscle also sends fibers to share in the formation of the conjoint longitudinal muscle (Fig. 1-4).

The muscle fibers of the pubococcygeus, while proceeding backward, downward, and medially, form an elliptical space called the "levator hiatus" (Fig. 1-7) through which the lower part of the rectum, prostatic urethra, and dorsal vein of the penis in men or vagina, and urethra in women pass. The intrahiatal viscera are bound together by part of the pelvic fascia which is more condensed at the level of the anorectal junction, and has been called the "hiatal ligament" by Shafik (Fig. 1-8).[22] He believes that the function of this "ligament" is to keep the movement of the intrahiatal structures in harmony with the levator ani muscle.

According to Shafik, the crisscross arrangement of the anococcygeal raphe prevents the constrictor effect upon the intrahiatal structures during levator ani contraction, and causes a dilator effect.[22] The puborectalis and levator ani muscles have a reciprocal action: as one contracts, the other relaxes. During defecation there is puborectalis relaxation accompanied by levator ani contraction which widens the hiatus and elevates the lower rec-

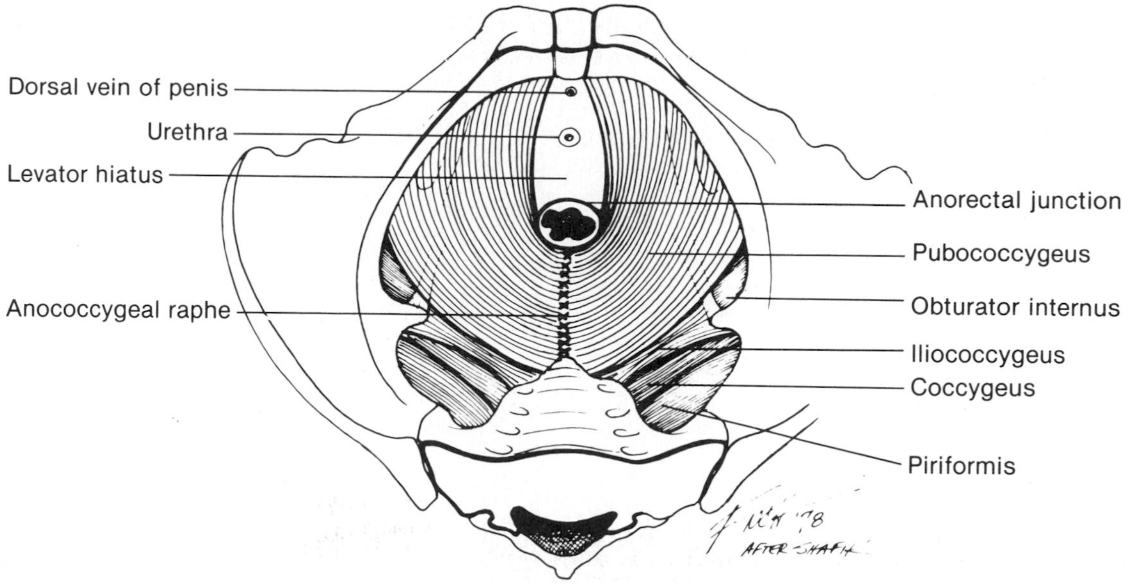

Dorsal vein of penis

Urethra

Levator hiatus

Anococcygeal raphe

Anorectal junction

Pubococcygeus

Obturator internus

Iliococcygeus

Coccygeus

Piriformis

FIGURE **1-7.** *The levator ani muscles and the levator hiatus.* (*Modified from Shafik, A.: Invest. Urol.,* **13:**175, 1975).

tum and anal canal. In an upright position, the levator ani muscle supports the viscera.

*Puborectalis.* This muscle arises from the back of the symphysis pubis and the superior fascia of the urogenital diaphragm, runs backward alongside the anorectal junction, and

joins its fellow muscle of the other side immediately behind the rectum where they form a U-shaped loop which slings the rectum to the pubes.

*"Anorectal ring",* a term coined by Milligan and Morgan, denotes the functionally impor-

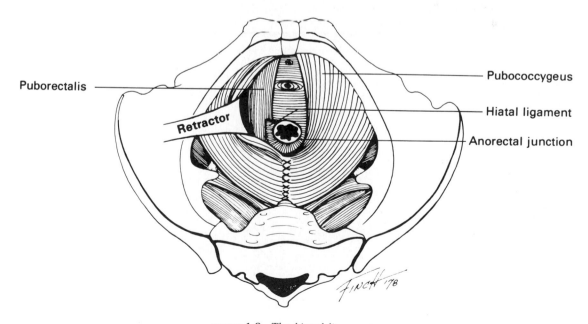

Puborectalis

Retractor

Pubococcygeus

Hiatal ligament

Anorectal junction

FIGURE **1-8.** *The hiatal ligament.*

tant ring of muscle which surrounds the junction of the rectum and anal canal.[16] It is composed of the upper borders of the internal and external sphincters, and the puborectalis muscle. It is of paramount importance during the treatment of abscesses and fistulae because division of this ring will inevitably result in anal incontinence.

## ANORECTAL SPACES

Certain potential spaces in and about the anorectal region are of surgical significance and will be briefly described (Fig. 1-9, 1-10).

*Perianal space,* which is also referred to as the marginal space, is in the immediate area of the anal verge surrounding the anal canal. Laterally, it becomes continuous with the subcutaneous fat of the buttocks, or may be confined by the conjoined longitudinal muscle, while medially, it extends into the lower part of the anal canal as far as the dentate line. It is continuous with the intersphincteric space. It contains the lowest part of the external sphincter, the external hemorrhoidal plexus, branches of the inferior rectal vessels, and lymphatics. The radiating elastic septa divide the space into a compact honey-comb ar-

rangement which accounts for the severe pain produced by collections of pus or blood.

*The ischiorectal fossa* is a pyramid-shaped space. The apex is formed at the origin of the levator ani from the obturator fascia, and the inferior boundary is the skin of the perineum. The anterior boundary is formed by the superficial and deep transversus perinei muscles, and the posterior boundary of the perineal membrane. The posterior boundary is made up of the sacrotuberous ligament, and the lower border of the gluteus maximus muscle. The medial wall is composed of the levator ani and the external sphincter muscles, including the fascia that covers them. The lateral wall is nearly vertical, is formed by the obturator internus muscle, where it lies on the ischium, and by the obturator fascia. In the obturator fascia, on the lateral wall, is Alcock's canal which contains the internal pudendal vessels and pudendal nerve. The contents of the ischiorectal fossa include a pad of fat, the inferior rectal nerve, coursing from the back of the ischiorectal fossa forward, and medially to the external sphincter, inferior rectal vessels, portions of the scrotal nerves and vessels in men and labial in women, the transverse perineal vessels, and the perineal branch of the

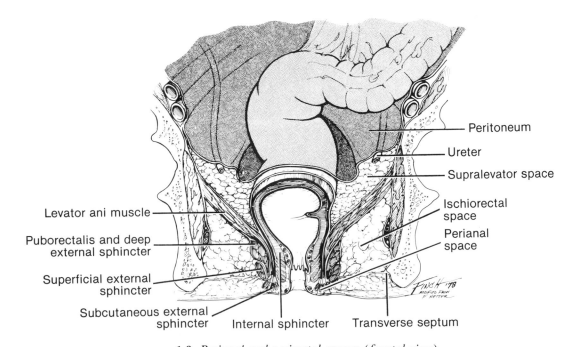

FIGURE **1-9.** *Perianal and perirectal spaces (frontal view).*

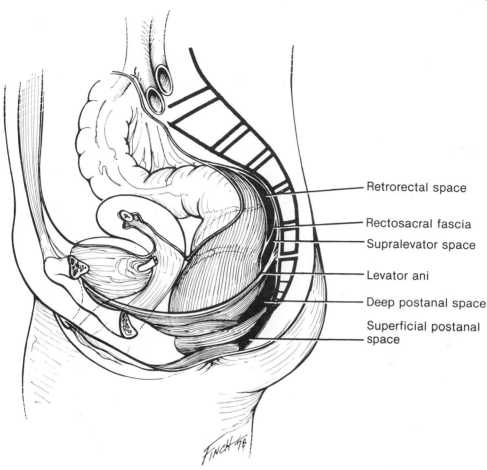

Retrorectal space

Rectosacral fascia

Supralevator space

Levator ani

Deep postanal space

Superficial postanal space

FIGURE **1-10.** *Perianal and perirectal spaces (lateral view).*

fourth sacral nerve running to the external sphincter from the posterior angle of the fossa.[5] Anteriorly the ischiorectal space has an important extension forward, above the urogenital diaphragm, which may become filled with pus in cases of ischiorectal abscesses.

*The Intersphincteric space* lies between the internal and the external sphincter muscles, is continuous below with the perianal space, and extends above into the wall of the rectum.

*The Supralevator space* is situated on each side of the rectum, bounded superiorly by the peritoneum, laterally by the pelvic wall, medially by the rectum, and below by the levator ani muscle. Sepsis in this area may occur due to upward extension of anal glandular origin or from pelvic origin.

*The Submucous space* lies between the internal sphincter and the mucosa. It extends distally to the dentate line, and proximally becomes continuous with the submucosa of the rectum. It contains the internal hemorrhoidal plexus. Although abscesses have been described in this space, they are probably of little clinical significance, and have been mistaken for what, in fact, were intersphincteric abscesses.

*The Superficial postanal space* connects the ischiorectal fossae with each other posteriorly, under the ano-coccygeal ligament.

*Deep postanal space (space of Courtney).* The right and left ischiorectal spaces are continuous posteriorly, above the ano-coccygeal ligament, but below the levator muscle, through

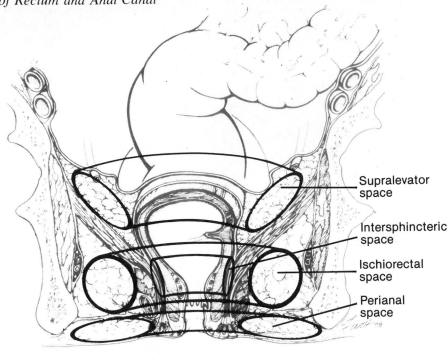

Supralevator
space

Intersphincteric
space

Ischiorectal
space

Perianal
space

FIGURE **1-11.** *"Horseshoe" connection of anorectal spaces.*

the deep postanal space or the retrosphincteric space of Courtney.[7] This postanal space is the usual pathway for purulent infection to spread from one ischiorectal fossa to the other resulting in the so-called *horseshoe fistula* (Fig. 1-11).

*The Retrorectal space* lies between the upper two-thirds of the rectum and sacrum above the rectosacral fascia. It is limited anteriorly by the fascia propria covering the rectum, posteriorly by presacral fascia, and laterally by the lateral ligaments (stalks) of the rectum. Superiorly, it communicates with the retroperitoneal space, and inferiorly, is limited by the retrosacral fascia which passes forward from the S4 vertebrae to the rectum, 3 to 5 cm. proximal to the anorectal junction. Below the rectosacral fascia is the supralevator space, a horseshoe shaped potential space, limited anteriorly by Denonvillier's fascia, and below by the levator ani (Fig. 1-10, 16-1). The retrorectal space contains loose connective tissue. The presacral fascia protects the presacral vessels which lie deep to it. The presacral veins are part of the extensive vertebral plexus, and responsible for the major bleeding problems encountered in this area during operation. In addition to the usual tissues from which neoplasms can arise, this is an area of embryological fusion and remodeling; thus, the site for persistence of embryological remnants from which neoplasms can also arise.

## CIRCULATION
### Blood Supply of Rectum and Anal Canal

*The superior rectal (hemorrhoidal) artery* is the continuation of the inferior mesenteric artery which, after crossing the left common iliac artery, changes its name to superior rectal artery (Fig. 1-12). It descends in the sigmoid mesocolon where, at the level of the third sacral segment, it bifurcates into right and left branches with the right branch further dividing into a right anterior, and right posterior branch. Further branches pierce the muscular coat, and in the submucosal plane reach the anal columns, where they terminate above the anal valves as a capillary plexus. This vascular distribution may account for the prominence of hemorrhoids in the three major positions.

*The middle rectal arteries* arise from the anterior divisions of the internal iliac arteries and reach the lower portion of the rectum anterolaterally at the level of the levator ani muscle. They have been described as not traversing the lateral stalks as previously believed.[4] They supply the lower part of the rectum, and upper anal canal.

*The inferior rectal arteries* arise from the internal pudendal arteries (in Alcock's canal) which in turn arise from the internal iliac. They traverse the ischiorectal fossa supplying the anal sphincter muscles.

*The middle sacral artery* (median sacral artery) arises from the back of the aorta, 1.5 cm. above its bifurcation descends over the last two lumbar vertebrae, sacrum, and coccyx, and behind the left common iliac vein, the presacral nerve, and the superior rectal vessels

to suply the lower portion of the rectum. The surgical significance of this vessel is that during rectal excision it is exposed on the front of the sacrum, and when the coccyx is disarticulated this vessel may give rise to troublesome bleeding.

There is some controversy as to the various anastomoses of the three supplying vessels. It has been stated that the anastomoses of the gut wall are so extensive that the middle and inferior rectal arteries can supply the entire rectum if the inferior mesenteric artery is ligated.[1,13] Goligher believes that the middle rectal arteries anastomose with the superior and inferior rectal arteries, as well as the inferior rectal artery communicating with its namesake of the opposite side.[12] On the other hand, Boxall, stated that there is no evidence of an anastomosis between the superior and inferior rectal arteries.[4]

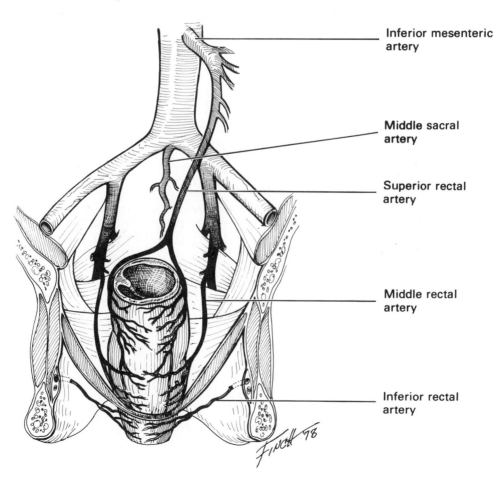

FIGURE **1-12.** *Arterial supply of the rectum and anal canal.*

## Venous Drainage of the Rectum and Anal Canal

Blood return from the rectum and anal canal is via two systems: portal and systemic (Fig. 1-13). The superior rectal, or hemorrhoidal, vein drains the rectum and upper part of the anal canal into the portal system via the inferior mesenteric vein. The middle rectal veins drain the lower part of the rectum and upper part of the anal canal into the systemic circulation via the internal iliac veins. The inferior rectal veins drain the lower part of the anal canal via the internal pudendal veins which empty into the internal iliac veins; hence, into the systemic circulation. The veins accompany the corresponding arteries.

There are differing opinions as to the anastomoses formed by these three systems. Some researchers believe a communication between the superior and middle rectal veins forms an important anastomosis between the portal and systemic systems.[12] The anastomosis of the inferior rectal veins, with the middle and superior rectal veins, constitute another portal systemic anastomosis. Tributaries of the superior, middle, and inferior rectal veins communicate at the level of the rectal, or hemorrhoidal, plexus in the submucosa of the columns of Morgagni. Dilatation of this plexus, for whatever reason, is one theory for the causation of internal hemorrhoids.

## Lymphatic Drainage of the Rectum and Anal Canal

The lymphatic vessels follow the arterial blood supply. Lymph from the upper and middle parts of the rectum ascends along the superior rectal artery and, subsequently, to the inferior mesenteric lymph nodes. The

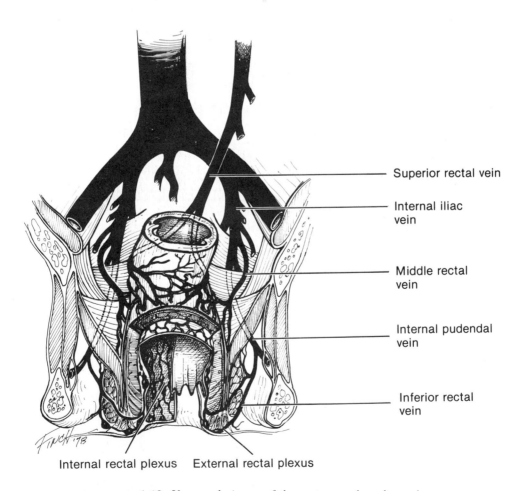

Superior rectal vein

Internal iliac vein

Middle rectal vein

Internal pudendal vein

Inferior rectal vein

Internal rectal plexus    External rectal plexus

FIGURE **1-13.** *Venous drainage of the rectum and anal canal.*

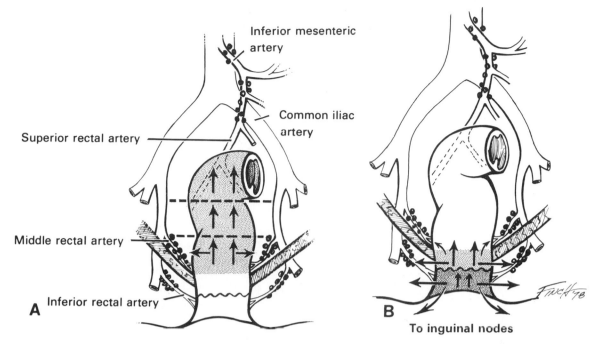

FIGURE **1-14.** (*A*) *Lymphatic drainage of the rectum.* (*B*) *Lymphatic drainage of the anal canal.*

lower part of the rectum drains cephalad, via the superior rectal lymphatics, to the inferior mesenteric nodes, and laterally, via the middle rectal lymphatics, to the internal iliac nodes (Fig. 1-14A).

Lymphatics from the anal canal above the dentate line drain cephalad, via the superior rectal lymphatics, to the inferior mesenteric nodes, and laterally, along both the middle rectal vessels and inferior rectal vessels through the ischiorectal fossa to the internal iliac nodes (Fig. 1-14B).[12] Lymph from the anal canal, below the dentate line, usually drains to the inguinal lymph nodes; however, it can drain to the superior rectal lymph nodes, or along the inferior rectal lymphatics, to the ischiorectal fossa if obstruction exists (Fig. 1-14B).[12]

Studies in women have shown that when dye is injected 5 cm. above the anal verge, spread occurs to the posterior vaginal wall, uterus, cervix, broad ligament, fallopian tubes, ovaries, and cul de sac. When dye was injected at 10 cm. above the anal verge, spread occurred only to the broad ligament and the cul de sac; whereas, injection at 15 cm. showed no spread to the genital organs.[3] It has been generally agreed that metastases to the lymph nodes, below the level of a carcinoma of the rectum (retrograde lymphatic spread), occurs only after there has been extensive involvement of perirectal structures, serosal surfaces, veins, perineural lymphatics, and proximal lymphatic channels.[20] This information is obviously helpful in planning a curative operation for a patient with a rectal or anal canal malignancy.

## INNERVATION OF RECTUM AND ANUS

The large intestine, including the rectum, is innervated by the sympathetic and parasympathetic systems. The external anal sphincter and the lining of the anal canal, below the dentate line, are supplied by somatic nerves. The following account draws heavily from the description by Goligher.[12]

### Rectum

*The sympathetic fibers* to the rectum are derived from the first three lumbar segments of the spinal cord, which pass through the ganglionated sympathetic chains, and leave as

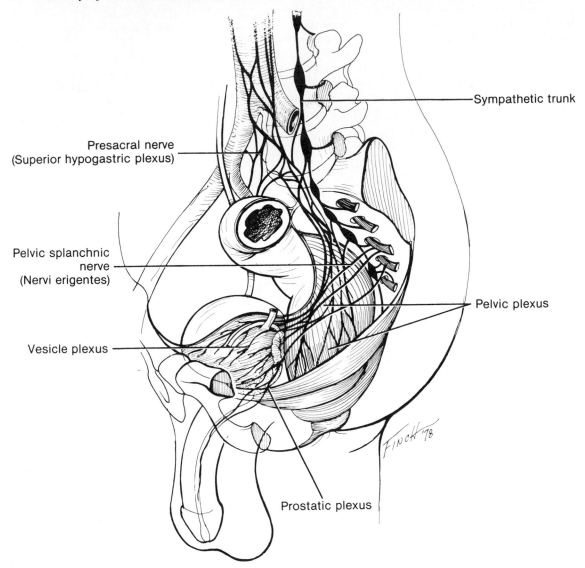

**FIGURE 1-15.** *Nerve supply to the rectum (lateral view).*

a lumbar sympathetic nerve which joins the preaortic plexus. From here, a prolongation extends along the inferior mesenteric artery, as the inferior mesenteric plexus, and reaches the upper part of the rectum.

The presacral, or hypogastric, nerve arises from the aortic plexus and the two lateral lumbar splanchnic nerves (Figs. 1-15 & 1-16). The plexus thus formed divides into two branches which separate, and pass to each side of the pelvis, where they join branches of the sacral parasymphatetic nerves, or nervi erigentes, to form the pelvic plexuses (Fig. 1-16). These

supply the lower rectum, anal canal, urinary bladder, and sexual organs. This distribution does not follow the course of blood vessels.

The presacral nerve lies behind the inferior mesenteric vessels between the two ureters but is closely applied to the iliac vessels and lumbar vertebrae (Fig. 1-16). The two branches of the presacral nerve descend, closely attached to the postero-lateral aspect of the rectum, and unless special attention is given to brush them off the bowel, they are liable to injury during rectal mobilization. Once the divisions of the presacral nerves have reached the pelvic side-wall, and joined the parasympathetic nerves, they are probably less liable to injury; although, they may be cut if the lateral ligaments are drawn-in excessively or divided unduly, laterally, or if dissection of the internal iliac lymph nodes was undertaken.

*The parasympathetic nerve supply* is from the nervi erigentes, which originate from the second, third, and fourth sacral nerves, on either side of the anterior sacral foramina, and pass laterally forward, and upward, to join the pelvic plexuses on the pelvic side-walls, from where fibers are distributed to the pelvic organs (Fig. 1-15).

Both parasympathetic and sympathetic nervous systems are involved in erection. The nerve impulses from the parasympathetic nerves which lead to erection produce arteriolar vasodilatation and increased blood in the cavernous spaces of the penis. Activity of the sympathetic system inhibits vasoconstriction of the penile vessels; thereby, adding to vascular engorgement and erection. Moreover, sympathetic activity causes contraction of the ejaculatory ducts, seminal vesicles, and prostate, with subsequent expulsion of semen into the posterior urethra.[2] Depending upon which nerves have been damaged certain deficiencies may occur, including incomplete erection, lack of ejaculation, or total impotence.

**Anal Canal**

*Motor Innervation.* The internal sphincter is supplied by both the sympathetics and parasympathetics which presumably reach the muscle by the same route as that followed to the lower rectum. The sympathetic is motor, and parasympathetic inhibitory to the sphincter. The external sphincter is supplied by the inferior rectal branch of the internal pudendal, and the perineal branch of the fourth sacral nerve. Levator ani muscles are supplied, on their pelvic surface, by twigs from the fourth sacral nerves, and on their perineal aspect,

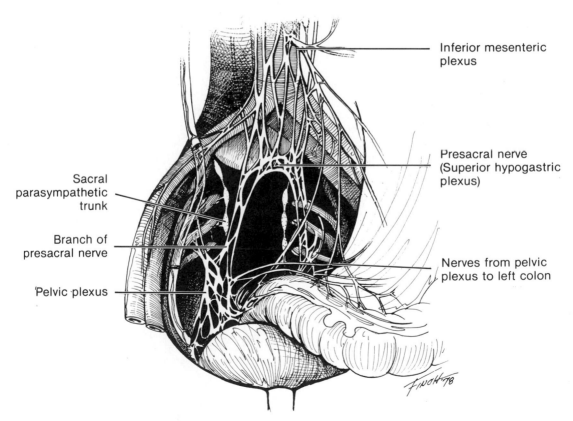

Inferior mesenteric plexus

Presacral nerve (Superior hypogastric plexus)

Nerves from pelvic plexus to left colon

Sacral parasympathetic trunk

Branch of presacral nerve

Pelvic plexus

FIGURE **1-16.** *Nerve supply to the rectum (frontal view).*

by the inferior rectal, or perineal branches, of the pudendal nerves.

*Sensory Innervation.* The cutaneous sensation, experienced in the perianal region and wall of the anal canal below the dentate line, is conveyed by the afferent fibers in the inferior rectal nerves; hence, can be abolished by an inferior rectal nerve block.[10] A poorly defined dull sensation, experienced in the mucosa above the dentate line, in response to touching with forceps or injection of hemorrhoids, is possibly mediated via the parasympathetic nerves.

# REFERENCES

1. Ault, G. W., Castro, A. F. and Smith, R. S.: Clinical study of ligation of the inferior mesenteric artery in left colon resections. Surg. Gynecol. Obstet., *94:*223, 1952.

2. Babb, R. R. and Kieraldo, J. H.: Sexual dysfunction after abdominoperineal resection. Dig. Dis., *22:*1127, 1977.

3. Block, I. R. & Enquist, I. F.: Lymphatic studies pertaining to local spread of carcinoma of the rectum in female. Surg. Gynecol. Obstet., *112:*41, 1961.

4. Boxall, T. A., Smart, P. J. G. and Griffiths, J. D.: The blood supply of the distal segment of the rectum in anterior resection. Br. J. Surg., *50:*399, 1962.

5. Brasch, J. C. (ed.): Cunningham's Manual of Practical Anatomy. 12th ed. 1958 London Oxford University Press.

6. Chiari, H.: Uber die Nalen Divertikel der Rectumschleimhaut und Ihre Beziehung zu den Anal Fisteln. Wien Med. Press *19:*1482, 1878.

7. Courtney, H.: Posterior subsphincteric space. Its relation to posterior horseshoe fistula. Surg. Gynecol. Obstet., *89:*222, 1949.

8. Crapp, A. R. and Cuthbertson, A. M.: William Waldeyer and the rectosacral fascia. Surg. Gynecol. Obstet., *138:*252, 1974.

9. Dukes, C. E. and Galvin, C.: Colloid carcinoma arising within fistulae in ano-rectal region. Ann. Roy. Coll. Surg. Engl., *18:*246, 1956.

10. Duthie, H. L. and Gairns, F. W.: Sensory nerve endings and sensation in the anal region of man. Br. J. Surg., *47:*585, 1960.

11. Fine, J. and Lawes, C. H. W.: On the muscle fibres of the anal submucosa, with special reference to the pecten band. Br. J. Surg., *27:*723, 1940.

12. Goligher, J. C.: Surgery of the Anus, Rectum and Colon. Springfield, Illinois, Charles C Thomas, ed. 3. 1975.

13. ———: The blood supply to the sigmoid colon and rectum. Br. J. Surg., *37:*157, 1949.

14. Goligher, J. C., Leacock, A. G. & Brossy, J. J.: The surgical anatomy of the anal canal. Br. J. Surg., *43:*51, 1955.

15. Grinvalsky, H. T. and Helwig, E. B.: Carcinoma of the anorectal junction. I. Histological considerations. Cancer, *9:*480, 1956.

16. Milligan, E. T. C., and Morgan, C. N.: Surgical anatomy of the anal canal with special reference to ano-rectal fistulae. Lancet, *2:*1150, 1934.

17. Morson, B. C., and Dawson, I. M. P.: Gastrointestinal Pathology. Oxford, Blackwell Scientific Publications, 1972.

18. Oh, C. and Kark, A. E.: Anatomy of the external anal sphincter. Br. J. Surg., *59:*717, 1972.

19. Parks, A. G.: Pathogenesis and treatment of fistula-in-ano. Br. Med. J., *1:*463, 1961.

19a. Parks, A. G.: The surgical treatment of hemorrhoids. Br. J. Surg., *43:*337, 1955.

20. Quer, E. A., Dahlin, D. C. and Mayo, C. W.: Retrograde intramural spread of carcinoma of the rectum and rectosigmoid. A microscopic study. Surg. Gynecol. Obstet., *96:*24, 1953.

21. Shafik, A.: A new concept of the anatomy of the anal sphincter mechanism and the physiology of defecation—III. The longitudinal anal muscle: anatomy and role in anal sphincter mechanism. Invest. Urol., *13:*271, 1976.

22. ———: A new concept of the anatomy of the anal sphincter mechanism and the physiology of defecation—II. Anatomy of the levator ani muscle with special reference to puborectalis. Invest. Urol., *13:*175, 1975.

23. ———: A new concept of the anatomy of the anal sphincter mechanism and the physiology of defecation—the external anal sphincter: A triple-loop system. Invest. Urol., *12:*412, 1975.

24. Walls, E. W.: The anatomy of the Colon, Rectum and Anal Canal. In Morson, B. C. (ed.): Diseases of Colon, Rectum and Anus. London, William Hememann Medical Books, 1969.

# 2

# Anorectal Physiology

The physiology of the anorectal region is a very complex matter, and only recently have there been any detailed investigations which would allow us a better understanding of its functioning. Kerremans declared that the anorectal functions of fecal continence, and defecation, are the result of the combined physiological activity of both dynamic and static mechanisms, each being related to a specific morphological apparatus.[27]

Connell stated that much morbitidy results from disorders of the anal closing mechanism, such as difficulties in defecation and fecal incontinence.[27] In recent years, techniques have become available which allow a systematic and fundamental study of the mechanisms of anal continence. These involve manometric and electrophysiological studies, as well as radiological observations. Furthermore, there are new, and valuable, pharmacological agents which allow a fuller explanation of smooth muscle responses. From all these sources, a clearer picture of the reactions of the skeletal, and the smooth muscle of the lower rectum and anal canal has evolved. Observations on disordered physiology can now be made on a firmer scientific basis.

## ANAL CONTINENCE

The definition of normal anal continence is difficult. Complete control, or complete lack of control, are easy to define, but varying degrees of lack of control of flatus, and fecal soiling may present major disabilities to some patients, while they are not even mentioned by less fastidious individuals. Moreover, the consistency of the stool is important because patients who have weakened mechanisms may be continent for a firm stool but incontinent for fluid feces. In addition to the consistency of stool, the rate of delivery of feces into the rectum is important.

From a review of the works of several investigators, one realizes that maintenance of anal continence depends upon a highly integrated series of complicated events, upon which there is not uniform agreement. A number of theories have been proposed as being important anosphincteric mechanisms of continence, and these are briefly listed and discussed below. Most likely, all the factors mentioned play some role in the overall maintenance of continence.

### Mechanisms of Anal Continence
RESERVOIR FUNCTION
  Mechanical
  Physiological
SENSORY COMPONENTS
  Intrinsic sensory receptors of the anal canal
  Extrinsic sensory receptors
  Neuropathways
SPHINCTERIC FACTORS
  Basal Tone
    pressure zone
    resistance to opening
  Structural Considerations
    angulation between rectum and anal canal
    "flutter valve"
    "flap valve" theory
    forces around the anal canal
    "triple loop system"
REFLEXES
CORPUS CAVERNOSUM OF THE ANUS

## Reservoir Function

*Mechanical.* Adaptive compliance in the colon, and retentive mechanisms in the rectosigmoid, normally maintain the distal rectum empty and in a collapsed state. Mechanically, the lateral angulation of the sigmoid colon and the valves of Houston retard progression of material. The weight of stool tends to accentuate these angles and enhance their barrier effect (Fig. 2-1).[40]

*Physiological.* Motor activity is more frequent, and contractile waves are of higher amplitude, in the rectum than in the sigmoid.[6] This reversed gradient provides a pressure barrier resisting caudad progression of stool. This mechanism probably accounts for the cephalad movement of retention enemas or suppositories (Fig. 2-2).[40] Differences in pressure patterns between the distal, and proximal levels, of the anal canal result in the development of a force vector in the direction of the rectum. This continuous, differential activity may be of importance in controlling the

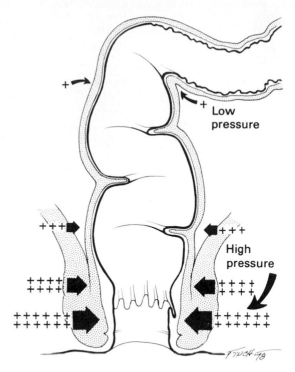

**FIGURE 2-2.** *Physiological Reservoir Function.*

retention of small amounts of liquid matter, and flatus in the rectum.

## Sensory Components

Rectal sensation is important to give awareness of the arrival of material into the rectum. Anal canal sensation may contribute to the discrimination of the nature of the material.

*Intrinsic Sensory Receptors of the Anal Canal.* Duthie and Gairns carefully plotted the sensory nerve endings within the anal canal.[9] They found an abundance of conventional nerve endings which denote pain (free intraepithelial), touch (Meissner's corpuscles), cold (Krause-end-bulbs), pressure or tension (corpuscles of Paccini and Golgi Mazoni), and friction (genital corpuscles), together with unnamed conventional receptors in the anal canal of adults, distal to the dentate line, and to a point 0.5 to 1.5 cm cephalad to this level. These receptors are responsible for fine sensory discrimination. No receptors were found in the rectal mucosa, although nerve trunks and Meissner's plexus of ganglion cells were identified. The rectum is insensitive to stimuli other than stretch (Fig. 2-3).

Stephens and Smith feel that the findings by

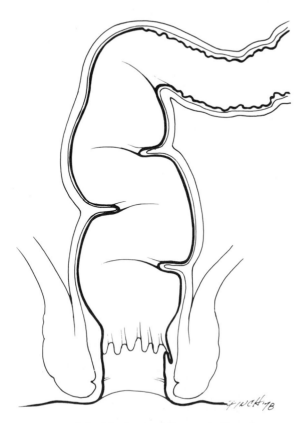

**FIGURE 2-1.** *Mechanical Reservoir Function.*

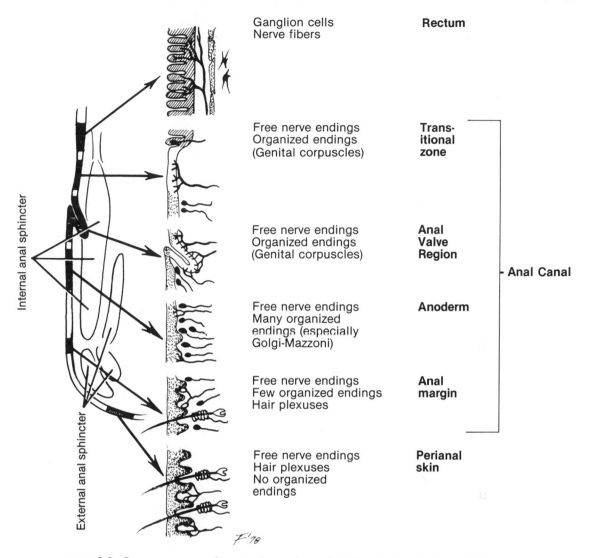

Ganglion cells
Nerve fibers — **Rectum**

Free nerve endings
Organized endings
(Genital corpuscles) — **Trans-itional zone**

Free nerve endings
Organized endings
(Genital corpuscles) — **Anal Valve Region**

Free nerve endings
Many organized
endings (especially
Golgi-Mazzoni) — **Anoderm**

Free nerve endings
Few organized endings
Hair plexuses — **Anal margin**

Free nerve endings
Hair plexuses
No organized
endings — **Perianal skin**

Internal anal sphincter

External anal sphincter

**Anal Canal**

FIGURE **2-3.** *Sensory nerve endings in the anal canal. (After Duthie, H. L., and Gairns, F. W.: Br. J. Surg., 47:585, 1960)*

Duthie, and Gairns of keen intrinsic receptiveness of the short, skin-lined anus to distention, temperature, friction, etc., alone create a warning which is too late, and hence ill-timed.[44] They feel that the sleeve and sling muscles (puborectalis and levator ani) are the chief instruments of continence.

*Extrinsic Sensory Receptors.* There are several bits of evidence to suggest that sensory receptors are located in the puborectalis, and surrounding pelvic musculature. Stephens and Smith suggested that the initial signal of dis-

tention of the rectum may not come from the rectal mucosa alone.[44] Since patients gain a large measure of control following surgical construction of an anal canal with the puborectalis sling only, they consider that this extrinsic muscle has both fine sensory, and motor function essential to continence. Goligher and Hughes, from studies of patients following pull-through operations, concluded that the response to distention probably arose in structures surrounding the bowel.[16] Parks, et al, and Porter, in studies of the pelvic floor muscles in rectal prolapse, suggested that the receptors

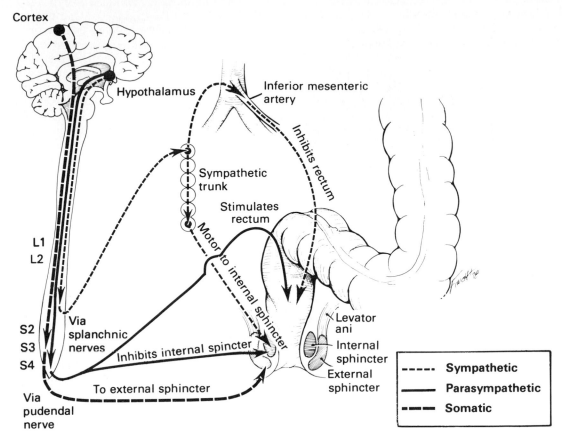

Cortex

Hypothalamus

Inferior mesenteric
artery

Inhibits rectum

Sympathetic
trunk

Stimulates
rectum

Motor to internal sphincter

L1
L2

S2
S3
S4

Via
splanchnic
nerves

Inhibits internal spincter

To external sphincter

Via
pudendal
nerve

Levator
ani
Internal
sphincter
External
sphincter

| ----- | **Sympathetic** |
| ——— | **Parasympathetic** |
| ▬▬▬ | **Somatic** |

FIGURE **2-4.** *Innervation of the rectum and anal canal.*

lay in the rectal wall and surrounding pelvic floor muscles.[36,38] Kiesewetter and Nixon, by their anatomical and physiological studies of rectal sensation in patients following surgical correction of anorectal malformations, considered that sensory receptors responsible for a measure of rectal sensation were probably present in the puborectalis.[28] Holschneider believes that the increase of activity in the puborectalis muscle during speaking, coughing, taking a deep breath, or touching the rectum, shows that the puborectalis is a much more sensitive receptor for alterations in pressure than the rectum.[24] Because the receptors for this proprioceptive reflex mechanism lie in the parapuborectalis tissues, this reflex remains intact even after amputation of the rectum, or low anastomoses.

*Neuropathways.* The internal sphincter is supplied by a dual innervation containing a motor supply from the sympathetic outflow through the hypogastric nerve, and an inhibitory supply from the parasympathetic outflow (Fig. 2-4). Contrary to former beliefs, it has been shown that an intact rectum is not necessary to elicit sphincter responses.[31] In the unique physiological situation where the colon has been anastomosed to the upper anal canal, distention of this portion of the colon usually results in essentially normal responses, with inhibition of the internal sphincter, and an initial excitation followed by inhibition of the external sphincter. The most likely explanation for the restoration of the internal sphincter reflex is the regeneration of the intramural network of nerves across the anastomosis. It is likely that the external sphincter reflexes are initiated by receptors which lie, not in the gut, but probably, in the levator muscles. For good functional results to be obtained, it is essential that the anatomical relationships not be distorted by pelvic sepsis.

Gunterberg, et al reported that anorectal

function in patients following major sacral resections, which resulted in bilateral loss of sacral nerves, was seriously impaired.[17] Preservation of the first and second sacral nerves, bilaterally, was not sufficient for discrimination between different qualities of rectal content passing the anal canal. The sensation of rectal distention was also impaired. The reflex pattern of the internal sphincter was intact. The external sphincter displayed a weak spontaneous myoelectrical activity in patients who had at least one second sacral nerve intact. The normal transient increase of myoelectrical discharge, from the external anal sphincter, in response to rectal distention, could not, however, be elicited. In patients with unilateral loss of the sacral nerves no significant impairment of anorectal function was noted. Total one-sided denervation implied deficient sensibility of the anal canal, unilaterally, but no disturbance of sphincter function, as judged from the reflex response of the internal and external sphincters, to the rectal distention. It can be assumed that receptors for this external sphincter response lie either in or near the rectal mucosa, since the reflex disappears after application of cocaine to the mucosa (Fig. 2-4).

### Sphincteric Factors

*Basal Tone.* PRESSURE ZONE. The most commonly accepted explanation of anal continence is that the higher *pressure zone* in the anal canal at rest (average 25 to 120 mm Hg) provides an effective barrier against pressure in the rectum (average 5 to 20 mm Hg).[7] Both the internal and external sphincter contribute to the resting tone. The zone of elevated pressure in the anal canal may extend from 3 to 7 cm from the anal margin (an average of about 4 cm), with the peak pressure being found about 2 cm from the anal verge. Floyd and Walls demonstrated continuous tetanic activity at rest in the levator ani, and external sphincter muscles, even during sleep.[11,38] Parks, et al showed this tone to be constantly fluctuating, to balance postural changes with increased tone, in the upright position.[34] In this regard, the external sphincter is unique: other striated muscles are electrically silent at rest. This sphincter is further unique in that it does not degenerate even when separated from its nerve supply. Deep inspiration, and the Valsalva maneuver, result in a sharp in-

crease in activity, which is accompanied by increases in the intraluminal pressure or force in the anal canal.[5] Another physiological function that has an influence on the external anal sphincter is micturation. When the external urethral sphincter is inhibited, during the passage of urine, the myoelectrical activity of the external anal sphincter is likewise diminished. The activity is augmented on perianal stimulation (anal reflex), on increases in intra-abdominal pressure, such as coughing or sneezing, and on distention of the rectum. Response of the skeletal muscle to rectal distention is twofold: with initial small volumes, activity is increased; but, with a large volume, an urge and desire to defecate occurs. Reports of response to bearing down have varied from inhibition to little change in activity, and slight increase.[38,27,39]

Continuous electrical potentials have been recorded from the internal sphincter at rest, and these appear to play the dominant role in the development of the high pressure zone in the anal canal.[2,27] This continuous electrical potential is believed to arise from a fused tetanus, resulting from the summation of successive twitches of one fiber, and from the spatial summation, and coordination, of the activity of multiple fiber bundles of the internal sphincter.

There is not entire agreement on the importance played by each of the internal and external sphincters in maintaining anal continence. This variance is due to the overlapping of the sphincters. However, when the external sphincter is paralyzed, the pressure is not materially altered, so that the resting pressure would seem to be largely due to the internal sphincter.[10]

Although it has been demonstrated that activity is always present in the external anal sphincter, and pelvic floor muscles, these muscles can only be contracted voluntarily for periods from 40 to 60 seconds; thereafter, both the electrical activity, and pressure within the anal canal, return to basal levels.[36,38]

*Resistance to Opening.* Harris and Pope proposed that the pressure recorded in the anal canal depends not so much on the ability of the muscles to squeeze around the anal canal, but rather on their ability to resist the opening of the anal canal.[23] The adhesion of the moist surfaces of the mucosal lining of the anal canal would have to be broken to allow the potential space to be opened.

## Structural Considerations

ANGULATION BETWEEN RECTUM AND ANAL CANAL. The lumen of the anal canal in the normal resting state is occluded by the puborectalis sling, and by the resting tone of the internal and external sphincters. The angulation of the anorectal system, due to the continuous tonic activity of the puborectalis, is without doubt the most important mechanism for the conservation of gross fecal continence. This angle, of 80 degrees between the axis of the rectum and the anal canal, is present except when the hips are flexed more than 90 degrees, or during defecation. Radiographic studies have elucidated changes in this angle during defecation (Fig. 2-5).[3,37]

"FLUTTER VALVE." As a result of manometric and radiologic studies, Phillips and Edwards sugested that additional protection could be afforded by intra-abdominal pressure being transmited at the level of the levator ani, laterally to the side of the anal canal at the level of the anorectal junction. The anal canal is an anteroposterior slit, and pressure could compress it in a fashion similar to a *flutter valve*. However, this hypothesis, albeit attractive, cannot exclude the action as being due to the puborectalis. In addition, although this mechanism may protect against an elevated intra-abdominal pressure, it would not protect against an increase in intrarectal pressure (Fig. 2-6).

"FLAP VALVE THEORY." *The "flap valve" theory*, advanced by Parks, et al is basically an extension of the fluter valve theory.[35] It suggests that continence is achieved by virtue of the flap of anterior rectal mucosa, which comes to lie over the upper end of the anal canal, functioning as an occlusion produced by the pull of the puborectalis at the anorectal angle. Any incresed intra-abdominal pressure (weight lifting, straining, laughing, coughing) tends to accentuate the angulation, and force the anterior rectal mucosa more firmly over

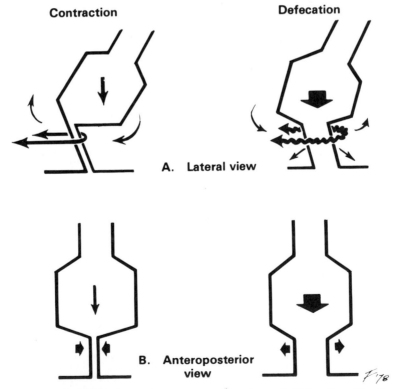

**Contraction**     **Defecation**

A.  Lateral view

B.  Anteroposterior view

FIGURE 2-5. *Angulation between the rectum and anal canal. (After Ihre, T.,: Scand. J. Gastroenterol. Suppl., 25:10, 1974)*

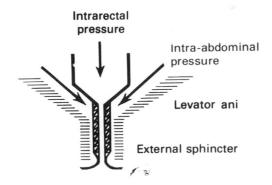

FIGURE **2-6.** *The "flutter" valve theory. (After Kerremans, R.: Press. Acad. Europ., Bruxelles, 1969).*

the upper anal canal, producing the flap valve effect. For defecation to occur, the flap valve must be broken. This breakage takes place by lengthening of the puborectalis, descending of the pelvic floor, and obliterating the angle (Fig. 2-7).

"FORCES AROUND THE ANAL CANAL." *Forces around the cephalad portion of the anal canal* are maximal posteriorly, less laterally, and minimal anteriorly.[5] This finding is compatible with the combined action of the puborectalis sling and the internal sphincter. Because they are more caudad the internal and external sphincters together provide the force which is greater laterally than anteroposteriorly. The external anal sphincter provides the final voluntary guard (Fig. 2-8).

A peristaltic wave creates tension in the sling and thus results in a contraction, in order to arrest a peristaltic movement, as in resisting the passing of flatus. Greater efforts to resistance may be accompanied by colic, until such time as it is convenient to permit the evacuation of the rectal contents. It is considered that the sleeve-and-sling can differentiate between flatus, solid, or fluid feces, and has the ability to permit one to escape with or without the other.[44]

Conjoined longitudinal fibers, being derived partly from the pubococcygeus muscle, and partly from the involuntary muscle of the rectum, actively produce an *ectropion* of the anus during the peristaltic phase of expulsion of a bolus of feces. This function is predisposing to cleanliness of the skin-lined part of the anal canal. The external sphincter supplements the sling action in arresting defecation.

It has a resting tone, which when forced open by flatus under high pressure, exhibits a flutter valve action with the accompanying characteristic noise. Stephens and Smith feel that neither the internal nor external sphincter account for the minute to minute, day and night, fecal continence which appears to be the function of the sleeve-and-sling.[44]

Any operative procedure, and postoperative complication, involving the anorectal angle may result in loss of anal continence. Procedures for restoration of the angular architecture of the anorectal junction with skeletal muscles cannot bring about any unconscious sphincteric activity. These transposed skeletal muscles cannot maintain a continuous tonic activity because they consist primarily of phasic motor units.

"TRIPLE-LOOP SYSTEM." A new concept of the mechanism of action of the external sphincter in anal continence during defecation was described by Shafik as the *triple-loop system*.[42] He distinguished three main "loops": the top, consisting of the puborectalis and deep portion of the external sphincter; the intermediate, consisting of the superficial portion of the external sphincter, and the base, consisting of the subcutaneous

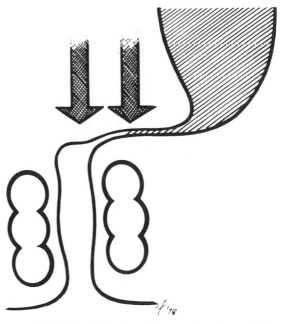

FIGURE **2-7.** *The "flap" valve mechanism. (After Parks, A. G.,: Proc. R. Soc. Lond. 68:24, 1975).*

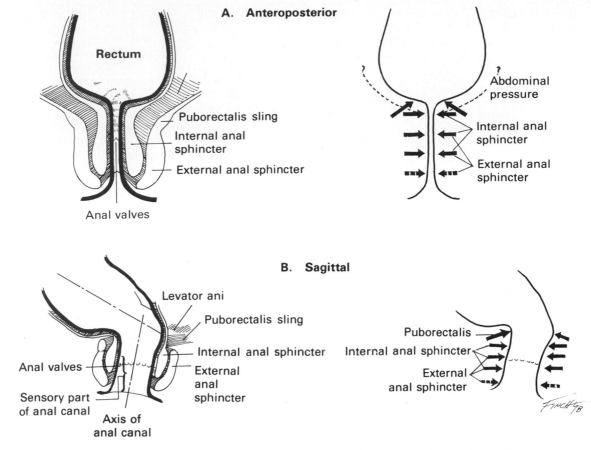

FIGURE **2-8.** *Forces around the anal canal.* (*After Duthie, H. L.,: Gut. 12:844, 1971*).

loop of the external sphincter. An air-tight occlusion of the anal canal could be achieved by the triple-loop system in that the top loop pulls upward and forward, the intermediate loop horizontally and backward, and the base loop downward and forward. It is suggested that unless all three loops are destroyed, any single loop can act as a sphincter which maintains continence to solid stool, but not necessarily to fluid ones or flatus (Fig. 1-6).

### Reflexes

Duthie suggested that rectal distention results in transient relaxation of the internal sphincter, and simultaneous contraction of the external sphincter (Fig. 2-9). This decrease in anal canal pressure would be sufficient to momentarily allow the rectal content to reach far enough into the anal canal to contact the very sensitive receptors, and thus aid in recognition of the physical state of the threatening material, whether solid, liquid, or gas.[8] This is not only a conscious recognition of the nature of the content, but also subconscious since flatus can be passed safely during sleep. When flatus is to be evacuated, without the passage of feces, it is done by keeping the ampullar pressure high from abdominal pressure, and holding the anal canal closed due to high voluntary phasic activity. The internal sphincter will then be constantly relaxed, and the tonic activity in the striated muscles will have ceased. A further increase in ampullar pressure will expel the gas, despite the phasic activity, at the same time as the anal opening will be too small to permit the escape of feces.[25]

The reflex contraction of the external sphincter, which is synchronous with relaxation of the internal sphincter, maintains continence during the time that the stimulating material reaches this sensitive sensory area, and allows time for impulses to reach conscious awareness so that having determined the nature of the material, the individual can decide what he wants to do about it, and then take appropriate action. Voluntary contraction of the external sphincter can extend the period of continence, and allow time for compliance mechanisms within the colon to provide for adjustment to increased intrarectal volumes. As the colon accomodates to its new volume, stretch receptors are no longer activated, and afferent stimuli and the sensation of urgency disappear.[41] Further rectal distention leads to inhibition of the external sphincter.[38]

Although the internal sphincter reflex is initiated only by rectal distention, external sphincter response may be initiated by a number of stimuli such as voluntary effort, postural changes, perianal scratch, rectal distention, increased intra-abdominal pressure, and anal dilatation.

### Corpus Cavernosum of the Anus

Stelzner postulated that the vascular architecture in the submucosal, and subcutaneous tissues of the anal canal, really represent what he called a corpus cavernosum of the rectum.[43] This tissue, with its physiological ability to expand and contract, could take up the so-called slack, and thereby contribute to the finest degree of anal continence. This

theory might be supported by the fact that certain patients, after a formal hemorrhoidectomy, have minor alterations in continence, a situation which may arise due to the excision of this corpus cavernosum.

## DEFECATION
### Usual Sequence of Events

The stimulus to the initiation of defecation is distention of the rectum. This, in turn, may be related to a critical threshold of sigmoid, and possibly, descending colon distention. As long as fecal matter is retained in the descending, and sigmoid colon, the rectum remains empty, and no urge is felt for defecation. This reservoir type of continence does not depend on sphincter function. Distention of the left colon initiates peristaltic waves, which propel the fecal mass downward, into the rectum.

This process normally occurs one or several times a day. The timing of the act is a balance between environmental factors, as this urge may be suppressed by a complex cortical inhibition of the basic reflexes of the anorectum. In many people, a pattern is established so that the urge is felt either upon rising in the morning, or in the evening, or following food or drink. This balance can be altered by travel, admission to hospital, or by alterations in diet.

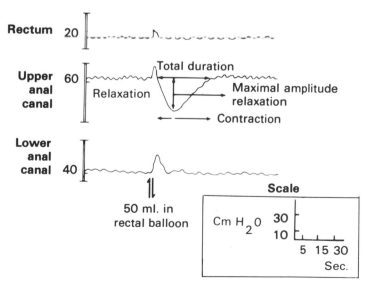

FIGURE **2-9.** *The anorectal reflex. (After Martelli, H., et al.: Gastroenterology. 75:614, 1978).*

Normally, rectal distention induces relaxation of the internal sphincter. This, in turn, triggers contraction of the external sphincter, thus, sphincter continence is induced. If the decision is made to accede to the urge, the subject takes up the squatting position. In doing so, the angulation between the rectum and the anal canal is straightened out. The second semivoluntary stage is the performance of the Valsalva maneuver, which overcomes the resistance to the external sphincter, by voluntarily increasing the intrathoracic and intra-abdominal pressure. The pelvic floor descends, and the resulting pressure on the fecal mass in the rectum increases intrarectal pressure. In this manner, pressures as high as 100 to 200 torr can be generated.[18] Inhibition of the external sphincter permits passage of the fecal bolus. Once evacuation has been completed the pelvic floor, and anal canal muscles, regain their resting activity, and the anal canal is closed.

### Responses to Entry of Material into the rectum

Reviewing his extensive studies upon the dynamics of the rectum and anus, Duthie concluded that most dynamic changes in the anorectum are in response to two stresses: the change in intra-abdominal pressure, and entry of material from the colon into the rectum.[7] The rate and timing of the entry of feces and flatus into the rectum vary greatly in different individuals. Colonic transit is accelerated by physical activity and by eating meals. Local reflexes may be inhibited by cortical inhibition which is a feature of social training. Afferent nerve impulses, that signal the entry of material into the rectum, proceed at a subconscious level, with the accomodation, and sampling responses taking place reflexly. In support of this contention is the clinical finding that patients admitted to routine clinical examination of the rectum often have a considerable amount of feces in the rectum unknown to them.

*Accomodation Response.* After inflation of a rectal balloon (about 10 ml) the external anal sphincter shows a transient increase in electromyographic activity, while in the internal sphincter a similar short-lived reduction in its pressure activity can be measured within the lumen. With persistent inflation of the balloon, an increase in pressure within the rectal ampulla is maintained, for one to two minutes, and then decreases to preinflation level (Fig. 2-10). This is known as the accomodation response, and is said to consist of receptive relaxation of the rectal ampulla to accomodate the fecal mass. With increasing volume there is a gradual step-wise increase in rectal pressure, and, depending upon the age of the patient, an urge to defecate is experienced. This urge, however, abates in a few seconds as the rectum accomodates the stimulus. When volume increases rapidly, over a short period, the accomodation response fails, and leads to urgent emptying of the rectum.

The afferent nerve endings for the accomodation reflex are in the rectal ampulla and in the levator ani muscle. The nerve center for the spinal part of the reflex is in the lumbosacral cord with higher center control to permit suppression of the urge to defecate.

*The sampling response* consists of transient relaxation of the upper part of the internal sphincter, which permits rectal contents to come into contact with the somatic sensory epithelium of the anal canal to assess the nature of the content (Fig. 2-10). Conscious sampling is done by slightly increasing abdominal tension, and maintaining, by voluntary control, an increase in the activity of the external sphincter. Thus, solids can be retained where gas can be passed, thereby relieving the intrarectal pressure. If fluid is present in the rectum contact with the sensory area in the anal canal excites conscious activity of the external sphincter to maintain control, until the rectal accomodation response occurs, and so continence is maintained.

### Commencement of Defecation

The method of commencement of the act of defecation varies from person to person. If one is exerting anal control during an urge, merely relinquishing this voluntary control will allow the reflex to proceed. On the other hand, if the urge abates, voluntary straining with increased intra-abdominal pressure is necessary before defecation can begin. Once begun, the act may follow either of two patterns. Expulsion of the rectal contents, accompanied by mass peristalsis of the distal colon, clearing the bowel in one continuous movement can occur, or the stool is passed piecemeal with

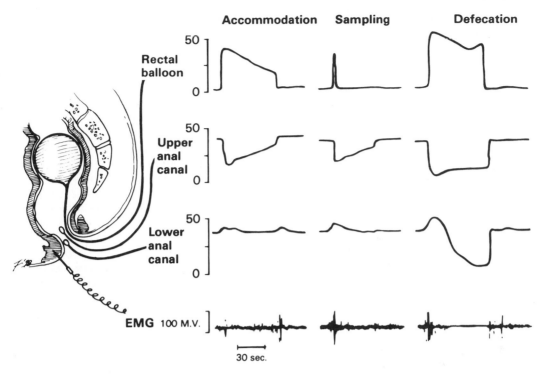

**FIGURE 2-10.** *The accommodating and sampling responses. (After Duthie, H. L.,: Glin. Gastroenterol. 4:469, 1975).*

several bouts of straining. The habit of the individual, and the consistency of the feces, largely determines which pattern is followed.

### Urgent Defecation

If large volumes are rapidly introduced into the rectum, the accomodation response may be overcome, cortical inhibition may be unavailing, and the urgency can be controlled for only 40 to 60 seconds by the voluntary external sphincter complex. This time may be long enough to allow some accomodation. If not, leakage will temporarily relieve the situation.

### Neuropathways

Defecation involves the simultaneous action of voluntary and involuntary muscles, is susceptible to derangement by emotional stimuli, and, although capable of autonomous regulation by intrinsic nerves, is seriously impaired by complete extrinsic denervation.

Cerebral influences on defecation are exerted by neurons of the motor cortex. A center in the mid-brain affects tonus of the rectal muscles, and a medullary center gives rise to straining, and the evacuation of stool. Sympathetic impulses from the thoracolumbar outflow (through inferior mesenteric ganglia, hypogastric nerves, and inferior hypogastric plexus) exert an inhibitory effect on the rectal muscle, and a variable one on the internal sphincter. The internal sphincter was found to be independent of cerebral influence at rest as well as during rectal distention.[12,13] Parasympathetic nerve centers in sacral segments of the spinal cord are responsible for the contraction of the rectum, and the relaxation of the sphincter. The voluntary nerve supply to the external sphincter and levator ani (pudendal nerve) originates in the same spinal segment from which the pelvic splanchnics derive. This facilitates reflex integration of the action of the sphincter muscles.

Rectal distention initiates impulses which pass through visceral afferents, and the dorsal root ganglia, to the respective spinal segment, where they are distributed by at least three routes.[1] The first route is by ascending tracks to the sensory cortex, to elicit the necessary voluntary actions, which are the closure of the glottis, the contraction and fixation of the diaphragm, and the contraction of the abdominal wall muscles. The second route is through connector neurons dorsal to ventral horn cells to mediate reflex relaxation of external sphincter, and reflex contraction of abdominal, perineal, and hamstring muscles. The third route is by neuronal connections to the pelvic autonomic nerves, which stimulate the circular, and longitudinal muscles of the rectum, to expel contents. In addition, the internal sphincter is also altered through local intrinsic ganglia to dilate (Fig. 2-4).

## Pathological Conditions

During the period of "spinal shock", which supervenes for some weeks immediately following transection of the spinal cord above the origin of the lumbar sympathetic nerves, the rectum and sphincters are completely paralyzed, and the patient is incontinent.[1] Frenckner revealed in these patients a cessation of all electrical activity from the striated muscles in response to rectal distention, and also a less pronounced inflation reflex.[12] Thereafter, the tonus of the sphincter returns, and defecation occurs, reflexly, from the lumbosacral center through pelvic and pudendal nerves. Since voluntary contraction of the external sphincter is no longer possible, and since distention of the rectum is no longer perceived, the patient has no control over the act of defecation. In paraplegics this poses a difficult problem, which is managed generally by the regular use of enemas, and digital evacuation of the rectum. In some of these patients, the defecation mechanism can be triggered by a stimulus to the somatic innervation, such as stroking the thigh or the perianal region.

When the cord lesion involves the cauda equina, with destruction of the sacral innervation, the reflexes are abolished, and defecation then becomes automatic (i.e., dependent entirely on intrinsic nervous mechanisms). In these circumstances, the rectum still responds, though with little force to distention, and the reciprocal relaxation of the already patulous sphincters enables feces to be extruded.

Internal sphincter relaxation has been found to persist with spinal cord transection, and occurs if the presacral sympathetic nerves are stimulated. One possible explanation of this mechanism is that it is some form of local muscular reflex.[7]

The accumulation of a large mass in a greatly dilated rectum, occurring especially in the elderly, is suggestive of the abnormal condition known as *rectal dyschezia,* which results from a loss of tonicity of the rectal musculature. It may be due to a longstanding habit of ignoring or suppressing the urge to defecate, or to degeneration of nerve pathways concerned with defecation reflexes. When further complicated by weakness of the abdominal muscles, defecation becomes a chronic problem. In these cases, evacuation may be obtained only by a mechanical washing-out of the mass with enemas, or by the administration of cathartics which keep the stools semiliquid.

Painful lesions of the anal canal, such as ulcers, fissures, and thrombosed hemorrhoids, impede defecation by exciting a spasm of the sphincters, and by voluntary suppression to avoid the resulting pain.

Constant urge to defecate in the absence of appreciable content in the rectum may be caused by external compression of the rectum, by intrinsic neoplasms, and, particularly, by inflammation of the rectal mucosa. This mucosa, normally insensitive to cutting or burning, when inflamed, becomes highly sensitive to all stimuli, including those acting on the receptors mediating the stretch reflex.

## CLINICAL APPLICATION OF ANORECTAL PHYSIOLOGY

Electromyographic and manometric studies of the anorectal region play an increasing part in the diagnosis and management of a number of anorectal disorders. Schuster pointed out that rectosphincteric studies can be employed *1)* to investigate physiology and pathophysiology; *2)* as a sensitive tool to detect functional abnormalities which represent early signs of disease; *3)* for the differential diagnosis of clinical disorders; *4)* to assess immediate response to some clinical modality; *5)* to evaluate long-term progress; and, *6)* as an integral part of treatment itself (as in operant conditioning).[40]

Treatment of a disorder may be empiric or rational. Rational treatment relies on the understanding of the basic physiology and pathophysiology. With this in mind, specific applications and potential clinical implications are discussed.

## Fissure-in-Ano

Hancock found elevated anal pressures in patients with fissures.[19] Keighley found increased anal pressures occur only in patients with acute fissures.[26] In patients with anal fissures, Nothmann and Schuster demonstrated an "overshoot" contraction of the internal sphincter which follows immediately after a normal relaxation.[33] Successful treatment of a fissure results in disappearance of this contraction. The overshoot, recorded in the internal sphincter, suggests that the anal spasm, which accompanies the anal fissure, is due to a pathological motor response in the internal anal sphincter. A lateral internal spincterotomy would therefore appear to be a rational physiological treatment of this abnormality.

## Hemorrhoids

Anal motility in normal subjects is characterized by slow pressure waves. The frequency is fastest in the distal anal canal, and this frequency gradient may represent a normal mechanism to keep the anal canal empty. Kerremans feels that the internal sphincter plays a role in the reflux from the internal venous plexus in a cephalad direction, by originating differential motility at the distal and proximal level of the anal canal, resulting in antiperistaltic movement.[27] From a theoretical point of view, it is, therefore, conceivable that dysfunction of the internal sphincter may contribute to venous stasis, and impaired emptying of the internal hemorrhoidal plexus, and consequently, may intervene in the pathogenesis of internal hemorrhoids. This hypothesis is supported by electrophysiological and manometric investigations in patients with internal hemorrhoids, in whom ultraslow pressure waves, with spiking activity, and long tetanic contractions, as well as the disappearance of the normal antiperistaltic activity of the internal sphincter, have been found. He believes that this preliminary data concerning the pathogenesis of internal hemorrhoids will allow an earlier diagnosis of the disease (i.e., before irreversible dilatation of the hemorrhoidal plexus has occurred). Moreover, these findings may, perhaps, serve as a starting point for the investigation of pharmacological agents which can inhibit sphincteric dysrhythmia, or which can regulate sphincteric contractions, thus reversing, or at least preventing, progression to a state of "decompensation".

The internal anal sphincter responds in different ways to pharmacological agents in its proximal and distal parts, and the mechanism of action is under investigation at the present time.[15] The proximal part has alpha adrenergic stimulatory, and beta adrenergic inhibitory, receptors.[27] Acetylcholine will cause a contraction exactly as in the rectum, and in the rest of the alimentary tract, and noradrenaline will cause relaxation. Parks found the distal part contracts to acetylcholine, and relaxes to nicotine, but Kerremans found acetylcholine will cause no reaction, and adrenaline will cause a contraction.[34,27] All the fibers show muscarinic inhibitory receptors which are thought to mediate the anorectal reflex.[27]

Intraluminal pressure studies by Hancock suggested that the internal sphincter may be more active in patients with hemorrhoids.[19,21] He subsequently recorded ultraslow pressure waves in 42 per cent of patients with hemorrhoids, but in only 5 per cent of normal subjects. This finding was attributed to a synchronous contraction of the whole internal sphincter.[20] Keighley found increased anal pressure only in painful secondary hemorrhoids.[26] Lane also found patients with hemorrhoids to have a significantly higher resting pressure, but suggested that the raised anal canal pressure in these patients may be the result of the presence of the hemorrhoidal masses, rather than any internal sphincter abnormality.[30]

## Anal Incontinence

Some factors which disturb the normal control mechanisms are: *1)* central nervous system or spinal cord injury; *2)* disturbance or loss of the afferent sensory component of the rectosphincteric reflexes as occurs with proctectomy; *3)* diseases that impair smooth or striated muscles, such as scleroderma or polymyositis, respectively; and, *4)* direct muscle damage which can occur with perianal disease or surgical trauma.[40]

Lane stated that one method of defining incontinence is to divide it into three distinct groups: *1)* True incontinence is the passage of feces without the patient's knowledge (i.e., sensory deficit), or without adequate voluntary contraction (i.e., mechanical deficit), or both; *2)* Partial incontinence is the passage of flatus or mucus per anus, without the patient's knowledge, or without voluntary contraction, or both; and *3)* "Overflow" incontinence is the result of distention of the rectum with relaxation of the anal sphincters, as occurs, for instance, with simple fecal impaction when mucus and liquid feces leak past solid impacted feces.[29]

True incontinence implies impairment of both internal and external sphincters, but combined electromyographic and manometric studies suggest that gross incontinence is more often related to dysfunction of the external sphincter, which has a low resting tone in the basal state.[29,41] A normal external sphincter exhibits a good excitatory response for one minute.[36] The maximal normal resting anal canal pressure ranges from 70 to 100 cm of water. This can be doubled during a contraction effort. A negligible resting pressure denotes an incompetent internal sphincter. The continuous high pressure contributed by the tonically contracted internal sphincter serves the function of guarding against incontinence of small amounts of liquid.

### Constipation

Many investigators have demonstrated that following rectal distention there is a temporary relaxation of the internal sphincter, but no mechanism has been established to explain this rectosphincteric reflex. In the normal patient, gradual increments of rectal distention result in corresponding falls in anal canal pressure, which returns after a few seconds. The rectal pressure is altered little, reflecting the normal capacity to accomodate increasing volumes. Ihre demonstrated that patients with constipation as the only diagnosis have a reduced ampulla and impaired sensibility to filling. Callaghan first demonstrated the absence of the rectosphincteric reflex in patients with Hirschsprung's disease.[4] This disease is the only condition in which the reflex does not occur. Such physiological data suggest that internal sphincterotomy be incorporated into the primary operation for this condition.

Dysfunction of the internal sphincter may produce long-term constipation. Although the rectosphincteric reflex is present, the pressure returns to the initial baseline after one to two seconds. Pressure in the distal anal canal may fall with rectal distention, but there is no alteration in baseline pressure from the proximal anal canal.[29] It is possible that the reason these patients are constipated is because the internal sphincter fails to relax long enough to allow

rectal contents to pass into, and through, the anal canal. This condition, referred to by Kerremans as "dyschesia of unknown origin", occurs more commonly in women.[27] It has been little recognized in the past, and the logical aim or treatment would be to overcome this internal sphincter resistance by a procedure such as internal sphincterotomy (Chap. 21).

### Rectal Prolapse

Patients with rectal prolapse differ from normals in the following ways: *1*) they have a diminished sensitivity to rectal distention, and require larger volumes of distention before the urge to defecate is appreciated; *2*) straining produces immediate inhibition of the electrical activity, whereas in normals this is increased; *3*) reflex recovery of muscle tone after straining may be delayed or grossly diminished; *4*) distention of the anal canal produces inhibition of the electrical activity, and relaxation of the sphincter muscles, whereas in normal people distention produces an increase in sphincter activity; and, *5*) using rectal balloons, Freckner and Ihre found maximal anal pressure at rest was lower in the incontinent patients than the continent ones, and the former had significantly smaller relaxation of the internal sphincter upon rectal distention.[7,35,14] The increase in anal pressure during voluntary squeezing, a function of the external sphincter, did not differ significantly, compared to the healthy subjects, in either incontinent or continent patients. On the basis of these findings it was concluded that the function of the internal sphincter is impaired in incontinent patients since the maximal anal pressure at rest is mainly due to the activity of the internal sphincter. Thus, with persistent straining, the rectal wall bulges into the anal canal, where it is perceived as a mass that induces further straining, and ultimate protrusion. Further relaxation of the sphincter muscles produces further prolapse. Incontinence in these patients is attributed to the sphincteric relaxation induced by this mechanism.

Recordings by Kerremans of electromyographical activity of the skeletal anal musculature, during straining, distinguished two groups of people in the population.[27] Twenty per cent showed an inhibition of the electromyographical activity during straining, while the other 80 per cent showed an increase in this activity. The results of cineradiography demonstrated that in people who can start defecation at will, the distal part of the anal canal remained closed during the initial stage of defecation, allowing filling of the rectal and anal funnels. Only after complete stretching of the funnel walls did relaxation of the distal canal appear and allow evacuation.

The first group is not trained for socially acceptable defecation, perhaps because of special circumstances which allow them to respond immediately to each call to stool (i.e., autonomous defecation). The electromyographical investigations in these people showed that striated muscles of the pelvic floor, including the sphincters, relax in response to a minimum degree of rectal distention. Also, when asked for straining, the striated sphincters relax at once. Nevertheless, they cannot easily perform voluntary defecation, since failure to meet resistance at the level of the anal canal results in the funnel walls not being stretched, and hence, the fecal mass is not evacuated.

The second group includes people who are trained for socially acceptable defecation. They contract the subcutaneous external sphincter for a few seconds in order to close the distal canal during the initial effort to defecate. The simultaneous relaxation of the pelvic floor musculature allows the filling of the funnels by increased intra-abdominal pressure, provided that the rectum is sufficiently filled with feces. The stretch organs within the rectal wall in these people are more or less adapted to prolonged rectal distention, and therefore, a larger distention of the rectum is needed for inhibiting the striated sphincters. This finding means that these people are habituated to retain feces in the rectum, but are also able to start defecation at will.

The first clinical consequence resulting from these data concerns the etiopathology of rectal procidentia. From a theoretical point of view, it may be assumed that the contraction of the subcutaneous portion of the external sphincter during voluntary straining is an adequate mechanism which prevents procidentia. As a consequence, procidentia may occur in people who are not trained for voluntary defecation because their anal sphincter relaxes immediately, and completely, on starting the straining procedure. Therefore, constipation is potentially hazardous for those people, since this condition necessitates prolonged straining.

## Anorectal Malformation

Electromyographic techniques can be used preoperatively to determine the location of the external sphincter muscle in infants with imperforate anus, and can thus assist in appropriate placement of the rectum if a pull-through operative procedure is necessary. In postoperative patients who are incontinent, circumferential probing around the newly placed rectum may demonstrate the absence of activity in one or more quadrants, thus indicating possible misplacement of the rectum.

## Rectocele

Cinefluoroscopic studies in women with rectocele demonstrated a blind pouch which, during effort at defecation, fills like a hernial sac.[27] In some patients evacuation may be unsuccessful since the contents fill the rectocele rather than moving caudad. This is due to the fact that in women the anterior wall, resting against the vagina, does not provide adequate supportive resistance. This condition may be enhanced by the prevailing tendency to perform socially acceptable defecation as described with rectal prolapse.

## Solitary Ulcer Syndrome

Rutter recorded characteristic electromyographical findings in patients with solitary ulcers. Instead of the puborectalis becoming inhibited during a bearing down effort, there was considerable overactivity. He postulated this to be a major predisposing factor in the development of this condition, whereby, the anterior rectal wall is repeatedly, and forcefully, thrust down onto a solid bar of muscle, resulting in mucosal trauma and ulceration. Treatment of this condition should consist of breaking the vicious cycle, by counselling cessation of continued straining, to allow the ulcer to heal. Otherwise, the puborectalis will eventually give way, resulting in perineal descent.

## Aging

Neuman and Freeman performed balloon studies in 130 patients with normal rectums to determine defecatory sensation.[32] There was a progressive rise, with age, in the threshold for the factors such as rectal pressure, rectal diameter, and rectal tension. Rectal sensitivity to distention was lower in the constipated patient than in those who were not constipated. Evidence from measurements of pressure-volume relationships suggest a decrease in elasticity in elderly patients.[40] This decrease leads to smaller volumes in rectal distention, resulting in defecation.

## Miscellaneous

In scleroderma, smooth internal sphincter muscle may fail to relax in response to rectal distention, while the striated muscle response is normal. By contrast, with dermatomyositis, the internal sphincter may be intact, but there is impaired external sphincter response.[40] In the irritable bowel syndrome the internal sphincter spasmodically relaxes in synchrony with spasmodic rectosigmoid contraction.[40]

# REFERENCES

1. Bachrach, W. H.: Functional and Diagnostic Aspects of the Lower Digestive Tract. The CIBA collections of Medical Illustrations. Vol. 3 Digestive System Part II Lower Digestive Tract, by Netter, F. H., pp. 87–88, 1962. Published by CIBA Pharmaceutical Co. NJ, 1962.

2. Bennett, R. C., and Duthie, H. L.: The junctional importance of the internal anal sphincter. Br. J. Surg., *51:*355, 1964.

3. Broden, B., and Snellman, D.: Procidentia of the rectum studied with cineradiography; a contribution to the discussion of causative mechanism. Dis. Colon Rectum, *11:*330, 1968.

4. Callaghan, R. P., and Nixon, H. H.: Megarectum: Physiological observations. Arch. Dis. Child., *39:*153, 1964.

5. Collins, C. D., Duthie, H. L., Shelly, T., and Whittaker, G. E.: Force in the anal canal and anal continence. Gut., *8:*354, 1967.

6. Connell, A. M.: The clinical physiology of colonic muscle. Proc. R. Soc. Med. *57:*283, 1964.

7. Duthie, H. L.: Dynamics of the rectum and anus. Clin. Gastroenterol., *4:*467, 1975.

8. Duthie, H. L., and Bennett, R. C.: The relation of sensation in the anal canal to the functional anal sphincter; a possible factor in anal continence. Gut., *4:*179, 1963.

9. Duthie, H. L., and Gairns, F. W.: Sensory nerve endings and sensation in the anal region of man. Br. J. Surg., *47:*585, 1960.

10. Duthie, H. L., and Watts, J. M.: Contribution of the external anal sphincter to the pressure zone in the anal canal. Gut., *6:*64, 1965.

11. Floyd, W. F., and Walls, W.: Electromyography of the sphincter externis in man. J. Physiol., *122:*599, 1953.

12. Frenckner, B.: Function of the anal sphincters in spinal man. Gut., *16:*638, 1975.

13. Frenckner, B., and Ihre, T.: Influence of autonomic nerves on the internal anal sphincter in man. Gut., *17:*306, 1976.

14. ———: Function of the anal sphincters in patients with intussusception of the rectum. Gut., *17:*147, 1976.

15. Friedmann, C. A.: The action of nicotine and catecholamines on the human internal anal sphincter. Am. J. Dig. Dis., *13:*428, 1968.

16. Goligher, J. C., and Hughes, E. S. R.: Sensibility of the rectum and colon; its role and mechanism of anal continence. Lancet, *1:*543, 1951.

17. Gunterberg, B., Kewenter, J., Petersen, I., and Stener, B.: Anorectal function after major resections of the sacrum with bilateral or unilateral sacrifice of sacral nerves. Br. J. Surg., *63:*546, 1976.

18. Hagihara, P. F., and Griffin, W. O.: Physiology of the colon and rectum. Surg. Clin. North. Am., *52:*797, 1972.

19. Hancock, B. D.: The internal sphincter and anal fissure. Br. J. Surg., *64:*92, 1977.

20. ———: Measurement of anal pressure and motility. Gut., *17:*645, 1976.

21. Hancock, B. D., and Smith, K.: The internal sphincter and Lord's procedure for hemorrhoids. Br. J. Surg., *62:*833, 1975.

22. Hancock, B. D. and Smith, K.: The internal sphincter and hemorrhoids. Br. J. Surg., *61:*919, 1974.

23. Harris, L. D., and Pope, C. E.: "Squeeze" verses resistence; an evaluation of the mechanism of sphincter competence. J. Clin. Invest., *43:*2272, 1964.

24. Holschneider, A. M.: The problem of anorectal continence. Prog. Pediatr. Surg., *9:*85, 1976.

25. Ihre, T.: Studies on anal function in continent and incontinent patients. Scand. J. Gastroenterol., *25*, 1974, Suppl.

26. Keighley, M. R. B., Arabi, Y., and Alexander-Williams, J.: Anal pressures in hemorrhoids and anal fissure. Br. J. Surg., *63:*665, 1976.

27. Kerremans, R.: Morphological and Physiological Aspects of Anal Continence and Defecation. Bruxelles, Presses Académiques Europeenes, S.C., 1969.

28. Kiesewetter, W. B., and Nixon, H. H.: Imperforate anus: 1. Its surgical anatomy. J. Pediatr. Surg., *2:*60, 1967.

29. Lane, R. H. S.: Clinical application of rectal physiology. Proc. R. Soc. Med., *68:*28, 1975.

30. Lane, R. H. S., Casula, G., and Parks, A. G.:

Anal pressure before and after hemorrhoidectomy. Br. J. Surg., *63:*158, 1976.

31. Lane, R. H. S., and Parks, A. G.: Function of
the anal sphincters following colo-anal anastomosis. Br. J. Surg., *64:*596, 1977.

32. Newman, H. F., and Freeman, J.: Physiologic
factors affecting defecatory sensation: Relation
to aging. J. Am. Geriatr. Soc., *22:*558, 1974.

33. Nothmann, B. J., and Shuster, M. M.: Internal
anal sphincter derangement with anal fissures.
Gastroenterology, *67:*216, 1974.

34. Parks, A. G., Fishlock, D. J., Cameron, J. D. H.
and May, H.: Preliminary investigation of
the pharmacology of human internal anal
sphincter. Gut., *10:*647, 1969.

35. Parks, A. G., Porter, N. H., and Hardcastle,
J. D.: The syndrome of the descending perineum. Proc. R. Soc. Med., *59:*477, 1966.

36. Parks, A. G., Porter, N. H., and Melzak, J.:
Experimental study of the reflex mechanism
controlling the muscles of the pelvic floor. Dis.
Colon Rectum, *5:*407, 1962.

37. Phillips, S. F., and Edwards, D. A. W.: Some
aspects of anal continence and defecation.
Gut., *6:*396, 1965.

38. Porter, N. H.: A physiological study of the pelvic floor in rectal prolapse. Ann. R. Coll. Surg.
Engl., *31:*379, 1962.

39. Rutter, K. R. P.: Electromyographic changes in
certain pelvic floor abnormalities. Proc. R.
Soc. Med., *67:*53, 1974.

40. Schuster, M. M.: The riddle of the sphincters.
Gastroenterology, *69:*249, 1975.

41. Schuster, M. M., Hendrix, T. R., and Mendeloff, A. J.: The internal anal sphincter response: Manometric studies on its normal physiology, neuropathways, and alteration on bowel
disorders. J. Clin. Invest., *42:*196, 1963.

42. Shafik, A.: A new concept of the anatomy of
the anal sphincter mechanism and the physiology of defecation, the external anal sphincter; a
triple loop system. Invest. Urol., *12:*412, 1975.

43. Stelzner, F.: The morphological principles of
anorectal continence. Prog. Pediatr. Surg., *9:*1,
1976.

44. Stephens, F. D., and Smith, E. D.: Anorectal
malformations in children. 28. Chicago Year
Book Medical Publishers, 1971.

# 3

# Diagnosis of Anorectal Disease

## HISTORY: MECHANISM OF SYMPTOMS

As in the diagnosing of any medical problem, the history is a most important facet which assists the physician in the diagnosis of anorectal pathology. Often we are able to make the diagnosis on the basis of history alone and need only confirm it with our examination.

### Pain

*Anorectal pain* which occurs during and following a bowel movement, and is described as sharp in nature, is usually associated with an anal fissure or an abrasion in the anal canal. Tenesmus is a discomfort frequently associated with inflammatory or neoplastic conditions of the anorectum, and it is a symptom complex of straining and the urge to defecate. One must keep in mind that the lower anal canal obtains its innervation from the somatic nervous system, and therefore, any pain-producing lesion in the anal canal is likely to be described as sharp, burning or stinging. The pain associated with a perianal abscess is usually described as throbbing in nature. The pain associated with an intersphincteric abscess is often associated with an increase in intensity when the patient coughs or sneezes. Pain which is not associated with the passage of a stool is rarely anal in origin. Anorectal pain may be referred to the sacral region, and here one must be very careful in eliciting the history as it relates to a bowel movement. The classic history of levator ani muscle spasm, better known as proctalgia fugax, is frequently misdiagnosed as hemorrhoidal or fissure pain (Chap. 30). Referred pain to the rectum may occur from aneurysmal dilatations in the pelvic vascular tree or from retrorectal tumors. Usually this condition is described as a fullness in the area. Coccygeal pain is rarely anal in origin. Most patients complaining of this type of pain have sustained some trauma to the ligaments or periosteum of the coccyx. Occasionally when a presacral cyst is inflamed the pain may be referred to the coccyx.

*Abdominal pain* of colonic origin may be crampy in nature when related to an intramural lesion, or excessive colonic contraction, or distension, or may be associated with peritoneal irritation when related to any inflammation in the colon. Patients may complain of discomfort in the right, lower quadrant due to a distended cecum. When the mesentery of the colon is stretched, pain will be appreciated, and this can be duplicated in the process of performing a proctosigmoidoscopic or colonoscopic examination. Peritoneal pain may be secondary to colonic disease when there are adhesions between the colon and the parieties.[7]

The sites of referred pain to the body surface are determined by the same principles as referred pain elsewhere. Pain from the colon is referred to just above the symphysis pubis, and that from the rectum can go directly to the sacral area.

Abdominal pain may be a manifestation of anorectal disease when the supralevator space is involved. Because this space has peritoneum as its "roof", a suppurative process may result in signs of peritoneal irritation.[9]

## Bleeding

The differential diagnosis of an anorectal condition can frequently be made by the accurate delineation of the type of bleeding experienced by the patient. One must determine whether the patient is passing clots, or if it is true melena; whether the blood is mixed with the stool, or separate from the stool; whether the blood appears on the toilet tissue, or it drips into the toilet bowl. Blood which drips into the toilet bowl, and is bright red in nature, and free, and separate from stool, is frequently associated with bleeding internal hemorrhoids. Blood which is on the tissue tends to be associated with anal fissures or an abrasion of the anal canal. Melena, obviously, can be caused by any pathological processes higher up in the gastrointestinal tract. The association of blood and mucus usually is seen with a low-lying carcinoma or, more frequently, with an inflammatory condition such as ulcerative colitis or Crohn's disease. The passage of blood clots is usually associated with a source of colonic origin. A rare cause of "bleeding" which is frequently misdiagnosed is that which is associated with the eating of fresh beets. Betacyanins are violet-red pigments that are the main coloring matter in beets and can mimic blood in the toilet water.[10]

## Mucus and Discharge

Mucus is the product of the goblet cells of the colonic mucosa, and may be seen in the stool under many different circumstances. It may be the result of normal production of mucus; it may be the early sign of a villous adenoma of the bowel or an early colitic condition. A great deal of mucus is produced by chemical irritations. The packaged phosphosoda enemas can elicit a tremendous response from the bowel, and one is immediately impressed with the amount of mucus seen upon endoscopic examination of the bowel following administration of just such an enema. If the mucus is associated with bleeding, it may be the sign of a neoplasm or inflammatory process.

## Bowel Habits

Change in bowel habits is a difficult symptom to define. The normal defecatory patterns of patients are so varied, and multifactorial, that any suggestion of a change must be investigated completely. When searching out a history of constipation one must ask if the patient is referring to a hard stool, a stool that is difficult to pass, or an infrequent stool. A similar definition must be elicited from the patient regarding the frequency and consistancy of a diarrheal stool. Tenesmus is usually associated with a lesion in the distal colon and rectum, such as colitis, or a neoplastic lesion. Operative procedures such as vagotomy, cholecystectomy, or small bowel resection may alter gastrointestinal motility, absorption, and secretion, and consequently, alter bowel habits.

Patients who have had a jejunoileal bypass for morbid obesity are subject to a great number of anorectal problems associated with diarrhea. When a patient presents with a history of incontinence, following a previous anorectal surgical procedure, the details of this procedure certainly must be elicited in order to fully evaluate his complaints. A good obstetrical history regarding the nature of the episiotomy, and any complications associated with it, should be obtained, as well as the nature and type of delivery.

## Flatulence

Because everyone passes gas per rectum, one must inquire as to whether this is an excessive passage of flatus or an unusual sense of awareness of the normal passage. The majority of patients with increased flatulence are found to have a dietary indiscretion, in the form of excessive intake of gas-producing substances, rather than any specific malady of the gastrointestinal tract. Patients are unaware that fermentation is taking place all the time. A simple test for a patient is to ask him to go on a clear liquid diet for 24 hours, and observe the amounts of flatus following this therapeutic test. Frequently, he will learn that very little gas is formed when there is not an excessive amount of food in the gastrointestinal tract. Another simple test is to ask him if he was troubled with flatus on the day he was prepared for the barium enema study. Often he will tell you that he was free of flatus for the first time when he was cleaned out for the x-ray study. Elegant studies by Levitt have shown that hydrogen, and methane, are produced solely by bacteria, and not a product of human cellular metabolism.[6] He has also shown that hydrogen production is negligible in the fasting state, and it appears that colon bacteria are dependent upon ingested fermentable substrates (carbohydrates) for hydrogen production. Certain vegetables, particularly legumes, contain a high concentration of indigestible oligosaccharides which are nonabsorbable, even by normal subjects, and these oligosaccharides account for the notorious gaseous properties of legumes. Carbon dioxide can be produced by bacterial fermentation or by the reaction of bicarbonate and acid. Digestion of an average meal could theoretically produce several hundred mEq of acid, thus yielding 4,000 cc of carbon dioxide. While excessive gas is assumed to be a common cause of "functional abdominal complaints", there is almost no hard data to support this assumption.[6]

Passing gas per vagina, or per urethra, is usually indicative of a fistula to the gastrointestinal tract. Occasionally gas-forming organisms in the bladder may give rise to pneumaturia without a fistula, but this is rare except in the diabetic patient. A complete gastrointestinal evaluation is mandatory if a history of pneumaturia or flatus per vagina is obtained.

### Perianal Swelling

One must always ascertain whether the swelling is painful or not, and whether it has discharged blood or pus. The swelling also might be intermittent as one would expect with a prolapsing, hypertrophied anal papilla. In the event that this swelling is associated with fever and chills, one would certainly be suspicious of an anorectal abscess. The common swelling at the anal verge is usually a thrombosed external hemorrhoid, which comes on rather quickly, and is associated with pain, and occasional bleeding, if ulcerated.

### Pruritus

Pruritus ani is a common symptom associated with anorectal pathology. Most commonly, pruritus ani occurs in patients who have loose stools, and are unable to cleanse their anal canals in a proper fashion. Pruritus also may be associated with the healing phase of an anal condition. The patient who has a healing anal fissure may present with a symptom of itching. Severe pruritus ani is usually associated with a mucoid discharge, which may be blood tinged due to the open ulceration of the perianal skin. One must always question the patient regarding the use of antibiotics since they may be the cause of pruritus ani. Enterobius vermicularis (pin worms) is a rare cause of pruritus ani in the adult (Chap. 10).

### Prolapse

In questioning the patient who presents with a protrusion from the anal aperture, one might inquire as to whether the prolapse occurs only at the time of defecation, or whether it will occur independently. Independent prolapsing is more suggestive of a hypertrophied anal papilla, or a complete rectal procidentia. Does the prolapse spontaneously reduce itself or must it be replaced manually? This may suggest the magnitude of the problem. The patient can frequently give you an idea of the relative size of the prolapsing mass, and the amount of prolapse will often be very helpful in the diagnosis. The most common prolapsing condition is certainly rectal mucosal prolapse associated with prolapsing hemorrhoids. This must be differentiated from true procidentia of the rectum. Large hypertrophied anal papillae are also known to prolapse from the anal canal. Polyps in the rectum can prolapse; however, this is usually seen in a child with juvenile polyposis, or in the elderly patient with a massive villous adenoma.

### Exposure

In taking a history one must also be cognizant of the fact that the patient may have recently returned from a tropical country, and may have been exposed to certain parasitic diseases, especially in this day and age of jet travel. A history of sexual exposure will be important, especially if the patient has had anal intercourse (Chap. 12).

### Associated Medical Conditions

Inflammatory bowel disease is well known for its associated anorectal problems. A history of this condition should be pursued in any patient with an anorectal complaint. Diabetes mellitus is occasionally associated with nocturnal diarrhea. The patient with peptic ulcer disease may be taking antacids, which increase the firmness of the stool, and may cause anorectal pain and bleeding, while other antacids may cause loose stools.

### Family History

Often a patient's bowel habits will be very similar to those of his parents. It is amazing how frequently one will get a familial history of hemorrhoids in patients who are suffering from a rectal mucosal prolapse. A pertinent cancer history should be sought.

### Medications

The use of laxatives is commonplace, therefore, one must ascertain the medications that a patient is ingesting, both prescribed and over-the-counter, in order to fully evaluate his symptoms. A detailed laxative history is mandatory for any patient with a bowel complaint. As with any medical history, a complete history of drug allergies should be obtained.

### Bleeding Tendency

If a surgical procedure is necessary, a history of a bleeding tendency should be ruled out.

## EXAMINATION

The proctosigmoidoscopic examination may be uncomfortable, and, to the sensitive patient, it may be a source of acute embarrassment. Patient cooperation can be secured by simple explanation and reassurance. The proper performance of the examination requires suitable equipment: usually a few simple instruments will suffice. It is essential that the endoscopist be thoroughly familiar with the use of these instruments.

### Examination Room and Equipment

Endoscopic examinations can be carried out with the patient in the left lateral, or in the prone, jackknife position. The use of a tilting table has distinct advantages; however, an adequate examination can be carried out in the left lateral position with the patient on a flat table. It is important that instruments be within easy reach of the surgeon, but an attempt should be made to keep them covered, and out of view of the patient, since instruments can be a source of unnecessary anxiety. A good suction apparatus is mandatory.

*Table.* The prone jackknife position has the advantage of the negative pressure, which is created by the viscera sliding out of the pelvis, and thereby, less insufflation is required for viewing the bowel. The patient should be properly positioned on the table. The knee rest should be elevated so that the abdomen hangs freely, and a hand may be slipped comfortably beneath it. In the event that the examination is done in the left lateral position, care should be taken that the buttocks extend over the edge of the examination table. Proctosigmoidoscopic examination can be carried out quite well at the bedside, utilizing the left lateral position.

*Digital Examination.* Digital examination can be performed with either a latex glove, or a finger cot, using a water soluble type of lubricant. In most situations, a finger cot is adequate protection. Some surgeons prefer to lubricate the anal canal with a small, cotton-tipped, applicator prior to the digital examination. This procedure permits the surgeon to brush aside the anal hairs so that they will not be "dragged" into the anal canal with the examining finger. Under no circumstance should the patient experience pain due to the examination. With an acutely painful anorectal condition, digital examination may be performed with the aid of cocaine or other topical anesthetic agents, or alternatively, the patient may require examination under anesthesia.

*Suction and Swabs.* A good facility includes excellent suction. Some surgeons prefer the plastic suction tip so that there is no interference with electrocoagulation. Some proctosigmoidoscopes have a built-in suction tip for evacuation of gas at the time of electrocoagulation. In the past, cotton-tipped swabs have been used to remove blood and stool. This practice should be discouraged in favor of a repeat-packaged enema, and suction, as the latter is more efficacious and aesthetic. Cotton swab pressure may be used to control minor bleeding.

*Endoscopes.* Many different types of endoscopes have been developed. The most common one utilized is the *distal lighted fiberoptic proctosigmoidoscope* made by Welch Allyn (Fig. 3-1). It comes in various sizes, and the availability of a complete range of scopes is beneficial. The 19 mm by 25 cm scope is probably the most universally used instrument, especially in the event of polyp removal or biopsy, and electrocoagulation. Because it is a bit smaller, permitting a more comfortable ex-

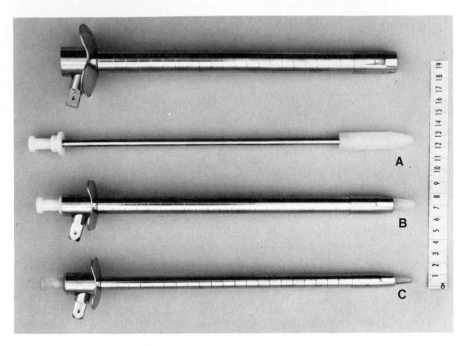

FIGURE **3-1.** *Proctosigmoidoscopes. (A) 19 mm. × 25 cm. scope. (B) 15 mm. × 25 cm. scope. (C) 11 mm. × 25 cm. scope.*

amination, some surgeons prefer the 15 mm by 25 cm proctosigmoidoscope for routine diagnostic examination. An 11 mm by 25 cm stricture scope, which is important for examining patients with a stricture of the anal canal, should be available.

Some models are adapted with built-in smoke tubes to which suction can be directly applied. There are several types of window apparatuses. Most surgeons prefer the removable taper window, as opposed to the hinged window, which has a tendency to lose its tight fit with usage. The distal illumination is an advantage; however, in certain circumstances when blood collects at the end of the proctosigmoidoscope; the examiner may have difficulty viewing the bleeding point, and wish he had a proximal light source at that time.

The larger diameter proctosigmoidoscopes rarely are needed, except in the operating room, for removal of large rectosigmoidal polyps. A 35 cm proctosigmoidoscope can be used; however, with the recent advent of the flexible fiberoptic sigmoidoscope, the need for the long rigid instruments is diminishing.

The Vernon-David modification of the Ives anoscope, which is only three inches long, is excellent for diagnostic work. It is small in caliber, and is well tolerated by patients (Fig. 3-2). The Hirschman anoscope has also been used for anal examinations, and especially for ligation of hemorrhoids. The Hinkel-James anoscope is an excellent instrument for banding and injection procedures (Fig. 3-3). Newer innovations have included the addition of a fiberoptic light source to the anoscope; however, these may actually be more cumbersome with the attached light cord than without. For this part of the examination most experienced colon and rectal surgeons seem to prefer a headlamp which can be directed onto the perianal area or into the anoscope. An overhead spotlight may serve the same function adequately. A long-bladed nasal speculum such as the Cottle or the Killian may come in handy in examining a patient with a severe anal stricture.

Since the advent of *flexible fiberoptic colonoscopy*, various instruments have been developed. The 60 cm flexible sigmoidoscope

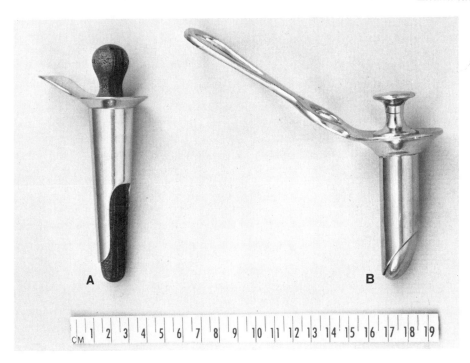

FIGURE **3-2.** (*A*) *Vernon-David anoscope.* (*B*) *Hirshman anoscope.*

has four-way movement of the tip, and a large channel for suction, biopsy, and polypectomy. The indications for its use have been under considerable discussion. Several authors have suggested that the primary use be in the training of endoscopists: to allow them to gain an early skill in handling a fiberoptic instrument in preparation for developing the necessary skills to handle the longer instrument, although, this has not been our experience. The routine use of this instrument in place of the rigid sigmoidoscope has been suggested by others. A flexible instrument may be inserted further, causing the patient less discomfort, while significantly increasing the yield of pathological conditions. These authors point out that the instrument can be used without prolonging the length of examination time, and in almost all cases, with greater comfort to the patient.[7] These examinations are usually accomplished as an outpatient procedure, following the administration of one packaged phosphosoda enema. The patient may be examined either in the prone jack-knife, or the left lateral, position. Among the disadvantages in the use of the fiberoptic colonoscope are the time required to clean the instrument (approx-

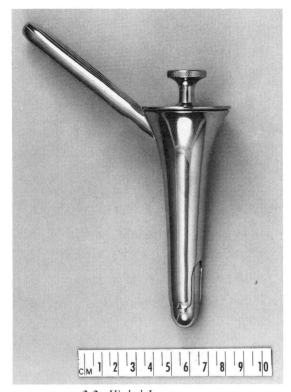

FIGURE **3-3.** *Hinkel-James anoscope.*

imately five to ten minutes), and an inadequate view of the rectum compared to that obtained using the rigid sigmoidoscope. In addition, the instrument is somewhat expensive, ranging from $2–5,000. The early results with the 60 cm flexible sigmoidoscope definitely have exceeded the diagnostic yield of the routine proctosigmoidoscopic examination, and the flexible sigmoidoscope diminishes the discomfort associated with rigid proctosigmoidoscopy. The optics are excellent, and the shorter length makes the distal tip responsive to small amounts of torque applied to the control head. The examination as an office or out-patient procedure has been found to be uniformly safe, but one must remember that the trials have been conducted by accomplished endoscopists. It can be performed quickly, without extensive preparation, and no sedation. The flexible fiberoptic sigmoidoscopes can be inserted nearly two to three times further than the rigid instrument. More patients prefer the use of this instrument. Nevertheless, as yet, this instrument has not found its place as standard office equipment.

*Cautery.* Any facility for proctosigmoidoscopy should have electrocautery capability. This may be of the unipolar or bipolar variety. For cutting currents, low voltage (200–400 V) is used with higher frequency.[2] Coagulation currents are damped, lower frequency, higher voltage currents. Blended currents are a combination of both, the damping being varied to give appropriate hemostasis. Cutting currents

result in an arcing, ionizing, or vaporizing of tissue and tissue water. Coagulation is more of a denaturing of tissue, and a slower process.

Two basic power generators are used in this type of equipment: the spark gap generator, and the radio-frequency oscillator. Of the two, the spark gap generator, which is an electromechanical device, is less dependent on patient parameters. The basic system is a bipolar system. A unipolar system would dispense with the indifferent electrode as such.

Care must be exercised not to use electrosurgical equipment in an unclean bowel for fear of explosion and perforation.[8] Familiarity with the equipment, and the depth, and width of heat produced is mandatory in order to minimize the risk of a bowel perforation. Carbon dioxide insufflation is not necessary to prevent explosion, if suction is frequently applied to eliminate the bowel gas.

A series of tips with ball points or needles are available. Most surgeons prefer the ball tip (Fig. 19-2).

*Probes.* A fine probe may assist the surgeon in evaluating a fistulous track, but this should be discouraged, except in the operating room where the track can be probed without hurting the patient. The probes pictured here are used in the operating room for fistula surgery (Fig. 3-4).

*Biopsy Instruments.* The Buie biopsy forceps (Fig. 3-5) is an excellent instrument for removal of polyps. It must be kept sharp, and

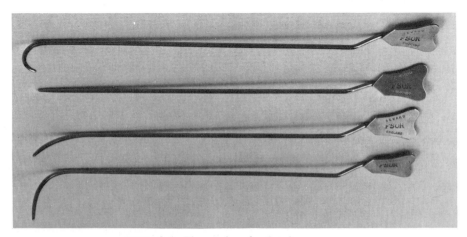

FIGURE **3-4.** *The probes for fistula surgery.*

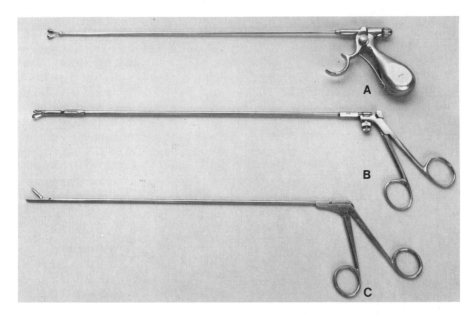

FIGURE **3-5.** (*A*) *Buie biopsy forceps.* (*B*) *Turell biopsy forceps.* (*C*) *Alligator forceps.*

handled with care. Minimal bleeding is obtained in removing mucosal lesions with this forceps. The Turell angulated rotating biopsy forceps has the advantage of turning the cutting jaws 360° without changing the position of the hand. It is used to biopsy larger neoplastic lesions. Alligator forceps for retrieval of polyps or foreign bodies should be available.

All of the electrosurgical companies make snares for snaring polyps. The requirements for a good snare include freedom from breakage, and malleability (Fig. 19-3). A second snare wire should always be available in the room.

*Ligation Equipment.* Ligation equipment including ligator, O-ring, and forceps should be available for immediate use (Fig. 3-6). Several forceps have been advocated for this technique; however, an Allis forceps may suffice.

*Sclerosing Equipment.* Sclerosing techniques for hemorrhoids are still common. A loaded syringe (Fig. 6-4.) with 5 percent phenol and vegetable oil, or quinine and urea hydrochloride should be readily available.

*Resuscitation Equipment.* In any medical facility basic resuscitation equipment should be available, especially where minor surgical procedures are being performed.

**Position**

Proctosigmoidoscopy is greatly facilitated by placing the patient in the inverted position. The four positions that have been used for this examination are the prone jackknife, the left lateral, the lithotomy, and the knee-chest.

*Prone Jackknife.* (Fig. 3-7) The prone jackknife position is probably the best method for examining the lower bowel. It has the advantage in the fact that gravitation of the intestine, out of the pelvis, occurs when the patient is in the inverted position. It has the disadvantage, however, of putting patients in an unfamiliar and insecure position. Care must be taken to have the patient properly positioned on the table so that his knees are gently separated, and that there is space between the abdomen and the table. The head-rest should be set at a comfortable angle for each patient, and the knee-rest should be elevated, or lowered, in order to make the patient completely comfortable. There is no need to invert the patient on the tilting table completely until the proctosigmoidoscope has been introduced to the level of the rectosigmoid. A mild tilt to the table is all that is necessary during the preliminary phases of the examination. Another advantage of this position is that any mucus present within the bowel will, by gravity, fall

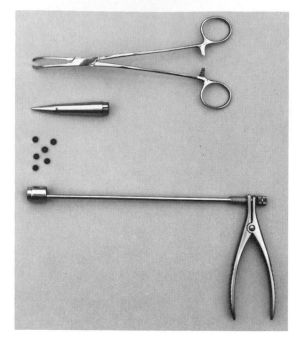

FIGURE **3-6.** *Rubber band ligation equipment.*

away from the field of vision, and very little insufflation is required to distend the bowel because of the negative pressure created by the viscera sliding away from the rectum.

*Left Lateral Position.* The left lateral position is a satisfactory position for the performance of an adequate proctosigmoidoscopic examination. It is very comfortable for most patients, and requires no special, expensive tilt table. The secret of the left lateral position is to project the buttock slightly beyond the edge of the examining table (Fig. 3-8). It is a position which lends itself to good use in doing a proctosigmoidoscopic examination on a patient sick in bed. It has the disadvantage of requiring a considerably greater amount of air to be insufflated to properly visualize the bowel.

*Lithotomy.* The lithotomy position is rarely utilized for proctosigmoidoscopy. Occasionally this position is used in the operating room, but, as a routine method of outpatient examination, most surgeons would prefer the left lateral or the prone jackknife positions.

*Knee-Chest Position.* This position may be used for proctosigmoidoscopic examination; however, it is most uncomfortable for the patient, and without a good tilt table, most surgeons would prefer the left lateral position.

**Anesthesia**

Anesthesia is rarely indicated for the routine examination of the anorectum. Many patients with anal fissures may be examined with a small diameter stricturescope without general

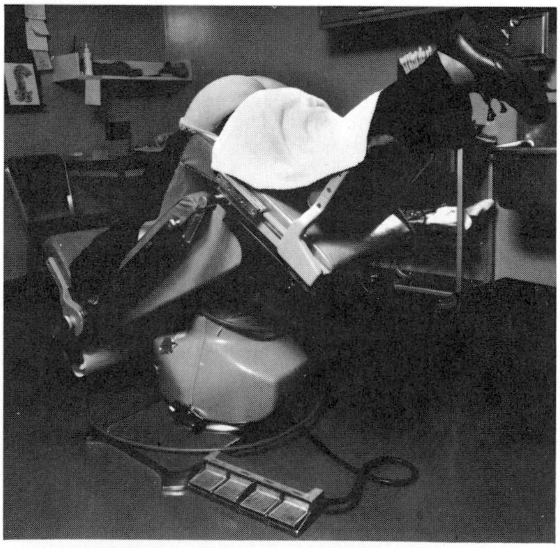

FIGURE **3-7.** *Prone jackknife position on examination (Ritter) table.*

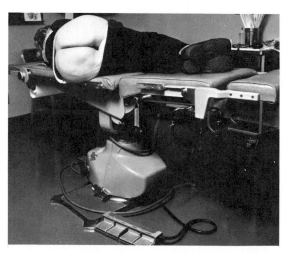

FIGURE **3-8.** *Left lateral position* (*note that the buttock projects slightly beyond the edge of the examining table*).

or regional anesthesia. However, if the patient has a very painful fissure, or an intersphincteric abscess, or is unable to tolerate any intra-anal manipulation, endoscopy should be deferred until the fissure has healed, or the appropriate anesthetic has been instituted. "Vocal anesthesia" which was perfected by Buie is the anesthetic of choice for most proctosigmoidoscopic examinations.[1] Occasionally the local application of cocaine crystals to a painful anal fissure may be necessary in order to proctosigmoidoscope the bowel, and rule out the presence of an inflammatory bowel disease. Injecting a local anesthetic, with a 27 or 30 gauge needle, into the perineum, and blocking the anorectum, may also be done when the patient has a painful anorectal condition. Usually the sequence of events is best handled by examining the patient under anesthesia in the operating room, and proceeding with the necessary surgical procedure. The electrocoagulation of rectal polyps in a patient with multiple polyposis of the rectum can be a painful procedure, even though the rectal mucosa is innervated by the autonomic nervous system, and is supposed to be insensitive to the pain of electrocoagulation. Frequently, these patients can feel pain in the presacral area, and may require an anesthetic for this electrocoagulation treatment.

### Examination Technique and Approach

It is always good to keep the endoscopic instruments under cover, especially when the patient is entering the examining room. This simple foresight will assist in lessening the patient's apprehension.

The surgeon should be careful to instruct his patient as to what to expect, and what is happening, as the examination progresses. These efforts on the part of the examining physician nearly always pay dividends in greater patient confidence, better patient cooperation, and avoidance of defense reaction stimulated by unexpected maneuvers.

It is not necessary for the patient to remove all of his clothing. The patient is usually instructed to kneel on the knee rest, and then drop his undergarment. Women patients are draped for the examination.

As the patient's head is lowered on the table, he is instructed that he will not fall, and that he may get a bit "light-headed." The examining surgeon may want to check the abdomen to see if there is room for the abdomen to "hang," and in addition, he may encourage the patient to let his back sag or be in a "sway-back" fashion. The object of these details is to allow the sigmoid colon to fall out of the true pelvis. This is facilitated by the inverted position.

There are four main steps in the examination technique: inspection, palpation, sigmoidoscopy and anoscopy.

*Inspection.* With adequate light, the perianal area is inspected, and the patient is instructed that he will feel the physician's hand. Visual scrutiny of the perianal region, lower back, and sacrococcygeal region is performed. Visualization of the lower anal canal is carried out in a very gentle manner, looking for fissuring of the perianal skin which is visualized by a gentle separation of the anus. External openings of fistulae, and the excoriations or lichenification, of pruritus ani may be noted. A point to be made at this time concerns the recording of findings. A plea is made to dispense with the use of the face of the clock as a means of describing the location of anal pathology. The examiner should describe his findings in an anatomic fashion, using the terms anterior, posterior, left lateral, and right lateral. One only has to think of the confusion that arises when terminology which refers to the clock face is used. The lithotomy position and the jack-knife position are 180° apart; in the left lateral position the 12 o'clock position would be 90° different from the 12 o'clock position in the prone jackknife position. Needless to say, anatomical description circumvents all the confusion.

*Palpation.* Adequate visualization of the anal and perianal skin, and the medial surfaces of the buttocks necessitates the retraction of the anal canal and buttocks, and enhances the "laying on of hands." Examiners should develop the habit of explaining briefly to the patient each step of the procedure. "I am now going to lubricate the anal canal and it may feel a bit cold." The digital examination should be carried out in a slow, and gentle, fashion. The patient may be asked to strain down against the examining finger which results in opening of the anal aperture. The other hand separates the perianal skin in order to assist introduction of the examining finger (Fig. 3-9). If a moderate degree of anal stenosis is present, it is not

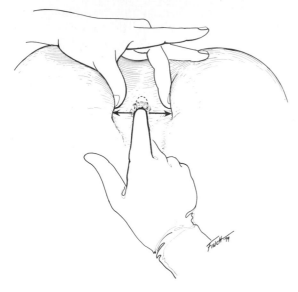

**FIGURE 3-9.** *Digital examination.*

mandatory to insert the entire digit into the anal canal. This may await complete examination under anesthesia.

If there is any question of a fistula-in-ano, a *bi-digital examination* of the sphincter muscle should be carried out, examining the muscle between the index finger and the thumb, in an attempt to ascertain if there is any thickened area of inflammatory tissue in the sphincteric mechanism. The presacral area can be a "blind area" with the sigmoidoscope, therefore, one must be very careful to examine it by palpation. With the finger in the rectum, the tone of the sphincter muscle and the puborectalis sling may be evaluated by asking the patient to voluntarily contract. With the examining finger, enlarged nodes in the retrorectal space can be palpated. The prostate should be evaluated, and a rectovaginal, or bi-manual examination may be required to properly assess any suggestion of pathology in the rectovaginal septum, or in the reproductive organs. The rectoabdominal examination, between the rectum and the abdomen, is impossible in the prone jackknife position; however, the left lateral position lends itself well to this type of synchronous examination. It is always important, when carrying out a digital examination, to start the examination away from the pathology. If a fissure is seen in the midline posteriorly, one should attempt to introduce

the examining finger over the anterior commissure.

*Proctosigmoidoscopy.* The instrument is advanced, utilizing a minimum amount of insufflation, just enough to encourage the retained mucus in the bowel to move out of sight. All of the folds of the rectum are flattened out in looking for neoplastic lesions. Often times one is only able to advance the instrument a distance of 12 to 16 cm. No attempt should be made to forcibly advance the instrument beyond this point. Air insufflation is used to best advantage during withdrawal of the endoscope to facilitate thorough inspection of all of its surfaces. When the proctosigmoidoscope reaches the level of the rectosigmoid the patient should be told that he may feel a cramp in the abdomen. You may tell the patient, "the cramp will disappear just as soon as I remove the instrument." You may also tell the·patient to breathe deeply, and slowly, through his mouth. This will relax the abdominal musculature and distract him long enough to allow the easy passage of the instrument. The proctosigmoidoscope will usually advance to the 15 cm level with ease. At this point the sigmoid colon usually curves to the patient's left, and special care must be exercised. The patient will notice cramping pains if the mesentery is placed under excessive tension. Warn the patient of possible cramps at this point. Frequently the mesentery is short, and the scope cannot negotiate the rather sharp bend, even in the most experienced hand. In this case, terminate further advancement and, above all, do not hurt the patient.

Ordinarily, the 19 mm proctosigmoidoscope will pass to the 25 cm level without difficulty in 30 to 50 per cent of cases. At this point, insufflation of air may allow the examiner to see another 1 to 5 cm ahead of the proctosigmoidoscope. Although insufflation is designed to allow distention of the bowel, throughout the examination its use should be limited, since excessive air may be traumatic and painful.

After advancing the proctosigmoidoscope as far as possible, tell the patient that the procedure is nearly complete, and that little or no discomfort should be experienced during withdrawal. However, it is at this point that the examination begins in earnest. All attention during advancement of the scope should be directed toward safe, and painless passage, whereas the most careful scrutiny of the bowel for pathology is carried out during withdrawal. Pull back slowly using a small, rotary motion in order to view all the mucosal surfaces. This motion is most essential in the rectum, where the lumen diameter is larger, and the posterior surface, coursing over the sacral convexity, is not always in view. Flatten each rectal valve ridge with the tip of the proctosigmoidoscope to visualize lesions on their superior surface. Always remember to release any air placed in the sigmoid just prior to removing the proctosigmoidoscope or cramps may follow the procedure. Finally, remember to remove residual lubricants from the buttocks with a tissue before the patient departs. If the examination has revealed nothing abnormal, be certain to tell the patient so. Do not limit yourself to indefinite terminology such as growths, tumors, and polyps. Patients want to know that they do not have cancer. If there have been positive findings it is wise to defer specific comments until the microscopic report is available.

A pitfall in which both the novice, and experienced, examiner frequently find themselves is the "blind pouch". The blind pouch is an apparent "dead end" segment of the bowel. The difficulty lies in the examiner's failure to withdraw the proctosigmoidoscope a short distance in order to obtain a better view of the lumen ahead. Any sudden movement by the patient when the proctosigmoidoscope is in place may result in a perforation. It is important not to make any sudden moves which may cause the patient to straighten up, and thereby result in a perforation. The incidence of perforation during proctosigmoidoscopic examination was found to be one per 20,600 examinations at the University of Minnesota.[3] During the examination, one must be aware of the nature of the mucosa and its submucosal vascular pattern, the appearance of the folds and, obviously, any neoplastic lesions. Any suspicious areas should be biopsied unless the surgeon plans to obtain a barium enema examination, in which case he may want to obtain the barium enema first, and remove the lesion at a later date. It is not uncomfortable for the patient and, in the hands of an experienced examiner, this procedure should take just a few minutes. It is only with additional procedures, such as a biopsy or a polypectomy, that sigmoidoscopy should require a longer time. One must keep in mind the anatomy of the pelvis, especially the peritoneal reflections, as the examination is carried out. The findings of the examination should be recorded as to the nature of the mucosa, and also as to the distance traversed. The presence of neoplastic lesions, their location, and gross description should likewise be recorded.

*Anoscopy.* The head of the table should be approximately 15° from level for the anoscopic examination. Some surgeons like to do this examination before proctosigmoidoscopy, while other surgeons prefer to do it following proctosigmoidoscopy because they may want to perform some minor procedure in the anal canal, and would do so only after knowing the proctosigmoidoscopic examination is completely normal. Several instruments are available for anoscopy. We have a preference for the Vernon-David modification of the Ives anoscope. It is of small diameter, and can be used in most patients, except those few who have a very painful or stenotic anal canal. Obviously it must be well-lubricated, and the instrument should not be rotated, except with the obturator in place. A frequent misdiagnosis made with an anoscope is that of bleeding associated with rectal mucosal prolapse. Often, when patients are examined in the prone jackknife position, physicians are not impressed with the magnitude of internal hemorrhoids, so it is important to ask the patient to "strain down" with the anoscope in place. One immediately becomes impressed with the ease with which the patient can bleed from internal hemorrhoids when this simple examination is performed. If the patient has no specific anal complaints, anoscopy may be omitted as part of a routine examination. However, if a patient has uncomplicated, bleeding, internal hemorrhoids, and sigmoidoscopy is negative, by performing the anoscopic examination at the completion of the proctosigmoidoscopy, one would be permitted the rubber band ligation, or injection of these hemorrhoids at that moment.

## Preparation for Examination

Preparation for a proctosigmoidoscopic examination should be very simple. Some ambulatory patients may be examined adequately with no preparation whatsoever. If the patient does not have any urge to defecate, more than likely, his rectum is free of stool. However, most surgeons prefer to have their patients prepared with one packaged phosphosoda enema. There is value in examining the patient, however, without prior preparation, especially when looking for an early colitis. Some patients get a very hyperemic bowel in response to the phosphosoda enema, and this can be indistinguishable from an early proctosigmoiditis. Blood, on the side of the bowel, which frequently indicates a lesion higher up in the bowel, may be washed away with a preparatory enema. Often patients who are bleeding can be examined without preparation, and if no significant pathology is noted, reexamined after preparation, in order to ensure a more complete examination.

Carbon dioxide-releasing suppositories have been used for preparation for proctosigmoidoscopic examination; however, they seem to hold no great advantage over a packaged phosphosoda enema given twenty minutes before the examination. Usually, one enema is all that is necessary for examining the patient with a standard proctosigmoidoscope. Examination with the 60 cm flexible sigmoidoscope may require two enemas. It certainly is not necessary to use castor oil, or any other oil cathartics, for routine proctosigmoidoscopy.

## DIAGNOSTIC TESTS
### Hemoccult, Guaiac

Since most cancers of the colon bleed, a screening sequence should begin with the testing for occult blood in the stool. Although a number of occult blood tests have been put forth in recent years, the one that is most reliable is the guaiac-impregnated paper slide test, introduced by Greegor, and known as Hemoccult.[5] Unlike tests using saturated guaiac, or tincture of guaiac solutions (50–60% false-positive reactions), or Hematest (a 30% false-positive rate), the Hemoccult test has a low false-positive rate, estimated to be less than 1 per cent in asymptomatic patients. Hemoccult false-negative rates are unknown, but are believed to be equally low. In addition, the usual guaiac tests are notoriously unreliable because of quality-control problems in the manufacturing of guaiac solutions, and on-shelf deterioration of the agent. Hemoccult, on the other hand, can be prepared with good quality control, and the reagent is stable. In a collaborative study of Hemoccult, involving the experience of 103 physicians, 139 cancers were detected (only 20 of which were within reach of the standard proctosigmoidoscopy), and only one patient who had followed the instructions had a false-negative result.[5] Moreover, in 47 cases of "silent", or asymptomatic, cancer revealed by Hemoccult testing, 85 per cent were found to be localized to the bowel wall, in sharp contrast with the usual 40 per cent. Although the Hemoccult test places on the patient the responsibility of preparing the slides, the task is esthetically simple (requiring only a thin smear of stool specimen put on the guaiac-impregnated paper with a wooden applicator), and the rate of patient compliance is usually very high. The procedure is as follows: at home, the patient prepares two slides from different parts of a stool each day for three days while on a meat-free, high bulk diet, which begins at least 24 hours before the first stool specimen is collected. Bulk and roughage must be included to stimulate bleeding in lesions, and so avoid the false-negative results that may occur on bland diets. Similarly, the intake of Vitamin C may also produce false-negative reactions, and therefore, should be avoided during the test period. On the other hand, tomatoes and cherries have been known to give a false positive result. In a study series, at the University of Minnesota Colon Cancer Control, of 48,000 participants of greater than 50 years of age, 23,500 of them have returned the Hemoccult slides: 525 participants have had one or more slides positive for occult blood in the stool, and 475 of them have come to University of Minnesota Hospitals for evaluation. Forty-seven gastrointestinal cancers were detected in 45 patients: 33 colon, 10 rectum, 2 stomach, 1 pancreas, 1 secondary colon.[4]

### Barium Enema: Air-Contrast

Barium enema examination is another essential technique in patients with colorectal symptoms. With the exception of emergency conditions, such as acutely obstructing lesions which are revealed by barium enema alone, the addition of air-contrast provides valuable diagnostic information. Lesions located in certain areas of the colon, particularly the flexures, may not be detected easily by radiographic examination. If symptoms persist, a negative barium enema examination should be repeated, and corroborated, by colonoscopy. With proper preparation of the patient (the colon must be completely clean), the air-contrast method will detect the majority of large lesions, but it will still miss many smaller lesions, for example the flat lesions of mild inflammatory bowel disease, and some polyps or cancers in patients with diverticular disease. It is also, of course, subject to errors of interpretation, as is any test.

## REFERENCES

1. Buie, L. A.: Practical Proctology. Springfield, Charles C. Thomas, 1960.
2. Curtiss, L. E.: High frequency currents in endoscopy. Gastrointest. Endos., *20:*9, 1973.
3. Gilbertsen, V. A.: Proctosigmoidoscopy and polypectomy in reducing the incidence of rectal cancer. Cancer, *34:*936, 1974 suppl.
4. Gilbertson, V. A., Williams, S. E., Schuman, L.: The earlier detection of Colorectal cancers. In Najarian, J. S., Delaney, J. P. (eds.): Gastrointestinal Surgery, pp. 593–599. Year Book Medical Publishers, Chicago, 1979.
5. Greegor, D. H.: Occult blood testing for detection of asymptomatic colon cancer. Cancer, *28:*131, 1971.
6. Levitt, M. D.: Volume and composition of human intestinal gas determined by means of an intestinal washout technique. N. Engl. J. Med., *284:*1394, 1971.
7. Marks, G., Boggs, H. W., Castro, A. F., Gathright, J. B., Ray, J. E. and Salvati, E.: Sigmoidoscopic examinations with rigid and flexible fiberoptic sigmoidoscopes in the surgeon's office: A comparative prospective study of effectiveness in 1,012 cases. Dis. Colon Rectum, *22:*162, 1979.
8. Mitchell, J. P., and Lumb, G. N.: The principles of surgical diathermy and its limitations. Br. J. Surg., *50:*314, 1962.
9. Nesselrod, J. P.: Clinical Proctology. Philadelphia, W. B. Saunders Co., 1964.
10. Paul, P. C., and Palmer, H. H.: Food Theory and Applications. New York, John Wiley and Sons, 1972.

# 4

# Pre- and Postoperative Management of the Anorectal Wounds

A full discussion of the mechanical and physiochemical aspects of wound healing is beyond the scope of this book; however, specific references will be made to facts that are known, and clinical observations that have been made, pertinent to the management of anorectal wounds. Many of the recommendations made will be policies adopted due to satisfactory clinical experience. These policies evolved through hit and miss trial of other techniques.

## PREOPERATIVE DISCUSSION

As with any well-timed, well-planned, elective operation, the patient should be given realistic expectations regarding the in-hospital stay, the postoperative time at home, and overall recovery time. In easy-to-understand terms, the patient and surgeon should review the anatomy involved, preferably by means of illustrative charts and diagrams, and discuss the goals of the operative procedure. The type of incision, extent of wounds to be created, and the possibility of decision-making at the time of operation should be outlined. Details as to how the wound will be repaired, average time for healing, as well as possible complications in healing, should also be discussed. The patient should be aware that suture material utilized will dissolve spontaneously, and will not require removal at a later date. This is reassuring to the patient because substantial postoperative pain may be experienced, and

With collaboration of Frederic D. Nemer

any unnecessary meddling in the perianal region will not be appreciated.

The patient should be made to understand that during the healing phase, symptoms such as itching, some bleeding, and some pain are usual. The degree of pain anticipated postoperatively, of course, varies with the individual patient, but reasonable expectations should be discussed. The patient should be reassured that all attempts will be made to keep him comfortable postoperatively, especially with the liberal use of pain medication, either intramuscularly, or by mouth. This practice gives the patient confidence that he will not be allowed to suffer unnecessarily. We have not seen patients abuse this privilege. Other adjunctive postoperative measures are comforting, as well. These include warm packs, warm baths, and most important of all, considerate and empathetic nursing personnel. If the operation is being done for a totally benign condition, the surgeon should stress this, thus reassuring the patient with "cancer phobia."

Certain details should be reviewed either in the office at the time of scheduling the procedure or preoperatively. Discussion should include the risk of incontinence from the operation, the chances for possible recurrence of the disease, and even the risks involved pertaining to anesthesia when applicable. Estimates as to the time off work, any disability that is to be expected (long or short term), when the patient may travel, drive a car, when sexual relations may be resumed, and all aspects of life pertinent to recovery should be discussed.

Post-operatively the anal sphincter tone is diminished temporarily, and the patient's sensation of the fecal bolus may not be normal. The two to three weeks of less than perfect continence should be explained as a condition that will return to normal, or near normal, so that the patient does not fret unnecessarily about permanent incontinence. Functional limitations, such as refraining from heavy lifting, straining, and excessive activities, immediately postoperatively, and for two weeks thereafter, should be outlined.

## PREOPERATIVE PREPARATION

The usual preoperative preparation of a patient for an anorectal procedure is quite straightforward, barring any serious medical condition. The laboratory screening is kept to a minimum. Chest radiograph, urinalysis, complete blood count (CBC), SMA12, and electrocardiogram suffice in most cases. In addition, if the patient is on any medications to prolong the normal bleeding time, coagulation studies should be performed to ensure a near normal range at the time of operation. Many patients undergoing anorectal elective surgery can be admitted the same morning, and some can go home the same day. In the case of the elderly person, it is probably prudent to admit the patient the day before operation, when a more leisurely evaluation and preparation period is allowed.

When the laboratory details have been attended to, the patient is allowed a regular meal the evening before operation. Stool softeners in the form of bulk producers (psyllium seed) are begun the night before operation, or preferably the whole day prior to operation, to ensure that the first stool coming through the repaired wound will be soft. A sodium phosphate enema is given one hour prior to the procedure itself. Antibiotics are rarely used, with the exception of patients with cardiac murmurs, prosthetic implants, or impaired immunological status. Two exceptions to this rule exist. One is the transanal excision of a villous adenoma, which is high in the rectum, with the possibility of perforation or subsequent intra-abdominal exploration being necessitated. This patient should have a complete bowel prep, including antibiotics, with

the possibility of intra-abdominal exploration explained thoroughly to him preoperatively if the lesion is high. The other exception is the use of extensive perianal flaps, such as an "S"-plasty for anal neoplasms or stenosis. Such flaps are composed primarily of fat and undermine extensive skin and soft tissue.

Almost all anorectal procedures can be performed satisfactorily without routine shaving of the perianal skin. The shaving not only creates minor cuts which are sometimes painful, and can become infected, but the itching and irritation following the shaving is most uncomfortable to the patient during the healing and regrowth period.

## POSTOPERATIVE CARE AND DISCHARGE INSTRUCTIONS

All the wounds should be hemostatically "dry" by the time the operation is completed. One should not accept oozing from any suture line while in the operating room. Wounds in the ischiorectal space, or spaces around the anorectum, seldom require packing or drains. However, for extensive fistulotomy or an ischiorectal abscess, utilization of a drain or packing for one or two days thereafter may be justified. Anal packing is not generally utilized as we prefer to be aware of any early bleeding, should it occur. In addition, such packing causes pain to the patient by creating spasm of both the internal and external sphincter, which then adds to the patient's discomfort. Rectal tubes similarly are not used.

The archaic practice of postoperative anal dilatation should rarely, if ever, be used. Utilizing the closed hemorrhoidectomy method, stressing fastidious operative technique with the conservative excision of anoderm, and utilizing methods for the proper reconstruction of the anal canal, mean that stricture should be a rare occurrence.[8,14,15,17]

The general postoperative management of most anorectal cases is quite routine and uncomplicated. Our emphasis is on the adequate relief of pain, prevention of constipation, and cleansing of the perianal wound. The "rubber doughnut", traditionally used postoperatively to decrease pain, may actually accentuate pain due to stretching of the perianal tissues. Sitz baths or tub baths are utilized primarily for cleansing, but are of great comfort, and are soothing to the patient. These baths may also allow the patient to void more easily by allowing sphincter relaxation when the reflex mechanism prevents spontaneous urination because of perianal pain.[9] Warm packs are used regularly, for comfort, in the perianal region. Stool softeners in the form of bulk "laxatives" are used routinely. Prior to the first bowel movement, a lubricant containing mineral oil is also used. Only mild laxatives, such as milk of magnesia, are used postoperatively, and, if the patient does not have a spontaneous bowel movement by the third postoperative day, a tap water enema instilled gently through a rubber tubing, or a packaged sodium phosphate enema is administered.

Voiding difficulties are frequently seen postoperatively.[6,9,17] In the elderly man, prostatic hypertrophy should be suspected preoperatively by a thorough history and physical examination. Intravenous pyelography may be indicated preoperatively. If the patient has difficulty voiding postoperatively, he is treated, initially, by allowing him to sit in a warm bath tub or sitz bath. Urecholine is given by mouth if not contraindicated. A Foley catheter is utilized only as a last resort when a palpable, distended bladder is present, and when the patient is uncomfortable. Many elderly men with borderline prostatic hypertrophy will decompensate postoperatively, require catheterization, and a subsequent work-up. Should straight catheterization with a persistently high residual volume be required more than two times in a 24-hour period, a Foley catheter is inserted, and left in place at least two days. The urine is cultured upon catheter removal, and appropriate antibiotics utilized when necessary. Bailey and others have pointed out that volume restriction of intravenous fluids given intraoperatively has dramatically reduced the incidence of bladder catheterization.[6,9] In a carefully controlled, prospective, randomized study of 500 patients undergoing anorectal surgery, Bailey and Ferguson were able to show a reduction of postoperative catheterization from 26 per cent to 3.5 per cent.[6]

The patient is helped to ambulate within several hours of operation following our preferred (caudal or general) anesthetic. Spinal anesthesia is avoided as many of these patients will need to remain in bed for eight hours or longer to minimize spinal headache.

The postoperative hospital stay for most anorectal procedures of an elective nature varies from one to four days.[8] The patient is discharged after a spontaneous bowel action occurs or a bowel movement occurs with an enema, when intramuscular pain relief is no longer required, and when the patient is comfortable enough to provide self care at home. A booklet of discharge instructions accompanies the patient for home use (see below). Discharge medications include a psyllium seed bulk stool softener, analgesic ointment for the anorectal wounds, and mild, usually noncodeine derivatives for oral pain medication. Rarely are codeine derivatives given to the patient and when they are he is cautioned carefully about the possible development of constipation. With regard to activity, the patient is allowed to resume all usual activity, including sexual relations, two weeks from the day of operation, but told to avoid heavy lifting during this period. Travel may begin when the patient desires. The patient is seen in the office ten days to two weeks postoperatively to examine the anal wounds. At the time of initial visit the wound is inspected, and a very gentle anal examination is performed. The patient is reviewed one month later and subsequently, as needed, to assure complete, satisfactory wound healing, at which time he is discharged from immediate care.

---

### POSTOPERATIVE INSTRUCTIONS
#### For Anorectal Surgical Patients

1. The following medicines or prescriptions will be sent home with you:
   Psyllium seed preparation—2 doses daily in ⅓ glass of liquid of your choice
   Analgesic—every three–four hours as needed for pain
2. Postoperative office visits are essential to insure proper healing of your anal wounds. Please call the office to make your first appointment as instructed.
3. Sitz baths, comfortably warm, should be taken three times a day, especially after bowel movements. Have the water as warm as can be tolerated. Bath should last no longer than 20 minutes.
4. Some bloody discharge, especially after bowel movements, can be expected after anorectal surgery. If there is prolonged or profuse bleeding, call us at once.
5. Bowel movements after anorectal surgery

are usually associated with some discomfort. This will diminish as the healing progresses. You should have a bowel movement at least every other day. If two days pass without a bowel movement, take an ounce of milk of magnesia and repeat in 6 hours if no results.

6. The use of dry toilet tissue should be avoided. After bowel movements use wet tissue or cotton or medicated pads to clean yourself, or if possible take a sitz bath.
7. A general diet is recommended, including plenty of fruits and vegetables. Try to drink 6 to 8 glasses of fluid a day.
8. No strenuous exercise or heavy lifting should be attempted until healing is well under way. Climbing stairs, walking and car riding and driving may be done in moderation.
9. If you have any questions about your postoperative care, feel free to call anytime.

## WOUND HEALING IN THE ANORECTUM

The cosmetic result achieved is important, but the comfort of the healed wound, and curing of the disease entity are the ultimate criteria upon which success in anorectal surgery is judged.

Fortunately, because of the abundant blood supply of the anorectum, primary healing of wounds in this area under normal, elective, operative conditions is not a problem. While Hippocrates' statement of centuries ago still holds true that the "best healing is by the apposition of healthy tissues", the medical literature has only a scant amount of research in anorectal wound healing, and most of what is understood about wound healing in this area is derived from clinical experience and observation.[12,18,32,42] Unless unusual circumstances are present, the external, perianal, or rectal wounds heal as any other soft tissue wounds. This healing takes place "naturally" if mechanical or chemical impediments such as packs, damaging drugs, improper use of sutures and drains, and improper handling of tissues are avoided.[12,18,32] Occasionally in chronically ill, debilitated patients, mineral or vitamin deficiencies may retard healing.[26] This is not to say that where indicated, small drainage wicks or packs cannot be utilized. Such drainage aids are beneficial where large, ischiorectal abscesses or horseshoe abscesses are found, and may be useful for short periods of time without impairing healing, by directing healing from above downward. Critical to the healing of anorectal wounds is the maintenance of the good blood supply, and respect for the tissues by gentle manipulation. By observing these two principles, anorectal wounds created electively can be closed primarily and will heal.[8,14,15,17]

Proper healing of anorectal wounds almost never requires antibiotics, including topical antibiotic ointments, most of which have not been shown to decrease healing time.[25] The fallacy of the argument that topical medication reduces inflammation, and combats infection, is apparent in view of the observed fact that mild or minimal infection of wounds is harmless because healthy cells not only are engendered with competent defense mechanisms, but also may have their healing ability actually stimulated by mild infection.[12,32] In certain instances the use of antibiotics is acceptable. Patients with diabetes or cardiac valvular disease, those undergoing flap procedures, and those who are immunosuppressed will be aided by the use of these drugs.

The rarity of perianal suppuration following elective anorectal surgery leads one to question whether or not this anatomical site has some sort of special environmental immunity. While such factors have not yet been elucidated, future studies may prove revealing. The primary healing of anorectal wounds depends upon the type of surgical procedure performed, gentleness in handling the tissues during the procedure, and maintenance of the excellent blood supply, rather than on any postoperative application of therapeutic agents, or the performance of any manipulation such as digital examination. Systemic processes such as diabetes mellitus, malignancy, or any form of immuno-incompetence, may severely retard normal anorectal wound healing and the overall host reaction to healing.[12,32]

### Primary Healing of Wounds

Primary closure of wounds in anorectal surgery has been performed for many years. Excision of anal fistulae and primary closure was supported in selected cases as long ago as 1903 by Cuthill.[18] At that time he emphasized the technical details to which one must adhere:

removing the fistulous track completely, and bringing the wall of the wound into firm apposition by chromic sutures. The method did not become popular, presumably, because it seemed unsound in theory, or because results of other surgeons were found to be unsatisfactory in practice. Suture of the fistula wound has been universally condemned, or ignored, by various authorities such as Goodsall, Miles, Gabriel, and Milligan.[18] In the 1950's, Starr of Sydney, Australia, reviewed this method of dealing with fistula and fissure wounds. By utilizing antibiotics orally, and systemically, for bowel antisepsis pre- and postoperatively, he claimed uniform success in securing uneventful primary healing.[18] Encouraged by Starr's experience, Leaper, Goligher, and others have undertaken studies with acute perianal and ischiorectal suppuration, utilizing systemic antibiotics, and closing the wounds primarily. The latter authors report primary healing in 60 to 70 per cent of these cases.[25] The fact that this method can be applied as an outpatient procedure with a recurrent fistula rate of approximately 10 per cent is encouraging. This work needs further clinical trial.

### Skin Grafts

The use of skin grafts in the perianal region has been recommended for decades.[16,18,21] Gabriel, in 1929, first utilized skin grafts to expedite the healing of anal wounds when he applied secondary Thiersch grafts, after the crevices and irregularities of the wound surface had evened out, with granulation tissue. In only one of the 21 cases so treated did the graft fail to take.[16] Other surgeons, such as Goligher, have found a much less satisfactory percentage of takes; so low, in fact, as to make them extremely doubtful whether it has even been worthwhile attempting.[18] Primary split thickness skin grafting was first used in 1944 in England by Ranck, who employed this method in the treatment of wounds resulting from excision of pilonidal sinuses.[18] In 1953, Hughes of Melbourne, Australia, utilizing colon antisepsis with penicillin-streptomycin therapy, applied primary grafting to anal wounds after laying open fistulae or excising fissures.[21] In certain instances where there was too much initial oozing of serum and blood from large, deep wounds to advise the immediate use of grafts, Hughes recommended delaying primary grafting for two or three days, and packing the wound with dry gauze in the meantime. The grafts may be nicked (''pie-crusted''), or meshed with scissors at many points, to facilitate the escape of serous fluid, and prevent them from being floated off. In the case of high posterior horseshoe fistulae, the wound may be a deep furrow. Firm pressure through molded pack is essential to assure good apposition in the difficult areas. The stent is retained in position for five to six days, at which time the sutures are removed, and the bowels opened by an enema or laxative. Healing of any remaining raw areas is completed under the regimen of baths, irrigation, and various dressings. Results by Hughes have been most impressive: 40 cases being treated by grafting with a virtual complete take in 30 and substantial, though incomplete, take in the others.[21] In Goligher's personal series, 50 to 70 per cent of the grafts succeeded primarily.[18] Anderson and Turnbull have recently reported good results in applying skin grafts to poorly healing perineal wounds in patients with Crohn's disease: forty-four out of forty-eight patients have achieved healing after grafting.[5]

The advantage of primary grafting in the anal region, if healing is successful, needs no emphasis. The patient leaves the hospital after approximately ten days with a healed wound, instead of having to spend several weeks healing by secondary intention. And yet, this procedure has not yet found much favor, primarily because of the extensive operation time necessary to prepare the grafts, and fix them in position. In addition, for most surgeons, it takes only one or two unsuccessful experiences with grafting to convince them that there may be more profitable uses of valuable operating room time. Although it is doubtful that substantial benefit will be reaped by employing skin grafts in the management of patients with fissures and fistulae, the application of a successful split-thickness skin graft to the perianal region following the excision of a perianal neoplasm or hidradenitis suppurativa, will undoubtedly expedite overall healing.

As an adjunctive development, Gordon and Sohn have independently described a technique of using an elemental diet and codeine to prevent the immediate evacuation of stool through newly closed primary anal wounds.[19,39] This technique may add to the effectiveness of primary healing, especially when skin grafts are employed.

Primary skin "covering" of large or small perianal wounds, either by immediate suture or grafting, is preferable to the delayed method of healing by secondary intention. Speaking to the point of closed primary wounds, and specifically about hemorrhoid operations, the Ferguson Clinic has demonstrated, in thousands of hemorrhoidectomies, that a closed technique offers the patient short healing time with minimal pain, and a brief hospitalization.[17] These results have been confirmed and reiterated by Buls and Goldberg.[8]

### Plastic Surgical Procedures in the Anorectum (Flaps)

The utilization of full-thickness, anoderm skin flaps is another means of achieving primary healing, and also achieving a smooth perianal orifice. Specifically, the use of the Y-V anoplasty can be adapted to many wounds and anal conditions. In addition to the full-thickness anodermal flaps, various buttock flaps in the form of rotating flaps for "S"-plasty of the anal canal can be utilized (Chap. 26).

### Healing by Secondary Intention (Granulation)

One of the major theoretical concerns, that our experience would contradict, is the fallacy that the patient will have sepsis if the wounds are closed primarily. For this reason, for hundreds of years, anorectal wounds were managed so that they would heal by secondary intention, thus supposing to resist infection until they granulated to satisfactory healing. This practice, in effect, meant that the wounds would be laid wide open at the time of operation; they would be kept open by a suitably applied dressing and dilatations; and, they would heal, only after time, by granulation. Epithelium would eventually cover the surface by growing from the periphery. This principle goes back to John Arderne, a 14th century surgeon.[42] His philosophy continues in this century under the teachings of several English surgeons: Lockhart-Mummery, Gabriel and Milligan-Morgan.[18] It is apparent from clinical experience that healing does take place reliably by secondary intention after treatment of hemorrhoids, fissures, fistulae, etc. However, there are significant, important disadvantages of leaving anorectal wounds open to granulate. First, is the length of time required to complete the healing, which may amount to as much as two or three months, or more in large horseshoe fistulae. Even an uncomplicated fistula or anal fissure (which is excised) seldom is healed in less than four to five weeks.[20,25] Second, is the scarring that has inevitably taken place following this type of healing may lead to troublesome stricture of painful scars. Today, with refined surgical techniques and suture materials, and with prudent utilization of antibiotics where indicated, it is appropriate to ask if sepsis or healing by granulation must still remain the hallmark of minor anorectal surgery. We should always strive for primary healing whenever this goal is attainable. Hemorrhoid and fissure surgery often lends itself to primary closure, whereas fistula surgery seldom provides an appropriate situation to favor primary healing.

Because of the excessive adipose tissue that exists in the ischiorectal and supralevator spaces, these areas, once infected, do not heal as well as primary wounds in the anorectum. Specifically, abscesses in these areas are most commonly treated by allowing healing by secondary intention (see exception as practiced by Leaper and associates[25]).

### The Role of Dilatation in Anorectal Wounds

During wound healing of the anorectum, the normal passage of well formed stools daily or every other day is enough, in most cases, to break up any superficial bridging or adhesions which may occur postoperatively. It appears that the frequent use of an anal dilator, or the index finger by the surgeon on the patient postoperatively is almost invariably necessitated by the complications resulting from a poorly conceived, or performed operative procedure, and is not required routinely. Occasionally anal dilatation in the office or operating room may be necessary. Indications for dilatation exist when, upon examination, the well lubricated index finger cannot be easily, and gently inserted into the healing anal canal. Dilatation with an anoscope can be done in the office during the first month postoperatively. Following the eventual healing of such wounds, the tissue generally lacks the elasticity or expansibility, that is essential in normal anorectal contraction. This deficiency often results in anal dysfunction, pain, or even narrowing, requiring a formal corrective operative procedure (Chap. 26).

## MANAGEMENT OF THE
## POSTERIOR SPACE

### Background

Management of the posterior space after proctectomy is a much discussed issue. It appears from a review of recent literature that primary healing can be achieved in the great majority of cases of proctectomy for malignant disease, and in about half the cases performed for inflammatory bowel disease.[3,11,22,24,30,31,33,37,43] Numerous authors have stated their technical preferences as to how to achieve the primary healing, and these will be enumerated.[3,4,7,23,28,30,35,37,38] The management of the posterior space, by allowing secondary healing to occur, is also a common, but perhaps over-utilized practice in the United States and elsewhere.[13,27,28,29,33] Proponents of this technique claim advantages such as less immediate postoperative pain and bleeding, and that the packing serves as a "dam". This dam prevents oozing or active bleeding in the postoperative period; however, prolonged healing time (up to three months or longer postoperatively) is the chief disadvantage of this technique.[13,27,28,29,38,41]

Perineal wound closure after rectal excision is a matter of great concern, and importance, for both the patient and surgeon. Various methods have been used in the past, such as packing of the wound, or partially closing the wound over a drain, with closure of the skin and levator muscles, with or without closure of the peritoneum, or using various types of suction catheters in primary closure of the perineal space.[3,18,22,23,29,30,31,43] Every surgeon has technical preferences regarding closure of the perineal wound, but the morbidity and delay in healing time with packing and partial closure is much greater than with the primary closure of the wounds.[3,7,22,23,30,31,43] Furthermore, the proponents of primary closure of the perineal wound claim greater patient comfort, simplified postoperative nursing care, and shortened length of hospitalization. However, special attention must be directed to maintaining patency of the suction catheters. Failure of this method of closure is most commonly attributable to hematoma formation followed by infection in the presacral space. To obviate this problem, Ruckley, in 1970, attempted to fill this space with a pedicled omental graft.[35] He reported complete healing within three weeks in one-half of the cases.

Other surgeons leave the pelvic peritoneum open so that the presacral space will be occupied by the small intestine.[18] Hulten, in 1971, managed 30 patients following rectal excision by primary closure of the wounds, and was successful in three-forths of the cases.[22] Altemeier, in 1974, reported primary wound healing in 92 per cent of his cases.[3]

Several types of drains, drainage systems, and catheters have been recommended when closing the posterior space primarily. Recently, the utilization of suction drains has been emphasized.[3,7,23,30,31] These drains are most often placed below the peritoneum which has been sutured. They exit the peritoneal cavity either transabdominally or through the perineum. After connecting these tubes, or drains, to various forms of suction, the cavity becomes "closed" by apposition of healthy tissues. Irrigation of the perineal space through these tubes, and use of antibiotic solutions, added to the decreased incidence of wound infection.[3,7,22,30] The decrease in hospital stay was statistically significant in the group undergoing primary closure of the wound, as compared to the group in which the perineal wound was managed by packing.[3,7,22,23,30,31,43]

### Healing of the Posterior Space

The major event in wound healing following proctectomy is obliteration of the pelvic cavity. This is not, as often taught, merely the result of allowing the open wound to "granulate in", nor does it follow contraction and fibrosis of the "pelvic coagulum" in wounds closed primarily. Rather, it is primarily the descent of the pelvic peritoneum, along with posterior displacement of the urogenital structures, and perhaps, upward shifting of the buttock soft tissues, which accomplish the process.[34,36,38]

### Adverse Factors in Perineal Wound Healing

Since descent of the pelvic floor is essential for wound healing, the following factors impede the process, and in so doing, predispose the patient to delayed healing, and a persistent perineal sinus.[4,11,35,38,40,41,43]

*The primary disease* has a definite effect on the outcome of perineal wound healing. Delayed healing, and persistent perineal sinus, are unquestionably more common following proctectomy for inflammatory bowel disease, whether the perineum is closed or not, and probably most common in patients with Crohn's colitis.[41,43] Several hypotheses have been offered to explain this difference: (*1*) better drainage afforded by wider resection for carcinoma, (*2*) pararectal inflammatory disease, and (*3*) more bowel resected in inflammatory bowel disease, and consequently less available to fill the pelvic space. Some authors feel that by not reconstructing the peritoneal floor, and allowing the bowel to fill the pelvic space, these factors can be overcome. While steroids have been implicated as a cause of delayed perineal healing, this theory has not been confirmed by several recent studies.[23,24,38]

*Contamination* of the perineal wound, either by inadvertent entry into the rectum, or by associated perianal abscesses or fistulae, has a definite adverse effect.[7,23] Chronic infection causes the walls of the cavity to become inflamed, rigid, and fibrotic, thus making them less likely to appose and heal.

*Extensive resection* of perianal skin, levator muscles, coccyx, and vaginal wall prolongs and retards obliteration of the pelvic space.[13] In an analysis of 50 patients undergoing proctectomy with open packing of the perineum, Eftaiha and Abcarian noted that all of the perineal wounds which had failed to heal within four months were in patients who had undergone radical perineal or pelvic dissection.[13]

*Hemorrhage and exudation of plasma* which stagnate in the pelvic space are detrimental to healing. Alexander and colleagues showed that blood and plasma which collect in surgical wounds not only progressively lose their ability to opsonize bacteria, but also interfere with access of phagocytic cells to them, and provide a fertile medium for bacterial growth.[1] Furthermore, if an infection does occur, a consumptive opsoninopathy develops, decreasing host resistance even further.[2]

*Packing* of the wound has been shown, by several authors, to delay healing.[13,23,24] The superiority of closed vacuum drainage systems is well recognized.[1] Not only is a potential portal of entry for exogenous bacteria obviated, but drainage is not dependent on patient position, thus, allowing more patient mobility, and the vacuum, theoretically, helps "pull down" the peritoneal floor. Irwin and Goligher, using a prospective randomized study comparing open packing with primary suture of the perineum, showed that at three months, only 30 per cent of wounds packed open were healed, as compared to 75 per cent of those closed primarily.[23] At six months, they found that while 80 per cent of wounds closed primarily had healed, only 60 per cent of those packed open had done so. Although Altemeier reported that 93 per cent of the patients who underwent abdominoperineal resection for carcinoma with primary closure of the perineum had primary healing, others using similar techniques have been less successful.[23] Most surgeons report failure of primary healing in 35 to 55 per cent of cases, although many series include patients with inflammatory bowel disease. Whatever the initial result, wounds closed primarily, which become infected and require drainage, heal just as quickly as those packed open initially, provided that they are drained early and adequately.

*Irradiation and systemic chemotherapy* are well recognized retardants of wound healing in the "posterior wound" as well as elsewhere.

## Method of Closure of Perineal (Posterior) Wound

One suitable method of perineal closure after proctectomy that we have found successful is as follows:

1. Mechanical bowel prep
2. Antibiotic bowel prep
3. Perioperative prophylactic systemic antibiotic
4. Mobilization of rectum with care to preserve wide peritoneal flaps (if curative resection is not compromised)
5. Pelvic peritoneal reconstitution without tension
6. Perineal phase (proctectomy) in prone position (unless done synchronously)
7. Copious intraoperative irrigation of posterior space with antibiotic solution
8. Closed drainage system through separate stab wound (of perineal surface—buttock, or transabdominal)
9. Closure of levators, ischiorectal fat in layers, and skin with absorbable sutures
10. Drains removed when clotted or output is less than 15 cc per day. Drains declotted

first 48 hours. Packing removed in 48 hours if used.
11. Wounds are left open and packed, if:
    a. gross contamination or infection
    b. unsatisfactory hemostasis
    c. inadequate tissue for closure

Reviewing our statistics of closure of the posterior wounds, we can say that approximately three-fourths of the perineal wounds closed for malignant disease healed primarily, and little over one-half of our wounds closed for inflammatory bowel disease have healed per primam.

## REFERENCES

1. Alexander-Williams, J., Korilitz, J., and Alexander N. S.: Prevention of wound infections: A case for closed suction drainage to remove wound fluids deficient in opsonic proteins. Am. J. Surg., *132:*59, 1976.
2. Alexander-Williams, J., McClennan, M. A., Ogle, C. K., and Ogle, J. D.: Consumptive opsinopathy; possible pathogenesis in lethal and opportunistic infections. Am. Surg., *184:*672, 1976.
3. Altemeier, W. A., Culbertson, W. R., Alexander, J. W., Sutorius, D., and Bossert, J.: Primary closure and healing of the perineal wound in abdominoperineal resection of the rectum for carcinoma. Am. J. Surg., *127:*215, 1974.
4. Anderson, R.: The dilemma of Crohn's disease: Management of the posterior wound after coloproctostomy. Dis. Colon Rectum, *20:*393, 1977.
5. Anderson, R., and Turnbull, R. B., Jr.: Grafting of the unhealed perineal wound after coloproctectomy for Crohn's disease. Arch. Surg., *111:*335, 1976.
6. Bailey, H. R., and Ferguson, J. A.: Prevention of urinary retention by fluid restriction following anorectal operations. Dis. Colon Rectum, *19:*250, 1976.
7. Braoder, J. W., Masselink, B. A., Oates, G. D., and Alexander-Williams, J.: Management of the pelvic space after proctectomy. Br. J. Surg., *16:*94, 1974.
8. Buls, J. G., and Goldberg, S. M.: Modern management of hemorrhoids. Surg. Clin. North Am., *58:*469, 1978.
9. Campbell, E. D.: Prevention of urinary retention after anorectal operations. Dis. Colon Rectum, *15:*69, 1972.
10. Clarke, J. S., Condon, R. E., Bartlett, J. G., Gorbach, S. L., Nichols, R. L., and Ochi, S.: Preoperative oral antibiotics reduce septic complications of colon operations. Ann. Surg., *186:*251, 1977.
11. Corman, M. L., Veidenheimer, M. C., Coller, J. A., and Ross, V. A.: Perineal wound healing after proctectomy for inflammatory bowel disease. Dis. Colon Rectum, *21:*155, 1978.
12. Dunphy, J. E. and VanWinkle, W., Jr.: Repair and Regeneration; The Scientific Basis for Surgical Practice: A Centennial Symposium. McGraw-Hill, New York, 1969.
13. Eftaiha, M., and Abcarian, H.: Management of perineal wounds after proctocolectomy: A retrospective study in which treatment by the open technique was used. Dis. Colon Rectum, *21:*287, 1978.
14. Ferguson, J. A., and Heaton, J. R.: Closed hemorrhoidectomy. Dis. Colon Rectum, *2:*176, 1959.
15. Ferguson, J. A., Mazier, W. P., Granchrow, M. E., and Friend, W. G.: The closed technique of hemorrhoidectomy. Surgery, *70:*480, 1971.
16. Gabriel, W. B.: Skin grafts for anal fistulae. Proc. R. Soc. Med., *71:*20, 1978.
17. Granchow, M. E., Mazier, W. P., Friend, W. G., and Ferguson, J. A.: Hemorrhoidectomy revisited—A computer analysis of 2,038 cases. Dis. Colon Rectum, *14:*128, 1971.
18. Goligher, J. C.: Surgery of the Anus, Rectum and Colon. 205–251, 256–274, 707–709. Springfield, Charles C. Thomas, 1975.
19. Gordon, P. H.: The chemically defined diet and anorectal procedures. Can. J. Surg., *19:*511, 1976.
20. Graham-Stewart, C. W., Greenwood, R. K., and Davies-Lloyd, R. W.: A review of 50 patients with fissure-in-ano. Surg. Gynecol. Obstet., *113:*445, 1961.
21. Hughes, E. S. R.: Primary skin grafting in proctological surgery. Br. J. Surg., *41:*639, 1953.
22. Hulten, L., Kewenter, J., Knutsson, V., and Olbe, L.: Primary closure of perineal wound after proctocolectomy or rectal excision. Acta Chir. Scand., *137:*467, 1971.
23. Irvin, T. T., and Goligher, J. C.: A controlled clinical trial of three different methods of perineal wound management following excision of the rectum. Br. J. Surg., *62:*287, 1975.
24. Jalan, K. N., Smith, A. N., Ruckley, C. B., Falconer, W. A., and Small, W. P.: Perineal wound healing in ulcerative colitis. Br. J. Surg., *56:*749, 1969.

25. Leaper, D. J., Page, R. E., Rosenberg, I. C., Wilson, D. H., and Goligher, J. C.: A controlled study comparing the conventional treatment of idiopathic anorectal abscess with that of incision, curettage and primary suture under systemic antibiotic cover. Dis. Colon Rectum, *19:*46, 1976.

26. Lee, P. W. R., Green, M. A., Long, W. B. III, and Gill, W.: Zinc and wound healing. Surg. Gynecol. Obstet., *143:*549, 1976.

27. Mayo, C. W.: The one-stage combined abdominoperineal resection for carcinoma of the rectum, rectosigmoid and sigmoid. Surg. Clin. North Am., *19:*1011, 1939.

28. McGainty, M. C., Mariory, C., and Walker, J.: Perineal wound healing after abdominoperineal resection. Am. Surg., *42:*206, 1976.

29. Miles, W. E.: A method of performing abdominoperineal excision for carcinoma of the rectum and of the terminal portion of the pelvic colon. Lancet, *2:*1812, 1908.

30. Mittal, V. K., Saharia, S., Khanna, S. K., and Yadov, R. V. S.: Management of perineal wounds following abdominoperineal resection. Am. J. Proctol., *19:*65, 1977.

31. Oates, D., and Alexander-Williams, J.: Primary closure of the perineal wound in excision of the rectum. Proc. R. Soc. Lond., (suppl), *63:*128, 1970.

32. Peacock, E. E., and Vanwinkle, W., Jr.: Surgery and Biology of Wound Repair. 583–586. Philadelphia, W. B. Saunders, 1970.

33. Remington, J. H.: Management of the posterior wound in the Miles resection. Proc. R. Soc. Med. (suppl), *63:*104, 1970.

34. Risberg, B., Kock, N. G., Myrold, H., and Nilson, A.: Topography of the reconstructed perineum following proctocolectomy. Dis. Colon Rectum, *17:*153, 1974.

35. Ruckley, C. V., Smith, A. N., and Balfour, T. W.: Perineal closure by omental graft. Surg. Gynecol. Obstet., *131:*300, 1970.

36. Saha, S. K., and Robinson, A. F.: A study of perineal wound healing after abdominoperineal resection. Br. J. Surg., *63:*555, 1976.

37. Schwab, P. M., and Kelly, K.: Primary closure of perineal wounds after proctocolectomy. Mayo. Clin. Proc., *49:*176, 1974.

38. Silen, W., and Glotzer, D. J.: The prevention and treatment of the persistent perineal sinus. Surgery, *75:*535, 1974.

39. Sohn, N., and Weinstein, M. A.: Use of total parenteral nutrition as a medical colostomy in management of severe lacerations of the anal sphincter. Dis. Colon Rectum, *20:*8, 1977.

40. ———: Unhealed perineal wound: Lavage with a pulsating water jet. Am. J. Surg., *134:*426, 1977.

41. Tolstedt, G. E., Bell, J. W., and Harkins, H. N.: Chronic perineal sinus following total colectomy for ulcerative colitis. Am. J. Surg., *101:*50, 1961.

42. Turell, R.: Diseases of the Colon and Anorectum. 1326–1340. Philadelphia, W. B. Saunders Co., 1969.

43. Warshaw, A. J., Ottinger, L. W., and Bartlett, M. K.: Primary perineal closure after proctectomy for inflammatory bowel disease. Am. J. Surg., *133:*414, 1977.

44. Watts, J. M., Bennett, R. C., Duthie, H. L., and Goligher, J. C.: Healing and pain after hemorrhoidectomy. Br. J. Surg., *51:*808, 1964.

# 5

# Principles of Anesthetic Management in Anorectal Surgery

The anesthetic management of patients presenting for anorectal surgery has received scant attention in the literature. This is surprising since the potential for complications during the conduct of these procedures is considerable. The aims of this chapter are to discuss the problems that may be encountered and to emphasize the principles that must be followed if good operating conditions are to be attained with a minimum of complications.

Not all the potential problems are related to the anesthetic techniques or agents used. Some may be primarily related to improper positioning of the anesthetized patient on the operating table. This is particularly true if the prone jackknife position is employed. Many operators prefer the prone jackknife position to the traditional lithotomy position because it provides better surgical access and less bothersome venous bleeding. To derive these benefits the abdomen and pelvis must be elevated from the operating table by a roll placed under the hips. Correct placement of the roll is essential. If the roll is placed under the abdomen, exposure of the operative field will be less than optimal. Further, compression of the inferior vena cava may result in increased surgical bleeding from back pressure transmitted to the hemorrhoidal veins.

The adverse effects of incorrect roll placement are not limited to the operative area. Ventilation may be reduced because pressure on the abdomen interferes with the respiratory excursions of the diaphragm. Circulation may also be adversely affected. Compression of the

inferior vena cava comprises venous return and predisposes to hypotension. This is particularly important since the homeostatic mechanisms which tend to support blood pressure when this occurs are interfered with both by general and regional anesthesia.

Many of the problems encountered with general and regional anesthesia can be avoided by using local infiltration anesthesia instead. Kratzer[31] has described considerable success using a local infiltration technique. Why this method is not more popular is unclear. One suspects an incidence of patient discomfort with the technique to be a contributing factor. At present it is more conventional to infiltrate the operative field only after general or regional anesthesia has been established. These techniques are now discussed. The advantages of supplementing general and regional anesthesia with local infiltration anesthesia are also discussed.

## LOCAL ANESTHESIA

Many anorectal operative procedures can be performed safely under local anesthesia. However, procedures that require relaxation of the puborectalis sling such as excision of villous adenomas of the mid-rectum or repair of transsphincteric or suprasphincteric fistulae-in-ano are not amenable to this technique. Patients' anxiety, discomfort related to the operative position, and the time required for the procedure are relative limitations. Local anesthetic infiltration is also a useful supplement to general and regional anesthesia.

With collaboration of Philip Juno

## Classification of Local Anesthetic Agents

Local anesthetic agents may be classified according to their intrinsic potency and duration of activity (Table 5-1). Procaine and chloroprocaine are relatively weak, short-acting drugs. Lidocaine, mepivacaine, and prilocaine represent agents of intermediate potency and duration of action. Tetracaine, bupivacaine, and etidocaine are highly potent, long-acting agents.[12]

## Action of Local Anesthetic Agents

Local anesthetic agents exert their primary pharmacological action by inhibition of the excitatory process in nerve endings or nerve fibers. They act at the nerve membrane, which is a highly lipid structure. Thus, the intrinsic anesthetic potency of different agents will be a function of their lipid solubility. Protein-binding is believed to be a primary determinant of anesthetic duration. The nerve membrane consists of proteins as well as lipids. The greater the binding affinity to nerve proteins, the longer anesthetic activity will persist.[12]

## The Use of Epinephrine in Local Anesthesia

All local anesthetic agents, except cocaine, cause peripheral vasodilatation by a direct relaxant effect on the musculature of the blood vessels. The degree of vasodilator activity appears related to intrinsic anesthetic potency. The more potent and longer-acting local anesthetic agents produce a greater degree and longer duration of vasodilatation.[12] Epinephrine incorporated into local anesthetic solutions constricts the blood vessels, thereby slowing absorption and minimizing any toxic reaction. Epinephrine accomplishes three purposes: 1) it reduces capillary bleeding, 2) it prevents rapid absorption of the local anesthetic agent and thus avoids a high blood level of the anesthetic agent while minimizing any toxic reaction, and 3) it prolongs the operating analgesia time.[36] Systemic toxic reactions may occur when the epinephrine has reached a high blood level. The common signs and symptoms are: pallor, tachycardia, perspiration, palpitation, apprehension, dyspnea, rapid respiration, and hypertension.[36]

## The Use of Hyaluronidase in Local Anesthesia

Hyaluronic acid found in interstitial spaces normally prevents the diffusion of invasive substances. Hyaluronidase, a mucolytic enzyme, allows anesthetic solutions to spread in the tissues by inactivating the hyaluronic acid.[9,36] It also tends to reduce swelling and increases the absorption of blood in the subcutaneous tissues. Hyaluronidase is not toxic to tissues and will not cause them to slough. Allergic reactions to hyaluronidase may occur but are insignificant.[36] The disadvantages are few. It may shorten the duration of analgesia. Toxic reactions to local anesthetic agents and vasoconstrictor drugs are more frequent when hyaluronidase is employed, but when it is incorporated in the anesthetic solution, smaller volumes of the solution may be used.[36] The dosage is 150 units in 50 ml of the anesthetic solution.

## Local Anesthetic of Choice in Anorectal Surgery

Because of their effectiveness and low incidence of toxicity,[36,39,44] we use either lidocaine (Xylocaine) 0.5% with 1:200,000 epine-

TABLE **5-1.** Classification of Local Anesthetic Agents

| AGENT | ONSET | DURATION (MINUTES) |
|---|---|---|
| *LOW POTENCY—SHORT DURATION* | | |
| Procaine | Slow | 60–90 |
| Chloroprocaine | Fast | 30–60 |
| *INTERMEDIATE POTENCY & DURATION* | | |
| Mepivacaine | Fast | 120–240 |
| Prilocaine | Fast | 120–240 |
| Lidocaine | Fast | 90–200 |
| *HIGH POTENCY—LONG DURATION* | | |
| Tetracaine | Slow | 180–600 |
| Bupivacaine | Intermediate | 180–600 |
| Etidocaine | Fast | 180–600 |

phrine (maximum dose of 500 mg), or bupivacaine (Marcaine) 0.25% with 1 : 200,000 epinephrine (maximum dose of 225 mg).

## Systemic Toxicity of Local Anesthetics

Allergic reactions to local anesthetics are extremely rare and are usually limited to ester linked agents such as procaine and tetracaine.[13] The vast majority of systemic reactions are due to an inadvertent intravenous injection of the anesthetic or to the extravascular administration of an excessive dose. The manifestations of systemic toxicity mainly involve the central nervous and cardiovascular systems (Table 5-2). Central nervous system excitation usually represents the earliest sign of local anesthetic toxicity. Excessive doses of local anesthetic agents may result in respiratory arrest and generalized central nervous system depression. They can also produce profound cardiovascular changes by direct cardiac and peripheral vascular action and indirectly by conduction blockade of autonomic nerve fibers.[12]

## Treatment of Systemic Toxic Reaction[36]

1. Clear airway—if unconscious.
2. Prevent aspiration.
3. Administer oxygen.
4. Intravenous fluid—for IV medication.

5. Stop convulsion:
   a. Oxygen alone may stop convulsion.
   b. If oxygen does not stop convulsion, use IV succinylcholine 2 ml (40 mg) and oxygenate patient; if recurs, may repeat after 6 to 8 minutes.
   c. If muscle relaxant is not available, give thiopental 50 mg over ½ to 1 minute.
6. Raise blood pressure—giving a vasopressive drug.
7. Cardiac massage if arrested.

## Rules to Be Remembered When Performing Local Anesthesia[36]

1. Do not exceed the recommended maximum dosage of the local anesthetic drugs.
2. Do not rely on premedication to prevent systemic toxic reactions.
3. Carefully observe patients after completion of injection.
4. Objectively evaluate any type of reaction no matter how mild. Do not treat a reaction without making a definite diagnosis; give only the necessary indicated therapy.
5. Be prepared to treat any type of reaction—convulsion, respiratory collapse, cardiovascular collapse, and so on.
6. Do not overtreat or undertreat the reaction. Some reactions require no treatment; on the other hand, intensive treatment and even closed cardiac massage may be necessary to save patients' lives.

## Technique of Local Injection in Anorectal Procedures

As a rule preoperative medication in the form of Innovar 1–2 ml one hour before the procedure, or diazepam 2.5–10 mg intravenously just before the procedure, is required. The skin at the perineal area is prepared with an antiseptic solution and is appropriately draped.

Using a 5–7.5 cm 25 gauge needle, the anesthetic solution is infiltrated around the perianal skin and the anal verge (Fig. 5-1). The anal canal is next injected subdermally and submucosally all around (Fig. 5-2). Complete sphincteric relaxation is achieved without having to inject the anesthetic solution directly into the sphincter muscles.[44] Some surgeons prefer to directly inject the muscle and/or the ischiorectal fossa but this is probably not necessary. In most cases 30–40 ml of the anesthetic solution are used.

TABLE **5-2.** Signs and Symptoms of Local Anesthetic Toxicity

| Mild | |
| --- | --- |
| CARDIOVASCULAR EFFECTS | CENTRAL NERVOUS SYSTEM EFFECTS |
| ↑ PR interval | Lightheadedness |
| ↑ QRS duration | Dizziness |
| ↓ Cardiac output | Tinnitus |
| ↓ Blood pressure | Drowsiness |
| | Disorientation |

| Severe | |
| --- | --- |
| CARDIOVASCULAR EFFECTS | CENTRAL NERVOUS SYSTEM EFFECTS |
| ↑↑ PR interval | Muscle twitching |
| ↑↑ QRS duration | Tremors of face and |
| Sinus bradycardia | extremities |
| AV block | Unconsciousness |
| ↓↓ Cardiac output | Generalized convulsions |
| ↓↓ Hypotension | Respiratory arrest |
| Asystole | |

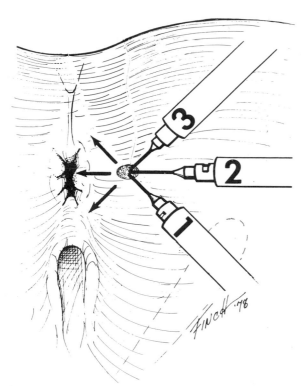

FIGURE **5-1.** *Infiltration of the perianal skin and anal verge.*

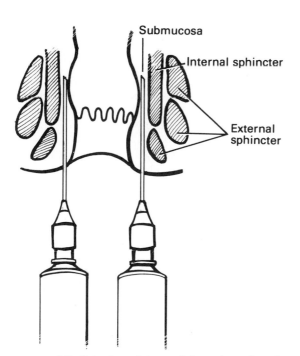

FIGURE **5-2.** *Injection into subdermal and submucosal tissue.*

## GENERAL ANESTHESIA

If the lithotomy position is used, general anesthesia for anorectal procedures rarely requires endotracheal intubation. If the prone jackknife position is employed, endotracheal intubation is mandatory. Few would disagree.

### Arguments for Intubation

To proceed without intubation may endanger the integrity of the airway in several ways. Surgical stimulation in the presence of light anesthesia may provoke laryngeal spasm. Secretions impinging upon the vocal cords may have the same result. Too deep a level of anesthesia may result in hypoventilation and airway obstruction. Precisely regulating the depth of anesthesia cannot be relied upon to prevent these problems from occurring. Should problems with the airway develop, they are more difficult to manage with the patient in the prone position. Proceeding without intubation therefore places considerable demands upon the anesthesiologist, and subjects the patient to unnecessary risk. Proponents of non-intubation claim that with judicious patient selection the risks are minimal.[4] Certainly airway problems are more common if the patient is obese, bull-necked, edentulous or suffers from nasal obstruction. However, even patients without these characteristics are vulnerable when subjected to general anesthesia in the prone position. The possibility of minor complications from correctly performed endotracheal intubation is a small price to pay for the protection of the airway which intubation affords.

The claim that ketamine anesthesia obviates the necessity for intubation is open to question. Ketamine has been recommended for this purpose by Alexander and colleagues,[5] primarily on the grounds that the pharyngolaryngeal reflexes which ensure integrity of the airway are unaffected by this drug. This is not always true. Both depression of these reflexes (resulting in airway obstruction and aspiration) and exaggeration of these reflexes (resulting in laryngeal spasm) are occasionally seen with ketamine.[8,10,48,53] The concurrent use of diazepam (to minimize the incidence of psychic disturbances associated with ketamine) frequently results in depressed ventilation and may also interfere with the ability of ketamine to maintain an unobstructed, protected airway.[8] Notwithstanding the report of Alexander, and colleagues,[5] documenting the safety of ketamine with and without diazepam in 200 patients undergoing anorectal surgery in the prone jackknife position, the above criticisms remain valid.

### Conduct of Anesthesia

Anesthesia is induced with thiopental, and a muscle relaxant is used to facilitate intubation. The application of a topical anesthetic prior to intubation will lessen the need for a deep general anesthetic. Thereafter anesthesia is maintained with nitrous oxide in oxygen and either a volatile inhalation agent (such as halothane or enflurane) or incremental doses of intravenous narcotic. If infiltration of the operative field with an epinephrine-containing solution is planned, halothane is probably best avoided since it sensitizes the myocardium to the action of catecholamines,[45] sometimes resulting in serious ventricular arrhythmias.[7,34] This risk may have been overemphasized in the past. Katz, and associates,[27] suggest that the injection of epinephrine during halothane anesthesia is safe "provided: (1) adequate ventilation is assured, (2) epinephrine in a solution of 1 : 100,000 to 1 : 200,000 is used, (3) the dose in adults does not exceed 10 ml of 1 : 100,000 epinephrine in any given ten-minute period nor 30 ml per hour." Nevertheless, it is wiser to choose an anesthetic other than halothane if adrenaline is to be utilized.

Once anesthesia is established the patient is placed in the prone jackknife position. Care is taken to avoid shoulder dislocation in the patient during transfer. Meticulous attention should be given to the position of the head and neck. The head is turned to one side. Undue twisting of the neck is avoided. Distortion of the endotracheal tube is not uncommon with the head and neck in this position; if it occurs, the patient's ventilation may be compromised. For this reason a non-kinkable tube is preferable. Care is taken to protect against corneal abrasion and compression of the eyeball. The arms are positioned so that radial or ulnar nerve injury does not occur. The roll must be correctly positioned under the hips.

Hypotension is not uncommon in the anesthetized patient when moved from the supine to the prone position because of depressed autonomic reflexes. If hypotension is present, in-

ferior vena caval compression must be ruled out. Hypotension not due to incorrect positioning of the roll is usually transient. On occasion a vasopressor may have to be administered. This is preferable to the infusion of large volumes of fluid which may contribute to postoperative urinary retention (see Chapter 24). If satisfactory ventilation and circulation are not rapidly established, the patient should be immediately returned to the supine position and the problem corrected. In most instances this maneuver will be all that is necessary. If this is successful, it is permissible to continue with the procedure, but it may now be prudent to do so with the patient in lithotomy, thereby avoiding recurrence of the original problem. Once satisfactory positioning and stability of the patient are established, infiltration of the operative field may be performed.

### Supplemental Local Infiltration

Infiltration of the operative field with a local anesthetic is a useful adjunct to general anesthesia. It provides better relaxation of the sphincters and, with the addition of epinephrine, a relatively dry field. It also limits the amount of general anesthesia required to that which is necessary to tolerate the endotracheal tube. If the procedure is short and particularly if a longer acting local anesthetic is used (e.g., bupivacaine 0.25 to 0.5% solution with epinephrine 1 : 200,000), a significant period of postoperative analgesia may also be gained.

Monitoring of the electrocardiogram is essential if local anesthetic solutions which contain epinephrine are used by the surgeon. Tachyarrhythmias and hypertension related to the use of epinephrine are minimized by using it in proper dilution (no stronger than 1 : 200,000)[32] and by taking precautions to prevent inadvertent intravenous injection. Should severe tachycardia result from the use of epinephrine, it can be controlled with the beta blocker propranolol; usually 0.5 to 1.0 mg of this drug administered intravenously will suffice. However, it must be emphasized that propranolol should not be used indiscriminately since possible side effects include bronchospasm, congestive failure, and atrioventricular conduction defects.[40] Johnston and associates,[26] showed that some general anesthetics, notably halothane, sensitize the myocardium to the development of arrhythmias following the injection of epinephrine. Other anesthetics such as enflurane and isoflurane are relatively safe in this regard. Johnston[26] also suggests that the concomitant injection of lidocaine with the epinephrine decreases the tendency of epinephrine to produce arrhythmia and thus will be safer than the use of epinephrine alone.

## REGIONAL ANESTHESIA

A variety of regional techniques may be used to advantage in anorectal surgery. The most commonly employed are caudal block and spinal (subarachnoid) block. Transsacral block is much less commonly used and is only mentioned for completeness. The interested reader is referred to Labat's Regional Anesthesia for a description of the technique.[2]

### Caudal Block

Caudal block is a form of extradural or epidural block. It provides excellent operating conditions. It is performed by injecting a suitable local anesthetic solution into the sacral (caudal) canal. For obvious reasons, infection in the area of intended puncture contraindicates use of the technique. This may be relevant in certain pilonidal sinuses and fistulae. If the prone jackknife position is used, the technique is best performed with the patient already on the operating table positioned for surgery.

*Reactions Following Intravenous and Subarachnoid Injections.* Inadvertent intravenous injection of the local anesthetic may result in severe systemic reactions including convulsions, syncope, and coma. Subarachnoid injection may result in an excessively high block, the so-called "total spinal," with profound hypotension, respiratory distress (progressing to apnea), and coma. In institutions where caudal anesthesia is practiced extensively, the reported incidences of these complications are very low. Massey Dawkins,[33] reviewing the world literature, reports that convulsions occur in 0.2 per cent of patients. Unrecognized dural puncture leading to an accidental "total spinal" occurs in 0.1 per cent of patients. If convulsions occur, oxygenation of the patient is the principal treatment. The administration of oxygen alone by bag and mask will usually arrest seizure activity.[37] However, it may be necessary to give small doses of a short-acting barbiturate (thiopental) or a short-acting muscle relaxant (succinylcholine) to control the convulsion and facilitate oxygenation. Laryngoscopy and rapid intubation will be necessary if there is any difficulty in maintaining an unobstructed airway, or to prevent aspiration should the patient vomit. In the event of a "total spinal," ventilatory support and support of the circulation with vasopressors and intravenous fluids will be necessary. In either event, immediately returning the patient to the supine position is essential to successful treatment.

*Delayed Systemic Reactions.* Systemic toxic reactions which follow intravascular injection manifest immediately. The high plasma levels of local anesthetic responsible for these reactions may also occur during absorption of the drug from its site of action. When this occurs it usually takes 5 to 30 minutes following injection for the critical plasma level to be reached.[36]

*Supplemental Sedation and Local Infiltration.* Once anesthesia is established, attention must be given to the prevention of positional discomfort, apprehension, anxiety, and restlessness. Supplemental sedation may be required.

Local infiltration of the operative field is apparently a useful adjunct to regional anesthesia. Certainly the presence of epinephrine in the solution provides the advantage of a relatively dry field. Kratzer[29] also claims that relaxation of the sphincters, particularly the internal sphincter, is superior with local infiltration. He attributes this observation to blocking of the "intrinsic nervous mechanism" which cannot be accomplished by regional techniques. Alexander and colleagues[4] agree that relaxation is superior, adding that "sufficient muscle tone remains for easy identification of the boundaries of the sphincter muscles."

Unsatisfactory results and failures in the performance of caudal block occur occasionally. In most instances failure is due to improper placement of the needle. This occurs most frequently when there is difficulty in locating the sacral hiatus, or when there is difficulty in advancing a needle into the sacral canal.[6] According to Massey Dawkins,[33] failure to identify the sacral hiatus occurs in 3.1 per cent of patients. A sacral hiatus too narrow to permit insertion of a needle may be encountered in 5 per cent of patients. Failures are least common in patients with easily identifiable landmarks.

## Spinal Block

Spinal or subarachnoid block also provides excellent operating conditions. Contraindications to the technique, as with caudal anesthesia, include the presence of infection in the area of intended puncture, coagulation defects, and neurological disease. With spinal anesthesia, technical difficulties and failures are much less frequent than with caudal block. In addition, spinal anesthesia can be administered without fear of systemic toxicity since very small doses of local anesthetic are required.[38] The risk of post-spinal headache is, however, a disadvantage.

*Etiology of Post-Spinal Headache.* There is considerable evidence that post-spinal headache is caused by leakage of spinal fluid at the dural puncture site.[19,52] When the rate of loss of spinal fluid exceeds its replacement by the choroid plexus, cerebrospinal fluid hypotension results. This in turn allows the brain to sag when the patient assumes the upright position. It has been suggested by Wolff[52] that when the brain sags, traction on the pain-sensitive supporting structures of this organ (blood vessels, meninges, dural sinuses) causes the headache.

Many factors determine whether dural puncture will be complicated by headache. Accordingly, the reported incidence of headache varies widely. The diameter of the needle used to perform the puncture and the number of punctures made appear to be the most important factors. This is not surprising; the larger or more numerous the holes in the dura, the more rapidly spinal fluid escapes. There are many studies which demonstrate the importance of needle size. Harris and Harmel[24] report an 8 per cent incidence of headache using a 20-gauge needle and a 3.5 per cent incidence using a 24-gauge needle. Tarrow,[47] reviewing several series, reports the incidence of headache as 1 per cent or less when a 25- or 26-gauge needle is used. Hatfalvi,[25] on the other hand, claims that the diameter of the needle may be less important than the angle at which it is introduced into the subarachnoid space. Age is also an important factor. The incidence of post-spinal headache is higher in young adults. The reason for this is uncertain. It is thought that the meninges and blood vessels of young individuals are more susceptible to dilatation traction.[16,41]

It has also been observed that the incidence of post-spinal headache is higher following anorectal surgery than following other surgical procedures. Whether it is actually the type of surgery which is responsible or whether other factors (such as age, fluid restriction and early ambulation) are more relevant, is difficult to determine.[35] Owen and associates[41] postulate that, "The high incidence of headache after . . . anorectal . . . surgery may be related to post-operative dilatation of the pelvic veins with compensatory collapse of the epidural veins and dilatation of the dural sac. This would reduce the amount of spinal fluid available for floating the brain and thus intensify spinal headache." Whatever the reason, the comparatively high incidence of post-spinal headache after anorectal surgery has caused the technique of subarachnoid block to fall into particular disfavor with many colorectal surgeons.

*Treatment of Post-Spinal Headache.* Therapy may be purely symptomatic (analgesics, recumbency). Rational treatment of post-spinal headache is aimed at restoring cerebrospinal fluid pressure to normal. This may be achieved by increasing the production of cerebrospinal fluid (hydration, nicotinamide, Pituitrin),[35] by preventing further losses through the hole in the dura (epidural blood patch),[1,14,15,20] or by decreasing the epidural space and compressing the dural sac (epidural injection of saline, application of abdominal binders).[35]

Many measures have proven disappointing. Severe protracted spinal headache not responding to conservative measures may be best treated by epidural blood patch. This involves the injection of up to 10 ml of unclotted autologous blood into the epidural space at the level of the previous dural puncture; strict asepsis is mandatory. This method of treatment is almost always successful, is usually immediately effective, and to date has proven free of any reported serious complications.[1,14,15,20]

*Urinary Retention.* Another criticism of spinal anesthesia has been that postoperative urinary retention occurs more frequently than with other types of anesthesia. Greene,[23] in describing the effect of spinal anesthesia on the ability to void, states that "the preganglionic parasympathetic nerves innervating bladder muscles and sphincters are particularly sensitive to local anesthetics and so may remain blocked when other types of nerve fibers have regained their function. As a result there may be prolonged periods of urinary retention when . . . sensory and motor functions of the lower extremities have returned."

Whether the incidence of urinary retention following spinal anesthesia is greater than that following other types of anesthesia is disputed.[18,30,43] A recent study by Prasad and Abcarian[43] concluded that the type of anesthesia used in anorectal surgery was not a significant factor in the development of urinary retention. In a study of over 300 patients at Mount Sinai Hospital in Minneapolis, who underwent anorectal procedures, catheterization was necessary in 9.3 per cent of patients given general anesthesia, in 10.4 per cent after caudal anesthesia, and in 13 per cent of patients following spinal anesthesia.

*Hypotension.* Hypotension is common following spinal anesthesia. Although hypotension is primarily the result of preganglionic sympathetic blockade, many factors affect the cardiovascular response to a given level of spinal anesthesia.[22] More pronounced hypotension occurs in the presence of old age, hypovolemia, and cardiovascular disease. Susceptibility to hypotension is also increased by subjecting the patient to positional changes following completion of the block. Winnie[51] has demonstrated this in patients presenting for pinning of fractured hips. The incidence of hypotension was reduced by two-thirds (from 35.5 per cent to 11.0 per cent) when he changed his technique to allow the block to be administered after the patient had been positioned on the fracture table. The same principle may be used to advantage in patients presenting for anorectal surgery. Employing a hypobaric saddle block technique eliminates shifting and turning of the patient since he is placed in the prone position for induction of the block and remains in it during the operation.[3]

*Neurological Sequelae.* Several reports indicate that permanent neurological damage may result from spinal anesthesia. Reported deficits include paraplegia and lesions of the cauda equina which may result in retention of urine, incontinence of feces, loss of sexual function and hypoesthesia of the sacral and lower lumbar nerves.[11,28] Several other reports indicate that the incidence of neurological complications in properly managed spinal anesthesia is extremely low.[17,42,46] Properly managed spinal anesthesia includes the careful selection of patients. Spinal anesthesia is contraindicated in patients with sepsis in the area of intended puncture. It is also contraindicated in patients with coagulation disorders. In these patients vascular trauma during puncture may produce uncontrolled epidural (or subarachnoid) bleeding resulting in compression of nerve roots or of the spinal cord.[49] Spinal anesthesia should be avoided in patients with neurologic disorders and disorders which may subsequently give rise to neurological manifestations even though its influence upon the course of these disorders is uncertain.[21,50]

SUMMARY: Advantages and Disadvantages of Different Types of Anesthesia in Anorectal Surgery

| TYPE OF ANESTHESIA | ADVANTAGES | DISADVANTAGES |
|---|---|---|
| *General Anesthesia* | 1. Better accepted by most patients<br>2. Excellent relaxation of anal canal and rectum | 1. Requires intubation in prone jackknife position<br>2. May have airway problem in obese, bull-neck patient (in prone position)<br>3. May be contraindicated in poor risk patients<br>4. May have postoperative nausea and vomiting |
| *Caudal Block* | 1. Excellent relaxation of anal canal and rectum | 1. Contraindicated when the area is infected<br>2. Systemic reaction may occur from inadvertent IV injection |

SUMMARY: (*Continued*) Advantages and Disadvantages of Different Types of Anesthesia in Anorectal Surgery

| TYPE OF ANESTHESIA | ADVANTAGES | DISADVANTAGES |
| --- | --- | --- |
| | | 3. Hypotension<br>4. Higher failure rate<br>5. May require large amount of IV fluid to maintain adequate blood pressure |
| *Spinal Block* | 1. Excellent relaxation of anal canal and rectum | 1. Spinal headache<br>2. Urinary retention?<br>3. Hypotension<br>4. May require large amount of IV fluid to maintain adequate blood pressure<br>5. Difficult in obese patient<br>6. Contraindicated if the adjacent area is infected<br>7. Neurological damage may result |
| *Local Anesthesia* | 1. Excellent relaxation of anal canal<br>2. Well tolerated by poor risk patients<br>3. No postoperative sequelae<br>4. Require negligible amount of IV fluid<br>5. Anesthesia complication is extremely rare at the recommended dose | 1. Not acceptable to a number of patients<br>2. Requires full cooperation and understanding<br>3. Not suitable in certain cases as in deep fistula-in-ano, intersphincteric abscess<br>4. Uncomfortable from the roll under the pubis in prone jackknife position |

# REFERENCES

1. Abouleish, E., de la Vega, S., Blendinger, I., and Tio, T. O.: Long-term follow-up of epidural blood patch. Anesth. Analg., *54:*459, 1975.

2. Adriani, J.: Labat's Regional Anesthesia: Techniques and Clinical Applications, 3rd ed. Philadelphia, W. B. Saunders, 1967, pp. 282–289.

3. Adriani, J.: Labat's Regional Anesthesia: Techniques and Clinical Applications, 3rd ed. Philadelphia, W. B. Saunders, 1967, pp. 361–362.

4. Alexander, R. M., McElwain, J. W., and MacLean, M. D.: Combined intravenous and local anesthesia in anorectal surgery. Dis. Colon Rectum, *6:*121, 1963.

5. Alexander, R. M., McElwain, J. W., MacLean, M. D., Hoexter, B., and Powers, H. J.: Intravenous ketamine hydrochloride and local anesthesia in anorectal surgery. Dis. Colon Rectum, *15:*11, 1972.

6. Bonica, J. J.: Principles and Practice of Obstetric Analgesia and Anesthesia. Philadelphia, F. A. Davis, 1967, pp. 597–598, 607.

7. Brindle, G. F., Gilbert, R. G. B., and Millar, R. A.: The use of fluothane in anaesthesia for neurosurgery. Canad. Anaesth. Soc. J., *4:*265, 1957.

8. Carson, I. W., Moore, J., Balmer, J. P., Dundee, J. W., and McNabb, T. G.: Laryngeal competence with ketamine and other drugs. Anesthesiology, *38:*128, 1973.

9. Clery, A. P.: Local anaesthesia containing hyaluronidase and adrenaline for anorectal surgery: Experiences with 576 operations. Proc. R. Soc. Med., *66:*680, 1973.

10. Corssen, G., Miyasaka, M., and Domino, E. F.: Changing concepts in pain control during surgery: Dissociative anesthesia with CI-581. Anesth. Analg., *47:*746, 1968.

11. Courville, C. B.: Untoward effects of spinal anesthesia on the spinal cord and its investments. Anesth. Analg., *34:*313, 1955.

12. Covino, B. G.: Pharmacology of local anesthetic agents. Surgical Rounds, July 1978. pp. 44–51.

13. de Jong, R. H.: Toxic effects of local anesthetics. JAMA, *239:*1166, 1978.

14. DiGiovanni, A. J., and Dunbar, B. S.: Epidural injections of autologous blood for postlumbar-puncture headache. Anesth. Analg., *49:*268, 1970.

15. DiGiovanni, A. J., Galbert, M. W., and Wahle, W. M.: Epidural injection of autologous blood for postlumbar-puncture headache. II. Additional clinical experiences and laboratory investigation. Anesth. Analg., *51:*226, 1972.

16. Dripps, R. D., and Vandam, L. D.: Hazards of lumbar puncture. JAMA, *147:*1118, 1951.

17. Dripps, R. D., and Vandam, L. D.: Long-term follow-up of patients who received 10,098 spinal anesthetics. Failure to discover major neurological sequelae. JAMA, *156:*1486, 1954.

18. Egbert, L. D.: Spinal anesthesia for anorectal surgery. Int. Anesthesiol. Clin., *1:*811, 1963.

19. Gilbert, J. J., Benson, D. F., and Patten, D. H.: Some observations concerning the post lumbar puncture headache. Headache, *11:*107, 1971.

20. Gormley, J. B.: Treatment of postspinal headache. Anesthesiology, *21:*565, 1960.

21. Greene, N. M.: Neurological sequelae of spinal anesthesia. Anesthesiology, *22:*682, 1961.

22. Greene, N. M.: Physiology of Spinal Anesthesia, 2nd ed. Huntington, N. Y., Robert E. Krieger, 1976, pp. 90–94.

23. Greene, N. M.: Physiology of Spinal Anesthesia, 2nd ed. Huntington, N. Y., 1976, Robert E. Krieger, pp. 171–172.

24. Harris, L. M., and Harmel, M. H.: The comparative incidence of postlumbar puncture headache following spinal anesthesia administered through 20 and 24 gauge needles. Anesthesiology, *14:*390, 1953.

25. Hatfalvi, B. I.: The dynamics of post-spinal headache. Headache, *17:*64, 1977.

26. Johnston, R. R., Eger, E. I., II, and Wilson, C.: Comparative interaction of epinephrine with enflurane, isoflurane, and halothane in man. Anesth. Analg., *55:*709, 1976.

27. Katz, R. L., Matteo, R. S., and Papper, E. M.: The injection of epinephrine during general anesthesia with halogenated hydrocarbons and cyclopropane in man. Anesthesiology, *23:*597, 1962.

28. Kennedy, F., Effron, A. S., and Perry, G.: The grave spinal cord paralyses caused by spinal anesthesia. Surg. Gynecol. Obstet., *91:*385, 1950.

29. Kratzer, G. L.: Relaxation of the internal sphincter in anorectal surgery. Dis. Colon Rectum, *2:*294, 1959.

30. Kratzer, G. L.: Local anesthesia in anorectal surgery. Dis. Colon Rectum, *8:*441, 1965.

31. Kratzer, G. L.: Improved local anesthesia in anorectal surgery. Am. Surg., *40:*609, 1974.

32. Löfström, B.: Clinical evaluation of local anesthetics. In Regional Anesthesia, ed. J. J. Bonica. Philadelphia, F. A. Davis, 1969, pp. 19–43.

33. Massey Dawkins, C. J.: An analysis of the complications of extradural and caudal block. Anaesthesia, *24:*554, 1969.

34. Millar, R. A., Gilbert, R. G. B., and Brindle G. F.: Ventricular tachycardia during halothane anaesthesia. Anaesthesia, *13:*164, 1958.

35. Moore, D. C.: Complications of Regional Anesthesia. Springfield, Charles C Thomas, 1955, pp. 177–196.

36. Moore, D. C.: Regional Block, 4th ed. Springfield, Charles C Thomas, 1978, pp. 19–43.

37. Moore, D. C., and Bridenbaugh, L. D.: Oxygen: The antidote for systemic toxic reactions from local anesthetic drugs. JAMA, *174:*842, 1960.

38. Moore, D. C., Bridenbaugh, L. D., Bagdi, P. A., Bridenbaugh, P. O., and Stander, H.: The present status of spinal (subarachnoid) and epidural (peridural) block: A comparison of the two techniques. Anesth. Analg., *47:*40, 1968.

39. Moore, D. C., Bridenbaugh, L. D., Thompson, G. E., Balfour, R. I., and Horton, W. G.: Bupivacaine: A review of 11,080 cases. Anesth. Analg., *57:*42, 1978.

40. Nickerson, M., and Collier, B.: Propranolol and related drugs. In The Pharmacological Basis of Therapeutics, 5th ed., ed. L. S. Goodman and A. Gilman. New York, Macmillan, 1975, pp. 447–452.

41. Owen, C. K., Owen, J. J., Sergent, W. F., and McGowan, J. W.: Twenty-six gauge spinal needles for the prevention of spinal headache. Am. J. Surg., *85:*98, 1953.

42. Phillips, O. C., Ebner, H., Nelson, A. T., and Black, M. H.: Neurologic complications following spinal anesthesia with lidocaine: A prospective review of 10,440 cases. Anesthesiology, *30:*284, 1969.

43. Prasad, M. L., and Abcarian, H.: Urinary retention following operations for benign anorectal diseases. Dis. Colon Rectum, *21:*490, 1978.

44. Ramalho, L. D., Salvati, E. P., and Rubin, R. J.: Bupivacaine, a long-acting local anesthetic, in anorectal surgery. Dis. Colon Rectum, *19:*144, 1976.

45. Raventós, J.: The action of fluothane—a new volatile anaesthetic. Br. J. Pharm., *11:*394, 1956.

46. Sadove, M. S., and Levin, M. J.: Neurological complications of spinal anesthesia. A statistical study of more than 10,000 consecutive cases. Ill. Med. J., *105:*169, 1954.

47. Tarrow, A. B.: Solution to spinal headaches. Int. Anesthesiol. Clin., *1:*877, 1963.

48. Taylor, P. A., Towey, R. M., and Rappaport,

A. S.: Further work on the depression of laryngeal reflexes during ketamine anaesthesia using a standard challenge technique. Br. J. Anaesth., *44:*1163, 1972.

49. Usubiaga, J. E.: Neurological complications following epidural anesthesia. Int. Anesthesiol. Clin., *13:*38, 1975.

50. Vandam, L. D., and Dripps, R. D.: Exacerbation of pre-existing neurologic disease after spinal anesthesia. N. Engl. J. Med., *255:*843, 1956.

51. Winnie, A. P.: Spinal anesthesia for hip pinning given with patient supine. JAMA, *207:*1663, 1969.

52. Wolff, H. G.: Headache and Other Head Pain, 2nd ed. New York, Oxford University Press, 1963.

53. Yeung, M. L., and Lin, R. S. H.: Laryngeal reflexes in children under ketamine anesthesia. Br. J. Anaesth., *44:*1089, 1972.

# 6

# Hemorrhoids

For centuries the human race has been plagued with a disease called "hemorrhoids," and yet the whole subject is still clouded by misconception and folklore. In his early writings, Maimonides pointed out that the composition of one's foods should always produce softening of the stools.[24] Considered as most valuable to those people who suffer from hemorrhoids was broth made from the flesh of fat chickens! In his treatise on hemorrhoids, a host of concoctions in the form of suppositories, ointments, and enemas were recommended for the alleviation, and even prevention, of the symptoms of hemorrhoidal disease. Currently available preparations are very reminiscent of such historical concoctions. Even then he regarded the operative excision of hemorrhoids with skepticism because, as he wisely recognized, surgery does not remove the underlying causes that produce hemorrhoids. It is the aim of this chapter to dispel such myths and to provide a rational and scientific approach to the diagnosis and management of patients with this disease.

## BACKGROUND
### Definition and Etiology of Hemorrhoids

A precise definition of hemorrhoids does not exist because the exact nature of the condition is not completely understood. Upon examination, a mass of vascular tissue is seen in the anal canal. Various theories have been proposed regarding the exact nature of this tissue.

With collaboration of John G. Buls

For many years these swellings have been considered varicosities of the hemorrhoidal plexus, but this is probably an oversimplification. An extension of this concept is that hemorrhoids are masses of dilated venules. Stelzner and associates demonstrated arteriovenous communication in the anal mucosa, and suggested that this tissue might be a "corpus cavernosum recti."[36] This observation is clinically supported by the finding of bright red arterial bleeding at the time of operation.

A more recent study has described the presence within the anal canal of specialized highly vascular "cushions" consisting of discrete masses of thick submucosa which contain blood vessels, smooth muscle, and elastic and connective tissue.[39] It is suggested that hemorrhoids are nothing more than a sliding downward of this part of the anal canal lining. Such cushions are present in everyone, and it is suggested that the term "hemorrhoids" be confined to situations where these cushions are abnormal and, as well as being present, cause symptoms. The presence of even very large cushions, in the absence of symptoms, is no cause for alarm, and is certainly not an indication for treatment.

Three cushions lie in constant sites: left lateral, right anterolateral, and right posterolateral. Smaller discrete secondary cushions may be present between the main cushions. The configuration is remarkably constant, and appears to bear no relationship to the terminal branching of the superior rectal artery, as previously thought. This vessel and its branches were found to reach the anal canal in a variety of ways. That this arrangement of anal cushions is the normal state of affairs is borne out by the fact that it is present in children, and can be demonstrated in the fetus, and even in the embryo. The function of such cushions is entirely speculative; however, many reasonable theories have been advanced. Because of their bulk, it is believed they aid in anal continence. During the act of defecation, when they become engorged and tense with blood, they cushion the anal canal lining. Because they are separate structures, rather than a continuous ring of vascular tissue, they allow the anal canal to dilate during defecation without tearing.

As noted in Chapter two, on anal physiology, there is a motility differential in the proximal, and distal anal canal, resulting in antiperistaltic movement of blood in the venous plexus. It is conceivable that dysfunction of the internal sphincter may contribute to impaired emptying of the internal hemorrhoidal plexus, and such venous stasis may lead to hemorrhoid formation.[22] Supporting the concept of an abnormality of the internal sphincter being etiologic in the formation of internal hemorrhoids was the demonstration, by Hancock, of increased activity of the internal sphincter in such patients.[18]

Return of blood from the anal canal is via two systems: the portal and systemic. A connection between the two occurs in the region of the dentate line. The submucosal vessels situated above the dentate line constitute the internal hemorrhoidal plexus from which blood is drained through the superior rectal veins into the inferior mesenteric vein, and subsequently into the portal system. Elevations in portal venous pressure may manifest as engorgement and gross dilatation of this internal hemorrhoidal plexus. Vessels situated below the dentate line constitute the external hemorrhoidal plexus from which blood is drained, in part through the middle rectal veins terminating in the internal iliac veins, but mainly through the inferior rectal veins into the pudendal veins which are tributaries of the internal iliac veins. The veins constituting this external hemorrhoidal plexus are normally small; however, in situations of straining, because communication exists between internal and external hemorrhoid plexi, they become engorged with blood. If allowed to persist, this condition can lead to the development of combined internal and external hemorrhoids.

## Incidence and Pathogenesis of Hemorrhoids

Although it is not possible to know precisely the incidence of this disease in our community, it is known that hemorrhoids are among the most common diseases of Western man. At least 5 per cent of the general population suffers from symptoms referrable to hemorrhoids, although, it is unusual under the age of 30 years, except in pregnant and post partum women.[29]

The incidence of hemorrhoids apparently increases with age, and it seems likely that at least 50 per cent of people over the age of 50 have some degree of hemorrhoid formation.[16] The disease is not confined to older individuals, and may be present at any age, including childhood. Men seem to be affected approximately twice as frequently as women.

Burkitt observed that the prevalence of hemorrhoids is highest in affluent countries in the Western world, lowest among people living traditionally in developing countries, and intermediate in countries with standards between these extremes.[8] The prevalence of hemorrhoids increases in non-Western countries after contact with Western culture. He postulates that fiber-depleted diets are the fundamental cause of constipation. Constipation results in straining during evacuation of firm feces causing engorgement of the hemorrhoidal plexuses.

With continued straining the normal supports of the cushions are stretched, and the tendency to prolapse below the dentate line, and hence outside the anal canal, exists. Early in its evolution this prolapse reduces spontaneously, but with repeated episodes manual replacement becomes necessary. In the advanced state of the disease prolapsing persists despite replacement. The normally lax rectal mucosa above the anal cushions is eventually stretched, and dragged along with the prolapsing anal cushion so that it adds to the bulk of what could now be described as a "classical hemorrhoid." The prolapsed cushions, lying outside the normally tonic anal sphincter ring, may become strangulated with possible thrombosis of the venous plexus. This condition, in turn, may result in gangrene with the risk of abscess formation, and rarely, pylephlebitis. It appears that the risk of these problems can be reduced substantially, and the early stage of the disease ameliorated by the addition of sufficient bulk to the diet.

## Predisposing and Associated Factors

Many factors have been implicated in the causation of hemorrhoidal disease, notably heredity, erect posture, the absence of valves in the hemorrhoidal plexi and draining veins, and obstruction of venous return due to raised intra-abdominal pressure. All the factors may be contributory in the causation of the disease, but these anatomical factors do not account for the differences found in epidemiological studies. Portal hypertension may lead to venous engorgement of the hemorrhoidal plexus, and on rare occasions, result in true varices in this area (as in the lower esophagus, retroperitoneum, and around the umbilicus). Pregnancy undoubtedly aggravates pre-existing disease, and by mechanisms ill-understood, predisposes to the development of disease in patients previously asymptomatic. Furthermore, such patients usually become asymptomatic after delivery, suggesting that hormonal changes, in addition to direct pressure effects, may be involved. Recently, it has been suggested that hyperfunction of the internal sphincter, co-existing with continued straining, may be the factor most responsible in initiating the disease state.[2,18] Straining in an attempt to overcome this problem will, in many cases, result in the appearance of hemorrhoidal symptoms. Paradoxically, diarrheal states also predispose to the development of hemorrhoids or to the aggravation of pre-existing disease. Patients with inflammatory bowel disease may, in fact, present with true hemorrhoidal symptoms or symptoms suggestive of hemorrhoidal disease. This fact must always be considered in the evaluation of all patients with hemorrhoids. Any patient with the combination of diarrhea and hemorrhoids should be viewed with suspicion, and all attempts made at excluding inflammatory bowel disease. Operative intervention in such patients will be frought with greater complications.

## Classification and Nomenclature of Hemorrhoids

For clarity of surgical description the various types and stages of hemorrhoidal disease will be defined.

*External skin tags,* as the name implies, are discrete folds of skin arising from the anal verge. Such tags may be the end result of thrombosed external hemorrhoids, or may be a complication of inflammatory bowel disease independent of any hemorrhoidal problem.

*External hemorrhoids* are the dilated venules of the inferior hemorrhoidal plexus which is located below the dentate line and covered by squamous epithelium.

*Internal hemorrhoids* are the symptomatic, exaggerated, submucosal vascular tissue located above the dentate line, and covered by transitional and columnar epithelium. It is possible to subdivide patients suffering from internal hemorrhoids. *First degree internal hemorrhoids* are said to be present when the hemorrhoids are seen to be bulging into the lumen of the anal canal, and produce painless bleeding. *Second degree internal hemorrhoids* are those which protrude at the time of a bowel movement but which reduce spontaneously. *Third degree internal hemorrhoids* are said to be present if protrusion occurs spontaneously or at the time of a bowel movement, and requires manual replacement. *Fourth degree internal hemorrhoids* are those which are permanently prolapsed, and irreducible despite attempts at manual replacement.

*Mixed hemorrhoids* are those in which elements of internal and external hemorrhoids are present. Multiple skin tags are often an accompaniment, and most frequently occur in the external hemorrhoids but may, on less frequent occasions, occur in the internal hemorrhoids.

*Strangulated hemorrhoids.* In circumstances where the prolapsed hemorrhoids, due to the spasm of the sphincter, have their blood supply cut off, strangulated hemorrhoids are said to exist. In the acute stage this will prove to be a rather spectacular event for the patient. Progression will result in gangrenous hemorrhoids.

Graham-Stewart has suggested that there are two main types of hemorrhoids, vascular and mucosal, classified by degree, according to the presence or nature of prolapse.[17] *Vascular hemorrhoids* are said to occur in young, muscular men in whom engorgement of the vascular cushions readily occurs, even in the absence of undue straining. When examined, these patients are seen to have large hemorrhoids which bleed readily with minimal trauma. Prolapse is not a prominent symptom. *Mucosal hemorrhoids* are those present in women, more often than men, who are older, asthenic patients in whom protrusion is the main problem. The protruding "hemorrhoid" consists of a vascular cushion pulling with it an enlarged, and redundant fold of rectal mucosa. Of course, combinations of these two clinical types are usual, and can occur at any age, in either sex.

## DIAGNOSIS AND TREATMENT
### Differential Diagnosis

The examiner should rule out certain disorders before diagnosing hemorrhoids. These are: rectal mucosal prolapse, hypertrophied anal papillae, rectal polyp, melanoma, carcinoma, rectal prolapse, fissure, intersphincteric abscess, and perianal endometrioma.

*Rectal mucosal prolapse* is a common condition which frequently is confused with prolapsing hemorrhoids. As the name suggests, patients with this condition present with prolapse of rectal mucosa below the dentate line. Bleeding may also occur due to trauma of this displaced vascular mucosa. The condition usually results from the same precipitating factors which lead to hemorrhoidal disease, especially chronic straining at stool; however, in many cases the hemorrhoidal cushions are small. Rectal mucosal prolapse may also occur for the same reasons that lead to complete rectal prolapse, and, in fact, may precede this latter condition by some months or even years. Anal sphincter dysfunction, which is primary or due to trauma, especially surgically induced as in internal sphincterotomy or maximal anal dilation, may also predispose to mucosal prolapse. It is important to recognize this condition as different from hemorrhoidal disease because the treatment, although similar, has to be modified by excision of a more proximal extent of rectal mucosa to achieve satisfactory results without the chance of recurrence.

*Hypertrophied anal papillae* are said to be present when one or more of the anal papillae, situated on the dentate line, enlarge. This condition may be secondary to underlying anorec-

tal disease, notably anal fissure, but in most instances no identifiable cause is apparent. The majority of patients with this condition are asymptomatic, and if enlargement is uniform and not gross, it should be considered as a variation of normal. Occasionally, a papilla will hypertrophy to large proportions and protrude below the dentate line. In such cases a pedicle is present and the term "fibrous anal polyp" is sometimes used; however, it must be remembered that this is in no way similar to the true colorectal polyps, and hence, it is suggested that this term "fibrous polyp" be abandoned.

Rectal polyps, melanoma, carcinoma, rectal prolapse, fissure, intersphincteric abscess, and perianal endometrioma must be considered in the differential diagnosis of hemorrhoids. These entities will be discussed in their respective chapters.

### External Hemorrhoids

Occasionally a patient with a thrombosed external hemorrhoid may present without pain, either primarily or sometime after the acute pain has settled. In this case, treatment should be non-operative, and consist of reassurance, the use of bulk forming agents, and watchful expectancy, since the condition will spontaneously resolve. Operative intervention is not necessary, is meddlesome and will cause pain where none exists.

Most patients with external hemorrhoids are asymptomatic until the complication of thrombosis supervenes. This complication presents, in the early stages, as severe pain in the area associated with a perianal swelling which comes on spontaneously or after straining. Examination reveals a tender subcutaneous lump. Treatment at this stage of the disease depends upon the severity of the pain (Fig. 6-1). If it is severe treatment consists of immediate excision under local anesthetic with electrocoagulation of any subcutaneous bleeding points (Fig. 6-2). The aim of this procedure is to relieve the severe pain. The excision is readily performed in the office or emergency room. Incision and evacuation of the thrombus is not recommended because the clots forming the palpable lump are usually intravascular and multiple, hence, some may be missed; effective control of bleeding points is difficult; redundant skin is not removed so the likelihood of a subsequent skin tag is high;

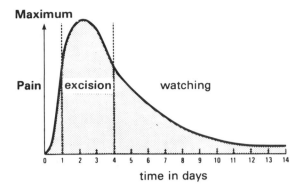

FIGURE **6-1.** *Timing of excision in thrombosed external hemorrhoids.*

and the external hemorrhoidal vessels which led to the thrombosis are not removed, hence, may subsequently re-thrombose.[12] Postoperative care in such cases is simple. It consists of frequent warm baths for comfort and cleanliness, the use of mild oral analgesics as required (although these are rarely needed as the symptomatic relief obtained by excision is dramatic), and the use of psyllium seed, bulk-forming agents to soften the stools so that further straining is prevented. The small wound which is created may be sutured primarily or

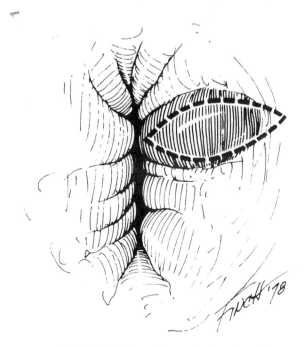

FIGURE **6-2.** *Elliptical excision of thrombosed external hemorrhoids.*

may be allowed to heal by secondary intention, which occurs rapidly. Sigmoidoscopy is indicated, but can be deferred until a follow-up visit.

The end result of many thrombosed external hemorrhoids is a skin tag. In the majority of patients it is entirely symptomless, and hence, requires no treatment. If it is troublesome, it is a simple maneuver to excise the offending tag under local anesthesia as an office procedure. The thrombosed hemorrhoid, which has progressed to ulceration and bleeding, but is painless, rarely requires treatment.

Multiple areas of thrombosis, recurrent episodes of thrombosis, and external hemorrhoids associated with symptomatic internal hemorrhoids, are indications for formal hemorrhoidectomy, sometimes on an emergency basis.

### Internal Hemorrhoids
### Symptoms

In the diagnosis of internal hemorrhoids several symptoms may be present.

*Bleeding* is classically bright red and painless, and occurs at the end of defecation. The patient complains of blood dripping or squirting into the toilet bowl. The bleeding may also be occult, resulting in anemia or guaiac positive stools. In such instances one must exclude other causes of bowel bleeding before these problems are attributed to hemorrhoids, even if gross hemorrhoidal disease exists.

*Prolapse* of the hemorrhoids below the dentate line usually occurs at the time of straining at defecation. In most instances spontaneous reduction occurs. Occasionally, manual replacement is necessary. In some advanced cases, the prolapse is irreducible. Chronic states of prolapse predispose to mucus and fecal leakage resulting in pruritus and excoriation of the perianal skin with accompanying discomfort.

*Pain,* per se, is not a symptom of uncomplicated hemorrhoids but indicates associated disease such as anal fissure, perianal abscess, or notably, an intersphincteric abscess. If thrombosis occurs, pain does become a marked feature of the disease. Prolapsed, strangulated hemorrhoids present as an acute problem with symptoms of pain associated with discharging, edematous, tender, irreducible hemorrhoids. Occasionally, when this state of affairs is left untreated for some time gangrene and infection with sloughing and secondary bleeding will occur. Because of the connection with the portal venous system, infection in this area of venous drainage is possible, and pylephlebitis, although exceedingly rare, is nevertheless a potential complication.

**Examination**

Examination of patients with suspected internal hemorrhoids should be aimed at several aspects.

*General patient assessment* to ascertain the general health status, and in particular to exclude associated disease, notably bleeding disorders and liver disease with portal hypertension, should be the first phase of examination.

*Inspection* will reveal gross and late stages of hemorrhoidal disease, and will exclude coincidental lesions.

*Digital examination* will exclude low-lying rectal and anal canal neoplasms, as well as enable the tone of the anal sphincter to be assessed.

*Anoscopy* is the definitive examination. It is performed to assess the extent of disease. With the anoscope in place the patient is asked to strain as if having a bowel movement so that the amount of prolapse can be assessed. During anoscopy it is also important to look for, and rule out, a co-existing anal fissure, especially in patients complaining of pain or those in whom anal sphincter tone is deemed to be excessive.

*Proctosigmoidoscopy* must be performed in all cases in order to visualize the rectum and lower colon so that co-existing conditions may be excluded, in particular, carcinoma and inflammatory bowel disease. This latter condition may produce symptoms similar to hemorrhoidal complaints, and, of course, it may also potentiate any hemorrhoids present.

*Barium enema* examination must be performed in any patient with unusual symptoms or in whom it is hard to attribute the symptom to the limited degree of hemorrhoidal disease found. This examination must be undertaken before any treatment is commenced since colon diseases beyond the range of the sigmoidoscope must be excluded first. Patients who fall into the age or family history category of being at risk for having colorectal neoplasms should also have a barium enema. For practical purposes, this age is arbitrarily set at 45 years.

*Colonoscopy* should be considered as an adjunct to barium enema examination in those patients with unusual symptoms, particularly if the study is questionable or in some cases even negative.

**Treatment**

Treatment is undertaken only after other causes of lower intestinal bleeding have been excluded. Various modalities are available.

*Medical.* The aim of this regime is to avoid straining on defecation. Dietary manipulation and education is all that is required in patients with first degree hemorrhoids with occasional symptoms of painless bleeding, especially if that bleeding is associated with straining to pass hard stools. It is important to assure that the patient has an adequate fluid intake, and that he increases his intake of bulk in the form of vegetable fiber or unprocessed cereal fiber (e.g., bran). Hydrophilic bulk-forming agents such as psyllium seed compounds may be prescribed to supplement these measures. Excess dairy products in the diet should be excluded because they may be constipating. It is important to impress upon the patient not to ignore the urge to defecate.

*Rubber band ligation* as described by Barron has proved to be a simple, quick, and effective means of treating most forms of uncomplicated hemorrhoidal disease (Fig. 6-3).[4] The basis of its success lies in the fact that it replaces the hemorrhoidal cushions in the normal position; it removes redundant rectal mucosa above the hemorrhoids; and, it decreases the size of the hemorrhoids by causing submucosal scarring and partial atrophy of the submucosal venous plexi. This technique is, therefore, the procedure of choice for patients with first degree hemorrhoids unrelieved by dietary means, all cases of second degree hemorrhoids, and cases of early or minimal rectal mucosal prolapse.[1,4] It is sometimes effective in patients with third degree disease, especially if they are unwilling or unfit for an operative procedure. Patients with prolapsed strangulated hemorrhoids are unsuitable for

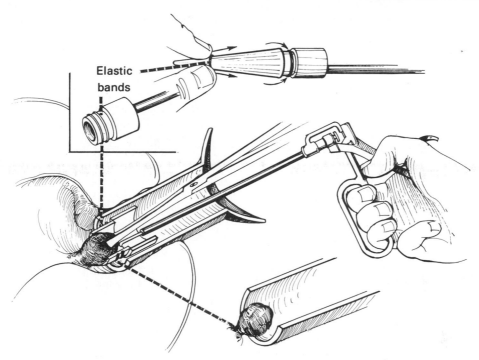

Elastic
bands

FIGURE **6-3.** *Rubber band ligation for internal hemorrhoids.*

this procedure. Rubber band ligation can be undertaken, with caution, in patients on a well-controlled anticoagulant therapy.

As an office or outpatient procedure, without special preparation, a constricting rubber band is placed on the most redundant portion of the rectal mucosa, at the level of the anorectal ring, immediately above the internal hemorrhoid. It is imperative that this area alone is treated since banding tissue at a lower level may result in severe pain. Anatomically, the area above the dentate line is innervated by visceral autonomic nerve fibers, and hence, "insensitive" to superficial pain. Below the dentate line, somatic nerves provide sensory stimuli which means that this region is very sensitive to pain. In practice this area of demarcation is not as precise as anatomists would have us believe. The area of somatic sensation may extend higher than the dentate line, therefore, to allow for this variation the upper limit should be identified. It is recommended that the level of the anorectal ring be used for banding procedures. If symptoms persist subsequent bands may be applied at levels close to the dentate line. Care should be exercised to avoid the underlying muscula-

ture. Success can further be assured by the use of double bands, since breakage of the rubber is possible, and a single band may not be totally constricting.

Incorporated tissue sloughs in approximately seven to ten days, leaving a limited area of inflammation, which results in scar and point fixation. This technique does not require anesthesia since any excessive discomfort indicates that the band has been placed too low and should be removed immediately. Although not acutely painful, this procedure may produce a sensation of rectal discomfort and fullness which persists for several days. The patient must be made aware of this fact. In a few patients considerable discomfort is encountered for 24 to 48 hours. Relief can be readily obtained by the use of a mild oral analgesic supplemented by warm baths. All patients should be started on bulk-forming stool softeners of the psyllium seed kind, because a hard stool in the presence of an area of sloughing mucosa may, on rare occasions, precipitate a massive bleed. Usually a trace of blood will occur with the sloughing, and may persist until the area heals. Massive bleeding, if it is to occur, will do so at approximately seven to ten days after banding. Control can be obtained readily by electrocoagulation or suture ligation of the bleeding area under direct vision. Rarely, blood replacement may also be required.

Banding procedures may precipitate acute thrombosis. It may be of the external hemorrhoid alone or of the combined hemorrhoid. In the former case, it may be treated by simple excision. In the latter case, a formal hemorrhoidectomy may be necessary.[1]

Because of the unpleasant sensation of rectal fullness, it is preferable to band only one or two areas at any one time, and so repeated applications may be necessary to totally relieve the patient's symptoms. Bleeding may persist for some time after the procedure, therefore, a period of four to six weeks to allow for complete healing should elapse before any further treatment is contemplated. If after this time bleeding continues, further banding is undertaken, and repeated at intervals as required. Post ligation activity is not restricted. Results using this technique have been most gratifying, and support the enthusiasm with which it was initially introduced.[1,4,5,21,35]

*Sclerotherapy* is also a simple and effective means to control minor degrees of hemorrhoidal disease. The technique is widely practiced with great success in Great Britain.[38] This method relies on the production of submucosal scarring which results in fixation, retraction, and partial atrophy of the hemorrhoidal cushions which returns them to their normal anatomical sites. Like rubber banding, it is indicated in patients with first degree hemorrhoids unrelieved by simpler means, all cases of second degree hemorrhoids, and cases of early or minimal rectal mucosal prolapse.

Injection therapy is undertaken as an office or outpatient procedure without special preparation. A sclerosing solution, such as 5 per cent phenol in vegetable oil, is injected submucosally above the internal hemorrhoids.[1,16] Usually 3 to 5 cc are placed in each involved area at the level of the anorectal ring. At this site no pain is experienced; however, if incorrectly placed at a site nearer to or actually into the hemorrhoid, severe pain may be induced.[11] Moreover, such low injection may precipitate acute thrombosis of the external hemorrhoids necessitating a semi-emergency hemorrhoi-

dectomy. A sensation of rectal fullness or pain may be experienced by patients. Such symptoms may persist for some days and can be readily relieved by mild oral analgesics supplemented with warm baths.

The procedure is facilitated by the use of a special needle with a shoulder 1 cm from the bevelled sharp end (Fig. 6-4). This prevents too deep a placement of the solution. The needle is introduced into the submucosal plane at an angle, and injection is commenced. A visible swelling is produced, and the mucosa over it is seen to become pale with its vessels readily visible. Because of the viscosity of the sclerosing solution, injection is, of necessity, slow. This process may be performed more quickly if the solution is warmed prior to use. If pain is experienced at the time of the procedure, the injection must be stopped immediately, since incorrect placement has occurred.

After injection, the patient is started on hydrophilic, bulk-forming agents. He is reviewed in four to six weeks time. If symptoms are still present, the therapy may be repeated; however, the number of times this procedure can be safely performed is limited as submucosal scarring precludes safe injection. The great drawback of this technique is the fact that it is imprecise, and produces diffuse submucosal scarring. Offsetting this problem, is the fact that in most cases sclerotherapy is effective and safe.

The procedure is contraindicated in patients with known inflammatory bowel disease, leukemia, lymphoma, or portal hypertension. It is of no value in prolapsed strangulated hemorrhoids, and should be used with caution in patients who already have diffuse scarring of the anorectum.

Complications of the procedure are related to incorrect placement of the sclerosing solution. Mucosal sloughing will occur if an intramucosal injection is given. This condition will be apparent at the time as an area of sharply

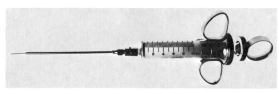

FIGURE 6-4. *Gabriel needle.*

demarcated pallor. If it is small, immediately recognized, and injection ceased, no untoward damage will ensue. Large areas of mucosal injection result in sloughing of the involved mucosa with the consequent production of a painful, bleeding rectal ulcer which may take a long time to heal. Extrarectal injection will produce scarring in the incorrect plane, and can result in stricture formation. More acutely, an abscess or fistula-in-ano may occur. Rarely, an oleoma may be produced, and occasionally an intravenous injection with oil embolus may occur. The onset of pain at the time of injection without submucosal swelling indicates that the needle is not in the submucosal plane, but rather extrarectal or intramuscular. Small volumes of sclerosing solution injected extrarectally usually do not cause any harm; therefore, if this misplacement is immediately recognized, the injection ceased, and the needle correctly repositioned, a satisfactory result will still be achieved.

*Manual dilatation of anus.* Although initially recommended by Récamier, anal dilatation for the treatment of various anal disorders also has been advocated by Lord.[23,28] The rationale for its use is the expectation of overcoming anal obstruction due to constricting bands, or anal sphincter dysfunction, or both. Such obstruction leads to straining at the time of defecation, resulting in engorgement of the internal hemorrhoidal venous plexuses, which causes further obstruction, thus setting up a vicious circle which ultimately results in bleeding and prolapse. It is claimed that if this vicious circle is broken, symptoms may be alleviated.

The procedure is usually carried out in the outpatient department under a general anesthetic in the lateral position. Gradually, and gently, the constricting bands are identified and disrupted by increasing dilatation and digital pressure to a maximum of eight fingers in the left and right lateral areas of the anus. The amount of dilatation will vary from patient to patient since it is imperative that the sphincter and overlying anoderm are not disrupted, particularly at the midline anteriorly and posteriorly, which are the weakest points. In men patients it is not usually possible to achieve an eight-finger dilatation without splitting the anoderm; hence, if one is unsure of the amount of dilatation required it is safer to do too little than too much, because the procedure may be

repeated at a later time, if required. A foam sponge is left in the anus and rectum for one hour after the end of the dilatation to minimize hematoma formation.[23]

After dilatation the patient is started on a bulk-forming stool softener, and further dilatation of the anus is carried out by the patient himself, with the use of a special grooved anal dilator. Dilatation is performed daily for two weeks, and at regular intervals for as long as six months.

Patients with any stage or degree of hemorrhoidal disease are said to be candidates for maximal anal dilatation.[23] This includes patients with late stage disease, prolapsed strangulated hemorrhoids, and, in particular, patients who have a combination of anal fissure and hemorrhoidal symptoms. However, one should be cautious in using this procedure in the elderly or other patients with known continence problems.[21,23] When the procedure is properly done, Lord claimed a low incidence of complications such as incontinence, hematoma formation, splitting, and mucosal prolapse.[23]

The main drawback of the dilatation method is the unpredictable amount of damage to the sphincter muscles with the danger of subsequent contraction necessitating prolonged use of a dilator after the treatment.[2] In a controlled study, manual dilatation of the anus for treatment of hemorrhoids showed no advantage over a simpler rubber band ligation.[19] Mucosal prolapse also remains untreated by manual dilatation.[9]

*Partial internal sphincterotomy* has become widely used for the management of patients with anal fissures where it is thought that the underlying problem is one of "hyperfunction" of the internal anal sphincter. It is claimed by some authorities that similar dysfunction accounts for the occurrence of hemorrhoidal disease.[2,18] Consequently, partial internal sphincterotomy has been advocated to overcome this abnormality.

Unlike maximal anal dilatation, partial internal sphincterotomy has the advantage of precise division of the sphincter under direct vision. This operation can be done under local, regional or general anesthesia. Incontinence, to varying degrees, occurs in 25 per cent of patients, and is minor in most instances. Prolapse of redundant mucosa is common, and usually requires further treatment. Recurrence of symptoms occurs in only 5 per cent of patients.[2] This procedure has no effect on external hemorrhoids and skin tags. Postoperative care is simple, aimed at patient comfort, and ensuring an early bowel movement.

Although it is a relatively simple technique, partial internal sphincterotomy for the routine treatment of hemorrhoids has not gained general acceptance, but it does have its advocates. In patients in whom an anal fissure accompanies the hemorrhoids, or in whom there is evidence of a hyperactive sphincter, there is no doubt that partial internal sphincterotomy should be part of the therapy undertaken. The controlled studies by Arabi and associates showed no advantage of internal sphincterotomy over rubber band ligation in the treatment of first and second degree hemorrhoids.[3]

*Cryotherapy.* Tissue destruction by freezing has long been a popular and effective method for dealing with certain dermatological conditions. More recently its use has been extended to deal with anorectal pathology, notably hemorrhoids. Specialized probes activated by carbon dioxide, nitrous oxide, or best of all, liquid nitrogen have been developed. Temperatures of $-180°$ C can be developed at the ends of the probe. Effectiveness of the procedure, however, depends on the rapid lowering of the temperature of the tissue to be destroyed. The critical temperature to destroy tissue is accepted to be $-20°$ C. The term cryotherapy for hemorrhoids involves destruction of deep and highly vascularized structures.[26] If the critical temperature cannot be achieved, deep freezing will not occur, and all that is achieved is superficial tissue destruction, resulting in painful lesions without resolving the hemorrhoidal problem.

The procedure is performed in the office or outpatient department. Although the actual freezing is not painful, at best the patient is quite uncomfortable, so it is recommended that local anesthetic infiltration be used. This addition results in anal sphincter relaxation, and removes any unpleasant sensations that the patient may experience. In some patients a general anesthetic is required.[32] Under direct vision, the cryosurgical probe, which is flat and rectangular, is placed in firm contact with the long axis of the hemorrhoidal cushion to be treated. Upon activation of the probe, freezing

begins immediately, and is maintained for one to three minutes. This procedure is then repeated in all areas requiring treatment; however, care is needed to preserve bridges of anoderm and mucosa between the hemorrhoids by visual control of ice formation.

Patients may be discharged within a few minutes after treatment. Oral analgesic tablets are prescribed as severe pain will occur once the local anesthetic has worn off. Frequently, warm baths are encouraged for comfort and cleanliness since the major problem encountered is that of profuse foul discharge, which begins almost immediately and continues at least two weeks (generally until all the frozen tissue necroses and sloughs). Early bowel movement is encouraged by the use of bulk-forming agents.

Because of the pain and discharge, few patients are able to resume activities immediately, and it is not uncommon for patients to miss work for as long as two to three weeks.[15] Healing of the area takes at least six weeks.[15] Secondary hemorrhage occurs in about 3 per cent of patients so treated.[32] Although Savin had an excellent result from cryotherapy, other series had disappointing results.[32] In Goligher's series, only 70 per cent of patients, after a prolonged healing time, have, what could be considered, a satisfactory result.[15] Some of the 30 per cent of patients who do not secure satisfactory results might conceivably be helped by repeat cryosurgery, but the discomfort associated with the first treatment has tended to militate against a repetition of this form of therapy. Even in those patients in whom internal hemorrhoidal symptoms are relieved, large skin tags are commonly produced as a result of the irregular and unpredictable tissue destruction. These tags may require surgical excision unless they are symptomless. In a controlled study comparing cryotherapy of hemorrhoids with closed dissection hemorrhoidectomy on the same patient, Smith found the latter to be far superior.[34]

It appears that cryotherapy for hemorrhoids has many problems and hazards, and therefore, has failed to gain widespread use and acceptance. Although there are proponents of the technique, they are few, since a procedure which depends on necrosis, gangrene, and sloughing has little to recommend it. It is possible to combine rubber banding with cryotherapy, whereby, the tissue incorporated in the constricting band is immediately frozen and the rubber band is removed.[30] It is claimed that this combination hastens the whole process, which it may do, but at the expense of turning a very simple office procedure into an unnecessarily complex and cumbersome one.

## CLOSED HEMORRHOIDECTOMY

Since the adoption of the widespread use of bulk-forming agents and rubber band ligature techniques for the treatment of early stages of hemorrhoidal disease, the need for hemorrhoidectomy has greatly decreased. In general, hemorrhoidectomy should be reserved for patients having unrelenting symptoms of prolapse, pain, or bleeding, or in whom large hemorrhoids are found to be associated with other anorectal pathology requiring operative management. The most frequent indication for hemorrhoidectomy in modern surgical practice is severe rectal mucosal prolapse associated with mixed hemorrhoids. Pain associated with hemorrhoids is most commonly due to thrombosis, although one must be aware that acute anal fissures may also be present. Rarely, an intersphincteric abscess may be misdiagnosed as a hemorrhoidal problem. When thrombosis is extensive, formal hemorrhoidectomy is indicated, although, the majority of solitary, painful, thrombosed hemorrhoids can be managed by simple excision of the entire hemorrhoidal complex under local anesthesia.

### Pre-Operative Evaluation

All patients undergoing hemorrhoidectomy must have a sigmoidoscopy performed at the time of their first examination. In the situation of painful prolapsed hemorrhoids, this examination should be deferred until the anesthetic has been given. If the patient is beyond the age of 45 years, or his symptoms suggest additional pathology, a barium enema examination, and possibly colonoscopy, are indicated. Special care must be taken to exclude the possibility of undiagnosed inflammatory bowel disease in any patient who has a history of diarrhea. One must remember that Crohn's disease is a relative contraindication to hemorrhoidectomy. Patients with known portal hypertension, leukemia or lymphoma, or

bleeding diathesis, should also be excluded. Past history of bleeding diathesis should be sought and, in all cases, the usual laboratory tests to rule out a bleeding diathesis should be obtained if there is any clinical doubt.

The patient is informed that he will be in the hospital for four to five days, although complete healing may not occur for three to four weeks. Complications related to the operation requiring further operative intervention occur in about 1 per cent of patients. Preoperative preparation is kept simple. One disposable packaged phosphated enema is given the evening before surgery and another approximately one hour before operation. In cases of severe pain due to extensive thrombosis, the enemas can be withheld. No perineal shaving is performed, and laxatives or antibiotics are unnecessary.

### Operative Procedures

Many operative procedures have evolved for the treatment of hemorrhoids. The principles for all excisional procedures include removing diseased tissue (i.e., internal and external hemorrhoids as well as redundant rectal mucosa), leaving minimal scarring of the anal canal, avoiding interference with the sphincteric mechanism, and resulting in an anal orifice ample for a normal bowel movement without discomfort. Although there are many variations, all hemorrhoidectomy operations basically employ the excision and ligature techniques. The method of handling the perianal skin differentiates various techniques. In some, the mucous membrane is closed up to the dentate line, but the external wound is left open.[31] Other techniques employ primary closure of the hemorrhoidectomy wound.[10,14]

The proponents of closed hemorrhoidectomy claim this operation offers: (*1*) effective removal of hemorrhoidal tissue and redundant rectal mucosa, (*2*) prompt healing of wounds, (*3*) diminished drainage by avoiding an open wound, (*4*) minimal inpatient and virtually no outpatient care, (*5*) less postoperative discomfort, (*6*) minimal disturbance of continence, and (*7*) no need for anal dilatation.[6,7,10] An adequate, dissection-type, closed hemorrhoidectomy may be carried out on acute, prolapsed, thrombosed edematous hemorrhoids without fear of anal stenosis or stricture, if meticulous dissection and preservation of anoderm are accomplished. Such a technique may safely be combined with other operative procedures, such as fissurectomy, internal sphincterotomy, fistulotomy, or excision of hypertrophied anal papillae.

**Operative Technique**

*Position of Patient.* Traditionally, anorectal procedures have been performed with the patients in the lithotomy position. Routine use of the semi-prone or jackknife position, with soft rolls under the hips and ankles of the patient ensuring that the patient is comfortable on the table, has many advantages, and we highly recommend it. It affords greater access to the operative field, and allows greater comfort for the operating surgeon, the assistant surgeon, and scrub nurse. Any bleeding which occurs will drain independently away from the operative field, and so enhance exposure.

*Preparation of the Area.* The operative area is not shaved. Adhesive tapes are applied to the buttocks to provide lateral traction, and so further expose the anus. Prolonged skin prep is unnecessary. A mild antiseptic solution will ensure cleanliness, and is all that is required.

*Anesthesia.* The prone position lends itself well to general, regional or local anesthesia. In all cases infiltration with local anesthesia and epinephrine is used to facilitate hemostasis during the operation and to provide pain relief in the immediate postoperative period.

*Fluids.* It is important to minimize the volume of intravenous solutions administered during operation, ideally, to less than 100 cc. By keeping the patient partially dehydrated in the intraoperative period, one insures that his bladder is not distended. This precaution results in spontaneous voiding sometime later; usually within 24 hours. By using this regime, urinary catheterization is required in only 10 per cent or less of patients undergoing hemorrhoidectomy.[7]

*Exposures.* Following the introduction of the local anesthetic agent, the anal canal is examined digitally, and then visually, by the use of a Pratt bivalve anal speculum. The specific hemorrhoidal areas are examined carefully, and the operation is planned in greater detail. The largest hemorrhoidal complex is removed first. The aeras involved are usually the left lateral, right posterolateral, and right anterolateral. After examining the

anus, a Fansler operating anoscope is introduced. Small, 7.5 cm², opened, gauze sponges, which fit through the operating scope, are used as an alternative to suction.

*Operation.* Dissection is started on the perianal skin. A narrow, elliptical incision is made with fine dissecting scissors removing skin and hemorrhoidal tissue down to the underlying internal sphincter muscle. No attempt is made to remove all the tissue in one motion. The redundant rectal mucosa is excised up to the level of the anorectal ring. If rectal mucosal prolapse is a major problem, excision may be extended to the level of the lowest rectal valve. The bleeding which occurs comes mainly from the submucosal vessels which can be easily identified, and individually electrocoagulated (Fig. 6-5).

At this point the anoderm and mucosa are elevated so that hemorrhoidal tissue may be dissected, and excised from beneath these flaps. Further hemostasis is achieved by electrocautery. After dissecting and excising the secondary hemorrhoidal tissues from beneath the raised flaps, and controlling the bleeding, the wound is closed, starting at the apex, utilizing a running suture of 3-0 chromic catgut, polyglycolic acid, or polyglactin sutures. The mucous membrane is sutured down to the underlying sphincter muscle in an attempt to create a longitudinal scar which will prevent further prolapse. Trimming of excess skin is carried out, but it is essential that the wound be closed without tension. The procedure is repeated in the other major areas, and in as many additional areas as necessary. In certain cases of prolapsed thrombosed hemorrhoids, as many as four areas may be excised and primarily closed. It is recommended that hemorrhoidectomy excision, ideally, should not be performed in the anterior or posterior commissure, unless plastic flap procedures are planned, because in this location there is a greater tendency to fissure formation.

If the anal canal does not accept the operating anoscope easily, a partial internal sphincterotomy is carried out in the base of a wound, usually in the left lateral area. At the completion of the operation all areas are examined carefully, and blood clots are removed. No packing or dressing is placed in the anal canal or perianal area. The average operating time is 30 to 45 minutes for surgeons experienced in this technique.

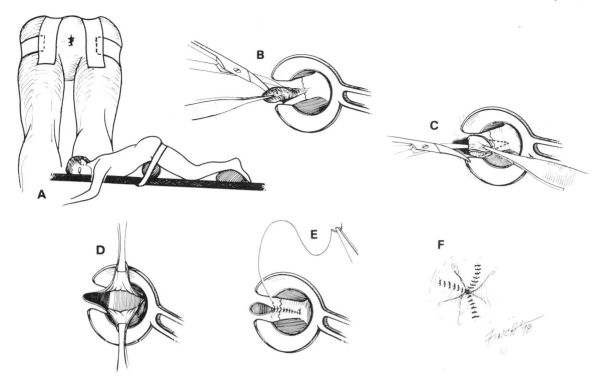

**FIGURE 6-5.** *Technique of closed hemorrhoidectomy.* (**A**) *Positioning of patient.* (**B**) *Exposure of the hemorrhoid using Fansler operative scope.* (**C**) *Elliptical excision starting at the perianal skin to anorectal ring.* (**D**) *Submucosal hemorrhoidal plexuses dissected from the internal sphincter, anoderm and mucosa.* (**E**) *The wound is closed with running suture.* (**F**) *At completion of the procedure.*

It is important that all excised tissues are properly labelled, and submitted separately for microscopic examination. Occasionally, unsuspected malignancy or inflammatory bowel disease may be so diagnosed. The results of such examination will be available before the patient is discharged so that appropriate treatment can be undertaken.

### Follow Up

Patients return for examination 10 to 14 days following operation, and are examined carefully. Anoscopy and digital examination may be carried out to assess the wound healing. In a recent survey of 500 patients managed in the way described it was found that: the hospital stay averages 4.3 days; the total healing time averages 4.1 weeks; primary healing occurred in one-third of patients.[7] In the remaining two-thirds some or all of the sutured wounds broke down, and healing occurred by secondary intention; however, the majority of patients falling into this category had partial breakdown only so that healing progressed at a rapid rate.

Complications related to a closed hemorrhoidectomy are few. Bleeding, which is a potential problem with all forms of hemorrhoidectomy, occured in 4 per cent of patients.[7] In the majority of patients this bleeding was of a secondary nature, presenting on or about the tenth postoperative day, and generally being minor in nature with spontaneous resolution. In 1 per cent of patients, hemorrhage was severe enough to require a return to the operating room for hemostasis. Most of these patients experienced bleeding while still in the hospital, and so, this should be regarded as primary in nature. Other complications which can occur are listed below.[7] It should be noted that abscess formation is rare, and did not occur in this series. Acute retention of urine can be kept to a minimum by deliberately limiting fluid intake as earlier described.

*COMPLICATIONS: 500 CONSECUTIVE CLOSED HEMORRHOIDECTOMIES*

| | |
|---|---|
| ABSCESS FORMATION | 0.0% |
| FISTULA-IN-ANO | 0.4% |
| ANAL FISSURE | 0.2% |
| ANAL STENOSIS | 1.0% |
| INCONTINENCE | 0.4% |
| SKIN TAGS | 6.0% |
| FECAL IMPACTION | 0.4% |
| THROMBOSED EXTERNAL HEMORRHOID | 0.2% |
| ACUTE URINARY RETENTION | 10.0% |

Fistula and fissure formation may be a complication of operation, or related to poor wound healing. Operative treatment may be required if symptomatic. Fistula-in-ano, if it does occur, is usually superficial and readily treated. Skin tags may result from any operative procedure on the perianal area; no greater incidence occurs with the closed hemorrhoidal technique. A large skin tag can be removed under local anesthesia at the time of the first postoperative review. It is not necessary to remove small skin tags since these act as a "pleat" so that the patient does not split the perianal skin when the anal canal opens at the time of defecation.

Anal stenosis and anal stricture occur rarely after the closed hemorrhoidectomy technique. In most cases when they do occur they are of a minor nature and improve with time. More permanent problems arise from the removal of too much normal perianal skin (e.g. fissure). With attention to detail such problems are minimized.

## OTHER FORMS OF HEMORRHOIDECTOMY

There are many other ways of surgically removing hemorrhoidal tissue. Most commonly used is the ligature and excision operation described in 1937 by Milligan and colleagues.[25] This operation is done with the patient in lithotomy position. After adequate perineal preparation and draping, the three main areas of hemorrhoidal disease are grasped in artery clamps, and pulled out of the anal canal. Each area, in turn, is then excised, leaving a proximal pedicle which is ligated. Further hemo-

stasis is achieved by electrocoagulation. The wounds are left open to heal by secondary intention. Using this technique one runs the risk of excision of excess amounts of perianal skin, but this can occur with any form of hemorrhoidectomy. The anal canal distortion, which is part of the exposure of the hemorrhoids, increases the possibility of this complication. If it occurs anal stricture formation is likely. The open wounds probably lead to increased postoperative discomfort, although this is difficult to prove.

The submucosal dissection of hemorrhoids described by Parks differs slightly from the technic just described.[27] In this operation the anoderm and the rectal mucosa are incised, and the submucosal vascular plexuses are dissected out, along with the perianal skin. The wound is then closed. His result is excellent, and the complications are low.

The Whitehead operation, whereby all the hemorrhoidal tissue is excised, and the rectal mucosa is sutured to the dentate line, was popular in years gone by. The operation, although effective in relieving hemorrhoidal problems, may lead to a "wet" anus deformity if performed incorrectly. The rectal mucosa continuously leaks mucus so that patients are

| *Suggested Rational Plan of Management* | |
|---|---|
| 1st degree hemorrhoids | Exclusion of other causes of bleeding, diet, psyllium seed, rubber band ligation sclerotherapy |
| 2nd degree hemorrhoids | Rubber band ligation |
| 3rd degree hemorrhoids | Rubber band ligation, closed hemorrhoidectomy |
| 4th degree hemorrhoids | Closed hemorrhoidectomy |
| Prolapsed strangulated hemorrhoids | Emergency closed hemorrhoidectomy |
| Thrombosed external hemorrhoids | Painful—excise: local anesthesia  Painless—observe |
| Perianal skin tags | Excise under local anesthesia if symptomatic |
| Hypertrophied anal papillae | Asymptomatic—no treatment  Symptomatic—excise |

subject to constant discharge and subsequent pruritus.

Other techniques of clamp and ligature have not achieved widespread popularity.

Techniques utilizing a clamp and cautery are mentioned to be condemned. These methods belong in the annals of surgical history, and not in modern surgery.

## HEMORRHOIDS OCCURRING IN SPECIAL SITUATIONS

### Pregnancy

Hemorrhoidal symptoms commonly occur, and intensify, during pregnancy and delivery. In most instances, however, hemorrhoids which do intensify during delivery resolve. Hemorrhoidectomy is indicated in pregnancy only if the complication of acute prolapse and thrombosis occurs. Prolapse and thrombosis of hemorrhoids occurring during delivery is an indication for operation in the immediate post partum period. Similarly, operation is indicated in patients in whom hemorrhoidal disease has been symptomatic prior to pregnancy, aggravated during pregnancy, and persists after delivery. In such patients hemorrhoidectomy is best performed in the immediate post partum period.[33]

### Inflammatory Bowel Disease

Ulcerative colitis, ulcerative proctitis, or Crohn's disease may be associated with hemorrhoidal symptoms. In most cases this association is due to, or aggravated by, a diarrhea state which if controlled leads to improvement of hemorrhoidal symptoms. Jefery and colleagues reviewed the cases of 42 patients with ulcerative colitis, and 20 patients with Crohn's disease, who were treated for hemorrhoids at St. Mark's Hospital between 1935 and 1975.[20] Both surgical and conservative treatment of hemorrhoids in patients with ulcerative colitis had low complication rates (four complications after 58 courses of treatment). In Crohn's disease the complication rate was high (eleven complications after 26 courses of treatment). One of the 42 patients with ulcerative colitis, and six of the 20 with Crohn's disease, required rectal excision for complications apparently dating from the treatment of hemorrhoids. The complications remained high even when they were treated before the diagnosis of Crohn's disease was made. These results suggest that treatment of symptomatic hemorrhoids is usually safe in patients with ulcerative colitis but is relatively contraindicated in those with Crohn's disease.

Anal inspection and proctosigmoidoscopy are essential in patients with rectal bleeding, even if the history suggests hemorrhoids as the cause. A biopsy specimen of the rectal mucosa must be obtained if the examination suggests the possibility of inflammatory bowel disease.

### Portal Hypertension

Although the hemorrhoidal plexuses communicate with the portal system, significant bleeding from the hemorrhoids is rarely a problem in portal hypertension.[16,37] A few patients may require hemorrhoidectomy, which should be performed only after correction of any coagulopathy. Our limited experience suggests that hemorrhoidectomy should be done one quadrant at a time, at one to two week intervals. Local anesthesia would be the method of choice, and a more lasting suture (Polyglycolic acid or Polyglactin) is recommended.

### Leukemia or Lymphoma

Patients with these problems or other causes of immunosuppression may present with hemorrhoidal disease. In these circumstances treatment is difficult as the risks from operative intervention are great; poor wound healing, and abscesses can readily supervene.

Patients with strangulated and thrombosed hemorrhoids may be candidates for hemorrhoidectomy after correction of any coexisting clotting disorder. Although complete healing may not occur, a small, clean anal wound is probably more comfortable, and easier to manage, than bleeding, discharging, and painful hemorrhoids. One must be aware that anal lesions similar to hemorrhoids, or other anorectal pathology, may be a feature of local leukemic or lymphomatous infiltration. Direct operation on these can lead to disaster.

### Intestinal Bypass for Obesity

Anorectal disease is a frequent occurrence following such procedures. In most cases the problems are non-specific and are related to the chronic diarrhea. Control of this problem, in most cases, leads to improvement of the hemorrhoids. In early stages of the disease rubber band ligation should be tried, reserving hemorrhoidectomy for only third degree hemorrhoids.

## Hemorrhoids in Association with Other Anorectal Disease

If hemorrhoids are associated with other anorectal problems, such as anal fissures or fistulae-in-ano, hemorrhoidectomy combined with sphincterotomy or fistulotomy can be done without added morbidity.[13] There is no data regarding the advisability of hemorrhoidectomy in conjunction with the operative treatment of condylomata accuminata of the perianal skin, or the anal canal.

## REFERENCES

1. Alexander-Williams, J., and Crapp, A. R.: Conservative management of haemorrhoids. Part I: Injection, freezing and ligation. Clin. Gastroenterol., *4*:595, 1975.

2. Allgöwer, M.: Conservative management of haemorrhoids. Part III: Partial internal sphincterotomy. Clin. Gastroenterol., *4*:608, 1975.

3. Arabi, Y., Gatehouse, D., Alexander-Williams, J., and Keighley, M. R. B.: Rubber band ligation or lateral subcutaneous sphincterotomy for treatment of haemorrrhoids. Br. J. Surg., *64*:737, 1977.

4. Barron, J.: Office ligation treatment of hemorrhoids. Dis. Colon Rectum, *6*:109, 1963.

5. Bartizal, J., and Slosberg, P. A.: An alternative to hemorrhoidectomy. Arch. Surg., *112*:534, 1977.

6. Bautista, L. I.: Hemorrhoidectomy—How I do it: Complications of closed hemorrhoidectomy. Dis. Colon Rectum, *20*:183, 1977.

7. Buls, J. G., and Goldberg, S. M.: Modern management of hemorrhoids. Surg. Clin. North Am., *58*:469, 1978.

8. Burkitt, D. P.: Hemorrhoids, varicose veins and deep vein thrombosis: Epidemiologic features and suggested causative factors. Can. J. Surg., *18*:483, 1975.

9. Editorial: To tie; to stab; to stretch; perchance to freeze. Lancet, *2*:645, 1975.

10. Ferguson, J. A., Mazier, W. R., Ganchrow, M. I., and Friend, W. G.: The closed technique of hemorrhoidectomy. Surg., *70*:480, 1971.

11. Gabriel, W. B.: The Principles and Practice of Rectal Surgery. 131. London, H. K. Lewis and Co., 1963.

12. Ganchrow, M. I., Bowman, H. E., and Clark, J. F.: Thrombosed hemorrhoids: A clinicopathologic study. Dis. Colon Rectum, *14*:331, 1971.

13. Ganchrow, M. I., Mazier, W. P., Friend, W. G., and Ferguson, J. A.: Hemorrhoidectomy revisited—A computer analysis of 2,038 cases. Dis. Colon Rectum, *14*:128, 1971.

14. Goldberg, S. M.: Closed Haemorrhoidectomy. *In Operative Surgery; Colon, Rectum and Anus.* London and Boston, Butterworth and Co., 1977.

15. Goligher, J. C.: Cryosurgery for hemorrhoids. Dis. Colon Rectum, *19*:213, 1976.

16. ———: *Surgery of the Anus, Rectum and Colon.* 116–167. Springfield, Charles C. Thomas Co., 1975.

17. Graham-Stewart, C. W.: What causes hemorrhoids? A new theory of etiology. Dis. Colon Rectum, *6*:333, 1963.

18. Hancock, B. D.: Internal sphincter and the nature of haemorrhoids. Gut., *18*:651, 1977.

19. Hood, T. R., and Alexander-Williams, J.: Anal dilatation versus rubber band ligation for internal hemorrhoids. Methods of treatment in outpatients. Am. J. Surg., *122*:545, 1971.

20. Jeffery, P. J., Ritchie, J. L., and Parks, A. G.: Treatment of haemorrhoids in patients with inflammatory bowel disease. Lancet, *1*:1084, 1977.

21. Jones, C. B., and Schofield, P. F.: A comparative study of the methods of treatment for haemorrhoids. Proc. R. Soc. Med. *67*:51, 1974.

22. Kerremans, R.: *Morphologic and Physiological Aspects of Anal Continence and Defecation.* Arscia, S. A. (ed.) Bruxelles, Presses Académiques Europeenes, S.C., 1969.

23. Lord, P. H.: Conservative management of haemorrhoids. Part II: Dilatation treatment. Clin. Gastroenterol., *4*:601, 1975.

24. Maimonides, M.: *Treatise on hemorrhoids.* Rosner, F. and Muntner, S. (trans.) Philadelphia, J. B. Lippincott, 1969.

25. Milligan, E. T. C., Morgan C. M., Jones, L. E., and Officer, R.: Surgical anatomy of the anal canal, and the operative treatment of haemorrhoids. Lancet, *2*:1119, 1937.

26. O'Connor, J. J.: The role of cryosurgery in management of anorectal disease: a study of cryosurgical techniques. Dis. Colon Rectum, *18*:298, 1975.

27. Parks, A. G.: Haemorrhoidectomy. Surg. Clin. North Am., *45:*1305, 1965.

28. Récamier, M.: *Quoted by* Maisonneuve, J. G.: Du traitement de la fissure à lánus par la dilatation forcée. Gaz d'hôp 3rd series, 1, 220, 1849.

29. Robbins, S. L.: Pathology. 869. Philadelphia and London, W. B. Saunders, 1967.

30. Rudd, W. W. H.: Hemorrhoidectomy—How I do it: Ligation with and without cryosurgery in 3000 cases. Dis. Colon Rectum, *20:*186, 1977.

31. Ruiz-Moreno, F.: Hemorrhoidectomy—How I do it: Semiclosed technique. Dis. Colon Rectum, *20:*177, 1977.

32. Savin, S.: Hemorrhoidectomy—How I do it: Results of 444 cryorectal surgical operations. Dis. Colon Rectum, *20:*189, 1977.

33. Schottler, J. L., Balcos, E. G., and Goldberg, S. M.: Postpartum hemorrhoidectomy. Dis. Colon Rectum, *16:*395, 1973.

34. Smith, L. E., Goodreau, J. J., and Fouty, W. J.: Operative hemorrhoidectomy versus cryodestruction. Dis. Colon Rectum, *22:*10, 1979.

35. Steinberg, D. M., Liegois, H., and Alexander-Williams, J.: Long term review of the results of rubber band ligation of haemorrhoids. Br. J. Surg., *62:*144, 1975.

36. Stelzner, F., Staubesand, J., and Machleidt, H.: Das Cavernosum Recti—Die Grundlage der Inneren Hammarrhoiden. Langenbecks Arch. Klin. Chir., *299:*302, 1967.

37. Taylor, F. W.: Portal tension and its dependence on external pressure. Ann. Surg., *140:*652, 1954.

38. Thomson, J. P. S.: Hemorrhoidectomy—How I do it: Current views in Britain. Dis. Colon Rectum, *20:*173, 1977.

39. Thomson, W. H. F.: The nature of haemorrhoids. Br. J. Surg., *62:*542, 1975.

# 7

# Fissure-in-Ano

A fissure-in-ano may be defined as a painful, linear ulcer, situated in the anal canal, and extending from just below the dentate line to the margin of the anus. It is a very common disease which causes suffering out of all proportion to the size of the lesion. In the acute phase, it is often a mere crack in the epithelial surface, but nevertheless, may cause much pain and spasm.

## FACTORS THAT CONTRIBUTE TO CORRECT DIAGNOSIS
### Clinical Features

The lesion is usually encountered in the younger, and middle-aged adult, but also may occur in infants, children, and the elderly. Fissures are probably equally common in both sexes. Although there is probably no difference in incidence, the site of fissure differs slightly. In men the fissure is usually located in the midline posteriorly, and rarely, in the anterior midline. Anterior fissures are more common in women than in men, accounting for 10 per cent of all fissures in the former, while accounting for only 1 per cent in the latter.[11] Occasionally, patients may develop anterior and posterior fissures simultaneously. In any event, the length of each fissure is remarkably constant, extending from the dentate line to the anal verge. This length corresponds roughly with the lower half of the internal sphincter, a point of practical importance when it comes to considering operative therapy.

One of the remarkable features of fissure-in-ano is that it is nearly always located in the midline posteriorly. An explanation for this usual location is the elliptical arrangement of the external sphincter fibers posteriorly. This arrangement offers less support to the anal canal during the passage of a large fecal bolus. Consequently, a tear develops more easily than elsewhere in the circumference of the anus.

### Pathology

Fissures usually heal promptly under conservative treatment, but may show considerable reluctance to heal. If the acute fissure does not heal readily, certain secondary changes develop. One of the most striking features is swelling at the lower end of the fissure, forming the so-called "sentinel pile". This is presumably due to a low-grade infection, and lymphatic edema, and often the tag has a very inflamed, tense, and edematous appearance. Later, it may undergo fibrosis, and persist as a permanent fibrous skin tag even if the fissure heals. At the proximal end of the fissure, at the level of the anal valve, swelling due to edema, and fibrosis occurs. This condition is referred to as a hypertrophied anal papilla. In addition, long-standing cases develop fibrous induration in the lateral edges of the fissure. After several months of nonhealing, the base of the ulcer, which is the internal sphincter, becomes fibrosed, resulting in a rather spastic, fibrotic, tightly-contracted internal sphincter. At no time, does the fissure lie in contact with the external sphincter.

At any stage, frank suppuration may occur,

and extend into the surrounding tissues, forming an intersphincteric abscess or a perianal abscess which may discharge through the anal canal, or burst spontaneously, externally to produce a low intersphincteric fistula. Usually, the external opening of this fistula lies close to the midline, and a short distance behind the anus.

### Etiology

All the factors in the causation of anal fissure have not been resolved. Why certain fissures readily heal with no problem, while others linger on creating long-standing problems, is not well understood. However, it is generally agreed that the initiating factor in the development of a fissure is trauma to the anal canal, usually in the form of the passage of a large, hard fecal bolus.

### Predisposing Factors

Secondary fissures may occur as a result of either an anatomical anal abnormality or inflammatory bowel disease, particularly Crohn's disease.[5] Previous anal surgery, especially hemorrhoidectomy, may result in anal scarring, skin loss, and stenosis. Fistula-in-ano surgery may result in distortion of the anal canal with scarring and fixation of the anal skin. This decreased elasticity of the anal canal may then predispose to fissure formation. Some of the anterior fissures occurring in women result from childbirth. Perineal trauma leads to scarring and abnormal tethering of the anal submucosa, thus rendering it more susceptible to trauma because of its loss of laxity and mobility. Individuals with long-standing, loose stools, usually on the basis of chronic laxative abuse, may develop an anal stenosis with scarring, and again, predisposing to fissure formation. The association of Crohn's disease with anal fissures is well recognized. Hemorrhoids are not likely a predisposing factor, but more likely an abnormality of the internal sphincter predisposes to the formation of both hemorrhoids and fissures.

### Pathogenesis

If one accepts the concept that trauma to the anal canal is the initiating factor in the establishment of a fissure-in-ano, one must then ask why certain fissures proceed to, and persist in, a chronic state. Perpetuating factors might include things such as infection, but it is unlikely

since there is no more florid sepsis in long-standing, chronic fissures than in the acute ones. Persistently hard bowel movements, as well as the initiation of the process, may continuously aggravate the anal canal, and result in perpetuation of the fissure. This factor must be taken into account when planning treatment.

Recent studies have demonstrated that following the initiation of a tear in the anal canal, the chronicity is probably perpetuated by an abnormality in the internal anal sphincter. Pressure studies by Duthie and Bennett have revealed that resting pressures are the same in patients with and without anal fissures.[6] However, Nothmann and Schuster and Hancock found that resting pressures within the internal anal sphincter were higher in patients with fissures than in normal controls.[13,24] Arabi and associates found that maximal anal pressures were also higher in patients with anal fissures.[3] Nothmann and Schuster demonstrated that following rectal distension there is a normal reflex relaxation of the internal sphincter.[24] In patients with anal fissures, this relaxation is followed by an abnormal "overshoot" contraction (Fig. 7-1). This phenomenon could ac-

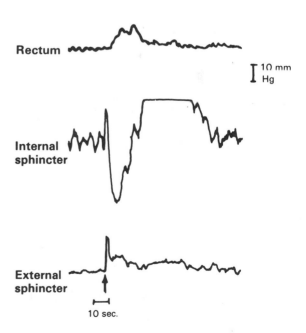

FIGURE **7-1.** *"Overshoot" contraction in a patient with an anal fissure. Compare with normal in Figure 2-10. (After Nothmann, B. J., and Schuster, M. M.: Gastroenterology, 67:218, 1974)*

count for the sphincter spasm, and explain the pain that results from rectal stimulation, occurring during defecation. Furthermore, they demonstrated that following successful treatment of the fissure, the abnormal reflex contraction of the internal sphincter vanishes. One must then also bear in mind this abnormality in the internal sphincter when trying to arrive at a rational treatment for the problem.

## Symptoms

The chief symptom of an anal fissure is pain in the anus during and after defecation. It is usually described as a sharp, cutting, or tearing sensation during the actual passage of stool. Subsequently, the pain may be less severe, and described as a burning or gnawing discomfort for several hours' duration.

Bleeding is very common with fissure-in-ano but is not invariably present. The blood is bright red in color, and usually scant in amount.

Some patients have a large sentinel pile which draws their attention to the anus. In such circumstances, patients usually complain of a painful external hemorrhoid.

Discharge may lead to soiling of the underclothes, and to increased moisture in the perianal skin with resulting pruritus ani, although pruritus may occur independent of any discharge.

Constipation is a frequent accompaniment as well as an initiating symptom.

Sometimes patients with a painful fissure develop disturbances of micturation, namely dysuria, retention, or frequency.

Although not usually a presenting complaint, dyspareunia may be caused by an anal fissure.

## Diagnosis

History alone usually makes the diagnosis of a fissure. The physical examination then confirms the suspicion, and rules out any other associated disease. The association between fissures and inflammatory bowel disease should always be remembered, and a careful history taken, followed, if indicated, by appropriate radiological, hematological and biochemical investigations.

Inspection is by far the most important step in the examination for anal fissure (Fig. 7-2). If properly sought, most fissures can be seen. Because anal fissures are such extremely pain-

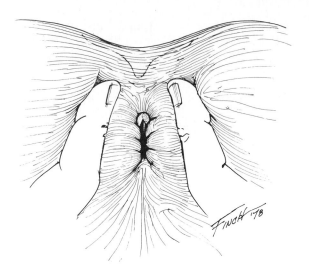

FIGURE 7-2. *Anal fissure.*

ful lesions, special care must be taken to make the examination as gentle as possible. It may help to apply a topical anesthetic to the fissure just prior to the examination. Gentle separation of the buttocks will usually reveal the fissure; however, spasm may keep the anal orifice closed, and indeed, the finding of spasm of a sphincter is suggestive of a fissure. The triad of a chronic anal fissure includes a sentinel pile, anal ulcer, and hypertrophied anal papilla. The first thing that will be noted is the sentinel pile posteriorly.

It cannot be too strongly stressed that in any patient in whom a fissure is noted to be off the midline, a specific systemic disease should be considered. A full differential of the possible diseases is included in the section on differential diagnosis.

Palpation is the next step in the examination, and confirms the presence of sphincter spasm. The digital examination will be uncomfortable with maximum tenderness usually elicited in the posterior midline. In fact, the pain may be so exquisite that a complete digital examination cannot be performed at the initial examination. However, it is essential that the examination be performed later in order to exclude other lesions of the lower rectum such as carcinoma or a polyp. With the chronic fissure, induration of the base, and the lateral edges, as well as a hypertrophied anal papilla may be palpable.

With the acute fissure, anoscopic examination is usually impossible due to the severe pain. With a chronic fissure, the ulcer itself will be noted as a triangular shaped slit in the anal canal with the floor being the internal sphincter. Just proximal to the ulcer, the hypertrophied anal papilla may be identified. Evaluation of the chronicity of the process is important. Once the entire internal sphincter is bared with scarring and fibrosis, in the face of a long-standing history of problems, the fissure is unlikely to heal without the benefit of an operation. It is also essential to anoscope the patient so that other conditions may be demonstrated such as internal hemorrhoids or proctitis.

Sigmoidoscopy, likewise, may be impossible to perform during the initial examination, but must be performed at a subsequent visit to rule out an associated carcinoma or inflammatory bowel disease.

One should finally state that any fissure that fails to heal after treatment should be biopsied. Such biopsy may reveal an unsuspected Crohn's disease or an implanted adenocarcinoma. Squamous carcinoma of the anal canal may be confused with fissure-in-ano.

## DIFFERENTIAL DIAGNOSIS

Most conditions presenting with anal pain, and swelling or bleeding, are usually easily distinguished. Thrombosed hemorrhoids or perianal abscesses are readily seen. Certain other conditions may require more careful discrimination (Fig. 7-3).

### Perianal Suppuration

Of greatest importance is the intersphincteric abscess which may closely mimic a fissure. An intermuscular, fistulous abscess without an external opening is usually situated posteriorly in the mid-anal canal, between the internal and external sphincter. It causes great pain which may last for many hours after defecation. Little, if anything, will be seen externally but, upon examination, exquisite tenderness will be elicited over the abscess which itself may not be palpable. This entity will be discussed further in Chapter Eight.

### Pruritus Ani

Pruritus ani with superficial cracks in the anal skin may sometimes prove to be a source

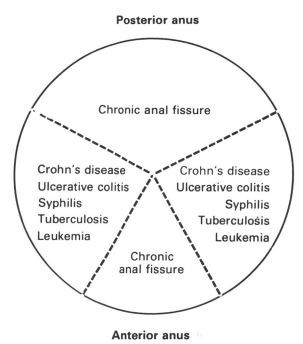

**FIGURE 7-3.** *Common locations of chronic anal fissure and other anorectal conditions. (After Goldberg, S. M., and Nivatvongs, S.: Principles of Surgery. Ed. Schwartz, S., I., p. 1240. N.Y., McGraw-Hill, 1979)*

of difficulty. The reason is that many cases of anal fissure develop pruritus due to the discharge irritating the perianal skin. However, the skin in pruritus ani shows only superficial cracks extending radially from the anus. These cracks never extend up to the dentate line, digital examination of the rectum does not elicit pain, and there is no true anal spasm or tenderness.

### Fissures in Inflammatory Bowel Disease

*Anal fissures associated with Ulcerative Colitis* are often situated off the midline, and may be multiple. These fissures, as well as being broad, are surrounded with inflamed skin.[11] This condition should put the surgeon on the alert for an associated proctocolitis which can be diagnosed if a view of the rectal mucosa can be obtained endoscopically.

*Anal and Perianal Ulceration Frequently Occurs with Crohn's Disease.* Here the ulcer is much greater than an idiopathic fissure, and often much more extensive. If a lesion is suspect, biopsy will frequently reveal the histological features of Crohn's disease. Sigmoidoscopy may, in fact, be normal as the involved intestine may be more proximal.

## Carcinoma of the Anus

Squamous cell carcinoma of the anus, or adenocarcinoma of the rectum, may involve the anal skin at which time considerable pain with defecation may occur. Palpation, however, may detect a greater degree of induration, and any lesion should be biopsied if suspect. (Chapter 14)

## Specific Infectious Perianal Conditions

*Syphilitic fissures* may be due to either primary chancres or condylomata lata. A chancre in its initial stage may closely resemble an ordinary fissure, but acquires a good deal of induration at its margin, and the inguinal lymph nodes become enlarged. A highly characteristic feature is the presence of a symmetrical lesion on the opposite wall of the anal canal. Suspect lesions can have the diagnosis made by the dark field examination. Anal condylomata lata may occur at the anal orifice, as well as in the perianal region, and may cause multiple anal fissures. Secondary skin lesions and mucous patches, however, are usually present, and the Wassermann reaction is strongly positive. Contrary to popular belief, syphilitic lesions in the anal region are not, by any means, always painless.

A *tuberculous ulcer* in the anal region is rare and, when it occurs, tends to enlarge, and develop undermined edges. It may be very difficult to differentiate this lesion from Crohn's disease; however, it is usually associated with pulmonary tuberculosis. Biopsy and guinea pig innoculations may have to be done. After antituberculous chemotherapy has been administered, these lesions may be treated the same as an idiopathic fissure.

## Hematological Conditions

Leukemic infiltration is extremely painful, and usually is the sign of the advanced phase of the malignant disease. No treatment is indicated except for drainage of abscesses.

An *anal abrasion* is a rubbing off, or scraping off, of the skin of the anal canal. It is a mild disorder which can be differentiated from a fissure by the features in listed below.

### Fissure-in-Ano vs. Anal Abrasion

| *Fissure* | *Abrasion* |
|---|---|
| deep ulcer | superficial ulcer |
| "sentinel pile" | none |
| anal papilla | none |
| overhanging edges | flat edges |
| associated scarring | none |
| rarely lateral | may be lateral |
| chronic condition | transient (1–2 days) |
| often surgical | not surgical |

When no local disease is found in the anal region other diagnoses should be considered, such as proctalgia fugax, coccygodynia, rectal crisis of tabes, or frank psychoneurosis.

Proctalgia fugax may cause severe pain, but usually awakens the patient at night, is of short duration, and is not necessarily related to bowel movements (Chap. 30).

## CONSERVATIVE TREATMENT
### Acute Fissure

Avoidance of constipation is probably the single most important item of conservative treatment. Patients should be reminded that they must maintain smooth bowel function, as bouts of hard stools will often result in a recurrence of an already healed fissure. The aim of treatment of an acute fissure-in-ano is to break the cycle of a hard stool, pain, and reflex spasm. This result can often be accomplished with simple measures such as warm baths to help relieve the sphincter spasm. Bulk-forming foods (e.g., adequate amounts of unprocessed bran) may be helpful. Alternatively, stool softeners, such as psyllium seed preparations can be used. This creates a soft stool which hopefully would not further tear the anal canal. An additional advantage of the large, bulky stool is that it may result in physiological dilatation of the anal sphincter.

Anesthetic ointments have been used with varying degrees of success. Application only in the perianal region would be of no help. One must have it inserted into the anal canal in order to have any effect. Many patients find this practice rather distasteful, as well as uncomfortable. In addition, a certain number of patients will develop a perianal dermatitis.

Anal dilators were strongly recommended

by Gabriel in 1948, and have continued to be used as the mainstay of treatment at St. Mark's Hospital.[9] However, the insertion of a cold metal anal dilator through an already exquisitely painful area, seems to be less than a kind form of therapy, and one which many patients will probably abandon because of the pain.

The injection of long-acting, local anesthetics enjoyed some popularity for a short period of time; however, because of the problems of sepsis leading to abscesses and fistulae that frequently followed these injections, this form of therapy was discarded. Also, the dosage required for the relief of pain resulted in temporary incontinence from the paralysis of the external sphincter. Furthermore, oleogranulomas may develop secondary to these injections. There is probably no place for such treatment today.

Currently, there are many suppositories available on the market for the treatment of fissure-in-ano. These contain, in different proportions, sundry combinations of anesthetics, analgesics, astringents, anti-inflammatory agents (usually hydrocortisone), and emollients, in a host of bases and preservatives. However, when the suppositories are inserted they rest well above the area of the fissure because they, by necessity, must rest above the puborectalis, and are therefore, not in direct contact with the fissure. Many patients complain that the insertion is painful. Credit claimed by the manufacturers for these various agents is probably due to the natural history of the healing of the majority of acute fissures with other measures such as warm baths, stool softeners, and a "tincture of time". Some suppositories may help because of their emollient function.

There are equally as many creams and ointments which generally contain the same variety of components as the suppositories. The comment regarding the unproven effectiveness of suppositories applies to these preparations as well.

### Chronic Fissure

It is of value to recognize the features of chronicity which include exposure of the internal sphincter, induration of the fissure edges, the development of a large "sentinel pile", and a hypertrophied anal papilla. Once these features are present it is unlikely that spontaneous healing will occur.

Condensed to the simplest form, the indications for operative repair of a fissure-in-ano are the presence of persistent pain and bleeding and, the lack of response to medical management, which is really a corollary of the first indication.

The clinical entity of a painless, non-healing fissure may prove annoying to both the patient and the treating physician. The patient may experience some bleeding from time to time but the symptoms may not be severe enough for the surgeon to recommend operative treatment. Such lesions should be biopsied, keeping in mind that it might be the prodromal sign of inflammatory bowel disease. Generally, operative treatment would not be entertained, but if symptoms warrant it, we would favor a lateral internal sphincterotomy.

## OPERATIVE TREATMENT

Once one has decided upon the necessity for operative correction, one must next consider the aims of treatment for a chronic fissure. Based on studies that have demonstrated an elevated "resting" pressure, as well as an exaggerated response to stimulation in people with fissures, the first aim should be to modify the function of the internal anal sphincter so that it cannot go into spasm. The potential diameter of the anal canal should be increased so that there would be less resistance to the passage of stool, thus reducing the degree of anal trauma associated with defecation. There is probably no need to remove either the fissure itself or the sentinel pile. A large skin tag may warrant removal for cosmetic or cleansing reasons. The function of the internal sphincter has been altered by manual dilatation of the anus, or by division of part of the sphincter.

Before advocating any one form of operative treatment certain factors must be assessed for each modality. Since the chief symptom is pain, one must first consider how effective a method is in the relief of this pain. The incidence of failure, or recurrence, as well as the incidence of impaired sphincter control are certainly of paramount importance. Also to be considered are the discomfort experienced by the patient during and after the procedure, and the healing time of both the fissure and the operative wound. Significant to both the patient and the treating physician are the number of follow-up visits required before healing is complete.

Over the years various operative procedures have been proposed for the treatment of a chronic or recurrent fissure. These include the classical excision of the fissure, with or without sphincterotomy, partial or complete; the V-Y anoplasty with sliding skin graft (advancement flap of anoderm); the anal sphincter stretch; and, internal sphincterotomy of the posterior and lateral varieties.

## Classical Excision

The classical excision of a fissure-in-ano is still used by many surgeons, and is usually associated with division of varying amounts of sphincter muscle. Excision of the anal fissure was popularized by Gabriel (1948), who excised the fissure along with a broad triangle of skin.[9] In addition, he divided the edge of the sphincter muscle, and also stretched the anal sphincters. Although his and other results were reported as good, it was not based on a detailed follow-up. The main criticism of this operation is that it leaves the patient with a large, rather uncomfortable, external wound that may be difficult to handle on an outpatient basis, and takes a long time to heal (Fig. 7-4).

Various complications have been described following excisional surgery for a fissure. These are problems which are common to almost any anorectal procedure and include bleeding, either immediate or delayed, abscess formation, stenosis and strictures, failure to heal, recurrence, and incontinence of varying degrees. Meticulous attention to surgical detail, and exacting postoperative care should help keep these complications at a minimum. (Chap. 4).

A modification of this operation was suggested by Hughes (1953) to expedite the healing, and shorten the convalescence.[18] He applied an immediate split-thickness skin graft to the fissure wound. The major disadvantage of this modification was that following this operation the bowels had to be confined for five or six days, and the patient had to remain in the hospital for at least a week.

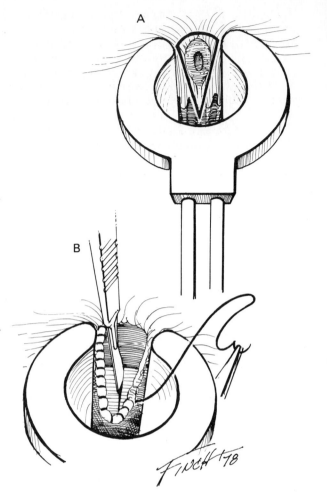

FIGURE **7-4.** *Fissurectomy.*

## V-Y Anoplasty (Advancement Flap Technique)

A method employing the use of excision of the fissure combined with an advancement flap of anoderm has been referred to as V-Y anoplasty. Using this technique, the fissure, and the adjacent crypt bearing hemorrhoidal tissue, are completely excised. A triangular skin flap based outside the anal canal is elevated in continuity with the excised fissure. One must ensure that there is a broad base with adequate blood supply to the flap. The flap is adequately mobilized to avoid tension on the suture line. Meticulous attention is paid to hemostasis, in order to prevent hematoma formation which increases tension, and the chance of infection.

The flap is then advanced, and the defect of the skin and anal canal is closed (Fig. 7-5).

Extensive experience using this technique has been reported by Samson and Stewart.[29] These authors state that excision of a chronic fissure-in-ano, and the coverage of the defect with a sliding, broad-based, skin graft offers several advantages over the classical excision: there is decreased postoperative pain; there is decreased postoperative wound care, both in the hospital and in the office; and, there is a decreased incidence of postoperative complications. Of 2,072 patients who were treated in this fashion, recurrent fissures occurred in ten patients, and there were only seven cases of mild anal stenosis. Postoperative bleeding occurred in two cases, and their slough rate was 2.4 per cent. The diameter of the anus is actually increased, and this is their procedure of choice for anal stenosis. An additional advantage to using this technique is that primary, as opposed to secondary, wound healing occurs, so that healing is more rapid, and there is decreased scar and resultant deformity.

The major disadvantages to this method are the facts that it involves considerable dissection, and requires an increased operative time. Contraindications to advancement flap technique include patients with an associated fistula and widespread undermining of the skin, as well as patients with friable, irritated skin.

In the past we have used this method in conjunction with a partial internal sphincterotomy (i.e., dividing an amount of sphincter which eliminates the scarred edge, and presents a smooth surface for the placement of the graft) with favorable results.

### Anal Stretch

Récamier (1838) is credited with first describing anal stretching.[27] The procedure was popularized in England by Goligher, and championed for various forms of anorectal disease by Lord.[10,20] This method is also referred to as manual dilatation of the anus, and involves the forceful stretching of the anal sphincter with as many as six or eight fingers. The effect on the internal and external sphincter is to produce a temporary paralysis, usually lasting several days or a week. There may be some incontinence during this time. By the nature of the procedure, sphincter fibers are torn, resulting in extravasation of blood leading to perianal bruising, and discoloration, which may be quite extensive.

Proponents of this method cite as advan-

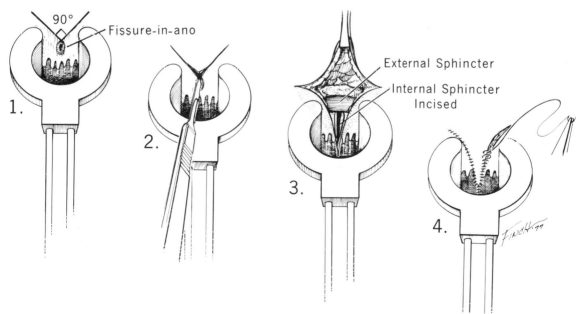

**FIGURE 7-5.** *V-Y Anoplasty. (After Goldberg, S., M., and Nivatvong, S.: Principles of Surgery. Ed. Schwartz, S., I., p 1241. N.Y., McGraw-Hill, 1979)*

tages that there is no anal wound, and that the patients have an early return to work, both enviable objectives. However, one must not overlook the significant disadvantages of this method: the incidence of persistent or recurrent fissures (16–28 %), and the disturbances of anal control. In 1965, Goligher reviewed 99 patients treated in such a fashion, and found relief of pain in 94.[10] Complications occurring included painful perianal edema within a few hours of the stretching in two patients, and one patient developed prolapsed thrombosed hemorrhoids. Consequently, it seemed as if this method should be avoided in cases with concomitant, large, internal hemorrhoids. Eleven patients complained of recurrent pain resulting in a total of 16 per cent unsuccessful treatment. Functional results include slightly imperfect control of flatus in 12 per cent, and of feces in 2 per cent, while 20 per cent noticed soiling of their underclothes.

Pressure studies have demonstrated an abnormality in the response of the internal sphincter of patients with fissures, thus, suggesting that a modification in its function is necessary in treating this condition. Nevertheless, until more evidence is available supporting this method, it would seem that a more controlled way of modifying the sphincter function should be utilized. An eight finger dilatation of the anus is hardly a delicate surgical operation! In addition, subsequent, prolonged use of an anal dilator is required, and this does not meet with a high degree of patient satisfaction.

## Internal Sphincterotomy

Internal sphincterotomy was originally performed for the surgical treatment of anal fissure under a complete misapprehension. Miles (1939) treated fissure-in-ano by pectenotomy which in retrospect was shown by Eisenhammer to be the lower fibers of the internal sphincter.[8,21] Credit for suggesting the treatment of anal fissure by internal sphincterotomy alone must rest with Eisenhammer (1951).[8] The method originally favored by him was division of the lower half of the internal sphincter in the posterior midline through the fissure itself. This procedure resulted in satisfactory results but had two significant disadvantages: the opened wound in the anal canal took a long time to heal, four weeks being the average period and six to

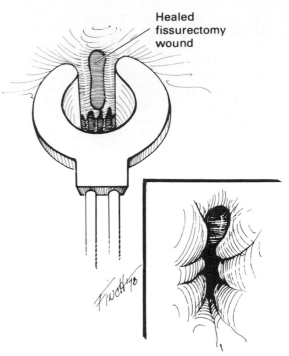

FIGURE **7-6.** *"Key-hole" deformity.*

seven weeks being common; and there was a disturbingly high incidence of minor imperfections of anal continence, as shown by occasional lack of control for flatus or feces, or inadvertent slight leakage of fecal matter, leading to soiling of the underwear. Lesser drawbacks included the prolonged postoperative pain, and prolonged hospitalization. Some of the fecal soiling and minor imperfections in continence are due to the "key-hole" deformity created by a posterior internal sphincterotomy. This abnormality is a groove in the area of the sphincterotomy along which fecal-stained mucus, and possibly stool, as well, escape (Fig. 7-6).

The possibility that a lateral sphincterotomy might cause a less prominent groove than a posterior one, and be followed by less disturbance of function was suggested by Eisenhammer (1959).[7] Parks strongly recommended lateral sphincterotomy.[25] There are variations in the exact details of current forms of lateral sphincterotomy. The procedure may be performed under local or general anesthesia. It may be performed open through a radial or circumferential incision, or it may be performed through a subcutaneous technique.

For those operations being performed by a subcutaneous technique, the muscle may be divided from medial to lateral, or from lateral to medial.

*Technique.* Patients may be operated under general, caudal, or local anesthesia. Our preferred position is the semiprone or so-called "jackknife" position. For those surgeons less familiar with the anorectal anatomy, or for those just starting to perform lateral sphincterotomy, the procedure is probably best performed open.

After anesthesia is administered, a Pratt bivalve speculum is inserted, and the anal pathology evaluated. The instrument is then rotated to the right or left lateral position, and a linear incision is made from the dentate line to just beyond the anal verge. The internal sphincter, and a few fibers of the external sphincter, will be exposed. Any bleeding is controlled with electrocautery. The full thickness of the internal sphincter from the level of the dentate line distally is then divided under direct vision. A definite "give" will be noted, and this should correct any element of anal stenosis, as well as cure the fissure. Any adjacent hemorrhoidal tissue can be excised as indicated. As a matter of fact, since prolapsing hemorrhoids are a recognized complication following lateral internal sphincterotomy, judicious use of concomitant hemorrhoidectomy should be employed, in cases of large hemorrhoids, in order to avoid this complication. In such cases, general or regional anesthesia would be preferable. The wound is then closed with a running, absorbable suture such as 3–0 chromic catgut, but may be left open if pre-

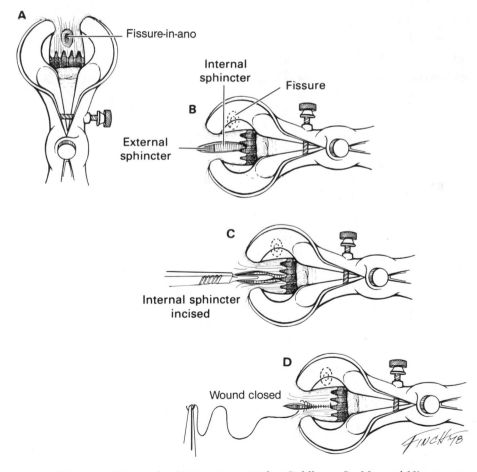

**FIGURE 7-7.** *Lateral internal sphincterotomy. (After Goldberg, S., M., and Nivatvongs, S.: Principles of Surgery. Ed. Schwartz, S., I., p 1241. N.Y., McGraw-Hill, 1979)*

ferred. The fissure itself need not be treated, but very large sentinel piles or prolapsing, hypertrophied anal papillae might be removed for cosmetic or cleansing purposes. A piece of fluff cotton is then placed between the buttocks to prevent soiling of clothes. Postoperatively, the patient is placed on a bulk-forming agent such as a psyllium seed preparation (1 tsp b.i.d.), frequent warm baths, and a mild analgesic (Fig. 7-7).

Parks described a subcutaneous technique, whereby, the sphincterotomy can be performed through a lateral skin incision.[25] Using one's anesthetic of choice, an anal retractor such as the one designed by Parks himself, or a Pratt bivalve, is inserted, and a 1 cm circumferential incision is made just outside the anal verge. The mucosa of the lower anal canal is lifted off the underlying internal sphincter, and the full thickness of the internal sphincter is divided from the level of the dentate line caudad. Hemostasis is obtained, and the wound is closed with two catgut sutures (Fig.

7-8). The great advantage of this method is that it avoids an intra-anal wound.

Even simpler, and more expeditious, is the technique of lateral, subcutaneous, internal sphincterotomy described by Notaras (Fig. 7-9).[23] This procedure leaves virtually no wound at all. The operation can be performed in the lithotomy, left lateral, or semiprone position, but we prefer the last. Anesthesia is achieved by a bilateral, inferior hemorrhoidal nerve block or local anesthesia. An anal speculum, such as the Pratt bivalve or Parks retractor, is inserted and, upon opening the blades, the anus is placed on a slight stretch. The intersphincteric groove and lower edge of the internal sphincter are now palpable. A narrow-bladed scalpel, flat side adjacent to muscle, is introduced through the skin in either lateral position and the tip advanced submucosally to the dentate line. The sharp edge of the blade is then turned toward the internal sphincter and the sphincterotomy performed. When this step is accomplished a

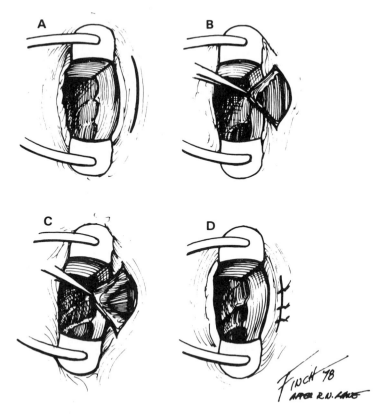

**FIGURE 7-8.** *Lateral internal sphincterotomy. (After Parks, A. G.: Hosp. Med. 1:738, 1967)*

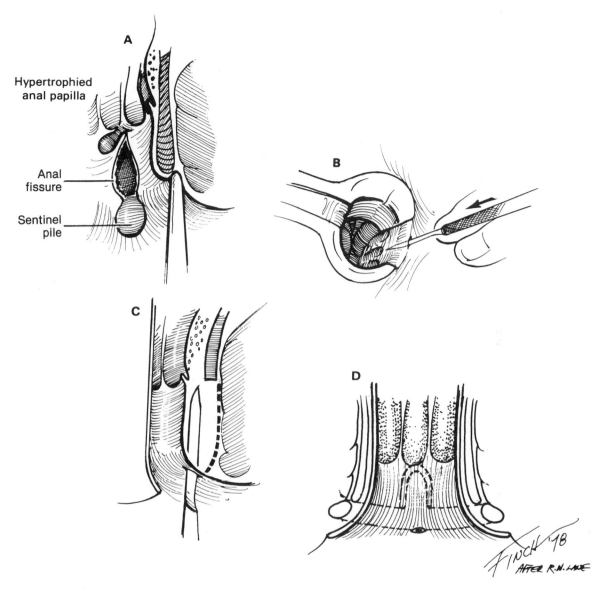

Hypertrophied
anal papilla

Anal
fissure

Sentinel
pile

FINCH 78
AFTER R.N. LANE

FIGURE **7-9.** *Lateral internal sphincterotomy. (After Notaras, M., J.: Br. J. Surg. 58:96, 1971)*

''give'' will result in release of the tension of the blades of the anal speculum. Pressure will arrest any bleeding, and the wound is left open to allow any drainage to escape. If one prefers, the scalpel blade can be advanced in the intersphincteric plane, and turned toward the lumen, thus accomplishing the sphincterotomy in this manner. Again, a large sentinel pile, and hypertrophied anal papilla, can be dealt with appropriately.

*Results.* Many reports on the results of internal sphincterotomy are now available (Table 7-1).[1,4,12,14–17,19,22,23,26,28] Early relief of pain is remarkable. Often pain (except for some soreness) disappears by the first bowel movement.

Although complications following internal sphincterotomy are known to occur, their numbers are few. These include ecchymoses and hemorrhage, perianal abscess, fistula-in-

TABLE 7-1. Lateral Internal Sphincterotomy

| | NO. OF PATIENTS | IMPAIRED CONTROL FOR | | FECAL SOILING | UNHEALED OR RECURRENCE |
| | | *FLATUS* | *FECES* | | |
|---|---|---|---|---|---|
| *Hardy & Cuthbertson (1969)*[15] | 17 | 29% T | 12% T<br>6% P | 47% | 18% |
| *Hawley (1969)*[16] | 24 | ? | 0 | 0 | 0 |
| *Hoffmann & Goligher (1970)*[17] | 99 | 6% | 1% | 7% | 3% |
| *Notaras (1971)*[23] | 82 | 2% | 1% | 6% | ? 10% |
| *Millar (1971)*[22] | 99 | 2% | 0 | 1% | 0 |
| *Ray (1974)*[26] | 21 | ? | ? | ? | 0 |
| *Abcarian (1977)*[2] | 125 | 30% T<br>0   P | 0 | 0 | 1.5% |
| *Hunter (1975)*[19] | 74 | 27%<br>T or P | 27%<br>T or P | 34% | 12% |
| *Rudd (1975)*[28] | 200 | 0 | 0 | 0 | 0.5% |
| *Gordon (1979 unpublished)*[12] | 79 | 2.5%<br>T or P | 0 | 2.5% | 1.3% |

T—Temporary
P—Permanent

ano, prolapsed hemorrhoids, and very rarely, minor alterations in continence. Clinical experience has shown that operative division of the internal anal sphincter may result in defects of fine anal continence. Bennett and Duthie attributed this condition to the demonstrated decrease in anal sphincter pressure following internal sphincterotomy.[6] Careful technique will reduce these complications to a minimum.

Abcarian[2] conducted a study in which he compared the results of lateral internal sphincterotomy to those of fissurectomy and posterior midline sphincterotomy. Each group contained 125 patients. By almost all the parameters studied, the lateral internal sphincterotomy group fared better. Hospital stay was shorter (2 days vs. 4 days), pain relief faster (1–2 week vs. 2–3 weeks), and wound healing quicker (2–3 weeks vs. 6–7 weeks). Persistent loss of control of flatus occurred in 5 per cent, while another 5 per cent experienced fecal soiling following fissurectomy and midline sphincterotomy, while none of the patients had this problem with the lateral internal sphincterotomy. However, using the lateral internal sphincterotomy, 1.5 per cent developed minor infections, a problem not encountered with the fissurectomy. The recurrence rate was found to be the same in both groups, 1.5 per cent.

*Advantages.* Many very definite advantages have been attributed to lateral internal sphincterotomy. The first is that hospitalization is generally not required. Whether the procedure is performed under local or general anesthesia, admission will probably not be necessary unless associated pathology, such as hemorrhoids, are being treated at the same time. There is quicker healing of both the fissure (avg. 3 weeks), and the operative wound (1 week). Less fecal soiling will occur. A major advantage is the fact that it can be performed under local anesthesia. Recurrence following this mode of therapy is uncommon. There will be less postoperative discomfort, and consequently, less time will be lost from work. All these factors result in the necessity for fewer follow-up visits. With the exception of two reports, it appears that of the various operative methods currently available for the treatment of idiopathic fissure-in-ano, the most convenient, and satisfactory, is the lateral internal sphincterotomy.[15,19]

## REFERENCES

1. Abcarian, H.: Lateral internal sphincterotomy: A new technique for treatment of chronic fissure-in-ano. Surg. Clin. North Am., *55:*143, 1975.

2. Abcarian, H.: unpublished, 1977.

3. Arabi, Y., Alexander-Williams, J., and Keighley, M. R. B.: Anal pressures in hemorrhoids and anal fissure. Am. J. Surg., *134:*608, 1977.

4. Bennett, R. C., and Goligher, J. C.: Results of internal sphincterotomy for anal fissure. Br. Med. J., *2:*1500, 1962.

5. Crapp, A. R., and Alexander-Williams, J.: Fissure-in-ano and anal stenosis, conservative management. Clin. Gastroenterol., *4:*619, 1975.

6. Duthie, H. L., and Bennett, R. C.: Anal sphincter pressure in fissure-in-ano. Surg. Gynecol. Obstet., *119:*19, 1964.

7. Eisenhammer, S.: The evaluation of internal anal sphincterotomy—operation with special reference to anal fissure. Surg. Gynecol. Obstet., *109:*583, 1959.

8. ———: The surgical correction of chronic anal (sphincteric) contracture. S. Afr. Med. J., *25:*486, 1951.

9. Gabriel, W. B.: Principles and Practice of Rectal Surgery. 250–252. Charles C Thomas, Springfield, Ill., 1963.

10. Goligher, J. C.: An evaluation of internal sphincterotomy and simple sphincter stretching in the treatment of fissure-in-ano. Surg. Clin. North Am., *42:*1299, 1965.

11. ———: Surgery of the Anus, Rectum and Colon. 889–890. Charles C Thomas, Springfield, Ill., 1975.

12. Gordon, P. H.: unpublished, 1979.

13. Hancock, B. D.: The internal sphincter and anal fissure. Br. J. Surg., *64:*92, 1977.

14. Hardy, K. J.: Internal sphincterotomy: An appraisal with special reference to sequelae. Br. J. Surg., *54:*30, 1967.

15. Hardy, K. J., and Cuthbertson, A. M.: Lateral sphincterotomy—an appraisal with special reference to sequelae. Aust. N.Z. J. Surg., *39:*91, 1969.

16. Hawley, P. R.: The treatment of chronic fissure-in-ano: A trial of methods. Br. J. Surg., *56:*915, 1969.

17. Hoffmann, D. C., and Goligher, J. C.: Lateral subcutaneous internal sphincterotomy in treatment of anal fissure. Br. Med. J., *3:*73, 1970.

18. Hughes, E. S. R.: Anal fissure. Br. Med. J., *2:*803, 1953.

19. Hunter, A.: Lateral subcutaneous anal sphincterotomy. Dis. Colon Rectum, *18:*665, 1975.

20. Lord, P. H.: Diverse methods of managing hemorrhoids: Dilatation. Dis. Colon Rectum, *16:*180, 1973.

21. Miles, W. E.: Rectal Surgery—A Practical Guide to the Modern Surgical Treatment of Rectal Diseases. London, 155. Cassell and Co., 1944.

22. Millar, D. M.: Subcutaneous lateral internal anal sphincterotomy for anal fissure. Br. J. Surg., *58:*737, 1971.

23. Notaras, M. J.: The treatment of anal fissure by lateral subcutaneous internal sphincterotomy—a technique and results. Br. J. Surg., *58:*96, 1971.

24. Nothmann, B. J., and Schuster, M. M.: Internal anal sphincter derangement with anal fissures. Gastroenterology, *67:*216, 1974.

25. Parks, A. G.: The management of fissure-in-ano. Hosp. Med., *1:*737, 1967.

26. Ray, J. E., Penfold, J. C. B., Gathright, J. B., and Roberson, S. H.: Lateral subcutaneous internal anal sphincterotomy for anal fissure. Dis. Colon Rectum, *17:*139, 1974.

27. Récamier, N. *Quoted by* Maisonneuve, J. G.: Du Traitement de la fissure à l'anus par la dilatation forcée. Gaz d'hôp 3rd series 1,220, 1849.

28. Rudd, W. W. H.: Lateral subcutaneous internal sphincterotomy for chronic anal fissure; an outpatient procedure. Dis. Colon Rectum, *18:*319, 1975.

29. Samson, R. B., and Stewart, W. R. C.: Sliding skin grafts in the treatment of anal fissure. Dis. Colon Rectum, *13:*372, 1970.

# 8

# Anorectal Abscess and Fistula-in-Ano

If one accepts the theory that both the abscess and the fistula-in-ano have a common cause, it seems convenient to consider the two conditions simultaneously. Indeed the term fistulous abscess has been used to describe this problem. The abscess is an acute manifestation, while the fistula is a chronic situation. A fistula may be defined as an abnormal communication between any two epithelial-lined surfaces. The fistula-in-ano is, then, an abnormal communication between the anal canal and the perianal skin. Many of these fistulae are easily recognized, and readily treated. However, some fistulae may be very complex, and correspondingly difficult to manage.

In a treatise on fistula-in-ano, in 1965, Percivall Pott wrote, "clear and precise definitions of diseases, and the application of such names to them as are expressive of their true and real nature, are of more consequence than they are generally imagined to be: untrue or imperfect ones occasion false ideas; and false ideas are generally followed by erroneous practice." Thus, the true understanding of a disease is only achieved when the exact cause is identified, and the mechanism of the disordered structure or function is established.

## GENERAL PRINCIPLES

### Anatomy

Understanding the anatomy of the pelvic floor is critical to appreciate the origin and ramifications of fistulae. Reduced to its simplest form, the pelvic floor consists of two funnel-shaped structures, one situated within the other. The inner structure is the lower end of the circular muscle of the rectum, which becomes thick and rounded, and is referred to as the internal sphincter. Surrounding this, there is a funnel of pelvic floor muscle formed by the levator ani, puborectalis, and external sphincter. Between the two structures is the intersphincteric plane. In the mid-portion of the anal canal at the level of the dentate line, the ducts of the anal glands empty into the crypts. The greatest concentration of these glands is in the posterior aspect of the anal canal. For further details regarding the anatomy, see Chap. 1 (Fig. 1-5).

### Etiology

Numerous conditions may play the etiological role in the formation of a fistulous abscess. These conditions might be classified as specific and nonspecific (*see list, below*). The specific inflammation associated with a fistula-in-ano will be mentioned in Chapter 11. Other causes will be listed in their respective chapters.

### Pathogenesis

Current evidence suggests that infection of the anal glands is probably the commonest cause of fistulous abscess.[6,7,28] In the acute form such infections present as an abscess, while in the chronic form the patient presents with a fistula-in-ano. As early as 1878 Chiari first described anal ducts and glands which discharged their contents at the mucocutaneous junction into the anal canal. His views were initially suspect because of the infrequency with which these structures were

**Etiologic Conditions in Fistulous Abscess**

Nonspecific—cryptoglandular origin
Specific
    Crohn's disease
    Chronic ulcerative colitis
    Tuberculosis
    Actinomycosis
    Foreign body
    Carcinoma
    Lymphogranuloma venereum
    Pelvic inflammation
    Trauma
        impalement
        enemas
        prostatic surgery
        episiotomy
        hemorrhoidectomy
    Radiation
    Leukemia—lymphoma

found, and because of their minute dimensions. Eisenhammer ascribed most anorectal abscesses and fistulae-in-ano to anal gland infection in the intersphincteric space, but unfortunately his papers did not contain patho-logical confirmation of his views.[6] However, specimens excised from patients with fistula-in-ano were carefully studied by Parks and Morson, who after tedious examinations, demonstrated infected anal glands in 70 per cent of cases, and histological evidence suggestive of this origin in another 20 per cent bringing the total which may be attributed to this etiology to 90 per cent.[27,28] Normal anatomy was studied by obtaining material at necropsy and following radical excision for carcinoma of the rectum. The anal glands were found to arise in the mid-anal canal at the level of the crypts and to pass into the submucosa, two-thirds continuing into the internal sphincter, while one-half penetrated into the intersphincteric plane (Fig. 8-1). Obstruction of these ducts, whether secondary to fecal material, foreign bodies, or trauma, will result in stasis and secondary infection. Morson believes that the chronicity of the condition is due to persistence of the anal gland epithelium in the part of the track joining the internal opening.[27] The presence of such persisting epithelium keeps the opening patent, and healing cannot take place.

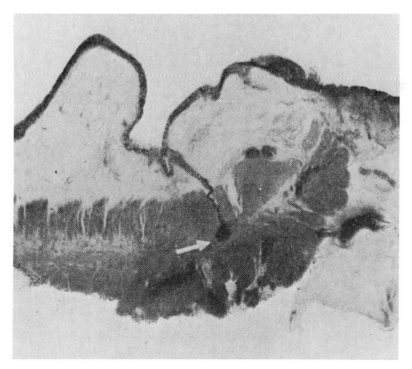

**FIGURE 8-1.** *Section through the anal canal showing the anal gland. (Br. Med. J. 1:465, 1961)*

The concept of cryptoglandular origin is not universally accepted. In a study of 60 patients with anorectal abscesses or fistulae-in-ano, Goligher and coworkers found intersphincteric abscesses in only 23 per cent, suggesting that this etiology is less often the precursor.[10] The theory of cryptoglandular origin is, however, supported by the fact that the primary internal orifice is found at the level of the pectinate line.

Several predisposing factors may be associated with the initiation of these fistulous abscesses. An acute episode of diarrhea can force liquid feces into the main duct of the intramuscular gland, and can cause an obstructive suppurative adenitis. Trauma, whether in the form of a hard stool or foreign body, may also be a contributing factor. Certain anatomic variations, such as large anal sinuses which collect material and are unable to empty properly because of the pressure on them in the anal canal, may initiate the pro-

cess. It has also been suggested that cystic dilatation may be a necessary precursor to infection as the disease may not start in a normal gland.

## Avenues of Extension

The commonest course for a fistula to pursue is from the mid anal canal downward in the intersphincteric plane to the anal verge. Infection may overcome the barrier of the external sphincter muscles thereby penetrating the ischiorectal fossa or it may extend upward in the intersphincteric plane either remaining in the rectal wall or extending extrarectally (Fig. 8-2).

In addition to tracking upward and downward, pus may pass circumferentially around the anus. This passage can occur in one of three tissue planes, the commonest of which is the ischiorectal fossa. This variety commences in the posterior midline of the anal canal, penetrates the sphincter mass, and then descends

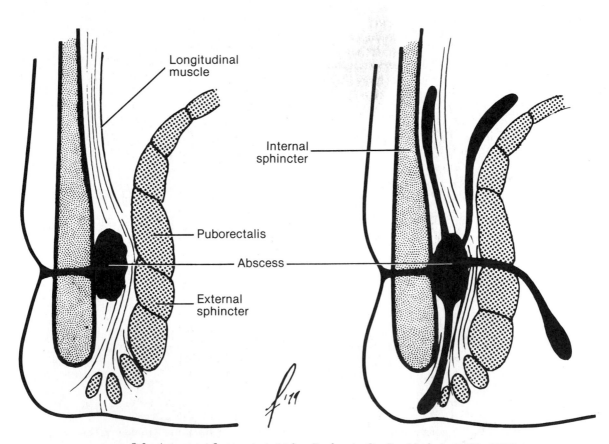

Longitudinal muscle

Internal sphincter

Puborectalis

Abscess

External sphincter

FIGURE **8-2.** *Avenues of extension. (After Parks, A. G.: Br. Med. J. 1:463, 1961)*

with two limbs, one in each ischiorectal fossa. This circumferential spread is referred to as horseshoeing. In addition, circumferential spread may occur in the intersphincteric plane or in the pararectal tissues above the levator muscles (Fig. 1-11).

## DIAGNOSIS

### History

A fistulous abscess may present either in the acute or the chronic phase. The patient with an abscess presents with acute pain and swelling in the anal region. Pain occurs with sitting or movement, and is usually aggravated by defecation and even coughing or sneezing. The clinical history may reveal a preceding bout of diarrhea. General symptomatology includes malaise and pyrexia.

In the uncommon, but very significant condition, of intersphincteric abscess, the importance of this condition as a cause of persistent undiagnosed anal pain must be stressed. The pain is generally throbbing in character, and remains continuous throughout the day and night. It is aggravated by defecation but may be so severe as to cause fecal impaction. In general, the pain is of longer duration than in patients with fissures. Minor anal bleeding may occur if the abscess is associated with an opening into the anal canal or a fissure. A discharge, when present, is due to small amounts of pus discharging into the anal canal.

In the chronic state, the patient will give a history of either an abscess which burst spontaneously or required drainage. The patient will notice a small discharging sinus or the discharge may cause skin excoriation and pruritus. There may be pain with defecation as well as bleeding due to granulation tissue in the region of the internal opening.

### Physical Examination

In the acute phase, the cardinal signs of inflammation are present with the rubor, calor, tumor, dolor, and functio laesa (redness, heat, swelling, pain, loss of function). Sometimes pus may be seen exuding from a crypt. The swelling may be in the immediate perianal region or in the ischiorectal fossa.

With the intersphincteric abscess there may be no swelling or induration in the perianal region. Rectal examination will be exquisitely painful or impossible, but in few cases a sug-

gestion of a mass is present. An opening into the anal canal, with or without a fissure, may be seen sometimes with pus exuding.[31] A point that might be helpful in the differentiation between an intersphincteric abscess and an acute fissure-in-ano is the fact, that with the abscess, inguinal lymph nodes may be enlarged and painful.

In the situation where pain is severe but the cause unknown, examination under anesthesia is not only justified but indicated. When the abscess is seen, it must be adequately drained. Neglect only allows extension of the abscess, and may lead to ischiorectal or supralevator abscesses, and possibly horseshoe extensions, each of these more difficult to manage than the simple intersphincteric abscess. If no abscess is found other pathology should be found, and it is usually an acute fissure. Treatment of this condition results in dramatic relief of pain (and many of these patients would probably not heal completely, spontaneously). We would like to draw the analogy to acute appendicitis where there is sometimes the dilemma whether or not to operate. By the same token that it is better to operate on a certain percentage of patients who turn out not to have acute appendicitis rather than expose them to the complications of perforation with abscess and the potential dire consequence of peritonitis, it is wiser to operate on patients suspected of having an intersphincteric abscess than to allow them to develop more complicated problems. In fact, these patients will usually demonstrate abnormalities amenable to surgical treatment.

With the supralevator abscess, the tender mass in the pelvis may be diagnosed by rectal or vaginal examination. Abdominal examination may reveal signs of peritoneal irritation because the pelvic peritoneum forms the roof of the supralevator space.

In the chronic state, an external opening can usually be seen as a red elevation or granulation tissue with purulent serosanguinous discharge on compression. Sometimes the opening is so small that it can only be detected when palpation around the anus expresses a few beads of pus from an otherwise inconspicuous opening. The internal crypt of the origin may not always be patent. The number of external openings, and their relationship to the anal canal, may reveal considerable information to the examiner. According to Good-

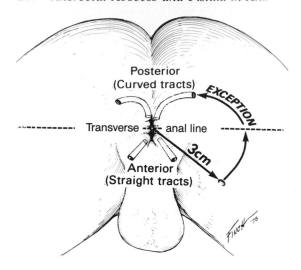

**FIGURE 8-3.** *Goodsall's rule. (After Goldberg, S., M., and Nivatvongs, S., Principles of Surgery. Ed. Schwartz, S., I., p 1243. N.Y., McGraw-Hill, 1979)*

sall's rule, if there is an opening posterior to the coronal plane, the fistula probably originates from the dorsal midline, but if anterior, probably runs directly to the nearest crypt. Openings seen on both sides of the anal canal are likely to arise from a midline posterior crypt with a horseshoe fistula (Fig. 8-3). An external opening adjacent to the anal margin may suggest an intersphincteric track while a more laterally located opening would suggest a transsphincteric one. The further the distance of the external opening from the anal margin the greater is the probability of a complicated upward extension.

The next step is to palpate the skin, since with a superficial fistula, a cord structure can be felt just beneath the skin leading from the secondary opening to the anal canal (Fig. 8-4). Further palpation may reveal circumferential extension which would be recognized by a ring of induration hugging the puborectalis sling in a horseshoe fashion. The supralevator spaces are then felt on each side.

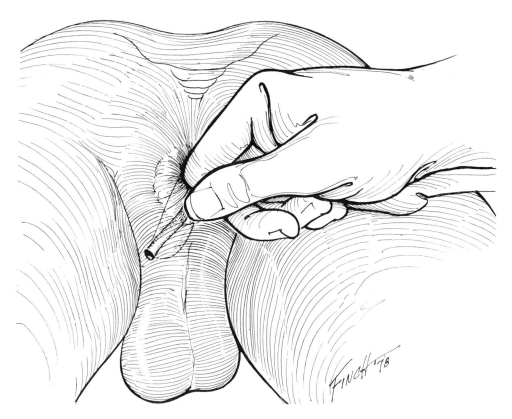

**FIGURE 8-4.** *Palpation of fistulous track. (After Goldberg, S., M., and Nivatvongs, S., Principles of Surgery. Ed. Schwartz, S., I., p 1244. N.Y., McGraw-Hill, 1979)*

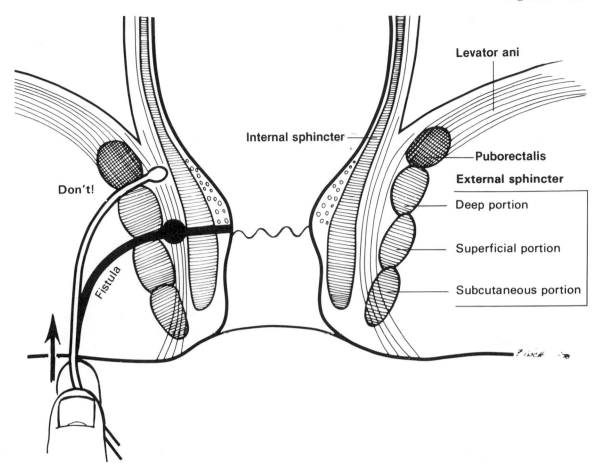

FIGURE **8-5.** *Probing fistula track. (After Goldberg, S., M., and Nivatvongs, S., Principles of Surgery. Ed. Schwartz, S., I., p 1242. N.Y., McGraw-Hill, 1979)*

In the anal canal one might be able to palpate a pit indicative of an internal opening. The crypt of origin is often retracted into a funnel by pulling the fibrous track leading to the internal sphincter. This condition is called the funnel or "herniation sign" of the involved crypt. The latter movement is, of course, performed in the operating room. Rarely is one able to feel a nodule due to a chronic intersphincteric abscess.

Probing, when done, must be performed with a feather-like touch in order to prevent false channels, therefore, it is best avoided outside the operating room. Even in the operating room, under anesthesia, great care must be taken to avoid the creation of false passages into the anal canal or into the rectum (Fig. 8-5). Following the gentle introduction of a probe into the track, a low fistula will pass toward the anus at an angle of approximately 30 degrees to the skin. Passage of the probe at an 80 degree angle to the skin or almost parallel to the anal canal, indicates the presence of a "high" fistula, or at least a supralevator or ischiorectal extension of a "low" fistula.

*Anoscopy and sigmoidoscopy* must be performed for at least three reasons. Anoscopy may help to identify the internal opening in the anal canal. Endoscopy may help distinguish between a rectal and anal canal opening. Sigmoidoscopy allows examination of the rectal mucosa in order to determine the presence of an underlying proctocolitis, should one exist.

## Radiographs

In the majority of patients who present with fistula-in-ano, radiographic examination is of limited value. A barium enema, however, is indicated in patients with a history of bowel symptoms or anyone with a recurrent fistula-in-ano. Some examiners feel that it is indicated in patients age 6 months to 25 years because, if active Crohn's disease is present, surgery may be hazardous.[33] Fistulography may be helpful in the delineation of extrasphincteric fistula of pelvic origin or in the evaluation of patients with recurrent fistulae.[29]

### Differential Diagnosis

A host of conditions might be included in the differential diagnosis of a fistulous abscess. The characteristics of these individual inflammatory processes are dealt with in their respective chapters. In any event, the acute abscess of any cause requires immediate incision and drainage as described later in this chapter, and the management of the chronic problem will depend upon the underlying cause.

---

**Differential Diagnosis of Fistulous Abscess**

Bartholin gland abscess
Sebaceous cyst
Hidradenitis suppurativa
Tuberculosis
Actinomycosis
Osteomyelitis of the bony pelvis
Fissure
Urethroperineal fistula
Carcinoma or epithelioma
Penetrating injuries
Pilonidal sinus
Retrorectal cyst
Folliculitis of the perianal skin
Pruritus ani

---

## ANORECTAL ABSCESS
### The Role of Antibiotics

There is probably little, if any, role for the use of antibiotics in the primary management of para-anal suppuration. Only in very rare exception will a cellulitis in this region be aborted by the use of antibiotics, and as a rule, operation will be required, so the sooner it is carried out the better. In patients with rheumatic or acquired valvular heart disease, antibiotic coverage would probably be indicated as an adjunct. Also, when soft tissue infection is unusually extensive as with involvement of the perineum, groin, thigh, or abdominal wall, antibiotics should be used. They are probably also indicated in diabetics with an extensive adjacent cellulitis. It is neither necessary nor wise to wait until fluctuation can be demonstrated, as delay in releasing the pus simply affords the inflammatory process an opportunity to extend and cause damage to the adjacent tissue, or more specifically, the anal sphincter mechanism.

---

**Classification of anorectal abscess**

Perianal
Ischiorectal
Intersphincteric
Supralevator

---

### Incidence

Anorectal abscesses are more common in men than women by a ratio of 2 to 1.[11] Since different authors use different classifications it is difficult to know the exact incidence of each kind. Nevertheless, the vast majority are of the perianal or ischiorectal variety. In a review of 50 consecutive abscesses seen by Gordon, the types of abscesses encountered were as follows: perianal, 26 per cent; ischiorectal, 54 per cent; intersphincteric, 16 per cent; supralevator, 4 per cent.[13]

In this review an unusually high incidence of intersphincteric abscess was noted. The reasons for this higher incidence may be explained by two factors. First, these statistics are from a referral practice and, second, if one is always conscious of this entity the diagnosis will be made before the septic process becomes more extensive and points in the perianal region, or bursts through the external sphincter and presents as an ischiorectal abscess. In other words, one has to seek out this diagnosis.

In a review of 200 abscesses by Ellis, the types of abscesses quoted were as follows: perianal, 54.5 per cent; ischiorectal, 39 per cent; submucous (or high intermuscular), 0 per cent; pelvirectal, 0 per cent; atypical, 6.5 per cent.[9] It can be seen that the distribution of perianal and ischiorectal abscess experienced by Ellis was an almost complete reversal of that seen by Gordon. No satisfactory explanation can be offered for this observed difference. Ellis' series also greatly underrates the incidence of what we refer to as the intersphincteric abscess.

## Treatment

Abscesses in the perineum are treated in the same manner as abscesses in other parts of the body; that is, they must be adequately drained. This drainage usually consists of making a cruciate incision or removing an elipse of skin over the abscess.

*A simple perianal abscess* almost always can be drained under local anesthesia in the office or outpatient department. Skin preparation with an antiseptic solution is probably not necessary. The most tender point is determined and in this region a 2 cm area of skin is anesthetized with one-half per cent lidocaine with 1 : 200,000 adrenaline. A cruciate incision is made which will readily allow free drainage of the pus. Skin edges must be excised be-cause, if only an incision is made, edges will readily fall together, seal, and the abscess may recur. In general, no packing is inserted as this only impedes the drainage of pus. Minor bleeding can easily be controlled by electrocoagulation. If cautery is unavailable, packing for a few hours may be necessary to control bleeding (Fig. 8-6).

*Ischiorectal Abscess.* The majority of ischiorectal abscesses may also be incised and drained under local anesthesia as an outpatient procedure. However, certain horseshoe abscesses or other more extensive abscesses might better be drained under a general anesthetic. Here loculations should be sought, and broken down, to ensure adequate drainage. The same principles of drainage and nonpack-

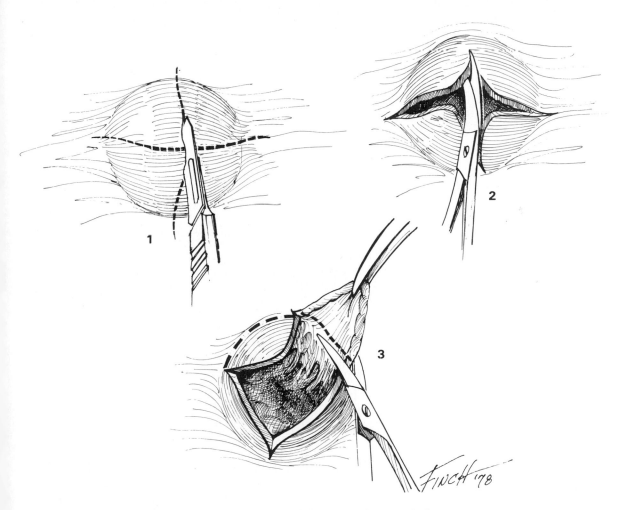

FIGURE **8-6.** *Incision and drainage of perianal abscess.*

ing are adhered to as with the perianal abscess.

Previous authors have stressed the importance of extensive unroofing by excision of enormous amounts of skin over each ischiorectal fossa. One need excise only that amount of skin which will allow adequate drainage and prevent the skin edges from falling together too rapidly, thus preventing the reformation of the abscess.

Hanley believes that the acute horseshoe abscess should be treated by drainage and primary fistulotomy.[14] McElwain is in agreement.[25] Using Hanley's technique, with the patient placed in a modified semi-jackknife position, caudal anesthesia is induced. The primary opening is usually located in a crypt in the posterior midline and sometimes pus can be seen draining from it. A probe inserted into the primary opening is directed toward the coccyx, thus passing into the deep post-anal

space. A fistulotomy performed at this stage (involving the division of the lower half of the internal sphincter and the lower portion of the external sphincter) decompresses the pus-filled post-anal space, and at the same time exposes the primary source of the infection. Para-anal incisions are made to drain the anterior extensions of the abscess in order to accomplish complete drainage of the abscess (Fig. 8-7). All ten cases treated by Hanley in this manner healed.[16]

For several reasons immediate fistulotomy is not performed. In the acute stage the tracks do not yet consist of hard fibrous tubes, and definitive fistula surgery would create greater separation of sphincter muscle. A significant number of properly drained abscesses will not result in fistula. If the patient is completely anesthetized, a modification of Hanley's technique is to accomplish adequate drainage by para-anal incisions, and divide only the lower

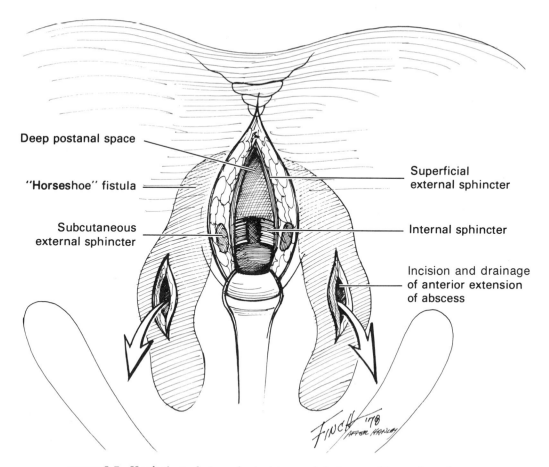

FIGURE **8-7.** *Hanley's technique for incision and drainage of horseshoe abscess.*

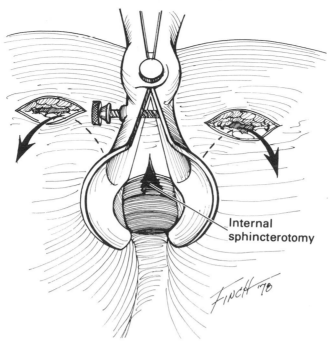

Internal
sphincterotomy

FIGURE **8-8.** *Modification of Hanley's technique for incision and drainage of horseshoe abscess. (After Goldberg, S., M., and Nivatvongs, S., Principles of Surgery. Ed. Schwartz, S., I., p 1245. N.Y., McGraw-Hill, 1979)*

half of the internal sphincter to eradicate the source of the infected gland. This procedure would preserve the external sphincter, and hopefully, result in better continence (Fig. 8-8).

*An intersphincteric abscess* will require a general or regional anesthetic since adequate exposure cannot otherwise be obtained. Treatment consists of laying open the abscess, with division of the fibers of the internal sphincter from its lower end up to the level of the dentate line, or higher if the cavity extends higher.

*Supralevator Abscess.* In a patient in whom a supralevator abscess is found, one must try to determine its origin prior to treatment. Such an abscess may arise in one of three ways. It may be due to the upward extension of an intersphincteric abscess, an upward extension of an ischiorectal abscess, or result from pelvic disease such as perforated diverticulitis, Crohn's disease, or appendicitis. If one has a supralevator abscess secondary to an upward extension of an intersphincteric abscess, then the supralevator abscess should be drained

into the rectum. If it is drained through the ischiorectal fossa, a suprasphincteric fistula will be formed and become a difficult problem to manage. If, however, a supralevator abscess arises secondary to the upward extension of an ischiorectal abscess, then the supralevator abscess should be drained through the ischiorectal fossa. Attempts at draining this kind of abcess into the rectum will result in an extrasphincteric fistula and become a much more difficult problem to handle (Fig. 8-9). In the drainage of supralevator abscesses of pelvic origin, one must take into consideration the original disease. These abscesses can be drained by three routes: into the rectal lumen; through the ischiorectal fossa; or through the abdominal wall. The choice of procedure would seem to depend upon the area to which the abscess points most closely, and the general condition of the patient.

Following the drainage of an abscess, it is wise to explain to the patient that this may not be definitive treatment. The patient is told that the abscess may heal and never trouble him again or it may continue to drain, in which case definitive repair of the fistula will be nec-

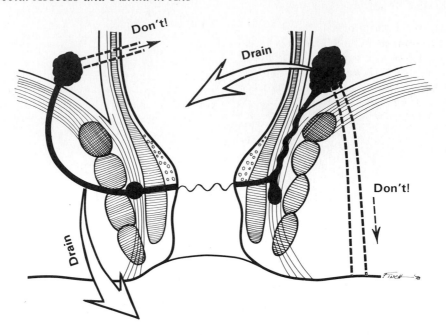

FIGURE **8-9.** *Incision and drainage of supralevator abscess.*

essary. He is also warned about possible re-currence of the abscess, in which case defini-tive surgery will also be required.

## FISTULA-IN-ANO
### Indications for Operation

The very presence of a symptomatic fistula-in-ano is an indication for operation. Spon-taneous healing of fistula-in-ano is very rare. Neglected fistulae may result in repeated abscesses and persistent drainage with its con-comitant morbidity. Very rarely, malignancy may supervene upon a long-standing fistula. Therefore, operation should be recommended unless there are specific medical contraindica-tions to anesthesia. In addition, patients with already compromised anal continence present a relative contraindication, since the further division of muscle required in the treatment of the fistula might render the patient totally in-continent. Anal fistulae are sometimes asso-ciated with active pulmonary tuberculosis, and the pulmonary disease must be controlled be-fore the tuberculous fistula is repaired. Since Crohn's disease is associated with anal fis-tulae, patients with any suggestive bowel symptoms should have their gastrointestinal tract investigated by both endoscopy and radiography. Control of active Crohn's dis-ease must precede any repair of an anal fistula associated with it (Chap. 11).

### Classification and Treatment

A number of authors have made significant contributions to the study of fistula anatomy. Eisenhammer stressed the importance of the intersphincter plane both in the pathogenesis and spread of fistulae.[7] Steltzner classified fistula-in-ano into three main groups: inter-muscular (between the internal and external sphincter), transsphincteric (spread across the external sphincter into the ischiorectal fossa), and extrasphincteric (a track passing directly from the perineal skin through the ischiorec-tal fossa, the levator ani muscles, and para-rectal fat into the rectum, outside all the sphincters).[35] Lilius further extended the con-cept of intermuscular spread, in particular, ex-tension upward into the rectal wall.[20] And fi-nally, Parks described the classification that will be presented below.[32]

Over the years, many classifications of fis-tulae, in and about the anorectal region, have been described. Some have been very simple but of no help in the treatment, while others have used terms which have different connota-tions to different surgeons. The aim of any such classification should be to help the surgeon in the operative cure of the disease. The classification which we are going to employ, although very detailed, gives an accurate description of the anatomical course of the fistulous tracks. This knowledge then acts as a guide to the operative treatment and one would, therefore, heartily endorse it. The full credit for its description goes to Parks, although some aspects of it were previously described by Steltzner.[32,35]

---

### Parks' Classification of Fistula-in-Ano

1. Intersphincteric
   a) simple low track
   b) high blind track
   c) high track with rectal opening
   d) rectal opening without a perineal opening
   e) extrarectal extension
   f) secondary to pelvic disease
2. Transsphincteric
   a) uncomplicated
   b) high blind track
3. Suprasphincteric
   a) uncomplicated
   b) high blind track
4. Extrasphincteric
   a) secondary to anal fistula
   b) secondary to trauma
   c) secondary to anorectal disease
   d) secondary to pelvic inflammation

---

The following discussion will elaborate on this classification and, with the aid of diagrams, deal with the treatment as we go along, in order to show the practicality of this detailed clasification.

### 1. Intersphincteric Fistulae

In the category of the intersphincteric fistula, the process involves only the intersphincteric plane. This fistula is the commonest of all types and is the intermediary form which leads to most of the other kinds of fistula.

*a) Simple Low Track.* After penetrating the internal sphincter at the level of the dentate line, the track passes from the primary abscess down to the anal verge. The treatment of this kind of fistula involves eradication of the primary source of disease in the mid anal canal by division of the lower half of the internal sphincter. This treatment seldom gives rise to

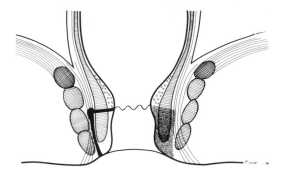

FIGURE **8-10.** *Intersphincteric fistula: simple low track.*

any disturbance of function. In the acute phase this fistula presents as a perianal abscess (Fig. 8-10).

*b) High Blind Track.* This kind, in addition to the downward extension, tracks proximally, resulting in a fistula between the internal sphincter and the longitudinal muscle of the upper anal canal and the rectal wall itself. Treatment consists of division of the internal sphincter for as high as the high blind track ascends. This procedure will unroof the infected anal gland as well as the blind extension. Little disturbance of continence will ensue because the edges of the sphincter are held together by fibrosis around the fistulous track. Failure to recognize this upward extension might be a cause for recurrence (Fig. 8-11).

*c) High Track with Rectal Opening.* This type is an extension of the previous variety with the fistula breaking back into the lower rectum. It should be noted that the whole of this track is intersphincteric, and the tissue

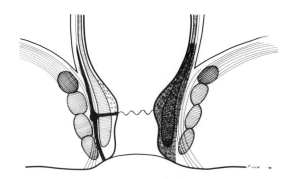

FIGURE **8-11.** *Intersphincteric fistula: high blind track.*

above it can usually be divided without risk. However, it is easy to mistake the track as passing outside the external sphincter. If the probe passes straight upward (i.e., parallel to the anal canal), this direction often helps in making the diagnosis. With experience it is not difficult to tell the two apart because in the case of an intersphincteric track, the probe passes close to the lumen of the anal canal. If old scarring and previous operations make the distinction difficult, an electromyographic needle placed into the tissue lateral to the track can be extremely helpful. A potential from the external sphincter will be registered if the fistula is intersphincteric, but not if it is an extrasphincteric. Alternatively, electrical stimulation can be used to demonstrate contractions in the external sphincter (Fig. 8-12).

*d) High Track Without a Perineal Opening.* Infection passes in the intersphincteric plane upward into the rectal wall, and terminates as a blind track or re-enters the gut through a high secondary opening. There is no downward extension to the anal margin, and no external evidence of a fistula. In the past this variety, in its acute phase, was referred to as a submucous abscess, but, since the track is deep to the internal sphincter, it is, in fact, an intersphincteric abscess. Treatment consists of simply laying the track open into the rectum. In addition, it is essential to incise the lower portion of the track in the mid-anal canal because it contains the primary source of infection, and if left behind recurrence will ensue (Fig. 8-13).

*e) Extrarectal Extension.* Infection may spread upward in the intersphincteric plane to

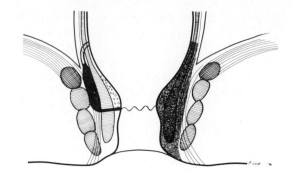

FIGURE **8-13.** *Intersphincteric fistula: high track without a perineal opening.*

reach the true pelvic cavity. Here it lies above the levator plate. This type is usually encountered in the stage of an acute abscess. Correct treatment is drainage into the rectum. One should note that any attempt to drain such an abscess through the ischiorectal fossa will result in the production of a suprasphincteric fistula which is a considerably more difficult problem with which to deal (Fig. 8-14).

*f) Secondary to Pelvic Disease.* The last category is a fistula which manifests itself in the perianal region but originates in the pelvis. Processes such as perforated diverticulitis or Crohn's abscess might be causative. The prime goal must be elimination of the abdominal source, for failure to do so makes cure of the fistula impossible. As a rule, no local treatment, other than possible curettage of the track, is necessary because they usually heal once the pelvic disease has been removed. This disorder is not a true anal fistula, and therefore, the division of muscle is both un-

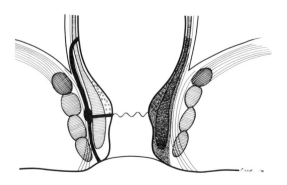

FIGURE **8-12.** *Intersphinteric fistula: high track with rectal opening.*

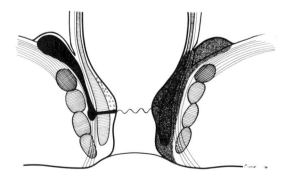

FIGURE **8-14.** *Intersphincteric fistula: extrarectal extension.*

necessary and potentially dangerous (Fig. 8-15).

2. Transsphincteric

*a) Uncomplicated.* In the uncomplicated variety the track passes from the intersphincteric plane, through the external sphincter, into the ischiorectal fossa, and then to the skin. The level at which the track crosses the external sphincter determines the ease or difficulty encountered in treatment. Most of them cross at a low level so that laying open the fistula will result in division of only the lower portion of the external sphincter and the lower half of the internal sphincter, consequently, disturbance of function is unlikely. The highest level is just below the puborectalis at which point all the external sphincter may have to be divided. Even so, the puborectalis is usually adequate to maintain near perfect continence. In order to preserve sphincter muscle, fistulae with tracks crossing at higher levels may be treated by division of the lower half of the internal sphincter, creating adequate drainage of the fistulous track, and dividing only a portion of the external sphincter. The external portion of the track may be curetted or "cored out" (Fig. 8-16, 8-25, and 8-26).

*b) With a High Blind Track.* The transsphincteric fistula with a high blind track is a most important fistula because of the dire consequences which might ensue if it is improperly treated. The track crosses the external sphincter but then divides into an upper and lower arm. The lower arm extends to the

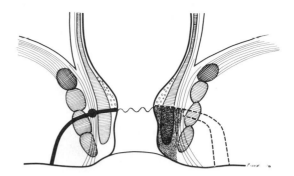

FIGURE **8-16.** *Transsphincteric fistula: uncomplicated.*

perineal skin; the upper arm may reach the apex of the ischiorectal fossa or even pass through the levator ani muscles into the pelvis. A high extension causes induration above the anorectal ring, and can be felt digitally through the rectum. If a probe is passed into the external opening it will go into the upper arm of the track and the originating extension from the anal canal will not be demonstrated. The great danger here is that the tip of the probe may pass through the rectal wall, thus, creating an iatrogenic extraphincteric fistula with its rather grave implications to be discussed below. The height and extent of a secondary track is not of paramount importance, provided that it has not ruptured into the rectum. The treatment of this variety consists of finding the primary track, which passes in the anal canal, and laying it open. The high extensions are then provided with adequate drainage. It is possible that a greater amount of external sphincter will require division, but the amount depends upon the level at which the fistula track crosses the sphincter. Otherwise, the same considerations pertain as with the uncomplicated variety (Fig. 8-17).

3. Suprasphincteric

*a) Uncomplicated.* With this variety, the fistula starts in the intersphincteric plane in the mid-anal canal and then passes upward to a point above the puborectalis. It tracks laterally over this muscle and downward between the puborectalis and the levator ani muscle into the ischiorectal fossa, thus, looping over the entire sphincter mass. Treatment of this fistula by a classic lay-open technique would result in division of all the external sphincter and puborectalis muscle, most likely rendering

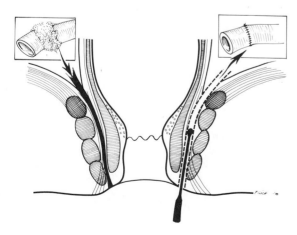

FIGURE **8-15.** *Intersphincteric fistula: secondary to pelvic disease.*

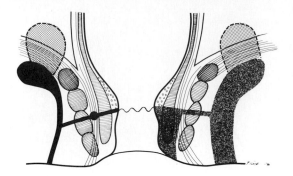

FIGURE **8-17.** *Transsphincteric fistula: high blind track.*

the patient incontinent. Therefore, it is best to use a modification of a lay-open method in which the sphincter mass is divided in successive stages. The fistula itself, fortunately, usually helps to provide a solution to the problem. As it passes over the puborectalis, fibrous tissue is created around it. This problem is treated by division of the lower half of the internal sphincter (to eradicate the anal gland of origin), creating adequate drainage of the secondary limb, and dividing variable amounts (about half) of the external sphincter. The use of a seton is encouraged, and division of contained muscle is performed in stages, if necessary. Functional results will be better if muscle can be preserved (Fig. 8-18).

*b) High Blind Track.* This fortunately very rare variant of fistula, in addition to the above path, sends an extension into the supralevator compartment. If this were not already complicated enough, there is a tendency for this variety to spread in a horseshoe fashion in the supralevator compartment. The horseshoe ex-

tension deposits fibrous tissue above the puborectalis, a structure which can be felt as a rather narrow, sharp ring resembling a crescentic knife edge. Since this fibrous band is above the puborectalis, if the muscle is cut beneath it the edges of the sphincter will not separate a great deal, and continence will probably be maintained. Treatment is similar to the uncomplicated suprasphincteric fistula, but adequate drainage of the abscess in the supralevator compartment must also be established. The supralevator abscess may be bilateral and requires corresponding drainage (Fig. 8-19).

#### 4. Extrasphincteric

Extrasphincteric fistulae are most conveniently classified according to pathogenesis. With this fistula, a track passes from the perineal skin through the ischiorectal fossa, the levator ani muscles, and finally penetrates the rectal wall. This route lies entirely outside the ring of sphincter muscle. Obviously, if this track is laid open, total incontinence will result.

*a) Secondary to Anal Fistula.* In this category, a transsphincteric fistula with a high extension may burst spontaneously into the rectum, although this is very rare. More commonly, a secondary opening above the puborectalis is iatrogenic due to the overenergetic probing of the surgeon during the repair of a transsphincteric fistula. Once established, this fistula has two factors causing its perpetuation. First, the focus of disease in the anal canal (i.e., the chronic infection of the anal gland in the intersphincteric plane), and

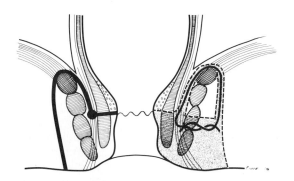

FIGURE **8-18.** *Suprasphincteric fistula: uncomplicated.*

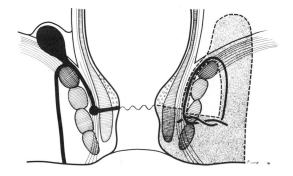

FIGURE **8-19.** *Suprasphincteric fistula: high blind track.*

second, the constant contamination of the rectal opening by high intraluminal pressures. These high pressures, which develop in the rectum, force mucus and fecal debris into the internal opening and become a major cause in the perpetuation of the fistula. Both these factors must, therefore, be eliminated before such a fistula will heal. The primary track in the anal canal must be eradicated by division of the lower half of the internal sphincter. The opening in the rectal wall is closed with two or three interrupted, nonabsorbable sutures such as wire. Adequate drainage of the fistulous track must be performed, with special attention paid to the elimination of pocketing at the apex of the ischiorectal fossa or supralevator extension. Occasionally, the rectal opening can be sutured without subsequent breakdown, but, more usually, it is necessary to perform a temporary, defunctioning colostomy to reduce rectal pressure before healing will be perfected. The colostomy may be closed three months later (Fig. 8-20).

*b) Secondary to Trauma.* A traumatic fistula may be caused in two ways. A foreign body may penetrate the perineum and enter the rectum; or, a swallowed foreign body (e.g., fish or chicken bone) may reach the rectum, straddle the sphincters, and be forced through the rectal wall, levator muscles, ischiorectal fossa, and reach the perineum. Treatment consists of removing the foreign body, establishing adequate drainage, and performing a temporary colostomy to reduce the rectal pressure. It is not necessary to cut any sphincter muscle (see Chap. 23) (Fig. 8-21).

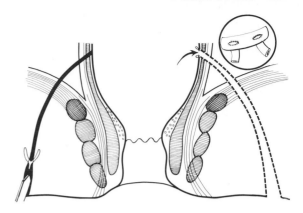

FIGURE **8-21.** *Extrasphincteric fistula: secondary to trauma.*

*c) Secondary to Specific Anorectal Disease.* Chronic ulcerative colitis, Crohn's disease, and carcinoma often result in gross and bizzare fistulization. They are not usually amenable to local treatment and one must treat the disease itself, usually in the form of a proctectomy (Fig. 8-22).

*d) Secondary to Pelvic Inflammation.* A pericolic abscess due to diverticulitis or Crohn's disease may spread through the levator muscles and discharge into the perineum. This type of fistula requires no local treatment, and will heal once the pelvic disease has been removed. Once again, no muscle requires division. The same principles pertain as in intersphincteric fistula secondary to pelvic disease (Fig. 8-23).

**Incidence**

Although it is more usual to mention this matter earlier in the discussion of fistulae, it is

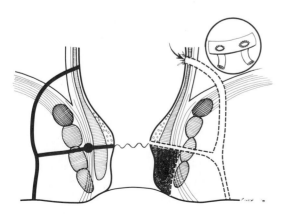

FIGURE **8-20.** *Extrasphincteric fistula: secondary to anal fistula.*

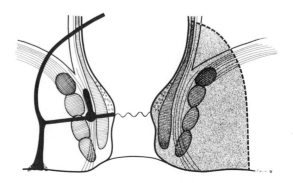

FIGURE **8-22.** *Extrasphincteric fistula: secondary to specific anorectal disease.*

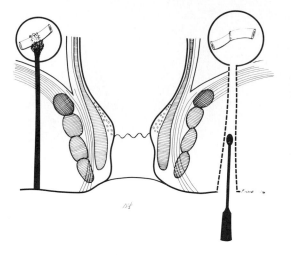

FIGURE **8-23.** *Extrasphincteric fistula: due to pelvic inflammation.*

being mentioned here because the classification which has just been presented has not been used by many authors, and it was felt that each type of fistula should be described prior to listing its frequencies. In a review of 400 fistulae by Parks and associates the following distribution was found: intersphincteric, 45 per cent; transsphincteric, 30 per cent; suprasphincteric, 20 per cent; extrasphincteric, 5 per cent.[32]

However, because of the highly selected patient population in this series, Parks estimated that a more representative incidence of the disease in the general population would be: intersphincteric, 70 per cent; transsphincteric, 23 per cent; suprasphincteric, 5 per cent; extrasphincteric, 2 per cent.

Marks and Ritchie reviewing a series of 793 consecutive fistulae treated at St. Mark's Hospital, London, including those patients reviewed by Parks, found the following distribution: superficial, 16 per cent; intersphincteric, 54 per cent; transsphincteric, 21 per cent; suprasphincteric, 3 per cent; extrasphincteric, 3 per cent; unclassified, 3 per cent.[22]

If one were to combine the superficial and intersphincteric fistulae in this series the statistics would roughly correspond to Park's estimated incidence of different varieties. These data suggest, with the appropriate early recognition and drainage of the intersphincteric abscess, that the incidence of fistula-in-ano should decrease.

## Technique

Prior to any operative treatment of fistula-in-ano, it is wise to ascertain whether the patient has normal continence. Fistula surgery has an unenviable reputation because of the risks of recurrence and impairment of anal continence. Therefore, extreme care must be exercised in order to keep these problems to a minimum. If one accepts the cryptoglandular origin of most fistulae, one realizes that a lay-open technique would require the division of portions of both the internal and external sphincter (Fig. 8-26). The key landmark as pointed out by Milligan and Morgan is the anorectal ring, as division of this portion of the sphincter mechanism will render the patient incontinent.

*Simple Low Level Fistulae.* With the patient under a light, general anesthetic, preferably in the prone jackknife position, the perianal region is prepared and infiltrated with a local anesthetic such as one-half per cent lidocaine with 1 : 200,000 epinephrine. An anal speculum such as a Pratt Bivalve is inserted in the anal canal, and any obvious internal opening is identified. A probe (we prefer a grooved, directional probe) is then inserted into the external orifice and passed along the distance of the track. In simple intersphincteric and low transsphincteric fistulae, the tissue over the track is divided by sliding a scalpel along the grooved probe director. Granulation tissue is then curetted and sent for biopsy. Careful examination is now made by inspection and probing of the granulating tracks to uncover any side or cephalad branches of the fistula track. Hemostasis is obtained using electrocoagulation. Marsupialization is then accomplished by approximating the skin edges to the edge of the track with a running absorbable suture, such as 3–0 chromic. This technique is preferred over trimming large amounts of skin and subcutaneous tissue, because it is our impression that the wounds heal more quickly. No packing is inserted. A loose, cotton dressing is applied to prevent soiling of clothes, and a T-binder or even underpants alone are used rather than tape since the latter is uncomfortable to remove, especially in hirsute patients (Fig. 8-24).

When the probe cannot be advanced along the full distance of the track, as was the case in 40 per cent of Parks' cases, a weak solution of

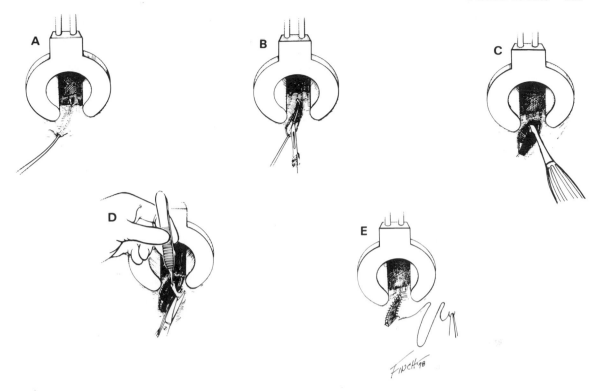

FIGURE **8-24.** *Technique for "simple" fistula.*

one part in 10 of Methylene Blue is injected. This additional method reduced the number of cases in which the internal opening could not be demonstrated to 10 per cent. Mazier stated the internal opening was found in 86.2 per cent of 1,000 cases.[24] When the primary opening is identified, the technique continues as described above. When no such opening can be found, the general direction of the fistulous tracks as shown by probing from the external opening, will indicate fairly clearly where the connection with the lining of the anal canal is located. The track can then be laid open and the procedure continued as above.

Patients with multiple secondary openings generally have tracks that communicate with one another, and with a single crypt of origin. Usually probing demonstrates this condition quite easily. It is uncommon for a patient to have entirely separate fistulae.

Parks described a conservative operation in which the lower half of the internal sphincter is divided to eradicate the causative infected anal gland and the peripheral fistula is managed by coring out, curettage, or incision and curettage. The major advantage of this technique is the preservation of the external sphincter. For fistulae crossing the external sphincter at a high level, the lower portion of this muscle will require division to allow adequate drainage and healing. It is in these "high" fistula that such a conservative approach is advantageous over the classical lay-open technique, and we fully endorse it (Fig. 8-25 and Fig. 8-26).

*Horseshoe Fistula.* Circumferential spread of the septic process results in the horseshoe fistula, which may demonstrate one or several secondary openings. Through probing it can be seen that these openings are connected to each other. When a complicated fistula is suspected a preoperative fistulogram may serve as a useful "road map" for the operating surgeon, thus reducing the risk of missing other tracks.

One commences by laying open a lateral limb of the horseshoe track. This procedure is followed by exposing the posterior extremity of the track, and then, the other lateral limb is

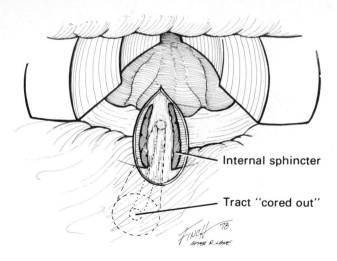

FIGURE **8-25.** *Parks' fistulotomy. (After Parks, A. G.: Br. J. Surg. 1:467, 1961)*

unroofed. Search is made for the opening into the posterior wall of the anal canal at the level of the dentate line so that the primary source of the fistula is exposed. It is important not to miss such an opening, for to do so inevitably results in recurrence, despite the wide unroofing of the secondary limbs. If no primary internal opening is discovered, but the tracks lead to the posterior midline, it is probably wise, based on the assumption that the initiating factor is infection of cryptoglandular ori-

gin, to divide the lower half of the internal sphincter posteriorly, to expose any such gland. Goligher recommends passing a director through the posterior wall of the anal canal from the main wound into the lumen at the level of the dentate line, and dividing the tissues below it. All tracks are curetted of their granulation tissue and carefully examined for further side tracks (Fig. 8-27).

This large wound can be handled in one of two ways. If feasible, marsupialization is at-

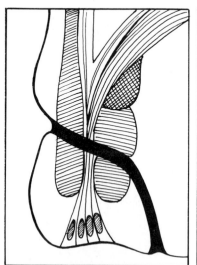
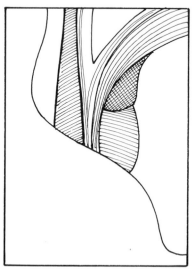
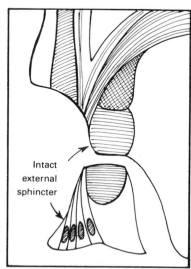

**Fistula-in-ano**      **Lay-open method**      **Park's fistulectomy**

FIGURE **8-26.** *Parks' fistulotomy vs. lay-open method. (After Parks, A. G.: Br. Med. J. 1:467, 1961)*

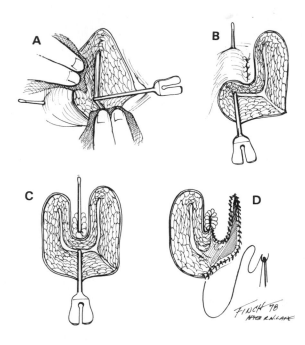

**FIGURE 8-27.** *Technique for horseshoe fistula. (After Goligher, J., C., Surgery of the Anus Rectum and Colon, p 233. Illinois, Charles C. Thomas, 1975)*

tempted, as this will markedly decrease the size of the wound and expedite healing. If this is not possible, the walls of the wound edges are trimmed of both skin and subcutaneous tissue.

A more conservative approach to the management of horseshoe fistulae was described by Hanley.[14] The technique for performing the fistulotomy of the portion of the track from the primary opening to the postanal space is the same as for the acute abscess. The tracks are readily identified by inspection and palpation of the cord-like structures. The single track, upon leaving the deep postanal space, may branch into superficial and deep branches, with numerous ramifications extending to the skin over the ischiorectal fossa, perineum, or scrotum, forming many secondary openings. When feasible, he recommends partial fistulectomy by excision of 1 to 1.5 cm of the T-shaped portion of the fistulous track in the deep postanal space.

The secondary openings are enlarged by incising the opening for 2 cm to permit thorough curettage of the tracks. In well healed tracks, complete fistulectomies are performed. Hanley cautions against division of the anococ-

cygeal ligament but Parks feels this would not affect anal function. Wounds are packed loosely, with fine gauze, and removed in 48 hours. All 31 cases so treated healed with minimal defect and no problems of incontinence.[16]

Once again, we feel fistulectomy is not necessary but agree with a conservative approach, that is laying open of the internal sphincter to eradicate the underlying focus of infection, and curettage and adequate drainage of tracks without the creation of extensive wounds. This procedure would also preserve the external sphincter, and result in better function (Fig. 8-28).

Anterior horseshoe abscesses or fistulae are very uncommon, but when they occur they are very difficult to manage, especially in women patients. The process may arise in a crypt in the anterior midline and, after penetrating the internal and external sphincter, lie deep to the transverse perinei muscles. In planning treatment, one must remember that anteriorly there is no puborectalis and, therefore, the patient would be rendered incontinent more readily by an immediate fistulotomy. In the acute stage, the abscess should only be drained. In the fistulous stage the primary source is handled in the anal canal by division of the lower half of the internal sphincter. Adequate drainage of the secondary track is then established, and a seton is inserted.

### Complications of Surgery for Fistulous Abscess

A long list of potential complications may ensue following operations for a fistulous abscess. Excluding urinary retention which occurred in 25 per cent of his patients, Mazier found that 5.4 per cent of patients developed complications.[24] These included hemorrhage, incontinence, acute external thrombosed hemorrhoids, cellulitis, inadequate drainage and pocketing, fecal impaction, recurrent fistulae, rectovaginal fistulae, persistent sinus, bridging, and stricture. However, with caution, these complications can be reduced to a minimum. It is our impression that avoiding primary fistulotomy will help reduce such untoward events.

### Causes of Recurrence

Anyone treating patients with a fistula-in-ano realizes that in certain instances, recurrences will occur despite the most careful op-

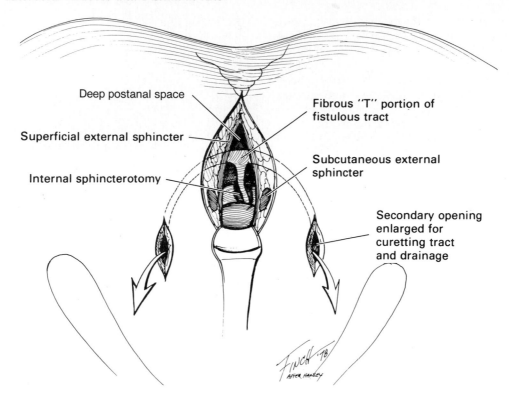

Deep postanal space

Superficial external sphincter

Internal sphincterotomy

Fibrous "T" portion of fistulous tract

Subcutaneous external sphincter

Secondary opening enlarged for curetting tract and drainage

**FIGURE 8-28.** *Modification of Hanley's treatment of horseshoe fistula. (After Hanley, P., et al.: Dis. Colon Rectum. 19:513, 1976)*

erative dissection. The commonest cause of recurrence of an anal fistula is failure to identify and treat the primary internal orifice. The result is that the causative infective anal gland in the intersphincteric space is not eradicated. Failure to detect and treat lateral or upward extensions may also be followed by recurrence. Failure to open the fistulous track for fear of causing incontinence may also result in recurrence. (This statement should not encourage operating with bold recklessness.) Of course, when the etiological factor of the fistula is a specific disease, such as Crohn's disease, recurrences are not infrequent.

### Causes of Anal Incontinence after Operation for Anal Fistula

*Division of the Anorectal Ring.* Complete severance of the anorectal ring will result in total incontinence. Division of lesser amounts of sphincter muscle may result in varying degrees of partial incontinence, depending upon the state of the sphincter muscle at the outset

and the location of the myotomy. Also, the age of the patient is a factor since the elderly, with a sphincter mechanism already weakened by age, are less likely to tolerate division of even smaller amounts of muscle.

*Severing a motor nerve to the sphincter mechanism* (inferior rectal nerve) will result in impaired continence, but control may be acceptable with only one nerve functioning. Damage to the nerves bilaterally will certainly render the patient incontinent.

*Prolonged packing* following anorectal surgery may be detrimental. Packing causes fibrosis of the sphincter and hard scar formation may result in some measure of incontinence. Mazier found that prolonged packing with iidoform gauze was a factor contributing to incontinence.[24]

### Postoperative Care

The postoperative care of the wound may be as important as the operative procedure. The primary goals are sound healing from the depths of the wounds and prevention of contact and premature healing of opposing skin edges. Patients are placed on a regular diet and analgesics are administered as needed. Some physicians prefer dressings soaked in solutions of sodium hypochlorite (Milton, Dakins, or Eusol), to keep the healing edges apart but, this procedure is not always necessary. Warm baths are taken three times a day. A bulk-forming agent is administered until wound healing has been completed, and an oil-emulsion lubricant is given orally until the first bowel movement. Some authors recommend the insertion of an anal dilator but one would think that this is rather harsh treatment. A large stool created by bulk-forming agents effects a physiological dilatation.

Because of the operative trauma and division of some muscle, patients may experience fecal leaks in the immediate postoperative period, especially if stools are liquid. However, if the anorectal ring has been preserved, after a week or ten days control approximates normalcy. The healing time required depends on the complexity of the fistula. Simple fistulotomy may heal in four to five weeks; while complex fistulae may take several months.

## Results

Results of fistula surgery vary considerably from surgeon to surgeon. Clearly, results will depend upon the complexity of the fistula treated.

In an excellent monograph on fistula-in-ano, Lilius reviewed the world literature up to 1964, and discovered an enormous difference in reported results of fistula surgery.[20] Reported recurrence rates varied from 0.7 per cent to 26.5 per cent, while reported disturbances in anal continence varied from 5 per cent to 40 per cent. Lilius' personal study of 150 patients operated upon for fistulae revealed a recurrence rate of 5.5 per cent, with disturbances of continence noted in 13.5 per cent of patients.

Bennett, in reviewing 108 patients, found a recurrence rate of just under 2 per cent, but questioning regarding functional results revealed considerable changes in anal continence.[2] Twelve per cent of patients complained of inadequate control of feces, 16 per cent of imperfect control of flatus, and 24 per cent of frequent soiling of underclothes. In all, 36 per cent suffered from one or more of these defects. The frequency and severity of poor control increased with fistulae at higher levels. Following operations for horseshoe fistula, one or more of these impairments occurred in 55 per cent. Thus, the classical methods of treatment are capable of affording cure in most cases, but impairment of control occurs in a significant percentage.

Marks and Ritchie reviewed 793 patients treated at St. Mark's Hospital, London, and found that follow-up of these patients revealed healing of almost all the fistulae.[22] However, the functional results were less satisfactory, with incontinence of loose stool in 17 per cent, of flatus in 25 per cent, and soiling in 31 per cent. They point out, though, that it must be borne in mind that there is a definite incidence of these three symptoms in a normal population.

Hanley, on the other hand, using techniques described earlier in this chapter, operated upon 31 horseshoe fistulae and reported no recurrences and no problems with control.[16] Mazier reported a 3.9 per cent incidence of recurrence in 1,000 patients.[24] Reportedly, only one of the 1,000 patients had a problem with control. Hill, reviewing a personal experience of 626 patients, reported a recurrence rate of less than 1 per cent with a 4 per cent incidence of difficulty with fecal control.[17] McElwain, reviewed 1,000 patients and found a recurrence rate of 3.6 per cent.[25] Problems with control were encountered in 7 per cent of patients up to two years and 3.2 per cent after two years. The recurrence rate in Parks' series was 9 per cent, but it must be remembered that his was a very selected series of patients.[30] There was an unusually high percentage of very complex fistulae in that study and, hence, the unusually high recurrence rate.

It is difficult to understand why there is such a great variation in the results of fistula surgery. Clearly, one factor is the difference in patient population, with some authors reporting the results of mostly simple fistulae, while others are reporting only the results of the treatment of complex fistulae. The skill of the individual operator is self-evident. Another factor is the thoroughness of reporting, or at least the intensity of interrogation of these patients during follow-up visits.

## SPECIAL CONSIDERATIONS
### Primary Closure of Anorectal Abscesses

An unconventional method of handling the perianal and ischiorectal abscess was described by Ellis.[8] After the purulent material is evacuated with the patient under general anesthesia, the abscess cavity is curetted and sutured primarily under systemic antibiotic cover. The rationale of curettage is that it is alleged to destroy the layer of granulation lining the abscess wall, thereby allowing the antibiotic to penetrate freely. Half an hour before operation, penicillin and streptomycin are given by injection. In a controlled trial of the conventional lay-open method compared with incision, curettage and suture, Goligher used ampicillin and cloxacillin, 500 mg each, intramuscularly with the premedication and orally for five days following treatment.[10] Primary healing occurred in 93 per cent of cases with a mean healing time of ten days as compared with 35 days for the open wounds. His follow-up was short (less than one year), but follow-up of Ellis' cases at two years revealed a 20 per cent incidence of fistulization.[10] Jones and associates described a series of patients in whom the antibiotics used were lincomycin with the premedication and clindamycin for four days postoperatively.[18] Patients were allowed to return home the same day. Follow-up results demonstrated a 14 per cent fistulization rate. Using the same technique, Wilson found 15 per cent developed recurrent abscesses and 7 per cent fistula-in-ano for an overall recurrence rate of 22 per cent.[36] Since experience with this technique has been limited, further evaluation will be necessary to confirm its efficacy (Table 8-1).

### "Superficial Fistulae"

There are a certain number of "low" fistulae which are not associated with anal gland infection. These are the submucous or subcutaneous fistulae which are associated with the bridging of fissure edges in the midline posteriorly or occur, occasionally, in a hemorrhoidectomy wound. The treatment is, very simply, lay-open technique or excision, and primary closure.

### Primary Versus Secondary Fistulotomy

There is some controversy as to whether a lay-open procedure should be performed at the same time as the incision and drainage of an ischiorectal abscess. There are certain advocates of primary fistulotomy.[1,14,25] However, since one-third of the patients will never have a further problem, it would seem that a primary lay-open technique would be unnecessary in the same proportion of patients.[33] In addition, if these abscesses are drained under local anesthesia, this temptation does not arise. Consequently, we do not recommend immediate fistulotomy and have the support of others.[21,32,33]

### How Much Muscle May Be Cut?

In simple intersphincteric or low transsphincteric fistulae, division of muscle caudad to the track usually does not significantly jeopardize anal continence. With the more complex fistulae, the dilemma is how to obtain adequate treatment of the fistulae without causing incontinence. It must be accepted, however, that to obtain healing in the more complex problems, some loss of muscle function is inevitable; the aim is to minimize it.

TABLE **8-1.** Reported Results of Primary Closure of Anorectal Abscesses

| AUTHOR | NUMBER OF CASES | ANTIBIOTICS | RECURRENCE RATE OF ABSCESS OR FISTULA |
|---|---|---|---|
| *Ellis, 1958*[9] | ? | Penicillin & Streptomycin | 20% |
| *Wilson, 1964*[36] | 100 | Lincomycin & Clindamycin | 22% |
| *Jones & Wilson, 1976*[18] | 23 | Lincomycin & Clindamycin | 14% |
| *Goligher, 1976*[12] | 110 | Ampicillin & Cloxacillin | 7% |

As a general rule, the whole of the internal, and most of the external sphincter, may be cut in the posterior quadrant, with the exception of the puborectalis muscle, without any serious loss of function.[32] Unfortunately, this is not true in all cases because all patients' sphincter function is not equal. For instance, in an elderly person with a weak external sphincter, division of only the internal sphincter may result in partial incontinence. For this reason, it is essential to assess the state of the sphincter muscles preoperatively. Where there is doubt regarding the competence of the sphincter, it is wise to divide it in stages at successive operations, a careful assessment being made of its state in the conscious patient after each stage. In women, division of a large amount of muscle, especially anteriorly, is more likely to result in loss of function.

### Fistulotomy Versus Fistulectomy

In performing fistula surgery, our very strong preference is a fistulotomy over a fistulectomy. There are several reasons for this. First, removal of the complete track and adjacent scar tissue will only result in appreciably larger wounds. Second, there would be a greater separation of the ends of the sphincter which would lead to a longer healing time and greater chance of incontinence (Fig. 8-29).

### Seton

This is simply the utilization of a nonabsorbable suture placed through the track to encircle the sphincter muscle below. The rationale for this maneuver is threefold. The first aim is the stimulation of fibrosis adjacent to the sphincter muscles so that when the second stage, which involves the laying open of the track is completed, the sphincter will not gape. This may have, in fact, already been accomplished by the fibrosis of the fistulous track. Another important benefit of the seton is that it allows the surgeon to better delineate the amount of muscle beneath the fistulous track. With the patient anesthetized, the pelvic floor is relaxed. One cannot always be sure of the amount of muscle caudad to the track. With the patient awake, reexamination may reveal that there is an adequate amount of muscle remaining not contained within the seton. A third advantage of the use of the seton is that it acts as a drain (Fig. 8-30).

This technique is especially helpful in deal-

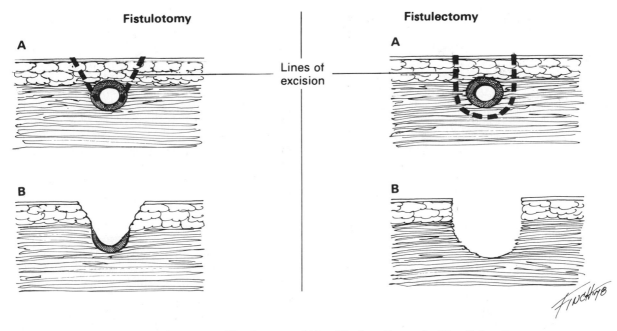

**Fistulotomy**

A

B

**Fistulectomy**

A

B

Lines of excision

FIGURE **8-29.** *Fistulotomy vs. Fistulectomy. (After Hanley, P., et al.: Dis. Colon Rectum. 19:513, 1976)*

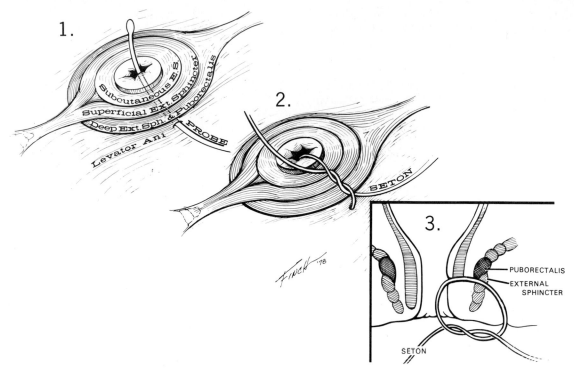

**FIGURE 8-30.** *Seton insertion. (After Goldberg, S. M., and Nivatvongs, S. Principles of Surgery, Ed. Schwartz, S. M., p 1245. N.Y., McGraw-Hill, 1979)*

ing with high level fistulae. With anterior fistulae, especially in women, where there is no puborectalis muscle, placement of a seton will help preserve continence. Setons are left in situ for six to eight weeks but may be left in place for several months. Residual muscle will require division after adequate fibrosis has occurred if fistula healing does not occur. If the wound does heal well, the seton can be removed without division of contained muscle.

Seton materials vary. A nonabsorbable suture, such as silk or nylon inserted and tied loosely, is commonly used. Numerous knots are tied to create a handle for manipulation of the seton. The patient is instructed to manipulate the seton to promote fibrosis.[15] Some surgeons prefer to use wire and twist it at intervals, thereby cutting through the muscle. Hanley recommends an elastic seton, tightened at two to three week intervals until it transects the muscle. This slow division and scarring ensures preservation of sphincter function.

Parks and Stitz found that assessment of

function in 68 patients in whom a seton was employed, revealed that 17 per cent of those having the seton alone complained of partial loss of control as compared with 39 per cent in the group that later had a division of the seton-enclosed muscle.[30] This finding emphasized the importance of conserving as much muscle as possible, even though it means extending the time taken for healing to occur. In view of such data we feel that it is most reasonable to run the higher risk of recurrence by not dividing the contained muscle in patients in whom the wound is healing satisfactorily.

Buls and colleagues* found a high degree of success utilizing a staged operation with setons in trans- and suprasphincteric fistulae.[4] They operated on 43 patients with excellent results in regard to continence, and there was no recurrences.

The level of the fistulous track is the critical factor in determining postoperative conti-

* Unpublished communication, 1977.

nence. Appropriate timing of transection of the sphincter subsequent to seton placement is essential for sufficient fibrosis to ensure sphincter function.

## Key Factors in Morbidity and Mortality

Significant morbidity and mortality may accompany anorectal infections for a number of reasons. First, a delay in diagnosis and treatment of any infection permits wider dissemination of the infection, and morbidity and mortality from infection are usually time and dose related.

Inadequate examination frequently leads to inadequate treatment. The diagnosis of a perianal or ischiorectal abscess is straightforward, but in the patient with severe pain who may be harboring an intersphincteric abscess, a general anesthetic may be required for adequate examination. When the differentiation between a fissure-in-ano and intersphincteric abscess is impossible, examination under anesthesia should be done to rule out the abscess.

Bevans and co-workers found a number of associated systemic diseases that were associated with anorectal suppuration.[3] The six disease processes most frequently noted were diabetes mellitus, blood dyscrasias, organic heart disease, chronic renal failure, hemorrhoids, and previous abscess or fistula.

In rare instances, anorectal suppuration may assume life threatening proportions. Abcarian has pointed out that this may be attributed to: delay in diagnosis and management; virulence of the organism, especially gas forming anaerobic bacteria; bacteremia and occurrence of metastatic infections; and, underlying disorders (e.g., diabetes mellitus, blood dyscrasias).[1]

The lethal potential of this disease was well described by Marks and associates in their report of 11 deaths related to fistula-in-ano with abscess, seven in the acute stage and four in the chronic form.[23] To prevent death, they recommend immediate incision and drainage, complete debridement ignoring form and function, adequate anesthesia, and preoperative antibiotic loading. These, of course, are cases of extensive suppuration which involved perineum, buttocks, thigh, and even abdominal wall. Death seemed to be associated with inanition and its complications, and therefore nutri-

tional support is demanded. Colostomy may be indicated in these cases. Repeated debridement under anesthesia may be indicated, and should be carried out without hesitation.

## Rationale of Repeat Examination Under Anesthesia

In the exceptional case where a fistula is complicated by high upward extensions to the apex of the ischiorectal fossa or the supralevator fossa, one must ensure that sound healing occurs from the apex caudad. To achieve this goal, one should not hesitate to reexamine the patient a week to ten days following the initial surgery, in the operating room, and under general anesthesia. If at these times healing is progressing satisfactorily, nothing needs to be done except the curettage of excessive granulation tissue which has formed. If pocketing has occurred, this can be corrected, or if further branched tracks are discovered, they can be opened. The upward extension of a track must heal soundly before the caudad part of the wound is allowed to heal. If at any point the surgeon is dissatisfied with the healing, especially if pus is found to be accumulating, examination in the operating room is indicated, and the wound may need to be enlarged and reshaped. Careful follow-up of extremely complicated fistulae may help prevent recurrence.

## Fistula-in-Ano and Cancer

Patients with long-standing fistulae or recurrent abscesses around the anus may, on exceedingly rare occasions, develop carcinoma. The rarity of this entity is further underscored by the fact that only 79 cases were reported in the literature up to 1975.[11] The commonest form of carcinoma to arise in a fistula is colloid carcinoma (44%), followed by squamous cell carcinoma (34%), and adenocarcinoma (22%).[19] It has been suggested that the colloid carcinomas arise in duplications of the lower end of the hind gut.[5] Should such a diagnosis be confirmed, abdominoperineal resection is required but the prognosis is nevertheless poor. In inoperable cases, radiotherapy may be of some value, especially in the cases of squamous epithelioma.

## Unnecessary Cryptotomy

In the past a frequently proposed adjuvant procedure has been the obliteration of the crypts along the dentate line. "Cryptotomy" or "cryptectomy" was carried out in the hopes of preventing development of inflammation, fissures, or abscesses. However, anyone with a sound understanding of the anatomical features of the anal canal and the pathogenesis of fistula, as described earlier in this chapter, readily realizes that such manipulation would not prevent disease but might, rather, contribute to it. We therefore feel that, since such procedures are in no way helpful and are potentially harmful, they should be abandoned.

### Associated Surgery

A hemorrhoidectomy may be performed in association with the treatment of fistula-in-ano. If, indeed, the patient has very large or prolapsing hemorrhoids, a hemorrhoidectomy would be indicated. However, one must individualize each case. It is also worth mentioning the complication of mucosal prolapse. It is not an infrequent consequence of extensive muscle division and is easily treated by injection, rubber band ligation, or operative excision.

### Septic Complications in Leukemic Patients

The occurrence of perianal complications such as ischiorectal abscess, fistula-in-ano, fissures, or infected thrombosed ulcerated hemorrhoids, in the leukemic patient poses a very special problem. Injudicious incision and drainage procedures in patients with acute leukemia or uncontrolled chronic leukemia can result in necrosis of the perineal area, accompanied by uncontrolled septicemia and hemorrhage, and may end up with sloughing of the whole buttock area and fecal incontinence. However, treatment with a small, well-placed incision should not be withheld if there is an obvious fluctuant abscess.

The policy evolved at Memorial Hospital for these extremely ill patients consists of two modalities of treatment.[34] The first combines radiation therapy consisting of 300 to 400 rads over one to three days and repetition a week later if induration persists or recurs, and symptomatic care consisting of sitz baths or warm compresses, stool softeners, analgesics, and broad spectrum antibiotics. This form of therapy is used in patients who have extremely depressed polymorphonuclear leukocyte counts, who are moribund, or whose lesions have established spontaneous drainage. The second mode of treatment combines radiation therapy, surgery, and symptomatic care. The most suitable candidates for surgical treatment are patients suffering from chronic forms of leukemia or acute leukemias which are in remission. Incision and drainage, fistulotomy, sphincterotomy, or hemorrhoidectomy can be performed in patients who have satisfactory white blood cell and platelet counts, although excessive bleeding may occur.

It is recommended that any leukemic patient who complains of pain in his perianal area should be assumed to have a perianal complication, and hence, started on precautionary measures including no rectal digital examination, instrumentation, or enemas. Symptomatic treatment should be instituted if he develops fever, redness, or induration.

### REFERENCES

1. Abcarian, H.: Acute suppurations of the anorectum. *In* Nyhus, L. M. (ed.): Surgery Annual. vol 8. 305. New York, Appleton Century Crofts, 1976.

2. Bennett, R. C.: A review of the results of orthodox treatment for anal fistula. Proc. R. Soc. Med., *55:*756, 1962.

3. Bevans, D. W., Westbrook, K. C., Thompson, B. W., and Caldwell, F. T.: Perirectal abscess, a potentially fatal illness. Am. J. Surg., *126:*765, 1973.

4. Buls, J. G. and Goldberg, S. M. (unpublished), 1977.

5. Dukes, C. E., and Galvin, C.: Colloid carcinoma arising within fistulae in the anorectal region. Ann. R. Coll. Surg. Engl., *18:*246, 1956.

6. Eisenhammer, S.: The internal anal sphincter and the anorectal abscess. Surg. Gynecol. Obstet., *103:*501, 1956.

7. ———: A new approach to the anorectal fistulous abscess on the high intramuscular lesion. Surg. Gynecol. Obstet., *106:*595, 1958.

8. Ellis, M.: The new treatment of ischiorectal abscesses. Univ. Leeds. Med. J., *2:*84, 1953.

9. ———: 1958 quoted by Goligher, J.C.: Surgery of the Anus Rectum and Colon. ed. 3. Springfield, Illinois, 1975.

10. Goligher, J. C.: Management of perianal suppuration. Dis. Colon Rectum, *19:*516, 1976.

11. ———: Surgery of the Anus, Rectum and Colon. Charles C Thomas Publisher, 3d. ed. Springfield, Ill., 1975.

12. Goligher, J. C., Ellis, M., and Pissidis, A. G.: A critique of anal glandular infection in the etiology and treatment of idiopathic anorectal abscesses and fistulas. Br. J. Surg., *54:*977, 1967.

13. Gordon, P. H.: unpublished data, 1977.

14. Hanley, P. H.: Conservative surgical correction of horseshoe abscess and fistula. Dis. Colon Rectum, *8:*364, 1965.

15. ———: Rubber band seton in the management of abscess-anal fistula. Ann. Surg., *187:*435, 1978.

16. Hanley, P. H., Ray, J. E., Pennington, E. E., and Grablowsky, O. M.: A ten-year follow up study of horseshoe-abscess fistula-in-ano. Dis. Colon Rectum, *19:*507, 1976.

17. Hill, J. R.: Fistulas and fistulous abscesses in the anorectal region; personal experience in management. Dis. Colon Rectum, *10:*42, 1967.

18. Jones, N. A. G. and Wilson, D. H.: The treatment of acute abscesses by incision, curettage, and primary suture under antibiotic cover. Br. J. Surg., *63:*499, 1976.

19. Kline, R. J., Spencer, R. J. and Harrison, E. G. Jr.: Carcinoma associated with fistula-in-ano. Arch. Surg., *89:*989, 1964.

20. Lilius, H. G.: Investigation of human fetal anal ducts and intramuscular glands and a clinical study of 150 patients. Acta Chir. Scand. (Suppl)., 383, 1968.

21. Lockhart-Mummery, H. E.: Anorectal Problems: Treatment of Abscesses. Dis. Colon Rectum, *18:*650, 1975.

22. Marks, C. G. and Ritchie, J. K.: Anal fistulas at St. Mark's Hospital. Br. J. Surg., *64:*84, 1977.

23. Marks, G., Chase, W. V. and Mervine, T. B.: The fatal potential of fistula-in-ano with abscess: analysis of 11 deaths. Dis. Colon Rectum, *16:*224, 1973.

24. Mazier, W. P.: The treatment and care of anal fistulas: A study of 1,000 patients. Dis. Colon Rectum, *14:*134, 1971.

25. McElwain, J. W., MacLean, M. D., Alexander, R. M., Hoexter, B. and Guthrie, J. F.: Experience with primary fistulectomy for anorectal abscess; a report of 1,000 cases. Dis. Colon Rectum, *18:*646, 1975.

26. Milligan, E. T. C. and Morgan, C. N.: Surgical anatomy of the anal canal with special reference to anorectal fistulae. Lancet, *2:*1213, 1934.

27. Morson, B. C. and Dawson, I. M. P.: Gastrointestinal Pathology. 609. London, Blackwell Scientific Publications, 1972.

28. Parks, A. G.: Pathogenesis and treatment of fistula-in-ano. Br. Med. J., *1:*463, 1961.

29. Parks, A. G. and Gordon, P. H.: Perineal fistula of intraabdominal or intra pelvic origin simulating fistula-in-ano; report of seven cases. Dis. Colon Rectum, *19:*500, 1976.

30. Parks, A. G. and Stitz, R. W.: The treatment of high fistula-in-ano. Dis. Colon Rectum, *19:*487, 1976.

31. Parks, A. G. and Thomson, J. P. S.: Intersphincteric abscess. Br. Med. J., *2:*537, 1973.

32. Parks, A. G., Gordon, P. H. and Hardcastle, J. D.: A classification of fistula-in-ano. Br. J. Surg., *63:*1, 1976.

33. Scoma, J. A., Salvati, E. P. and Rubin, R. J.: Incidence of fistulas subsequent to anal abscesses. Dis. Colon Rectum, *17:*357, 1974.

34. Sehdev, M. K., Dowling, M. D., Seal, S. H. and Stearns, M. W.: Perianal and anorectal complications in leukemia. Cancer, *31:*149, 1973.

35. Steltzner, F.: Die Anorectalen Fisteln. Berlin, Springer-Verlag, 1959.

36. Wilson, D. H.: The late results of anorectal abscess treated by incision, curettage and primary suture under antibiotic cover. Br. J. Surg., *51:*828, 1964.

# 9

# Pilonidal Sinus

In 1880, Hodges coined the term "pilonidal sinus" to describe the chronic sinus, containing hair, found between the buttocks (*pilus,* hair; *nidus,* nest).[4] He thought the basis of the condition was a congenital coccygeal dimple in which detached body hair and debris lodged. The average patient with pilonidal disease is a hirsute, moderately obese man in his second or third decade. However, people of both sexes and any age can be affected. There may be a history of repeated trauma to the gluteal region. Hairs are frequently found in the cyst or protruding from the sinus opening. This finding is pathognomonic of pilonidal disease and is responsible for its name.

## GENERAL PRINCIPLES
### Etiology

It was once thought that the etiology of pilonidal disease was congenital due to either ectodermal inclusions or remnants of the neural canal becoming separated.[7,9] However, King's research showed that hairs present in the sinuses have their roots nearest the opening; and Patey and Scarff described recurrent pilonidal sinus after wide and extensive excision, and the presence of pilonidal sinus in the interdigital cleft of barbers.[6,12] As a result of these findings the theory that the condition is acquired has become generally accepted. It is suggested that the rolling movement between the surface of the buttocks at the natal cleft may result in hair being twisted into a bundle

With collaboration of Steven E. Olchowski

which may drill its way obliquely into the skin. These hairs continue to grow, penetrate the skin and subcutaneous tissue, and eventually may become detached from the skin surrounding the opening. Unfortunately, on careful examination of the hairs usually found in a pilonidal sinus, the root end seems to be directed to the base of the sinus. Just how this occurs is not clear.

There are several aspects of the disease which are not explained adequately by the acquired theory: often the hair within the pilonidal sinus is much longer than the hair of surrounding skin; a pilonidal sinus may be produced in an almost hairless person. However, observations such as the isolated reports that pilonidal sinus occurs in unusual positions like the umbilicus, the healed amputation stump, and interdigital clefts, and the recurrence of the disease in an adequately excised area, all support the acquired etiology of this disease. Furthermore, pilonidal sinuses are more likely to occur in the hirsute patient. It is a very uncommon problem in the Chinese who have relatively little hair in the sacral region.

### Surgical Pathology

The main feature of a pilonidal sinus is the primary, midline tract which may be lined with squamous epithelium. This tract extends into the subcutaneous tissue for a variable distance, usually 2 to 5 cm. There may be small abscess cavities or branching tracts coming off the primary tract. These may rupture. The abscess cavity and secondary tract are usually lined with granulation tissue. Often hairs which are usually disconnected from the surrounding skin are seen projecting from the sinus opening. These hairs generally lie with their bases directed toward the depth of the sinus tract. It is uncertain whether hair follicles are present in the epithelial lining itself. Most pathologists would say they are absent or, at best, very difficult to find.

The pilonidal cavity is situated in the midline and has a longitudinal direction in most of the cases. It varies in length from 1 to 15 cm. The walls of the pilonidal cavity are composed of dense fibrous tissue.

Secondary tracts may lead from the pilonidal sinus cavity into the surrounding subcutaneous tissue, and may discharge onto the skin. Their openings have a different appearance from the primary midline ones in that they are marked by elevations of granulation tissue, partly covered by thin epithelium, and discharging seropurulent material. Secondary tracts extend laterally and may be bilateral. They may also extend in a cephalad direction or, occasionally, caudally toward the anus.

There have been isolated case reports of carcinoma developing in a pilonidal sinus or cavity.[3]

## Clinical Presentation

Pilonidal disease may present as an acute abscess at the base of the spine. It may rupture spontaneously or require incision by a physician. This process may recur many times. Eventually a chronic sinus develops with at least one, but usually multiple, openings. Often hair may be noted projecting from the opening. The area underlying the sinus opening is generally indurated and may be painful. The patient may present to the physician with either the complaint of acute pain and swelling in the sacrococcygeal region, which would be suspicious of a pilonidal abscess, or with chronic staining of his undergarments and a moderately or mildly painful area in the intergluteal fold. The patient may also state that this problem seems to wax and wane, which would lead one to suspect a pilonidal sinus. Other patients present with a totally asymptomatic sinus which periodically drains. Frankowiak and Jackman noted a special tendency for the disease to involve overweight men, and also observed that hirsute people were more likely to be affected.[2] In 85 per cent of cases of pilonidal infection, men are affected.[7] Pilonidal infections are rare in people under the age of 15 years, rise sharply to peak between 16 and 20 years, and remain high until age 25 when the incidence declines quickly.

*Pilonidal Sinus Complicated by Carcinoma.* Up to 1965 only 21 cases of pilonidal malignancy had been reported in world literature. Nearly all of them have been squamous cell carcinoma.[3] Another two cases were reported in 1973.[13] Treatment is consistent with the principles pertaining to carcinoma of the skin elsewhere (i.e., wide local excision).

## Diagnosis

Usually the diagnosis of this condition is made quite easily. The patient's history suggests the problem. A painful and fluctuant mass is the most common presentation of the acute process. In its earliest stage only a cellulitis may be present. In the chronic state the diagnosis is confirmed by the sinus opening in the intergluteal fold, approximately 5 cm above the anus. The sinus tract generally runs cephalad, but on occasion may run caudad and be confused with a fistula-in-ano or hidradenitis suppurativa. The differential diagnoses that must be considered include any furuncle in the skin, an anal fistula, specific granulomas such as syphilitic or tuberculous, and osteomyelitis with multiple draining sinuses in the skin. Actinomycosis in the sacral region has been described as virtually indistinguishable from pilonidal disease. When a pilonidal sinus is suspected, the diagnosis should be confirmed by the finding of a ray fungus in the smears of the discharge or in a culture.

## TREATMENT
### Incision and Drainage

The best treatment for the majority of patients with a pilonidal abscess is incision and drainage under local anesthesia. Simple incision and drainage is preferred over definitive treatment because of the presence of infection and marked hyperemia of adjacent tissues. With the patient in the prone or lateral position, 0.5 per cent lidocaine or 0.25 per cent bupivacaine with 1 : 200,000 epinephrine solution is injected with a fine needle into the skin overlying the fluctuant area. A cruciate incision is made over the most fluctuant or tender area. Specimens for culture and sensitivity may be obtained. The four corners of the cruciate incision are excised to allow more adequate drainage. Hemostasis is achieved by electrocoagulation when necessary, or light gauze packing. A dressing is applied, instructions in the proper technique of warm baths are given, and regular follow-up visits are discussed with the patient.

The abscess should be drained as soon as it is diagnosed. Antibiotics are not a substitute for surgical drainage, but occasionally may be indicated to treat accompanying cellulitis or other conditions in selected patients (diabetes, valvular heart disease, or immunodeficiency). If the abscess has not reached the fluctuant stage, the area of cellulitis which is most prominent should be drained. Relief of the pain is dramatic and patients may return to work as soon as they feel comfortable. If the situation is such that the abscess cannot be drained adequately under local anesthesia, the patient should be transferred to the operating room where a marsupialization of the abscess should be carried out.

The postoperative care of the patient with a pilonidal abscess consists of: examining him approximately every two weeks, shaving him, and having him abrade the wound with a washcloth during his daily shower. Once the wound is less painful, the surgeon can curette any excessive granulation tissue that has formed.

### Indications for Definitive Surgery

After adequate healing of the abscess has taken place, definitive surgery on the chronic pilonidal sinus may be performed. Many of these abscesses may not require definitive surgery since they will heal per primum. The need for definitive surgery can generally be ascertained at one to two months.

### Methods Available for Treatment of Chronic Pilonidal Sinus

*Marsupialization.* No one method of treatment of pilonidal sinus has proven completely successful. Because it is simple, and equally efficacious to other treatment modalities, the

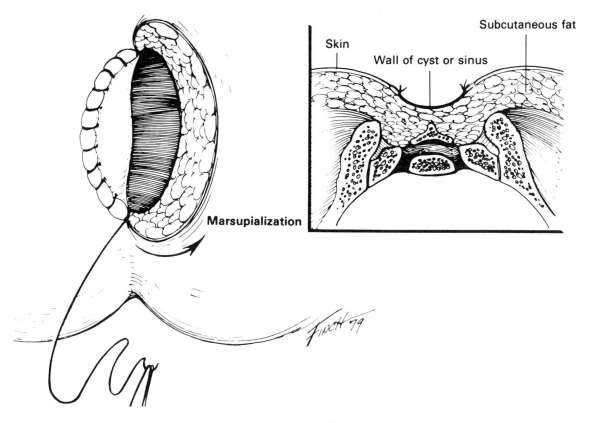

FIGURE **9-1.** *Marsupialization.*

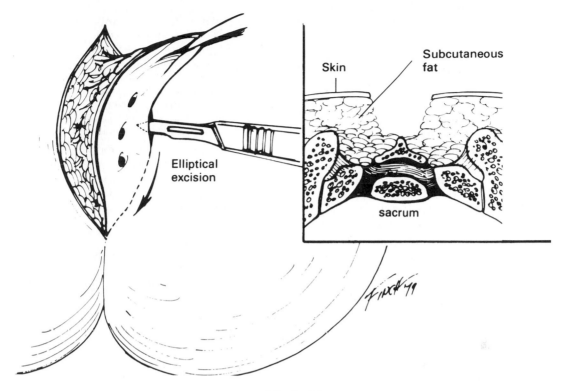

Skin

Subcutaneous fat

Elliptical excision

sacrum

FIGURE **9-2.** *Excision.*

preferential treatment for pilonidal sinus is the marsupialization technique. This surgical method of management was popularized by Buie, and consists of excising the anterior portion of the cyst wall and the overlying skin, or incising the tract and suturing the cut edges of the remaining cyst or tract to the adjacent skin edges (Fig. 9-1).[1] This procedure has been justified because of the observation that the remaining cyst wall lining undergoes re-epithelialization and soon assumes the characteristics of the adjacent skin epithelium. Lateral tracts are followed to their termination and are marsupialized in a similar fashion. Chromic catgut, polyglactin, or polyglycolic acid sutures work nicely for this procedure. The patient's hospital stay is usually limited to one, or at the most, two days. Indeed, many of the simpler pilonidal problems may be operated upon under local anesthesia on an outpatient basis. The advantages of this procedure are that it obviates an extensive wound, it reduces the period of convalescence, and reduces the percentage of recurrence. In a series

of 400 cases reviewed by Schottler, the hospital stay averaged 1.7 days for the patient who had a marsupialization versus an average stay of 3.4 days for the patient with block excision. The healing time was also shortened, and the incidence of recurrence was 3.2 per cent.*

*Complete excision of the sinus tract* and varying amounts of surrounding tissue is the technique used by many surgeons. It involves a wide elliptical incision surrounding the sinus tract and all of its branches and sharp scalpel dissection or electrocoagulation to the fascia overlying the sacrum and coccyx (Fig. 9-2). A common modification of this technique involves outlining the sinus tracts by simple incision over the probe in the main sinus tract and all of its branches, or by methylene blue injection. All of the diseased tissue is excised from the surrounding normal tissue, leaving a 0.5 to 1 cm cuff of normal tissue on the sinus tracts.

* Schottler, J. L.: unpub. data, 1975.

*Phenol Injection of Tract.* Maurice and Greenwood, in 1964, recommended a non-operative method of treatment.[10] With the patient anesthetized, the tract is injected with phenol. The phenol serves to destroy epithelium, sterilize the tract, and remove the imbedded hair. One or several milliliters of 5 per cent phenol are injected, taking great care to protect the patient's skin and the surgeon's eyes. The patient remains in the hospital for 36 hours. Following the injection there is soreness for a few days. The region may be kept shaved. Stephens and Sloane reported good results in 30 patients so treated and followed for six to twelve months.[16] Shorey reported similar good results using this method.[15]

## Postoperative Care

Using the open technique to manage the wound is very simple. The patient is instructed to keep a fluffy gauze dressing in place, to keep the edges separated, and the base as flat as possible. The dressings are maintained in position by the undergarment: this prevents skin irritation by frequent application of tape. Local hygiene is stressed. It is important that the wound edges be pulled apart. The wound must be kept from bridging over; but if it occurs, bridging is broken down with a cotton applicator. If there is excessive hair in the area, shaving may be necessary. Excessive granulation tissue is removed either with a curette or with silver nitrate applications. The wound must be followed regularly until complete healing has occurred. No antibiotics are necessary in the pre- and perioperative period when the open technique is used.

Primary closure is advocated by some authors in selected cases; however, we have found little application for this technique, which may result in delayed healing and possible re-infection.[11,15]

## The Unhealed Wound

Occasionally a patient is left with an unhealed wound. This may be handled by frequent curettage in the office or clinic. The technique advocated by Rosenberg of reverse bandaging, which keeps pressure on the wounds, has worked to promote the healing of their wounds.[14] A modification of this technique includes the use of montgomery straps.

The use of a Water Pik is simple and practical.[5] Skin grafting or Z-plasty has rarely been necessary to correct an unhealed wound. Some authors have advocated the use of zinc to promote wound healing.[8]

## Recurrent Pilonidal Disease

The treatment of a recurrent pilonidal sinus should be similar to the primary operation (i.e., marsupialization). It is as effective as any other treatment and is very simple. No attempt needs to be made to totally re-excise a recurrent pilonidal sinus and close the defect by suture or flaps.

## REFERENCES

1. Buie, L. A., and Curtiss, R. K.: Pilonidal disease. Surg. Clin. North Am., *32:*1247, 1952.

2. Frankowiak, J. J., and Jackman, R. J.: The etiology of pilonidal sinus. Dis. Colon Rectum, *5:*28, 1962.

3. Gaston, E. A., and Wilde, W. L.: Epidermoid carcinoma arising in a pilonidal sinus. Dis. Colon Rectum, *8:*343, 1965.

4. Hodges, A. M.: Pilonidal sinus. Boston Med. Surg. J., *103:*465, 1880.

5. Hoexter, B.: Use of Water Pik lavage in pilonidal wound care. Dis. Colon Rectum, *19:*470, 1976.

6. King, E. S. J.: Nature of pilonidal sinus. Aust. NZ. J. Surg., *16:*182, 1947.

7. Kooistra, H. P.: Pilonidal sinuses: Review of literature and report of 350 cases. Am. J. Surg., *55:*3, 1942.

8. Lee, P. W. R., Green, M. A., Long, W. P., et al: Zinc and wound healing. Surg. Gynecol. Obstet., *143:*549, 1976.

9. Mallory, F. B.: Sacrococcygeal dimples, sinuses and cysts. Am. J. Med. Sci., *103:*263, 1892.

10. Maurice, B. A., and Greenwood, R. K.: A conservative treatment of pilonidal sinus. Brit. J. Surg., *51:*510, 1964.

11. Notaras, M. J.: A review of three popular methods of treatment of postanal (pilonidal) sinus disease. Br. J. Surg., *57:*886, 1970.

12. Patey, D. H., and Scarff, R. W.: Pathology of post anal pilonidal sinus: Its bearing on treatment. Lancet, *2:*484, 1946.

13. Puckett, C. L., and Silver, D.: Carcinoma de-

veloping in pilonidal sinus: Report of two cases and review of the literature. Amer. Surg., *39:*151, 1973.

14. Rosenberg, I.: The dilemma of pilonidal disease: Reverse bandaging for cure of the reluctant pilonidal wound. Dis. Colon Rectum, *20:*290, 1977.

15. Shorey, B. A.: Pilonidal sinus treated by phenol injection. Br. J. Surg., *62:*407, 1975.

16. Stephens, F. O., and Sloane, D. R.: Management of pilonidal sinus: A modern approach. Surg. Gynecol. Obstet., *129:*786, 1969.

# 10

# Perianal Dermatology

Primary perianal dermatological conditions, as well as secondary perianal involvement in systemic diseases, may present with a variety of symptoms and macroscopic appearances. The most frequent symptom encountered, however, is pruritus.[2] Consequently, it serves as the basis for the following discussion and classification.

## PRURITUS ANI

### Definition

Pruritus ani is an unpleasant cutaneous sensation characterized by varying degrees of perianal itching. Men are affected over women in a ratio of four to one.[16] When no underlying etiology can be identified, the condition is referred to as 'Idiopathic Pruritus Ani'. This occurs in approximately 50 per cent of the cases.[6] The remaining cases are merely the symptomatic presentations of either localized or systemic diseases (e.g., hemorrhoids, diabetes, etc.).

### Clinical Features

*History.* Symptoms usually start insidiously, and are characterized by an occasional awareness of an uncomfortable perianal sensation. Often the patient is more aware of the problem at night, or in the hot humid weather, although this is not always the case. With time the condition may progress to an unrelenting, intolerably tormenting, burning soreness, compounded by the insurmountable urge to scratch, claw, and otherwise irritate the area in a futile effort to obtain relief. The severely afflicted patient is eventually completely exhausted, and more than a few have been driven to suicide as the only means of obtaining relief.

Poor anal hygiene is often a contributing factor; therefore, careful questioning about the patient's cleansing habits is important. The association of certain dietary ingredients, food allergies, neurogenic, psychogenic, and idiosyncratic reactions with pruritus, mandates interrogation along these lines whenever no other factor is readily identified (see specific etiologies below).[4,6,7] Inquiries as to diabetes, antibiotic utilization, vaginal discharge or infection, acholic stools or dark urine, or anal intercourse may readily establish the factor(s) responsible for the symptom.

*Physical Findings.* In the early stages of the condition examination may reveal only minimal erythema and excoriations. As the symptoms progress the perianal skin becomes thin, friable, tender, blistered, ulcerated, and "weeping." In the later stages the skin is raw, red and oozing, or pale and thickened (lichenified), with exaggeration of the normal radiating folds. Often there is a secondary bacterial or fungal infection present.

Careful local examination may rapidly distinguish an inciting factor, or a more detailed examination of the entire patient, including adjunctive laboratory and radiological testing, may be required to diagnose a primary cause (e.g., blood glucose, electrolytes or barium enema). If one embarks upon a complicated

With collaboration of John D. Nicholson

treatment program before ruling out the multiple factors which may result in pruritus, a primary etiology may be overlooked. Rather than decreasing the misery of the patient, the condition may be made intolerably worse.

*Histopathology.* Initially there is epithelial intracellular edema and vesiculation. This progresses to hyperkeratosis and subsequent atrophy of the outer layers of the epidermis, sebaceous glands, and hair follicles. Finally, ulceration may supervene.

## Etiology

In the following conditions, pruritus is merely a symptom of the primary disease. Treatment is directed to the specific disease, with adjunctive general modalities employed as discussed below.

*Poor Hygiene.* This is often associated with the remainder of the diseases discussed in this section. Not infrequently, this is the only factor identified with cases labelled as "idiopathic." This in part reflects the anatomy of the patient (e.g., a deep natal cleft rendering the perianal region inaccessible to proper cleansing). In other cases, the patient is less than fastidious in cleansing himself, and the retained mucus, sweat, and feces serve to initiate the process which is irritating the perianal skin. In a few patients crippling or disabling diseases such as arthritis, strokes or multiple sclerosis render the individual physically incapable of performing adequate perianal hygiene.

*Anorectal Lesions.* Any lesion in the gastrointestinal tract that can cause excessive moisture in the perianal region may result in pruritus. Hemorrhoids, anal fissures and fistulae, hypertrophied papillae, prolapse, and neoplasms are some of the more frequent offenders. Treatment should be directed to the pathology present, as discussed elsewhere in this book.

*Infections* can be caused by parasitic, viral, bacterial, and fungal and yeast sources. A discussion of the most common of these conditions, and their treatment is outlined below.

PARASITES. The most common cause of perianal itching in children is infestation with Enterobius vermicularis, or **pinworms.** The child, however, can be the source of infesting an entire family. The worms emerge from the anal canal at night, and consequently this is when the patient is most aware of the symptoms. The diagnosis is made by microscopically identifying Enterobius eggs on an adhesive cellulose tape swabbed on the perianal region. Treatment consists of piperazine citrate (anterpar elixir) in doses varied according to age and weight.

The **pediculosis pubis,** or louse, is a parasite visible to the naked eye; under magnification it appears similar to the crab. One can readily observe the nits embedded in the hair. Treatment consists of one or two showers with gamma benzene hexachloride (Kwell), and the complete sterilization of clothing and bedding by boiling.

*Scabies* is a parasitic infestation which is characterized by itching on the arms, legs and scrotum before the development of pruritus ani. As the parasite burrows, it creates dark punctate lesions, which are readily identified on the trunk, and particularly, between the fingers, and on front of the wrists. Treatment consists of Kwell showers, continued good hygiene, and cleansing of all clothing and bedding, again by boiling.

VIRAL. The most common viral infection in the perianal region is **condyloma acuminata,** and is discussed fully in Chapter 13.

Perianal presentation of *Herpes simplex* is rare, compared to its frequent presentation as "cold sores," fever blisters and genital infections. The mode of infection is usually sexual but the virus may be spread by direct contact from parent to infant or through the mouth and gastrointestinal tract.[15]

The incubation time is usually two to seven days, but may be up to three weeks, with prodromal symptoms consisting of minimal burning, irritation, or paresthesias. The infection is characterized by severe pain and pruritus with a serous or purulent discharge. Tenesmus and secondary spasm are common. The pain may radiate to the groin, thighs, and buttocks.

The initial lesion is a small vesicle with a surrounding erythematous areola. Within 24 to 48 hours the roof ruptures, and an ulcer results. This ulcer may become confluent, appearing as an ulcerating cellulitis. The lesions are distributed in equal frequency among the perianal skin alone, the anal canal alone, or both. If the patient has never had a herpes infection, systemic symptoms (e.g., fever, chills, malaise) are common.

The diagnosis is usually made by history and physical examination alone. Adjunctive methods include cytology, immunofluorescence, viral culture and serology.

The disease is usually self-limiting in one to three weeks if there is no secondary bacterial infection. Treatment is primarily symptomatic as discussed under idiopathic pruritus ani. Steroids are never used, as they may potentiate the infection. Specific treatment such as autoimmunization, vaccines, and idoxuridine (5-IOdO-2'-deoxyuridine) have been largely unsuccessful. Topical diethyl ether was recently shown to be ineffective in the treatment of genital herpes.[5] To date, photoinactivation with a heterocyclic dye (neutral red, proflavine 1%), and an incandescent light has been the most successful treatment.[10]

Lumbosacral dermatomes are involved in 11 per cent of patients with **herpes zoster**.[13] The causative virus is H-Varicellae with a variable incubation period. The first manifestations are fever, pain, and malaise. After three to four days the characteristic, closely-grouped, red papules appear, and they become vesicular quickly. Inguinal lymphadenopathy is common.

Sacral zoster may result in retention and sensory loss of both the bladder and rectum.[11] This can be seen even with unilateral skin involvement, which is somewhat perplexing in view of the fact that hemisection of the cord does not result in detectable sphincter dysfunction.

Treatment is mainly symptomatic. Complete spontaneous recovery over three to four weeks is the usual course. Postherpetic neuralgia is the most common sequela.

BACTERIAL. *Erythrasma* caused by Corynebacterium minutissimum, may affect the perianal and axillary regions, but is most common in the toe-webs. The characteristic pruritic perianal lesion is usually a large round patch, initially pink and irregular, but subsequently turning brown and scaly. The diagnosis is readily made by examining the lesions under ultraviolet light and observing the characteristic fluorescence secondary to porphyrin production by the bacteria. Treatment

consists of 250 mg of erythromycin, four times per day, for a 10 to 14 day period.[7]

Pruritus is caused in the patient with **syphilis** by the irritation secondary to exudates from the primary or secondary lesions. It is most uncommon in the tertiary stage, when there usually is no gross lesion.[4] This disease is more fully discussed in Chapter 12.

*Perianal tuberculosis* may present either as an ulcer with a sharp irregular outline and a grayish granular base, or as a purulent ulcerated verrucous lesion. It may also present as extensive perianal inflammation with areas of healing and breakdown, subcutaneous nodules, sinuses, and deformity. Pain is minimal, but soreness and pruritus are common. Generally the colon is also involved, and the diagnosis is made by having an antecedent history of tuberculosis, a positive chest radiograph, or identifying acid-fast organisms in scrapings from the lesions. With modern day treatment these lesions are relatively rare, and when they are present are readily conquered. The reader is referred to a standard medicine textbook for details of antituberculosis drug management.

FUNGAL AND YEAST. *Candida Albicans,* a saprophytic yeast, is normally present on the skin and in the gut. With a change in the patient's resistance or the normal environment (e.g., uncontrolled diabetes mellitus, prolonged antibiotic treatment, or prolonged use of steroids), these can become pathogenic. The skin appears moist, red, and macerated. Pustules form and become confluent, bright red, scaly, and sharp with well defined edges. Under microscopic scrutiny mycelial forms and spores can be identified from scrapings.

Treatment consists of mycostatin powder or ointment several times daily, along with controlling or eliminating the precipitating cause (e.g., control of diabetes, withdrawal of antibiotics and/or steroids).

*Epidermophyton and tricophyton rubrum* are fungal infections which usually present unilaterally with well marked, bizarre, or circinate edges, a scaly outline, and chronicity. Often, a similar lesion is seen between the toes. Diagnosis is confirmed by scrapings. Treatment is achieved with various fungicidal preparations, such as 0.5 per cent Whitfield's salicylic acid ointment or tinactin. It is important to eradicate any interdigital lesions to achieve a cure.

*Skin Diseases.* These lesions may be localized to the perianal region, or be systemic. It is imperative to examine the patient's entire body for evidence of further lesions whenever a dermatological condition is being investigated.

CONTACT DERMATITIS. These highly irritating, eczematous, ill-defined lesions are often the result of prolonged exposure to lanolin, neomycin, procaine, and "parabens." Topical anesthetics of the "caine" family may be especially irritating. Often the hand with which the patient applies the offending agent is similarly affected. The skin appears intensely erythematous and fragile, with thin perianal tissues.

The overuse of topical steroids is a particular problem, resulting in "steroid skin". The perianal skin develops marked striae. Overgrowth with candida is common, but can be prevented by limiting the duration and strength of the steroid ointment used. Prolonged use of the fluorinated steroid preparations results in atrophy of the perianal skin which leads to the symptoms for which the preparation was initially being prescribed.

PSORIASIS. This affliction has no known etiology. The lesion is usually a full, rich red color, sharply demarcated, often macerated, scaling plaque. The skin is thickened and pruritus is common. Because of the moisture in the intergluteal region the characteristic psoriatic plaque may not be present. Instead a paler, more poorly defined, non-scaling lesion may result. The lesions may be treated with fluocinolone acetonide 0.025 per cent cream (Synalar), flurandrenolone (Cordran), or fluocinolone cream in a coal tar base.[12]

LICHEN SIMPLEX. Lichenification is a thickening of all layers of the epidermis. Initially the skin appears red and edematous. In the later stages it evolves into a well-demarcated, erythematous, scaly thickened area. The diagnosis is confirmed by biopsy. There is no specific treatment other than the general symptomatic methods previously discussed.

LICHEN PLANUS. It is common for this dermatological condition to commence in the perianal region, and spread to more distant regions in its later stages. The lesions are shiny, flat-topped plaques with a darker pigmentation than is usually seen in the more distant lesions. Occasionally a more severe bullous form may occur, and be mistaken for secondary syphilis. The etiology is not known. Treatment is with bland, wet dressings, sitz baths, and a low concentration steroid cream.

LICHEN SCLEROSIS. This disease predominates in women over men in a ratio of five to one.[13] Etiology is unknown but often a preceding history of vaginitis is present. Ivory colored, atrophic papules frequently break down exposing a red, edematous, raw surface which leads to intense pruritus and soreness. As the edema subsides, it is replaced by sclerosis and chronic inflammation. The diagnosis is confirmed by skin biopsy. The condition is chronic, with exacerbations and remissions. There is no known effective cure. Estrogen-containing creams used in conjunction with the usual symptomatic treatments may aid in relieving the pruritus.

PEMPHIGUS VEGETANS. This variant of pemphigus may present either as early bullae later giving way to hypertrophic granulations studded with pustules and blisters, or early pustules later developing into warty vegetations. The former presentation is always accompanied by oral lesions and is known as the Hallopeau type. Both types are treated with oral steroids, the dosage being titrated to the response of the disease and the patient's tolerance.

*Diarrheal States.* Multiple loose stools can produce pruritus by causing a localized skin irritation secondary to the chemistry of the liquid stool itself. Also, trauma from frequent and vigorous cleansing further results in producing excoriating, weeping, itching lesions.

*Dietary.* Ingredients such as cola, coffee (decafeinated as well as cafeinated), chocolate, tomatoes, beer, and tea have been implicated as inciting factors of pruritus.[6] Certainly, individual allergies to certain foods can result in itching in various portions of the anatomy.[7] Occasionally, one finds that it is merely the volume of the ingredient ingested that produces loose watery stools and mucous discharge, rather than any inherent characteristic of the individual ingredient. This is seen more with liquids than with solids.

*Gynecologic.* Any inflammatory or ulcerative lesion of the vulva can lead to pruritus (e.g., Bartholin adenitis, lymphogranuloma venereum, Granuloma inguinale, syphilis, lichen sclerosis, or cancer). Kraurosis, a condition in which there is loss of the vulvar fat, is often characterized by scratching.[3] Irritation secondary to an increased vaginal discharge may also lead to pruritus, and mandate a work-up to identify the underlying cause (e.g., infection, foreign body such as an intrauterine contraception device, neoplasm, etc.).

*Antibiotics* may lead to pruritus either as a result of an allergic reaction or by altering the indigenous flora of the bowel or gynecological tract. This may result in an overgrowth of otherwise harmless bacteria or fungi, and lead to either diarrhea, increased vaginal discharge, or simply a perianal superinfection, particularly with monilia. Tetracycline is a notable offender.[7]

*Systemic Diseases.* Occasionally pruritus will be the presenting symptom of an otherwise distant or systemic disease. Severe jaundice from any cause is notoriously associated with itching. Diabetes, by virtue of its association with moniliasis, not infrequently has pruritus as its presenting symptom.

*Miscellaneous.* Any factor that results in irritation to the perianal skin can lead to pruritus. These may be quite apparent, such as postirradiation, or more nebulous, such as neurogenic, psychogenic, or idiosyncratic reactions.[4]

## Idiopathic Pruritus Ani

If after a comprehensive work-up no specific cause for pruritus can be identified, the condition is labelled as idiopathic. Often the only finding is increased moisture in the perianal region. Therapy is nonspecific and often involves multiple changes over the course of time, as outlined below.

*Treatment.* Whenever a specific disease entity is identified, therapy is directed toward that entity. Therefore, the remainder of this discussion is directed toward treating idiopathic cases.

REASSURANCE. Since, by definition, idiopathic pruritus ani has no identifiable primary etiology, treatment is mainly symptomatic and directed to decreasing moisture in the perianal area. Reassurance to the patient that there is no underlying pathology, particularly cancer, is often as effective in producing a "cure" as any of the physical or medicinal modalities employed. Often these patients have a long protracted course, and a sympathetic, reassuring approach is necessary to ultimately achieve success.

ADJUNCTIVE MEASURES. Patient education is very important. They are instructed to cleanse several times daily, especially after bowel movements. If infection is present, one-half ounce of Clorox added to a sitz bath may aid in relief.[16] Although cleanliness is stressed, the use of medicated soaps in the perianal region is discouraged. In the acute, excoriated, weeping, and crusting stage, warm wet packs may aid in debridement. The patient is then told to dry himself very gently with either a soft towel, or preferably, a hair-blower. A simple acid pH cream or lotion such as calamine or carbolic lotion 1 : 100 is then applied.[7] A dilute steroid such as .025 per cent fluocinolone acetonide (Synalar), or coal tar cream is utilized if lichenification is present. As the condition improves, or in the milder forms, creams and lotions are replaced with cornstarch powder or talc. A small wisp of absorbent cotton is tucked into the natal cleft to aid in keeping the area dry.

It has been suggested that coffee (including decaffeinated blends), tea, colas, chocolate, beer, and tomatoes are best avoided totally for at least two weeks, but such deletions are not universally helpful.[6] If the pruritus disappears, deleted foods are returned to the diet one at a time. If the pruritus recurs, the offending ingredient is immediately withdrawn. If the patient has "after leak," characterized by stinging, burning, or perianal "crawling" sensation superimposed on the itch following a bowel movement, he is instructed to irrigate the rectal ampulla with a bulb syringe. Following this procedure he is to cleanse the perianal area with a wet tissue while straining down and opening the anal canal. This process is continued until there is no brown stain left on the tissue.

Other nonspecific therapy includes shaving extremely hirsute patients. However, as the hair grows back, the short stubbles can be a source of irritation and increase the urge to itch, defeating the original gains. Extreme cases may require sedation and/or antihistamines such as Benadryl 25 mg four to six times per day. Estrogens may prove of some use in post-menopausal women.[16] Loose fitting clothes, and undergarments made of cotton may also be helpful. If a secondary bacterial or fungal infection is present, topical antibiotics or fungicides may be instituted based upon cultures and sensitivity.

In the past, various methods such as tattooing with mercury sulfide, sclerotherapy, radiation therapy, and surgical procedures have been used. These methods are now condemned, as they seldom result in a permanent cure.

FOLLOW-UP. Initially, patients with severe disease may require visits as frequent as twice per week. Reassurance and visible concern is often the most important part of therapy at this time. As symptoms improve, the time between visits can be gradually lengthened until the patient is seen once every three to four weeks. It is important not to discontinue seeing a patient using a steroid cream, as over-utilization can lead to the development of "steroid skin", superinfection, and a secondary pruritus (see above: contact dermatitis).

Often, there is a waxing and waning of symptoms, and achieving a cure is based more upon changing therapy, coupled with positive psychological reinforcement, than upon the actual agent(s) used. Constant re-iteration of the goals to be achieved and the methods to achieve them may be necessary. Finally, the physician should always be ready and willing to reassess the patient whenever there is any suggestion that there may be a more specific entity responsible for producing the symptom of pruritus.

## NON-PRURITIC LESIONS

Although pruritus ani is the most common presenting symptom of perianal dermatological conditions, many lesions do not present with pruritus, or this symptom is only of minor importance. In this section some of these diseases will be discussed.

### Infections

*Hidradenitis suppurativa.* This infection of the apocrine glands is more fully described in Chapter 30.

*Tropical Diseases.* LEPROSY. In patients with good resistance to microbacterium lepra, infection is often localized with lesions appearing as macules or plaques with healed central areas surrounded by erythematous or copper-colored extensions. The lesions favor the face, exterior surfaces of the limbs, the buttocks, and the back, and are often preceded by anesthesia secondary to early nerve damage.

If the individual has poor resistance, the skin lesions can occur anywhere including the perineum, and appear as small, circular, erythematous or copper-colored, smooth, shiny macules. Nerves are damaged late and, consequently, anesthesia always follows the development of the skin lesions.

The diagnosis is confirmed by skin biopsy scrapings from cutaneous lesions, or skin tests. Treatment is with diaminodiphenylsulfone (Dapsone, 4-4' diaminodiphenyl sulfone), clofazine, or rifampin (Rifamate). The reader is referred to textbooks on tropical medicine for further details.[3]

AMEBIASIS. This disease is caused by the protozoan, Entamoeba histolytica. Perianal manifestations consist of painful serpiginous ulcers with red vegetating bases covered by a white pseudomembrane. Therapy is instituted with metronidazole (Flagyl).[1,9,14] See Chapter 30 for further details.

ACTINOMYCOSES. This rare lesion is caused by Actinomyces hominas, an anaerobic, nonacid-fast fungus. A brawny, leathery infiltration of the skin accompanied by proctitis, abscesses, and fistulae is seen. The diagnosis is confirmed by identifying characteristic "sulfur" bodies with club-shaped rays in the discharges from the sinus. Treatment consists of penicillin and local symptomatic measures.

*Vegetating, Granulomatous and Stricturing Lesions.* LYMPHOGRANULOMA VENEREUM (LYMPHOGRANULOMA INGUINALE) is a disease caused by a sexually transmitted virus. In its advanced stage, the perianal region is deformed with widespread scarring and vegetating lesions. Periproctitis often results in a stricture 5 to 10 cm from the anal margin, around which fistulae develop. See chapter 12 for further details.

**Neoplastic Lesions**

Various neoplastic lesions are found in the perianal region. Several are mentioned below, but the reader is referred to Chapter 14 for their specific therapy.

*Acanthosis Nigricans.* This lesion is often associated with underlying bowel cancer. It appears as a velvety black, acantholytic papillomatous lesion, and is found in the axillary region as well as the perianal region. A complete gastrointestinal work-up is warranted to rule out any underlying neoplasm.

*Bowen's disease* is an intraepidermal carcinoma which it appears as a yellowish scale that is easily detached, leaving a reddened, granular surface. (see Chap. 14).

*Squamous Cell Carcinoma.* This lesion can be misdiagnosed as condyloma acuminata. It is a warty, nodular plaque that may or may not be ulcerated. Maceration and secondary infection is common, often masquerading the true nature of the disease. The diagnosis is confirmed by biopsy.

*Malignant melanoma* may occur in the perianal region, as well as the anus or rectum. The prognosis, even with abdominoperineal resection, is dismal.

*Perianal Paget's Disease.* This extramammary presentation of Paget's disease is rare. Grow et al report a 76 per cent association of perianal Paget's disease with subjacent or bowel carcinomas.[8] The lesion presents as a progressive, erythematous, eczematoid plaque. Because of the frequent association of underlying neoplasms, the prognosis is not good. However, if after wide excision no subjacent or bowel malignancy is found, the prognosis is good but local recurrence is not uncommon.

**Inflammatory Bowel Disease**

Anal lesions are present in approximately 25 per cent of patients with Crohn's ileitis and 75 per cent of patients with Crohn's colitis; they may precede the intestinal manifestation by several years.[13] Dusky, perianal sinuses with undermining ulcers or edema, indolent single or multiple fissures, and fistulae may be some of the early signs. The diagnosis can be made by biopsy, but extensive surgical procedures in the face of active disease are strongly condemned because the healing is notoriously poor. See Chapter 13 on Inflammatory Bowel Disease and Fistulae for further details.

## REFERENCES

1. Ahmed, T., Ali, F., and Sarnar, S. G.: Clinical evaluation of Tinidazole in amoebiasis in children. Arch. Dis. Child., *51:*388, 1976.
2. Alexander, S.: Dermatological aspects of anorectal surgery. Clin. Gastroenterol., *4:*651, 1975.
3. Bahr, Sir P. H. Manson: *Manson's Tropical Diseases.* 16 ed., London, Bailliere, Tindall and Cassell, 1966.
4. Buie, L.: *Practical Proctology,* 2 ed. Springfield, Charles C Thomas, 1960.
5. Corey, L., Reeves, W. C., Chiang, W. T., Ventuer, L., Remington, M., Winter, C., Holmes, K. K.: Ineffectiveness of topical ether for the treatment of genital herpes simplex virus infection. N. Engl. J. Med., *200:*237, 1978.
6. Friend, W. G.: The cause and treatment of idiopathic pruritus ani. Dis. Colon Rectum, *20:*40, 1977.
7. Goligher, J. C.: *Surgery of the Anus, Rectum and Colon,* 3 ed. Springfield, Charles C Thomas, 1975.
8. Grow, J. R., Kshirsagor, V., Tolentino, M., Gramling, J., and Schulte, A.: Extramammary perianal Paget's disease: A report of a case. Dis. Colon Rectum, *20:*436, 1977.
9. Islam, N., and Hanson, M.: Tinidazole in the treatment of intestinal amoebiasis. Curr. Ther. Res., *17:*161, 1975.
10. Jacobs, E.: Anal infections caused by herpes simplex virus. Dis. Colon Rectum, *19:*151, 1976.
11. Jellinek, E. H., and Tullock, W. S.: Herpes zoster with dysfunction of bladder and anus. Lancet, *2:*1219, 1976.
12. Lockridge, E., Jr.: Pruritus ani—Perianal psoriasis. South. Med. J., *62:*450, 1969.
13. Rook, A., Wilkinson, D. S., and Ebbing, F. J. G., (ed.): *Textbook of Dermatology.* Ox-

ford, and London, Blackwell Scientific Publications, 1969.

14. Seragg, J. N., Ribidge, C. J., and Protor, E. M.: Tinidazole in treatment of acute amoebic dysentery in children. Arch. Dis. Child., *51:*385, 1976.

15. Sheward, J. C.: Perianal herpes simplex. Lancet, *1:*315, 1961.

16. Sullivan, E. S., and Garnjobst, W. M.: Pruritus ani: A practical approach. Surg. Clin. North Am., *58:*505, 1978.

# 11

# Inflammatory Conditions of the Anorectum

The anorectum is an area frequently afflicted with a variety of inflammatory diseases. These may be nonspecific or specific conditions. Few conditions affect the anorectum exclusively; hence, in all cases the clinician should be alert to the fact that the disease process seen at the lower end of the alimentary tract may be a manifestation of a much more extensive intestinal or systemic illness.

## NON-SPECIFIC INFLAMMATIONS
## "Cryptitis and Papillitis"

Many patients present with a variety of vague, nonspecific symptoms referrable to their anorectum. Usually, on examination, no abnormality is found and all that is required in the way of treatment is reassurance, especially as to the absence of malignant disease. In some patients, normal-appearing but deep anal crypts and/or enlarged seemingly swollen anal papillae will be in evidence. In the past these patients have been diagnosed as having cryptitis or papillitis and the symptoms complained of have been ascribed to these apparent abnormalities. Indeed treatment, designed to destroy these "abnormalities", often with special instruments, has been advocated. It must be emphasized that these falsely labelled abnormalities are nothing more than normal anatomical variants and no relevance should be ascribed to their presence. At the same time, it should also be emphasized that cryptoglandular infection is the basis of the vast majority of

With collaboration of John G. Buls

perianal suppuration and fistula-in-ano.[19] The anal crypts may also be the site of specific infections, notably gonorrhea.

### Hypertrophied Anal Papilla

The anal papillae may enlarge in relation to diseases of the anal canal. Classically this occurs with a chronic anal fissure, but also may be part of hemorrhoidal disease.[21] Under such circumstances treatment is directed toward the underlying disease.

Nonspecific enlargement of anal papillae can also occur. This problem usually afflicts a single papilla which can become considerably enlarged. Patients present with a complaint of a lump in the anus, which often prolapses at the time of defecation. The precise cause for this condition is unknown. The disease is sometimes called fibrous anal polyp; however, it must be remembered that it is in no way associated with colorectal neoplastic polyps. No treatment is necessary, except if the patient is symptomatic, treatment consists of simple excision, usually as an office procedure done under local anesthesia. A very large hypertrophied anal papillae may require excision in the operating room.

### Anorectal Manifestations of Nonspecific Diarrhea

Any condition in which diarrhea is part of the problem will produce anorectal inflammations of a nonspecific type. Perianal excoriations, pruritus ani, and acute superficial anal fissures are very common. Proctosigmoidoscopy will often reveal minimally edematous and inflamed rectal mucosa. Similar appearances can be produced by enemas and vigorous bowel preparation. These changes are the result of the diarrhea, not the cause of it. Antibiotic therapy is a potent cause of diarrhea which, in the extreme, can be fulminating. Proctosigmoidoscopy in such instances usually shows nonspecific changes of varying severity. On occasion a pseudomembrane is formed; this is the classical abnormality of antibiotic related diarrhea (pseudomembranous colitis). This is readily recognized on proctosigmoidoscopy, and confirmed by biopsy and histopathology.[5]

Treatment of all these problems is obviously directed towards correcting the underlying disease which produces the diarrhea. In cases of antibiotic related diarrhea, cessation of the antibiotic is mandatory. In most situations the disease is self-limiting with spontaneous resolution occurring. Some patients require specific treatment such as vancomycin.[24] Resolution can take from a few days to several weeks; hence supportive care, especially nutrition and fluid, and electrolyte balance, is important. In all patients specific infection, notably amebiasis, should be excluded.

## SPECIFIC INFLAMMATIONS

The incidence of both specific and non-specific inflammations is very much related to geographical and social factors. In all developed areas of the world inflammations of the nonspecific variety are quite common, while those caused by specific infections are rare. In underdeveloped or developing areas the reverse is true: specific, and often seemingly exotic infections predominate.

### Nonspecific Mucosal Ulcerative Colitis

Nonspecific mucosal ulcerative colitis, a disease of unknown etiology, by definition, commences in, and almost always involves, the rectum. The resulting proctitis is, therefore, part of a spectrum of proctocolitis of varying extent and severity. Diagnosis of the condition is made on proctosigmoidoscopic observation and biopsy. A wide spectrum of appearances can be present. The mildest changes are those of edema, mucous discharge, and loss of the mucosal vascular pattern. More severe disease manifests as granularity, inflammation, and friability of the mucosa with contact bleeding. In extremely severe cases, the mucosa is denuded and spontaneous hemorrhage is evident. In all grades of the condition the changes commence at the dentate line and extend proximally into the rectum and colon in a continuous manner. By definition, colitis is present if the proximal extent of the changes cannot be seen on proctosigmoidoscopy. Macroscopic ulcers are rarely seen.

Anal and perianal disease is relatively common in this condition, but is of a nonspecific type, brought about by the diarrhea generated by the underlying proctocolitis. Perianal excoriations, acute anal fissures, and irritation or aggravation of hemorrhoidal disease are all commonly seen. In rare instances perianal suppuration and fistula-in-ano may also occur; however, under such circumstances one should suspect Crohn's disease which can mimic and be indistinguishable from nonspecific mucosal ulcerative colitis. Therapy for this condition varies depending upon the severity and extent of the disease. Most patients are managed by nonoperative means with a combination of medications including corticosteroids and sulfasalazine (Azulfidine). Fulminating patients, patients resistant to medication, or those with longstanding disease, require proctocolectomy for cure. This condition is premalignant, particularly in patients who have had the disease since a young age, have total colonic involvement, and who have carried the disease more than ten years.[10] In those in whom random rectal biopsy shows dysplasia, proctocolectomy is advisable as prophylaxis against colorectal carcinoma.

### Nonspecific Mucosal Ulcerative Proctitis

The mildest form of a wide spectrum of disease denoted as proctocolitis is nonspecific ulcerative proctitis. Patients present in good general health with episodic, bloody, mucous diarrhea. This condition may be aggravated by tenesmus of varying degrees. Quite often such patients are of nervous or anxious disposition, and clasically have exacerbation of their symptoms at times of particular stress. Examination reveals the same changes or proctitis that are discussed above; however by definition, the upper extent of rectal involvement is readily visible on proctosigmoidoscopy.

Management of these patients is relatively simple. If the upper extent of the disease is readily apparent, treatment can be undertaken immediately. If this is not so, or if there is doubt, a barium enema, possibly supplemented by colonoscopy and mucosal biopsy, is indicated to accurately document the extent of colonic involvement. It is important to distinguish this condition from ulcerative colitis as the prognosis and outlook are totally different. All patients must be reassured that the condition is one of proctitis, and that, although it is similar to colitis, it carries with it none of the commonly associated complications and stigmata. Classically the disease is characterized by spontaneous remission, therefore, assessment of treatment modalities is very difficult. At the present time the most popular form of therapy is short-term use of corticosteroid suppositories or retention enemas. These may be supplemented by the use of Azulfidine, but convincing evidence of its efficacy is lacking. Recent work has indicated that it is the salicylic acid component of Azulfidine which is effective in initiating remissions in cases of inflammatory bowel disease. As a consequence of this research, salicylic acid enemas are under trial for the treatment of this and other similar conditions. In a recent study it has been estimated that patients with ulcerative proctitis have a 10 per cent chance of the disease spreading to the proximal colon over a period of ten years.[6] There has been no information which would suggest that patients with this condition have a higher than usual chance of developing rectal cancer. Indeed the total prognosis of the condition is excellent; hence, it is very important to distinguish this disease from universal colitis with its inherent bad outlook.

### Crohn's Disease

Crohn's disease is a disease of unknown etiology which can afflict any portion of the alimentary tract. The anus and perianal areas are no exceptions. In 25 per cent of patients with small bowel involvement, 75 per cent of patients with colonic involvement, and almost all patients with rectal involvement, anal lesions of a variety of types will be in evidence at some stage during the patient's illness.[13] In 9 to 24 per cent of patients, the anal lesions preceded the onset of intestinal symptoms.[2,9,14]

*Manifestations*. Crohn's disease can cause problems in the anorectal area in a variety of ways. These should be considered as a spectrum of manifestations rather than separate disease entities. Even with severe and extensive disease elsewhere, the anorectum may be entirely spared.[12] One of the main intestinal disturbances brought about by the disease is diarrhea. As in other diarrhea states nonspecific anal problems can occur. These consist of perianal skin excoriation, often with pruritus ani; acute and usually multiple superficial anal fissures; and, initiation or aggravation of hemorrhoidal disease due to repeated straining. Direct involvement of the perianal skin produces a classical discoloration consisting of a blue cyanotic hue which, once seen, characterizes the disease. Further involvement results in areas of edematous perianal skin accompanied by large, fleshy edematous skin tags which usually take on the characteristic blue discoloration. Chronic anal fissures, or more correctly anal ulcers, are present in patients with more severe involvement. These ulcers may take on a variety of appearances. In many cases they may be indistinguishable from a nonspecific anal fissure. However, the classical lesion is large, eccentric, indolent, and often multiple. The edges are undermined and the skin changes described previously are usually also present. Some authors classify these lesions as painless. This is certainly not the case; however, the degree of discomfort and pain is sometimes less than would be expected from appearance of the lesion.

Perianal suppuration is another manifestation of the problem. This may take the form of a simple perianal abscess, but more often than not, more complex infection involving multiple tissue planes is present. Under such circumstances, associated lesions such as ulcers and/or fistulae often coexist. Unlike mucosal ulcerative colitis, Crohn's disease is a relatively common initiating cause of fistula-in-ano. Simple fistulae can, and do, occur but frequently the problem is one of complex fistulae (horseshoe) which may involve several perianal and perirectal tissue planes. Fistulization into surrounding organs is possible. The vagina, urethra, and bladder may be involved, as may the subcutaneous tissues at considerable distance from the anus. Such widespread sepsis and fistula formation can lead to destruction of the anal sphincter mechanism and result in incontinence. In certain patients, all the problems outlined can coexist. This would be regarded as the severest form of anorectal Crohn's disease.

Operative procedures which result in the production of anorectal wounds may bring covert Crohn's disease to light. Failure to heal hemorrhoidectomy, fistulotomy, or fissure operation wounds should alert the clincian to the possibility of underlying Crohn's disease. All patients who present with anorectal problems associated with diarrhea, even of a minor nature, must have inflammatory bowel disease excluded before any operation on the anorectal problem is undertaken.

*Management.* It is important when discussing this problem to emphasize that anorectal Crohn's disease should not be considered as a disease in isolation since it occurs as the sole manifestation of the whole problem in less than 5 per cent of patients. The backbone of therapy is one of conservatism.[12]

In all cases or suspected cases, it is imperative to accurately establish the extent of alimentary tract involvement. A complete history and physical are required to bring to light seemingly minor symptoms and signs of bowel disturbance. All patients need proctosigmoidoscopy and a barium enema. In many cases this procedure should be supplemented by an upper gastrointestinal series and small bowel follow through barium studies, often accompanied by colonoscopy. Further investigation, in the form of hematology and blood biochemistry is determined by the individual case.

Most patients with perianal problems related to the diarrhea of Crohn's disease can obtain relief when, and if, the diarrhea is controlled. This usually requires a variety of medications including corticosteroids, Azulfidine and antibiotics.[11] In severe cases bowel rest and total parenteral nutrition may be necessary. Operative treatment is undertaken if conservative therapy fails, or if a complication ensues. It is a commonly held belief that surgical excision of a segment of active disease, especially of the small bowel, will result in remission of anal Crohn's problems. This is true only in that in many cases the

excision results in control of diarrhea, hence nonspecific anal conditions will be ameliorated. There is no supported published evidence that excision of the more proximal bowel Crohn's disease will heal the anal lesions.[1]

PAINFUL ANAL FISSURE is a distressing problem. In all cases it is mandatory to control diarrhea by the most effective means suited to the case. Local anesthetic ointments may be used; however, these are usually ineffective. If it is considered that no other site of disease exists, in particular in the rectum, more active treatment may be undertaken. The simplest, safest, and most effective operation is that of lateral partial internal sphincterotomy. This is best performed as an open procedure. It must be remembered that one always runs the risk of the wound failing to heal, thereby making the situation worse. If one takes the precautions discussed previously, the chances of this occurring are reduced.

PERIANAL SUPPURATION occurs relatively commonly in the natural history of this condition. In all cases of abscess formation immediate incision and drainage are indicated. For the majority of patients this can be performed under local anesthesia as an office procedure. It is important to ensure a wide unroofing of the abscess cavity to provide adequate and complete drainage. A complex abscess (horseshoe) requires drainage under general anesthesia in an operating room. Such an abscess is often extensive, and widely infiltrative and destructive. Although there is a chance of the resulting wounds failing to heal, the problem of a painless, discharging wound is a better alternative to painful, often deep-seated perianal or ischiorectal infection. Only under rare circumstances, as with intersphincteric abscess, should it be necessary to divide any portion of the anal sphincter mechanism. Any degree of anal incontinence could make the already precarious situation far worse. Antibiotics alone have a limited role in the initial management of perianal suppuration. They are not indicated for the defined abscess. In cases of indolent disease there have been anecdotal reports of remissions induced by long term, low dose, broad spectrum, antibiotic therapy.[17] Although this is far from proven it would be recommended as a trial prior to operation being undertaken in cases where the alternative therapy is proctectomy.

FISTULA-IN-ANO is the chronic phase of perianal suppuration, and in patients with Crohn's disease is often complex, involving different tissue planes and causing varying degrees of sphincter involvement and destruction. Accepted radical treatment under such circumstances exposes the patient to the risk of inducing or worsening anal incontinence. At the same time, it must be emphasized that other patients with Crohn's disease suffer from simple and superficial fistula-in-ano. In these cases a fistulotomy is indicated for relief of symptoms. If no rectal disease exists the risk of worsening the situation is minimal. The majority of such fistulae are of the intersphincteric type; therefore, fistulotomy involves division of only the distal portion of the internal anal sphincter. The less common transsphincteric and the rare suprasphincteric fistulae create problems in management because fistulotomy for cure involves division of varying proportions of external anal sphincter. If the rectum is uninvolved a two-staged operation using a seton may be indicated. Such a procedure has the advantage of allowing the external component of the fistula to be unroofed and heal without division of the anal sphincters. Moreover, if this event occurs it indicates that the second stage of the operation, in which the sphincter is divided, would also, probably result in wound healing. However, as pointed out in Chapter Eight, the seton might be removed at this stage with little or no further division of the sphincter mechanism, thereby maintaining continence. If the healing process does not occur, the seton can be removed and the patient has not had further impairment of anal continence. Extrasphincteric fistula-in-ano associated with Crohn's disease invariably indicates active rectal involvement. For such patients proctectomy offers the only chance of control. If minimal symptoms result from such a situation then acceptance, along with medical therapy including antibiotics, may be satisfactory. This is usually a temporary measure as flareups and worsening will invariably follow, necessitating surgical excision. Supplemental therapy with elemental diet may be of benefit to some patients. Proximal diversion with loop ileostomy, or sigmoid colostomy may offer alternative forms of management.

RECTOVAGINAL FISTULA is yet another manifestation of Crohn's disease involving the rectum. If it is small it can be accepted without specific therapy.[25] More severe cases can be managed by bowel rest and total parenteral nutrition as an adjunctive treatment.[8] Medication including corticosteroids, Azulfidine, and low dose antibiotics may also be used.[11] In all cases, the disease is rarely kept in long term check by these means, and proctectomy is usually required. Surgical repair of such a fistula almost invariably breaks down, and usually results in worsening of the situation.[25] If such management is undertaken it may hasten acceptance of the necessary proctectomy.

SPHINCTER DESTRUCTION AND INCONTINENCE are the end result of progressive, severe perianal suppuration.[9] In most cases it accompanies continuing intestinal, usually rectal, Crohn's disease. The only sure way of relieving the situation is proctectomy with excision and drainage of the chronically infected perianal tissue spaces. In patients reluctant to accept this, particularly those in the difficult situation with minimal or no bowel disturbance, more conservative treatment may be considered. Total bowel rest with total parenteral nutrition supplemented by corticosteroids, Azulfidine and low dose antibiotics may result in amelioration and healing in some cases. This is a temporizing situation: recurrence invariably occurs. Proximal diversion with loop ileostomy or sigmoid colostomy may be offered.

PROCTECTOMY IN PATIENTS WITH INFLAMMATORY BOWEL DISEASE is rarely indicated as an isolated procedure. In almost all cases the procedure is performed as part of a total proctocolectomy and ileostomy. In the past there has been a reluctance to advocate proctectomy in young patients, particularly men, because of the fear of producing sexual disturbance by damaging the pelvic autonomic nerves. If the procedure is performed with this in mind and the techniques modified, the risk is minimal. In the cumulative data collected by Corman, the evidence of impotence is 4 per cent.[3] These results are obtained if the proctectomy is performed by staying close to the bowel wall during dissection in the pelvis. To prevent the creation of a large perineal wound a technique involving dissection of the anal canal in the intersphincteric plane, rather than encompassing the sphincter mechanism, has been advocated by Lyttle and Parks.[15] Packing or vigorous suction in the pelvis should be avoided. Such modification of technique is time consuming and may involve more than usual blood loss; however, the good results outweigh these objections. The problem of sexual dysfunction has not been studied in young, female patients and so this information is lacking. Another common problem after this operation is poor healing of the perineal wound. In 30 to 50 per cent of patients, healing will occur primarily if the wound is closed. Of the remaining patients, healing by secondary intention will occur in the majority, but it takes an average of 9 to 12 months. In a small proportion of patients complete healing does not occur, leaving them with a perineal sinus. Most patients with this problem accept it. In the few where it causes problems a variety of plastic procedures can be performed, but none has proved to be universally successful.

### Irradiation Proctitis

Irradiation proctitis is an iatrogenic condition which may affect patients undergoing irradiation therapy for diseases afflicting organs in close proximity to the rectum. The most common problem so treated is cancer of the cervix, but endometrial carcinoma and prostatic carcinoma are also managed in a similar way. The incidence of the problem is determined by several factors. The technique of irradiation therapy is important because radioactive implants which remain in situ for a long period of time are more likely to cause unavoidable irradiation damage to the adjacent rectum. Not only is the dose of irradiation critical in determining tissue effect, but also the time over which the dosage of irradiation is given has great significance.[18] The general health of the patient is another factor as patients with pre-existing vascular disease, notably atherosclerosis, hypertension, or diabetes,[4] are more likely to be affected.

The pathogenesis of the disease is ischemia. In the acute phase this is the result of nonspecific inflammation generated by direct radiation damage. This usually occurs a few days to several weeks after therapy began. In the chronic phase, obliterative endarteritis results in ongoing ischemia. Such changes may continue for many years after the initial radiation injury, and in fact, patients may not present with problems for a considerable period of time.

Symptoms in the acute phase are identical to those of any acute proctitis. These consist of rectal bleeding, diarrhea, and mucous discharge often associated with rectal pain and tenesmus. There may be associated irradiation enteritis with its accompanying profuse diarrhea. Late phases of the disease are characterized by ongoing proctitis often complicated by fibrotic rectal strictures and fistulae into the bladder or vagina.

Diagnosis of the condition can readily be made on proctosigmoidoscopy. It is important to know that the rectum has in the past been normal; hence, in all patients who are to undergo radiation treatment to the pelvis, a proctosigmoidoscopy should be part of the pretreatment work-up. Active disease is readily apparent as a proctitis of varying severity. The classical changes are maximal on the anterior rectal wall (the portion of the bowel in immediate proximity to the uterus or prostate). In most cases the changes are limited to the rectum; hence, an upper limit will be in evidence. The rectal mucosa may be edematous, erythematous, and friable. Mucosal necrosis with ulceration, especially anteriorly, is another common feature. More severe changes produce rectovaginal fistulae and strictures.[18] In such cases differentiation from malignancy is difficult, therefore, biopsy and histopathological examination are mandatory.

Treatment of patients with radiation proctitis is determined by the extent of involvement and severity of symptoms. In early phases of the illness, with minimal involvement and symptoms, all that is required is reassurance as most cases are self-limiting with complete spontaneous resolution. Patients with more severe symptoms may benefit from a short course of corticosteroid retention enemas or suppositories for seven days. As the disease is one of spontaneous remission the efficacy of steroid treatment is questioned. If these treatments fail to provide relief, a completely defunctioning end-sigmoid colostomy and mucous fistula in an area of non-irradiated bowel can be recommended.

After initial treatment, if the condition settles, re-establishment of bowel continuity is possible. In patients with complications such as rectovaginal fistula or rectal strictures, colostomy is frequently the only possible reliable operative procedure. Any definitive operation is difficult because of fibrosis and impaired blood supply to the bowel due to obliterative endarteritis. Resection and repair are fraught with danger of breakdown. In rare instances a very low coloproctostomy utilizing seemingly normal bowel is feasible. Adequacy of blood supply may be determined at the time of operation. If anastomosis is deemed possible it is made safer and more reliable by use of the end-to-end anastomosis (EEA) stapling device and a complementary colostomy. A proctectomy with a coloanal anastomosis and temporary, complementary transverse colostomy may also prove to be a satisfactory alternative.[20]

### Rare Perianal Infections

Rare perianal infections do occur in patients in North America from time to time and should always be considered when the clinical features of a particular anal complaint seem, in some way, to be atypical.

*Tuberculosis* affecting the anorectum as a primary disease is exceedingly rare even in areas where the disease is common. It can present in several ways but the most frequent is an anal fissure or ulcer.[23] This is classically large, eccentric and atypical. These patients invariably have coexisting gastrointestinal or pulmonary tuberculosis. Diagnosis is confirmed by demonstrating caseating granulomata and acid-fast bacilli in the lesion. More severe local involvement results in large, complex abscesses and fistulae. Treatment in these cases involves drainage of abscesses and commencement of specific antituberculosis chemotherapy. In all cases cultures must be set up for confirmation of the diagnosis and establishment of drug sensitivities. Such information may not be obtainable for several weeks. If fistulae remain symptomatic after adequate antituberculosis therapy has been administered, they may be treated under antituberculosis cover as fistulae of cryptoglandular origin.

*Actinomycosis* usually produces chronic perianal suppuration and complex fistulae and sinuses.[7,16] This rare condition is often difficult to diagnose definitively. Sulphur granules may or may not be present. Treatment consists of drainage of abscesses and administration of antibiotics. Penicillin is the drug of choice.

*Schistosomiasis* (*Bilharziasis*) is included for completeness. It can mimic any condition affecting the anorectum; hence, can be confused with common lesions, notably cancer and Crohn's disease.[22]

*Amebiasis* rarely involves the anorectum in isolation. It should always be excluded in all cases presenting as a proctocolitis by biopsy and histology rather than stool culture. Classically, the disease produces macroscopic ulcers with undermined erythematous edges seen on proctoscopy; however, any form of proctitis may be seen. Ameboma is a localized form of the infestation which presents as a mass lesion. In the rectum it can be confused with malignancy.

## REFERENCES

1. Alexander-Williams, J.: Surgery and management of Crohn's disease. Clin. Gastroenterol., *1*:469, 1972.

2. Baker, W. N. W., and Milton-Thompson, G. J.: The anal lesion as the sole presenting symptom of intestinal Crohn's disease. Gut., *12*:865, 1971.

3. Corman, M. L., Veidenheimer, M. C., and Coller, J. A.: Impotence after proctectomy for inflammatory disease of the bowel. Dis. Colon Rectum, *21*:418, 1978.

4. DeCosse, J. J., et al: The natural history and management of radiation induced injury of the gastrointestinal tract. Ann. Surg., *170*:369, 1969.

5. DuPont, H. L.: Etiology of antibiotic-associated colitis. Gastroenterology, *75*:913, 1978.

6. Farmer, R. G.: Long-term prognosis for patients with ulcerative proctosigmoiditis (ulcerative colitis confined to the rectum and sigmoid colon). J. Clin. Gastroenterol., *1*:47, 1979.

7. Fry, G. A., Martin, W. J., Dearing, W. H., and Cult, C. E.: Primary actinomycosis of the rectum with multiple perianal and perineal fistulae. Mayo Clin. Proc., *40*:296, 1965.

8. Harford, F. J., and Fazio, V. W.: Total parenteral nutrition as primary therapy for inflammatory disease of the bowel. Dis. Colon Rectum, *21:*555, 1978.

9. Homan, W. P., Tang, C. K., and Thorbjarnarson, B.: Anal lesions complicating Crohn's disease. Arch. Surg., *111:*1333, 1976.

10. Lennard-Jones, J. E., Morson, B. C., Ritchie, J. K., Shove, D. C., and Williams, C. B.: Cancer in colitis: Assessment of the individual risk by clinical and histological criteria. Gastroenterology, *73:*1280, 1977.

11. Lennard-Jones, J. E., and Powell-Tuck, J.: Drug therapy of inflammatory bowel disease. J. Clin. Gastroenterol., *8:*187, 1979.

12. Lockhart-Mummery, H. E.: Crohn's disease: Anal lesions. Dis. Colon Rectum, *18:*200, 1975.

13. ———: Anal lesions of Crohn's disease. Clin. Gastroenterol., *1:*377, 1972.

14. Lockhart-Mummery, H. E., and Morson, B. C.: Crohn's disease of the large intestine. Gut., *5:*493, 1964.

15. Lyttle, J. A., and Parks, A. G.: Intersphincteric excision of the rectum. Br. J. Surg., *64:*413, 1977.

16. Morson, B. C.: Primary actinomycosis of the rectum. Proc. R. Soc. Med., *54:*723, 1961.

17. Moss, A. A., Carbone, J. V., and Kressel, H. Y.: Successful treatment of Crohn's disease with broad spectrum antibiotics: initial and long-term results. Gastroenterology, *72:*83, 1977.

18. Novak, J. M., Collins, J. T., Donowitz, M., Farman, J., Sheahan, D. G., and Spiro, H. M.: Effects of radiation on the human gastrointestinal tract. J. Clin. Gastroenterol., *1:*9, 1979.

19. Parks, A. G.: Pathogenesis and treatment of fistula-in-amo. Br. Med. J., *1:*463, 1961.

20. Parks, A. G., Allen, C. L. O., Frank, J. D., and McPartlin, J. F.: A method of treating post-irradiation rectovaginal fistulas. Br. J. Surg., *65:*417, 1978.

21. Schulte, A. G., and Tolentino, M. G.: A second study of anal papillae. Dis. Colon Rectum., *14:*435, 1971.

22. Stock, F. E., and Li, F. W. P.: Granulomas of the large bowel simulating malignant disease. Br. J. Surg., *51:*898, 1964.

23. Tandon, H. D., and Prakash, A.: Pathology of intestinal tuberculosis and its distinction from Crohn's disease. Gut., *13:*260, 1972.

24. Tedesco, F. J., Napier, J., Gamble, W., Chang, T. W., and Bartlett, J. G.: Therapy of antibiotic-associated pseudomembranous colitis. J. Clin. Gastroenterol., *1:*51, 1979.

25. Tuxen, P. A., and Castro, A. F.: Rectovaginal fistula in Crohn's disease. Dis. Colon Rectum, *22:*58, 1979.

# 12

# Sexually Transmitted Diseases of the Anorectum

During recent years, the anorectal region has been a major site of the increasing incidence of sexually transmitted diseases. Almost any venereal disease that affects the genitalia can also involve the anorectum. Anal sexual practices among male homosexuals account for the majority of cases; however heterosexual females can also contract these conditions by the act of sodomy, which appears to be on the increase in our society. It is often difficult to recognize that these patients practice such sexual variations since only a few of them fall into the effeminate stereotype group commonly associated with such behavior. Diagnosis is made more difficult by the fact that anorectal venereal diseases, except for condyloma acuminata, frequently simulate other more common nonvenereal conditions. It must also be remembered that it is not unusual for the patients to acquire more than one venereal disease simultaneously. The diseases commonly seen in this country are condyloma acuminata, gonococcal proctitis, herpes simplex, syphilis and nonspecific proctitis. Other venereal diseases, common in tropical climates, such as lymphogranuloma venereum, chancroid and granuloma inguinale are rarely encountered in the United States or Canada.

With collaboration of John B. Buls

## COMMON DISEASES

*Condyloma acuminata* are the most commonly seen sexually transmitted diseases and are discussed fully in Chapter 13.

*Gonococcal proctitis* is due to infection by the bacterium Neisseria gonorrhea and is transmitted by anal intercourse. The incubation period is five to seven days, after which a proctitis and/or cryptitis result. Contrary to popular belief, most patients with this problem are asymptomatic. Symptoms which cause presentation include painless purulent or mucopurulent anal discharge often associated with rectal bleeding. Rectal pain and tenesmus may occur, but perianal abscesses are infrequent. Examination reveals a nonulcerating proctitis with thick, purulent material in the lower rectum. Such changes never extend proximal to 8 to 9 cm above the dentate line. The diagnosis is confirmed by culture of the mucopus on Thayer-Martin medium using a cotton-tipped swab in the area of the anal crypts prior to any application of lubricant jelly or ointment. Gram stain is unreliable because in most cases negative results are obtained. In all cases a serological test for syphilis must be obtained prior to initiation of appropriate antibiotic therapy.

Recommended treatment is a single dose of

*150*

aqueous procaine penicillin G, four to eight million units intramuscularly, half in each buttock. One gram of probenecid should be given orally one half hour prior to the penicillin. Patients in whom penicillin is contraindicated may be treated with oral tetracycline HC1, 1.5 grams initially, then 0.5 grams every six hours for four days (total dose 9.5 grams). Some patients are unreliable in that they will not complete a course of oral medication so an alternative is 4 grams of parenteral spectinomycin given as a single, intramuscular injection.[2] All patients should have a follow-up culture seven days after treatment as a test for cure since resistant organisms are now appearing. Changes to the appropriate antibiotics may be necessary. All sexual contacts to gonorrhea should be prophylactically treated with the same antibiotic schedule.

*Syphilis* is an infection caused by a spirochete, Treponema pallidum. The anal region is a common site of this condition as it occurs in the United States. The incubation period is usually three to four weeks but can vary from nine to ninety days.[1] The initial lesion (primary lesion) is a chancre at the anal margin or the anal canal, which unlike its genital counterpart, is usually quite painful and, hence, often mistaken for an anal fissure or ulcer.[1] Such lesions, however, are usually atypical in that they are eccentric, multiple, and strange in appearance. An ulceration that docs not have the characteristics of a typical chronic anal fissure should always arouse the clinician's suspicion. Characteristically, "mirror image" ulcers off the midline are present. A chancre will heal and regress spontaneously without treatment in about six weeks. Bilateral inguinal lymphadenopathy is present in the majority of patients while the chancre is present. At the primary stage of the disease, the diagnosis is confirmed by demonstration of the Treponema pallidium from the wound by darkfield microscopic examination.[1] The specimen is obtained prior to any application of lubricant jelly, by gently scraping the base of the chancre and pipetting up serum, free of red blood cells, for immediate examination. Serological tests for syphilis do not become positive until the primary chancre has been present for a few weeks.[1] The second stage of anal syphilis will appear in untreated patients six to eight weeks following the healing of the chancre as a rash and/or a condyloma latum. These are pale brown or pink, flat, wart-like lesions which are teaming with spirochetes, and are considered to be the most infectious form of syphilis. Diagnosis is established by demonstrating the organisms from the lesions. Serological tests for syphilis will be positive in almost all cases, often at a high titre.[1] Late stage or tertiary syphilis may mascarade as a perianal problem. Tabes dorsalis can produce anal sphincter paralysis or lancinating rectal or low pelvic pain. Gummata may produce a mass lesion which could simulate a malignancy; however, this is rare.

Treatment of patients with primary, secondary or early tertiary syphilis is with a single dose of benzathine penicillin G, 2.4 million units intramuscularly, in one injection. If allergy to penicillin is known or suspected, tetracycline or erythromycin in a dose of 0.5 grams four times a day for 15 to 20 days may be substituted. All sexual contacts to primary, secondary and early latent syphilis should be prophylactically treated with the same schedule.[5]

*Herpes simplex* is caused by infection with Herpes virus Type II. The lesions frequently develop four to 21 days after intercourse.[1] Patients usually present with mild irritation of the anal area followed by severe pain associated with constitutional symptoms of viremia. Examination usually reveals marked tenderness in the area, with small vesicles and aphthous type ulceration in the perianal skin, anoderm or lower rectum. Bilateral tender inguinal lymphadenopathy is a common associated feature. Diagnosis can be confirmed by viral culture of vesicular fluid. No specific treatment is available but the condition is self limiting with resolution occurring in one to three weeks.[3] Symptomatic relief may be obtained by the use of analgesic drugs and the local application of soothing agents.

The most effective treatment for herpes infection on exposed surfaces has been the photo inactivation of the virus once it has been exposed to a heterotricyclic dye such as neutral red or proflavine, in a 1 per cent solution. If vesicles are present, it is important to rupture and unroof them with a needle before this treatment. The lesions should be painted thoroughly with the dye, then exposed to a 150-watt incandescent or 15-watt fluorescent light, at a distance of 15 to 20 cm, for ten minutes. Exposure to light is repeated a few hours later and again in 24 hours. This method can bring about symptomatic relief within 24 hours to patients suffering from herpetic infections on the lips, penis, and labia, unfortunately it becomes difficult in practice to apply this to the very painful lesion within the anal canal.[3]

*Nonspecific venereal proctitis* is a condition related to nonspecific urethritis which is a common association. The etiology is unknown; however, Chlamydia oculogenitale and Mycoplasma hominis have been implicated.[1] Patients present with mild anal pain, irritation and anal discharge but culture of anorectal swabs is negative for pathogens. Treatment is empirical and consists of tetracycline or oxytetracycline, orally, at a dose of 250 mg every six hours for five or 10 days.[1]

## RARE DISEASES

*Enteric pathogens* may be transmitted as a possible consequence of oro-anal, anogenital and genito-oral contact either separately or in sequence. Giardiasis, shigellosis, amebiasis, and hepatitis B virus are being reported with increasing frequency in homosexual males.[4]

*Anorectal trauma* as a result of anal intercourse or other sexual practices is being seen more and more. Healing will take place if reinjury is avoided. In rare instances complete disruption of the anal sphincter may occur in which case repair will be required. Rectal ulcers, classically situated anteriorly and longitudinally directed may be confused with neoplasm.[4] These are the result of rectal trauma and are usually inflammatory in appearance. If any doubt exists, biopsy is necessary to exclude malignancy. In all cases gonorrhea and syphilis should be ruled out.

Treatment is directed toward avoidance of reinjury which can be induced by a variety of means such as anal intercourse, fist fornication, and insertion of all manner of foreign bodies including enemas for the purpose of sexual gratification.

*Lymphogranuloma venereum* is a rare disease in temperate climate and industrial countries with a high standard of living. It is caused by Chlamydia group of organisms.[1] Although primarily the disease of genital organs, it can occur in the anorectum, especially among homosexuals, and lead to an ulcerative proctitis. Rectal stricture is the sequela to perirectal lymphatic involvement or direct involvement of the infective agent on the anorectal mucosa. The stricture is usually situated low in the rectum. The diagnosis is confirmed by the Frei test or a more sensitive complement fixation test. Treatment is 500 mg of tetracycline every six hours for 10 to 14 days.[1] In early stricture dilatation by finger or dilator is recommended. In the case of complete obstruction, a colostomy is indicated.

## REFERENCES

1. Catterall, R. D.: Sexually transmitted diseases of the anus and rectum. Clin. Gastroenterol., 4:659, 1975.
2. Fiumara, N. J.: The treatment of gonococcal proctitis: An evaluation of 173 patients treated with 4 g of Spectinomycin. JAMA, 239:735, 1978.
3. Jacobs, E.: Anal infections caused by herpes simplex virus. Dis. Colon Rectum, 19:151, 1976.
4. Marino, A. W. M., and Mancini, H. W.: Anal eroticism. Surg. Clin. North Amer., 58:513, 1978.
5. Minnesota State Department of Health Venereal Disease Control Program: Recommended Treatment Schedule for Sexually Transmitted Diseases. June, 1975.

# 13

# Condyloma Acuminatum

Condyloma acuminatum is not usually a serious medical problem but frequently causes emotional distress to both patient and physician because of its marked tendency to recurrence.

## CLINICAL FEATURES

### Etiology

The causative agent in condyloma acuminatum is believed to be a papilloma virus which is auto-innoculable, filterable, and transmissable.[30] Oriel also demonstrated this virus in a case of carcinoma-in-situ arising from condyloma acuminatum.[30] However, Delap, et al were unable to demonstrate the presence of a distinct papova-like, circular DNA in human condylomata.[8] The incubation period for this virus is usually from one to six months but may be longer.

### Prevalence

The prevalence of condyloma acuminatum in the anorectal and urogenital regions points toward a sexual mode of transmission. They occur with greatest frequency in male homosexual patients. Swerdlow and Salvati reported that 46 per cent of their male patients with condylomata acuminata were homosexual.[36] Abcarian reported on an incidence of anal intercourse of 90 per cent in a series of 70 patients with condyloma acuminatum.[1]

A study by Carr and associates in a population of gay men in New York City revealed anal warts to be more frequent among men who practiced anal receptive intercourse.[4] Seventy two per cent of the patients had internal warts during the course of their illness. Anal warts were several times more common than penile warts in gay men. A possible explanation for this discrepancy may be that the moist, warm perianal area is more conducive to the growth of warts than the more dry, cool penile epidermis. Anal intercourse may introduce the virus into the anal region and concurrent local trauma may impair local defenses.

### Location

Locations in which condylomata are found include the perianal region and anal canal, as well as other parts of the perineum, vulva, vagina, and penis.

## PATHOLOGY

### Macroscopic

Condyloma acuminatum vary from pinhead size lesions to projecting cauliflower-like masses. Their surface is papilliform and they are pink or white in color. Individual warts may be sessile or pedunculated and have a tendency to grow in radical rows which may become confluent and form almost an entire sheet around the anal orifice. They are, almost invariably, multiple and may be so numerous as to obscure the anal aperture which is then found only with difficulty. Vulvar warts can grow so luxuriantly as to conceal the introitus. In addition, they frequently extend into the anal canal and even the rectum. Because of the moisture and warmth in the anal region, the warts may

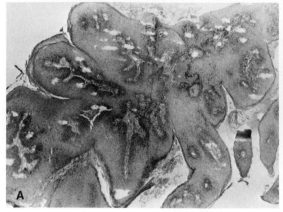
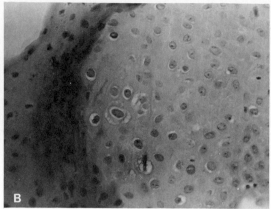
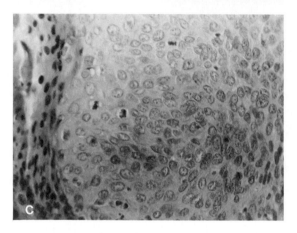

FIGURE 13-1.    (A) *In this* low power view of condyloma acuminatum (*mag.  40×*)
*marked papillomatosis and acanthosis of the epidermal surface with parakeratosis*
*of the tops of the papillae can be seen. Telangiectasia of stroma is also present.*
(B) *In the* high power view of acanthotic epithelium (*mag.  250×*) *surface parakera-*
*tosis with absence of the granular layer is noted. Enlargement of some prickle cells*
*due to uniform or compartmentalized cytoplasmic edema can be seen.* (C) *In this*
*view of* acanthotic ephithelium (*mag.  250×*) *tip superficial flattened papakeratotic*
*area with the subjacent hypercellular Malpigian cell layer showing increased nor-*
*mal mitotic figures and occasional edematous cells.* (*Microphotographs courtesy of*
*Dr. H. Srolovitz, Jewish General Hospital, Montreal*)

become sodden and white. This may produce
an irritating discharge with a disagreeable
odor. They are often soft and friable and,
therefore, may bleed.

### Microscopic

Microscopically, anal warts show marked
acanthosis of the epidermis with hyperplasia
of prickle cells, parakeratosis, and an underlying chronic inflammatory cell infiltration.[26]
Vacuolization of the cells of the upper prickle
layer is present (Fig. 13-1).[16]

## SYMPTOMS

Patients with condyloma acuminatum present
with relatively minor complaints.[1] Almost all
notice visible perianal warts. Two-thirds of the
patients experience pruritus ani which may be
due to the irritation of the warts or the patients' inability to properly cleanse themselves
after defecation. About half the patients experience some bleeding with defecation because of the friability of some of these warts.
Other patients complain of anal wetness, and a

minority experience discomfort or pain. Female patients may present with a vaginal discharge.

## DIAGNOSIS

In most cases, the clinical appearance of the lesions makes the diagnosis obvious. However, prior treatment with Podophyllin may alter the gross morphology of the lesions and this may mask the diagnosis. It should be stressed that all sexual contacts should be examined for the presence of warts.

It is important to determine the extent of the disease, since all lesions must be treated to minimize the risk of recurrence. Sohn et al found that half their male homosexual patients harbored condylomata.[35] In only 6 per cent were these confined to the perianal region, while in 84 per cent of the patients both perianal and intra-anal lesions were present. Eleven per cent had only intra-anal lesions. Thus, failure of the examiner to study the anorectum with an anoscope could have resulted in the failure to diagnose intra-anal lesions in 94 per cent of the patients.

Because of the free association of numerous diseases, and the frequency of condylomata acuminata, other sexually transmitted diseases must be excluded. Sohn stressed that in addition to the history and physical examination, proctosigmoidoscopy, stool cultures for bacterial pathogens, stool studies for ova and parasites, pharyngeal, rectal and uretheral smears for gonococci, and blood for syphilis serology should be considered.

Included in the differential diagnosis are condylomata lata, the lesions of secondary syphilis. However, these are usually fewer in number, smoother, flatter, whiter, and usually more moist. One must remember that the two lesions may occur concomittantly. A definitive diagnosis is made by the dark field examination which will demonstrate the spirochaetes.

Another condition that may require differentiation is the squamous cell carcinoma of the anus, but this is more indurated. A biopsy will establish this diagnosis.

## TREATMENT

A long list of methods of treating condylomata acuminata have been employed (see below).

These included the almost "non-treatment" of observation, "charming", and the unlikely use of hypnosis, or the applications of lime water or lemon juice. The few successful results of these methods are almost certainly examples of spontaneous regression. The topical application of more caustic agents such as Podophyllin or Bichloracetic acid has been used with varying degrees of enthusiasm. Various forms of local destruction have included surgical excision, electro-dissection, cryotherapy, and ultrasound. Attempts at systemic attacks on warts have included the use of Fowler's solution, autovaccine, vaccinia, and Bismouth sodium triglycollamate. Very rarely condyloma acuminatum may regress spontaneously.

---

*METHODS OF TREATING CONDYLOMA ACUMINATUM*
CAUSTIC AGENTS
  PODOPHYLLIN[6]
  BICHLORACETIC ACID[36]
FULGURATION[13]
SURGICAL EXCISION[37]
CRYOTHERAPY
  CARBON DIOXIDE SNOW[14,21]
  LIQUID AIR[12]
  LIQUID NITROGEN[14,21,27]
ANTITUMOR PREPARATIONS
  THIOTEPA[5,16]
  5-FLUOROURACIL[28]
  BLEOMYCIN[23]
IMMUNOTHERAPY[1,2,31]
UNUSUAL SUGGESTIONS
  OBSERVATION[21]
  LIME WATER[21]
  LEMON JUICE[21]
  "CHARMING"[21]
  HYPNOSIS[9,21]

---

Numerous therapeutic modalities have been utilized in the treatment of anal condylomata acuminata, all with a failure rate ranging from 25 to 70 per cent. There are several possible reasons why none of these approaches have been universally beneficial.[1] First, since the disease is probably the result of sexual contact, no matter what treatment is employed, the patients resume these contacts before therapy is completed. They may also change contacts and acquire new infections. The partners would have to be treated in order to obtain cures. The potentially long incubation period may cause reinfection of sexual partners or delayed recurrence of a new generation of warts. The relative isolation of a virus in the superficial layers of condyloma tissue may preclude its contact with the circulating lymphocytes.[1] Patients should be warned of the warts marked tendency to reappear.

## Podophyllin

The local application of podophyllin has often been effective treatment. It is a cytotoxic agent applied in a vehicle such as liquid paraffin or tincture of Benzoin, the latter having the advantage in that it adheres better to the warts. Various concentrations from 5 to 50 per cent have been used, but a 25 per cent suspension is probably to be recommended.

The method of application is to paint the warts accurately, avoiding the adjacent skin as podophyllin is intensely irritating. Dusting powder is then applied to the surrounding skin.

Patients are instructed to wash the treated area six to eight hours after each application to prevent damage to the surrounding skin. This treatment is repeated at weekly intervals as required. In some cases, this treatment must be abandoned because of the soreness and irritation of the perianal skin.

Credit for this mode of therapy has been given to Culp and Kaplan.[6] Of 200 patients so treated, 82 per cent required only one application, while an additional 15 per cent were cured by a second treatment. No one required more than four applications of the drug. It must be pointed out that most of these patients were troubled with penile warts. Unfortunately, other clinicians have been unable to obtain such excellent results with podophyllin in the treatment of anal canal warts.

Podophyllin has several disadvantages.[29] It is not a pure compound, and batches may vary in potency. It cannot be applied to perianal or anal warts by the patient himself so repeated visits to the office may be necessary. Local reactions may be severe, and penetration into keratinized warts is poor, so that only recently acquired lesions may respond. The application of large amounts of podophyllin may result in severe, systemic, toxic effects. Podophyllin poisoning has been associated with the treatment of condyloma acuminatum.[24] Finally, prolonged courses of treatment with podophyllin are probably undesirable since dysplasia has been produced. Moreover, it has also been

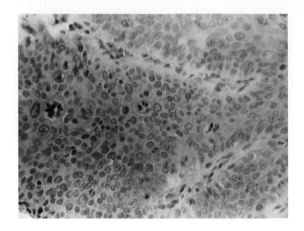

FIGURE **13-2.** *View of Podophyllin-treated condyloma (mag. 250×) showing epithelium as hypercellular and individual prickle cell nuclei with slight variation in size, shape, and staining quality. The presence of increased atypical mitotic figures, some with tripolar appearance should be noted. (Microphotograph courtesy of Dr. H. Srolovitz, Jewish General Hospital, Montreal)*

reported that treatment with Podophyllin may induce temporary changes that are difficult to differentiate histologically from carcinoma (Fig. 13-2).[25]

## Bichloracetic Acid

In the absence of a completely satisfactory mode of therapy, Swerdlow and Salvati proposed the use of another caustic agent, bichloracetic acid.[36] The technique involves cleansing and drying the perianal region with cotton and Witch Hazel. The caustic is applied with an applicator, taking care not to apply the chemical to adjacent skin as a burn will result. If too much acid is applied it should be wiped off, the area washed with water, and sodium bicarbonate applied as a local antidote if necessary. The lesions that are cauterized change from pink to a frosty white color. Lesions within the anal canal are treated similarly but dabbed gently with a cotton ball before the walls of the anal canal are allowed to fall back together.

Analgesics are prescribed routinely but necessary only when massive involvement is present. Patients are instructed to keep the area clean and dry. The caustic is applied at intervals of seven to ten days to get maximum benefit from the treatment. The patient's sexual partners should also be treated.

Approximately 25 per cent of Swerdlow and Salvati's patients had recurrences. They were treated with further short courses of therapy. The number of treatments needed varied according to the size and number of warts. They ranged from one to 13 treatments with most patients receiving four or less. Their feeling was that when patients treated with bichloracetic acid as an office procedure were compared to patients treated with other modes of therapy, they were more comfortable, did not develop post-treatment scars and strictures, and had prompt resolution of their warts without losing time from work.

**Electrocoagulation**

Electrocoagulation is an effective means of destroying these small lesions. It necessitates the use of local anesthesia. The benefits and complications vary with the skill of the operator who must control the depth and width of the wound. One must aim to obtain a white coagulum which generally corresponds to a second degree burn. Such wounds should heal without any significant scarring. However, a black eschar likely represents a third degree burn which will probably heal with scarring, and if such a burn is created circumferentially, a stricture may result. Working upon the vital anoderm must alert the operator to the potential problems of stenosis and damage to the underlying sphincter. Special care must be taken not to miss any of the warts lying in the anal canal. Extensive warts both perianal and intra-anal, might require the use of a general anesthetic. The postoperative care follows the conventional lines described in chapter 4 on postoperative care.

**Cryotherapy**

Another destructive method used recently is cryotherapy. Various techniques have been advocated including the use of liquid nitrogen, carbon dioxide snow, and liquified air. The depth and width of the wound, again, must be carefully controlled. The postoperative course is similar to that after electrocoagulation.

**Surgical Excision**

When massive involvement is present, surgical excision can be carried out using general or regional anesthesia. A simple enema the evening before is adequate bowel preparation.

The method avoids the use of cautery except for its use in controlling bleeding points.

A solution of 1:200,000 adrenaline in saline is injected subcutaneously and submucosally. This separates the warts and allows as much healthy skin and mucosa as possible to be preserved when the individual warts are removed using a pair of fine-toothed forceps and fine pointed scissors. Good judgment is necessary to gauge the amount of anoderm which may be removed and yet protect the underlying sphincter mechanism. The warts are similarly removed from the anal mucosa. The resulting small wounds heal rapidly but the severity of postoperative pain varies and prolonged convalescence is common. In the majority of patients, it is possible to remove all the warts on one occasion, but if there are too many, removal may be done in two stages at an interval of approximately one month.

Thomson and Grace reported the results in 75 patients upon whom this technique was used.[38] Over 75 per cent had lesions within the anal canal. In 80 per cent the warts were removed in one operation. Postoperative complications occurred in four patients: two bleeding, one hematoma, and one previously undetected coagulation defect. Relatively little discomfort was experienced, but a 42 per cent recurrence rate was noted.[38] In the majority of patients recurrent wart formation was detected by the end of the second postoperative month. Anal stenosis is a well-known risk following the removal of anal and perianal warts. If adequate normal skin and mucosa is left between the wounds, this complication should not occur.

A potential advantage over the electrocoagulation technique is that the postoperative wound weeps less, and as mentioned earlier, moisture is believed to enhance the growth of condylomata.

**Immunotherapy**

Because of the high recurrence rate following the treatment of condylomata acuminata by conventional means, Abcarian and co-workers reintroduced immunotherapy as an adjunctive treatment modality.[1] Because of the high recurrence rate, the utilization of immunotherapy may prove the logical choice in the treatment of extensive or recurrent disease.

The use of an autologous vaccine in the

treatment of condyloma acuminatum was first published by Biberstein in 1944.[2] Attention was next drawn to this mode of therapy by Powell, et al who presented a 95 per cent success rate with autogonous vaccine in 24 patients with persistent anorectal and urogenital condylomata.[31] Nel and Fourie reported 80 per cent favorable results with this technique.[28]

Using Abcarian's technique, at least 5 grams of tissue must be submitted for vaccine preparation. Once prepared, 0.2 ml. of the vaccine is injected subcutaneously in the deltoid area once a week for six consecutive weeks. No adverse reactions were seen in any of the patients receiving the vaccine. Total disappearance of condylomata occurred in 83 per cent of 70 patients studied by Abcarian.[1] All these patients remained disease free through a follow-up period averaging 26 months. In 11 per cent of patients, the great bulk of condyloma disappeared leaving only a small asymptomatic residual. Only 6 per cent of patients did not benefit from the vaccination. A second course of vaccination produced excellent results in half of the remaining patients. The mechanism of regression of warts has remained speculative.

The technique of immunotherapy produced an overall 94 per cent cure rate which represents a substantial improvement over conventional therapy. Abcarian and co-workers, therefore, feel that immunotherapy appears to be the treatment of choice in extensive persistent or recurrent condylomata acuminata.

## Post-Treatment Follow-up

Because of the frequency of recurrence, follow-up visits at monthly intervals for at least three months free of warts is recommended. Small recurrent warts are easily treated in the office.

## Duration Before Sexual Intercourse

With the proviso that condoms are used prophylactically, sexual activity may be resumed when the patient so desires. Without the use of condoms, sexual intercourse may probably be safely resumed after a three month disease-free period has elapsed.

TABLE 13-I. Treatment Modalities

| TREATMENT | ADVANTAGES | DISADVANTAGES | RESULTS |
|---|---|---|---|
| *Podophyllin* | EASE OF APPLICATION NO ANESTHESIA | SKIN BURNS CAN'T USE IN ANAL CANAL MULTIPLE VISITS DYSPLASIA WITH PROLONGED USE SYSTEMIC TOXICITY | DISAPPOINTING EXACT RECURRENCE RATE UNAVAILABLE |
| *Bichloracetic Acid* | EASE OF APPLICATION NO ANESTHESIA CAN USE IN ANAL CANAL | SKIN BURN MULTIPLE VISITS | 25% RECURRENCE |
| *Electrocoagulation* | SINGLE SESSION TREATMENT EFFECTIVE IN ANAL CANAL | ANESTHESIA REQUIRED POSTOPERATIVE PAIN | MAY REQUIRE REPEATED COAGULATIONS |
| *Cryotherapy* | SINGLE SESSION TREATMENT CAN BE USED IN ANAL CANAL | REQUIRES EXPENSIVE EQUIPMENT MAY REQUIRE ANESTHESIA | UNAVAILABLE |
| *Surgical Excision* | PRECISE REMOVAL TISSUE FOR PATHOLOGY | ANESTHESIA REQUIRED POSTOPERATIVE PAIN | 42% RECURRENCE |
| *Immunotherapy* | EFFECTIVE FOR EXTENSIVE WARTS | REQUIRES VACCINE PREPARATION REPEAT VISITS FOR VACCINE | 17% NON-RESPONSE |

## GIANT CONDYLOMA ACUMINATUM

Giant condyloma (Buschke-Lowenstein tumor) usually affects the penis or perianal region. Clinically it has the appearance of an aggressive, florid, fungating, squamous carcinoma, yet is histologically benign. Microscopically, differences between a Buschke-Lowenstein tumor and condylomata acuminata are primarily differences of degree. It shows marked papillary proliferation with extensive acanthosis and parakeratosis.[33] There is no evidence of invasion by carcinoma. These lesions have caused extensive erosion and destruction of adjacent structures by compression necrosis with invasion of the ischiorectal fossa, perirectal tissues, and even the pelvic cavity.

Until 1974, Fitzgerald and associates reported that only four cases of giant condylomata involving areas other than the penis had been reported.[10] One occurred in the perianal region, one inguinal, one rectal, and one involved the vulva and rectum.[7,15,17,22] However, Shah and colleagues in 1972 reported two additional cases in the perianal region.[33]

Giant condylomata represent one end of a spectrum of clinical behaviour, the other end of which is represented by the benign course of condyloma acuminatum. They do not respond to conservative treatment. The clinical course of this rare growth is one of relentless progression and expansion of the tumor by pressure necrosis of surrounding tissues. Carcinomas of the affected organs have been recorded. Litvack and associates reported giant condyloma acuminatum associated with carcinoma.[19]

Treatment by radiotherapy is not suitable. Natural anatomic and physiologic barriers are removed and any remaining tumor will expand by further pressure necrosis. Radical surgical excision at the onset offers the only hope of eradication of the tumor and permanent cure.[20]

## CONDYLOMA ACUMINATUM AND CANCER

The association of various benign anorectal conditions with carcinoma of the anus has been observed. One of these benign conditions is condyloma acuminatum. Sawyers reported the treatment of four patients with condylomata who had histologic evidence of squamous cell carcinoma arising in the venereal wart.[32] Those patients underwent abdomino-perineal resection. Buckwalter and colleagues have suggested the association of benign anorectal disease in the genesis of epidermoid carcinoma.[3] In particular, the association of malignancy with condylomata acuminata has been reported by several authors.[10,11,18,34]

Sufficient data is not available to ascertain the exact incidence of condyloma in association with squamous carcinoma. However, the isolated reports of the association of these two conditions makes the incidence very low.

## REFERENCES

1. Abcarian, H., and Sharon, N.: The effectiveness of immunotherapy in the treatment of anal condyloma acuminatum. J. Surg. Res., *22:*231, 1977.

2. Biberstein, H.: Immunization therapy of warts. Arch. Dermatol., *50:*12, 1944.

3. Buckwalter, J. A., and Jurayj, M. N.: Relationship of chronic anorectal disease to carcinoma. Arch. Surg., *75:*352, 1957.

4. Carr, G., and William, D. C.: Anal warts in a population of gay men in New York City. Sex. Transm. Dis., *4:*45, 1977.

5. Cheng, S. F., and Veenema, R. J.: Topical application of thiotepa to penile and urethral tumors. J. Urol., *94:*259, 1965.

6. Culp, O. S., and Kaplan, I. W.: Condylomata acuminata: Two hundred cases treated with Podophyllin. Ann. Surg., *120:*251, 1944.

7. Dawson, D. F., et al: Giant condyloma and verrucous carcinoma of the genital area. Arch. Pathol., *79:*225, 1965.

8. Delap, R., Friedman-Kein, A., and Rush, M. G.: The absence of human papilloma viral DNA sequences in condylomata acuminata. Virology, *74:*268, 1976.

9. Ewin, D. M.: Condyloma acuminatum: successful treatment of four cases by hypnosis. The Am. J. Clin. Hypn., *17:*73, 1974.

10. Fitzgerald, D. M., and Hamit, H. F.: The variable significance of condyloma acuminata. Ann. Surg., *179:*328, 1974.

11. Friedberg, M. J., and Serlin, O.: Condyloma acuminatum: its association with malignancy. Dis. Col. Rectum, *6:*352, 1963.

12. Gold, J. D.: Liquid air and carbonic acid snow: therapeutic results obtained by the dermatologist. N.Y. Med. J., 92:1276, 1910.

13. Graber, E. A., Barber, H. R. K., and O'Rourke, J. J.: Simple surgical treatment for condyloma acuminatum of the vulva. Obst. Gynecol., *29:*247, 1967.

14. Hall, A. F.: Advantages and limitations of liquid nitrogen in the therapy of skin lesions. Arch. Dermatol., *82:*9, 1960.

15. Judge, J.: Giant condyloma acuminatum involving vulva and rectum. Arch. Pathol., *88:*46, 1969.

16. Kerstein, M. D.: Thio-tepa in the management of anorectal condylomata acuminata: report of two cases. Dis. Col. Rectum, *20:*625, 1977.

17. Knoblich, R., and Failing, J. F. Jr.: Giant condyloma acuminatum (Bushke-Lowenstein tumor) of the rectum. Am. J. Clin. Pathol., *48:*389, 1967.

18. Kovi, J., Tillman, R. L., and Lee, S. M.: Malignant transformation of condyloma acuminatum. Am. J. Clin. Pathol., *61:*702, 1974.

19. Litvack, A. S., Melnick, I., and Lieberman, P. R.: Giant condyloma acuminata associated with carcinoma. J. Med. Soc. NJ., *63:*165, 1966.

20. Lock, M. R., Katz, D. R., Samoorian, S., and Parks, A. G.: Giant condyloma of the rectum: report of a case. Dis. Colon. Rectum, *20:*154, 1977.

21. Lyell, A.: Management of warts. Br. Med. J., *2:*1576, 1966.

22. Machacek, G., and Weakly, D.: Giant condylomata acuminata of Bushke and Lowenstein. Arch. Dermatol., *82:*41, 1960.

23. Mishima, Y., and Masahiro, M.: Effect of bleomycin on benign and malignant cutaneous tumors. Acta Derm. Venereol., *52:*211, 1972.

24. Montaldi, D. H., Giambrone, J. P., Courey, N. G., and Taefi, P.: Podophyllin poisoning associated with the treatment of condyloma acuminatum: a case report. Am. J. Obstet. Gynecol., *119:*1130, 1974.

25. Moriame, G.: Transformation maligne de végé- tations vénériennes de la verge. Arch. Belg. dermat. et. syph., *6:*175, 1950.

26. Morson, B. D., and Dawson, I. M. P.: Gastrointestinal Pathology. 623., Blackwell Scientific Publications, London, 1972.

27. Nahra, K. S., Moschella, S. L., and Swinton, N. W. Sr.: Condyloma acuminatum treated with liquid nitrogen: report of 5 cases. Dis. Colon. Rectum, *12:*125, 1969.

28. Nel, W. S., and Fourie, E. D.: Immunotherapy and 5% topical 5-Fluorouracil ointment in the treatment of condyloma acuminata. S. Afr. Med., *71:*234, 1978.

29. Oriel, D.: Letter to the editor. Proc. Roy. Soc. Med., *71:*234, 1978.

30. Oriel, J. D., and Almeida, J. D.: Demonstration of virus particles in human genital warts. Br. J. Vener. Dis., *46:*37, 1970.

31. Powell, L. C. Jr., Pollard, M., and Jenkins, J. L. Sr.: Treatment of condyloma acuminata by autogenous vaccine. South Med. J., *63:*202, 1970.

32. Sawyers, J. L.: Squamous cell cancer of the perianus and anus. S.C.N.A., *52:*935, 1972.

33. Shah, J. C., and Hertz, R. E. Giant condyloma acuminatum of the anorectum: report of 2 cases. Dis. Colon. Rectum, *15:*207, 1972.

34. Siegel, A.: Malignant transformation of condyloma acuminatum: review of the literature and report of a case. Am. J. Surg., *103:*613, 1962.

35. Sohn, N., and Robilotti, J. G.: The gay bowel syndrome, a review of colonic and rectal conditions in 200 male homosexuals. Am. J. Gastroent., *67:*478, 1977.

36. Swerdlow, D. B., and Salvati, E. P.: Condyloma acuminatum. Dis. Colon & Rectum, *14:*226, 1971.

37. Thomson, J. P. S.: Perianal and Anal Condyloma Acuminata Operative Surgery. 3 ed. Rob, C. and Smith, R. (eds.) Butterworth and Co., London, 1977.

38. Thomson, J. P. S., and Grace R. H.: The treatment of perianal and anal condylomata acuminata: a new operative technique. Proc. Roy. Soc. Med., *71:*180, 1978.

# 14

# Neoplasms of the Anal Canal

Malignancies of the anal canal are uncommon. They account for 3 to 4 per cent of all anorectal cancers.[33,47] Although the literature is replete with reports on this subject, there has been no uniform use of terminology and classification. Consequently it is difficult to interpret the results of treatment, since many malignant neoplasms of different behavior were grouped together.

## CLASSIFICATION AND TERMINOLOGY

The anal canal, which extends from the anorectal ring to the anal verge, is lined by different kinds of epithelium. Below the dentate line is squamous epithelium, whereas the epithelium above the dentate line is columnar. This junction is not abrupt: for a distance of 6 to 12 mm above the dentate line there is a gradual transition where columnar, cuboidal, transitional, or squamous epithelium may be found. This area, often referred to as the cloacogenic zone, has been considered to consist of "unstable" epithelium and, because of the diversity of this epithelium, gives rise to an interesting variety of neoplasms. These two areas of the anal canal not only have different routes of lymphatic drainage (see Chapter 1), but when the same type of neoplasm, develops in these areas, such as squamous cell carcinoma, a variety of behavior is evidenced. For these reasons, neoplasms of the anal canal should be divided into two categories in relation to the dentate line. We have, therefore, adopted the classification of Histological Typing of Intestinal Tumors used by the World Health Organization, and have used their standardized nomenclature.[30] In this classification the anal canal is arbitrarily divided into the area above the dentate line called "anal canal" and the area below the dentate line called "anal margin."

## NEOPLASMS OF THE ANAL MARGIN

1. Squamous cell carcinoma
2. Basal cell carcinoma
3. Bowen's disease
4. Perianal Paget's disease

### Squamous Cell Carcinoma

Squamous cell carcinomas of the anal margin resemble those occurring in skin elsewhere in the body. Macroscopically, they typically have rolled, everted edges with central ulceration.[39] Any chronic unhealed ulcer should be considered as a potential squamous cell carcinoma until proven otherwise by biopsy. They vary in size from as small as less than 1 cm to so large that they completely surround and obstruct the anal orifice. They are four times as common in men as in women, and occur at an average age of 63 years of age.[31] They are more common in under developed countries.

Histologically, they are usually well differentiated, with well-developed patterns of keratinization (Fig. 14-1). Local invasion oc-

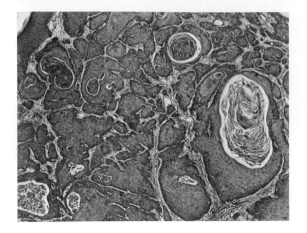

FIGURE **14-1.** *Squamous cell carcinoma.*

curs but the carcinoma is typically slow growing. Lymphatic spread from these carcinomas is to the inguinal lymph nodes.

Despite their surface location, the lesions are usually diagnosed late: over 50 per cent of cases are detected more than 24 months following the onset of symptoms.[29] The usual presentation is a lump, which has persisted and increased in size, mild but persistent bleeding, and itching. In the more advanced case, pain, tenesmus, and even incontinence may occur.[29]

*Treatment.* Since carcinomas of the anal margin are late to metastasize, adequate **local excision** for cure can be carried out. Adequate excision, for a lesion which is relatively mobile and does not encroach upon the dentate line, implies a 2 cm margin and a depth sufficient to achieve complete freedom from neoplastic infiltration.[4,7,23,41] Wolfe and associates noted that wide excision of these lesions, including a portion of the sphincter muscle, can be performed without loss of continence.[52]

For carcinomas which are extensive, involving the dentate line and deeply invading the underlying sphincter muscles, metastases proximally to the superior rectal nodes and laterally along the middle rectal nodes may occur. In such circumstances, **abdominoperineal resection** offers the best form of local control and best figures for survival.[4,41]

Papillon used **interstitial Curie therapy** (Radium Implantation) in selected patients with carcinomas of the anal margin and anal canal proper.[39] The five year survival in 64 pa-

tients was 68 per cent. Only four patients developed radionecrosis and these were due to faulty technique.

About 40 per cent of patients with carcinoma of the anal margin have metastases to the inguinal lymph nodes, consistent with the late discovery at the time of treatment.[31] For these patients, **groin dissection** should be performed.[4,47,50] Papillon recommended irradiation to the groin followed by dissection.[39] Examination of the groins at regular intervals is indicated because metastases to the groins are common even after excision of the primary lesion.

*Prognosis.* Because most authors have not adopted standard nomenclature the survival statistics are not all comparable. Of the available series, the overall five year survival is approximately 60 per cent.[7,16,28,33] Stearns reported a five year survival of 66 per cent in patients with anal margin lesions which did not invade the anal musculature treated by local excision.[47] If inguinal lymph nodes are involved at the time of surgery, the five year survival is less than 5 per cent.

### Basal Cell Carcinoma

Basal cell carcinomas of the anal margin comprise less than 1 per cent of anorectal neoplasms.[11,41] They occur three times as frequently in men as in women.

Macroscopically they are similar to cutaneous basal cell carcinoma found elsewhere in the body. They are characterized by a central ulceration with irregular and raised edges. They remain superficial, mobile and do not metastasize, although inguinal lymphadenopathy may occur from reactive inflammation.[11] Histologically they are similar to basal cell carcinomas of the skin elsewhere.[31] They are of long duration, have a low invasive potential, and must be distinguished from basaloid carcinomas (cloacogenic or transitional cell carcinomas) which have an entirely different origin and behavior. Patients may present with complaints of mild discomfort or mild bleeding. Metastases are rare.

*Treatment.* Local excision with adequate margins is the treatment of choice and the prognosis is excellent.[11,41] Adequate surgical excision virtually assures a cure.[41]

## Bowen's Disease

Bowen's disease of the perianal skin is a rare, slow growing, intraepidermal, squamous cell carcinoma (carcinoma in situ) most commonly occurring in the 50- to 60-year-old group.[18] Its proposed relationship to the simultaneous or subsequent development of internal malignancies is noteworthy.[13] Graham and Helwig reported that 70 to 80 per cent of patients with Bowen's disease, studied from the time of diagnosis to the death of the patient, had one or more primary internal malignancies, or primary cancer of the skin with metastases.[14] Further analysis of their data yielded about 10 per cent of patients with Bowen's disease developing invasive squamous cell carcinoma from the original lesion. About 35 per cent of these cases will develop metastases unless early adequate treatment is given. Furthermore 40 per cent or more of the patients with Bowen's disease will develop other cutaneous premalignant and malignant lesions, 6 or 7 years after the onset of Bowen's disease. In order of decreasing frequency, the respiratory tract, gastrointestinal tract, genitourinary organs, and reticuloendothelial system are most often implicated. Consequently, the need for continued observation of these patients is obvious.

*Clinical Features.* Macroscopically the lesions appear as discrete, erythematous, occasionally pigmented, non-infiltrating, scaly or crusted plaques, sometimes exhibiting a moist surface. Foci of ulceration indicate that an invasive carcinoma has developed a complication that occurs in 2 to 5 per cent of all cases.[13,48] Patients may complain of itching, burning, or spotty bleeding but only a biopsy will confirm this diagnosis. The histologic picture is that of an in situ squamous cell carcinoma which may have characteristic Bowenoid cells which are multinucleated giant cells with some vacuolization giving a "halo" effect (Fig. 14-2).[45]

*Treatment.* Wide local excision is the treatment of choice.[41,45] Frozen section study of the excised specimen may aid in achieving free margins. The defect so produced may be closed primarily, with the aid of rotation flaps, or split thickness skin grafts. Long term follow-up is imperative because of the high incidence of recurrence (20 per cent in 15 years

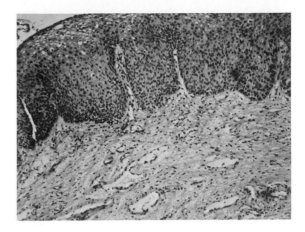

FIGURE **14-2.** *Bowen's disease. Atypical epithelial cells involve full thickness of the epidermis.*

follow-up).[13] Recently Raaf and colleagues reported a good response of these lesions to topical dinitrochlorobenzene and 5-Flurouracil.[43]

## Perianal Paget's Disease

Sir James Paget first described this disease in relation to the nipple of the breast in females. Extramammary Paget's disease may be found in the axilla and anogenital region (labia majora, penis, scrotum, groins, pubic area, perineum, perianal region, thigh and buttock). Ackerman and Rosai described Paget's disease of the perianal area as a malignant neoplasm of the intraepidermal portion of the apocrine glands with or without associated dermal involvement.[1] Morson stated that Paget's disease of the perianal skin has a long preinvasive phase but if the patient lives long enough an adenocarcinoma of apocrine gland type will develop.[32] It is more common in women than men with the highest incidence in the 7th decade.[16]

Grodsky reported the presence of an underlying carcinoma of one of the local apocrine glands in 50 percent of cases.[17] Helwig and associates reported that 85 per cent of patients with Paget's disease were found to have, or develop, a coexisting visceral carcinoma.[22]

*Clinical Features.* Intractable anal itching is usually present for many months.[16] Macroscopically it appears as an erythematous scaly or eczematoid plaque-like lesion similar to other cutaneous lesions, making clinical diagnosis difficult. A definitive diagnosis is made

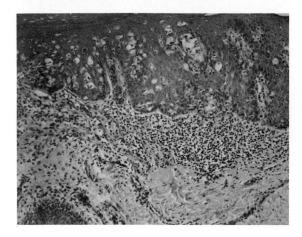

FIGURE **14-3.** *Perianal Paget's disease. Paget cells are present just above the basal layer.*

by biopsy which shows the characteristic Paget cells: large, pale vacuolated cells with hyperchromatic eccentric nuclei (Fig. 14-3). Some authors have considered them intraepidermal metastases from an underlying carcinoma. They invariably contain acid mucosubstances, an important feature in the differential diagnosis with melanoma and Bowen's disease.[1] Perianal Paget's disease is prone to be associated with malignancy elsewhere, such as carcinoma of the breast and the rectum.[3,22]

*Treatment.* Wide local excision is the treatment of choice for the localized lesion. Because of the high incidence of local recurrence it is of vital importance to obtain an adequate margin. A practical aid at the operating table is the use of supravital staining of the Paget cells. Using this technique the entire area of skin is washed with acetic acid 1 to 2 per cent. The whole area is painted with toluidine blue and once again washed with acetic acid. The nuclei of the Paget cells pick up the toluidine blue but the blue of the lesion is not washed away with the second washing of acetic acid. Then, multiple punch biopsies are done, 1 to 2 cm from the obvious lesion. If these are negative then this becomes the line of excision. If the lesion is small, a primary closure may be performed but with larger lesions a split-thickness skin graft may be required. In such circumstances, a colostomy is not necessary as the combination of a bowel preparation and the use of a chemically defined diet has been successfully employed under such circumstances.[12]

For more advanced lesions with an underlying carcinoma, an abdominoperineal resection, with inguinal lymph node dissection if positive lymph nodes are present, will be necessary. Because of the commonly delayed diagnosis (average 4 years), about 25 per cent of Paget's disease in this region had metastases.[16,22] The sites of metastases, in order of frequency, are inguinal and pelvic lymph nodes, liver, bone, lung, brain, bladder, prostate, and adrenal gland.[22] The prognosis is poor once metastases have occurred.

## NEOPLASMS OF THE ANAL CANAL

A. Carcinoma
  1. Squamous cell carcinoma
  2. Basaloid carcinoma
  3. Mucoepidermoid carcinoma
  4. Adenocarcinoma
    a. Adenocarcinoma of rectal type
    b. Adenocarcinoma of anal glands and ducts
    c. Adenocarcinoma within anorectal fistula
B. Malignant melanoma

### Squamous Cell Carcinoma

These carcinomas arise from the transitional zone of epithelium and are flat, ulcerating, non-keratinizing neoplasms which occur more frequently in women (4:3).[31]

*Clinical Features.* Presentation generally follows a long history of minor perianal problems, such as the bleeding which occurs in about half the patients.[4,47,50] Other symptoms include pain and an anal mass. Almost one-third of patients in Stearns' series had an initial mistaken diagnosis of benign or inflammatory disease.[47]

*Lymph Node Metastases.* At the time of treatment, squamous cell carcinomas of the anal canal have been found to metastasize, to superior rectal lymph nodes in 43 per cent of cases, and to inguinal lymph nodes in 36 per cent.[31]

*Prognosis.* In a series of 131 patients undergoing surgical treatment for squamous cell carcinomas of the anal canal the corrected five year survival was 49 per cent.[33] In Beahrs and

Wilson's series of 82 patients the five year survival was approximately 60 per cent following local excision or abdominoperineal resection, with or without radiotherapy.[4]

### Basaloid Carcinomas

These are a variant of squamous cell carcinomas that in some degree resemble basal cell carcinomas of the skin.[30] Basaloid refers to the histological appearance of palisading nuclei seen at the periphery of clumps of cells which characterize this malignancy (Fig. 14-4). Histologically they are unlike basal cell carcinoma in that there are areas of eosinophilic necrosis within clumps of the neoplastic cells. There is nuclear irregularity and the presence of giant cells, especially in the anaplastic variety. There is a slight female preponderance, and the average age of onset is 60 years with a spread from 40 to 80 years.

This type of carcinoma arises from the transitional zone above the dentate line and, therefore, Grinvalsky and Helwig proposed the term "transitional cloacogenic carcinoma".[15] Because of their similar behavior some authors group them together with squamous cell carcinomas as "epidermoid carcinomas of the anal canal".[47] The incidence of basaloid carcinomas is about 26 per cent of carcinomas of the anal canal with equal distribution between the sexes.[38]

The clinical features are similar to squamous cell carcinomas of the anal canal.

*Lymphatic Spread.* As in squamous cell carcinomas of the anal canal, about 50 per cent of patients already have regional lymph node involvement at the time of operation. Of the 27 patients treated by abdominoperineal resection, eight had superior rectal node involvement, four had both superior rectal and inguinal lymph node involvement, and two patients developed inguinal node involvement only.[38]

*Prognosis.* Morson classified these carcinomas on the basis of their histological differentiation, grading them according to the presence or absence of palisading and other cytologic characteristics. He found a good correlation between his classification and the five year survival rate. The five year survival for patients with well differentiated lesions is 90 per cent, moderately differentiated 60 per cent, and for anaplastic no five year survival occurred. The overall five year survival is 55 per cent.[38]

### Mucoepidermoid Carcinomas

These are another variant of the squamous cell carcinomas and have the same basic histological pattern except for the addition of mucin, which varies in amount from lesion to lesion, and even within different areas of the same lesion.[35]

There is a slight female preponderance, the average age of presentation being 55 years. The behavior and prognosis of these lesions are similar to squamous cell or basaloid carcinomas. Of the patients reviewed at St. Mark's Hospital, London, seven out of 21 had inguinal lymph node enlargement, and of those having abdominoperineal resection, 10 out of 18 had mesenteric lymph node involvement.[35]

### Adenocarcinomas

Carcinomas of the lower rectum occasionally extend downward to involve the anal canal, therefore it may be impossible to determine the origin of the lesion. One might also consider the very rare possibility of the secondary implantation of a carcinoma of the colon or rectum.

The ducts of the anal glands are lined by squamous epithelium close to their opening in the crypts, by transitional epithelium deeper, and in the depth of the gland by mucin secreting columnar epithelium.[15,36] The histologic picture of these lesions may, therefore, be one of adenocarcinoma, mucoepidermoid carcinoma, or transitional cell carcinoma.[36] The

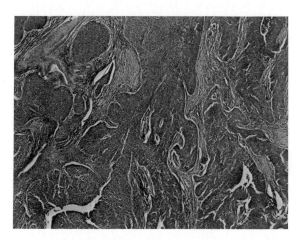

**FIGURE 14-4.** *Basaloid (cloacogenic) carcinoma.*

most characteristic feature of anal duct carcinoma is the extramucosal origin. If there is a break in the surface epithelium, as is often seen clinically, greater perianal involvement or deeper infiltration may be the only clue to the anal duct origin of these lesions.[19]

Patients usually present with complaints of pain and swelling in the anal area but no mass in the anal canal.[19,40,49] They may also present with a perianal or ischiorectal abscess or a fistula-in-ano.[36] Occasionally these are incidental findings in hemorrhoidectomy specimens.[36] The diagnosis is usually made late, and the disease has frequently spread beyond hope for cure.

Adenocarcinomas developing in long standing fistulae-in-ano have occasionally been reported.[10,24] It has been suggested that these carcinomas are due to chronic irritation on the epithelium around either the internal or the external openings of fistulae over a period of years.[10] Some authors, however, believe that carcinomas in fistulae are ductal in origin.[36]

### Treatment of Carcinomas of Anal Canal

*Local excision.* This form of therapy should be reserved for only those early lesions, or well differentiated lesions, which involve only the submucosa.[23,47] It may also be considered for individuals who are a poor risk for an extensive operation.

*Abdominoperineal resection.* In the majority of patients abdominoperineal resection, with wide excision of perineal tissue, forms the basis of treatment.[4,41,50] In women the posterior vaginal wall should also be excised because the incidence of invasion to this area is high (20%).[25]

In good risk patients, pelvic lymphadenectomy has been recommended by Stearns.[47] The extent of lymphadenectomy can be enlarged into the abdomen to include an aortocaval clearance. Advocates of this surgery feel that the five year survival rate of over 50 per cent is related to this radical approach.[44,47] However, Wolfe and associates reported that this type of radical clearance is not without significant problems, and the survival benefit was not confirmed in their series.[52] In a series reviewed by Fitzgibbons, the mortality was 30 per cent for patients beyond the age of 70 on whom this procedure was performed.[9] Stearns, reported a mortality of 1.7 per cent

for patient below the age of 70, compared to 8.5 per cent for those above the age of 70.[47] From the data available, it is difficult to determine the efficacy of radial lymphadenectomy, but, clearly, over the age of 70 it is certainly not indicated.

While abdominoperineal resection offers good macroscopic control of the carcinoma and may result in a cure, all too often local recurrence makes it clear that microscopic control was not achieved. In the series reviewed by Welch and colleagues, 43 patients were considered as having curative resections, but 17 had local or distant recurrent disease.[50] The five year survival following abdominoperineal resection lies between 50 to 58 per cent in the best series. Average survival figures are less than 40 per cent at five years. The results are far from ideal, especially when the operation of choice, in most cases, remains abdominoperineal resection.

*Irradiation.* Interstitial curie therapy (radium implantation) has been used successfully in selected cases of epidermoid carcinoma of the anal canal. Only small lesions without palpable nodes on the rectal wall are suitable for this approach.[39]

*Combined therapy.* In 1973 Nigro and colleagues reported three patients with squamous cell carcinoma of the anal canal treated successfully by a combined therapy of chemotherapy, and irradiation, followed by abdominoperineal resection.[37] The mode of treatment consisted of irradiation of 3000 r delivered to the pelvis for three weeks (15 treatments of 200 r each). The day after the irradiation, patients were started on 25 mg per kg of 5-FU, each 24 hours for five days. On the same day the patients also received mitomycin C, 4.5 mg per kg as a single bolus injection. Abdominoperineal resection was performed six weeks later. In their follow-up report, five of nine patients had no residual carcinoma after receiving preoperative treatment.[5] They suggested that in those patients with no residual found at biopsy after the preoperative treatment, no further surgery is necessary. This effective method of treatment for epidermoid carcinoma of the anal canal is also supported by Quan, et al.[42] Their chemotherapy protocol consisted of 1 dose of mitomycin C, 15 mg per square meter, intravenously on day one and 5-FU, 750 mg per square meter, daily by continuous infusion for five days. Radiotherapy was then commenced immediately after cessation of the 5-FU administration, and 3000 r were delivered to the pelvis to include the anal canal over a period of three weeks. Two or three weeks after completion of the radiotherapy (5 or 6 weeks after the first day of chemotherapy) the patient was subjected to surgical excision of the lesion. In four of ten cases there was, in fact, no microscopic evidence of residual cancer in the resected specimens. Because of these findings they were encouraged to do more local excisions for cure rather than proceeding with an abdominoperineal resection. Whether this effectiveness is from the radiation alone or from a combination of chemotherapy is not known. Only a randomized control study can give the answer.

*Inguinal lymph node dissection.* If prophylactic lymph node dissection were performed in all cases of carcinoma of the anal canal, the positive yield would lie somewhere between 10 to 30 per cent.[50] Inguinal lymph nodes are believed to become involved at some time during the disease process in 37 per cent of cases.[26] In the series reported by Stearns, et al, 61 of 82 patients having prophylactic groin dissections had negative glands.[47] Based on these statistics, because of the high morbidity and mortality, the risk of the added procedure outweighs the benefit and prophylactic groin dissection is not recommended.

The simultaneous appearance of inguinal metastases is an ominous sign. Only two of 14 patients survived five years.[47] In contrast, the subsequent appearance of inguinal metastases gives a better outlook. Fifteen of twenty such patients survived five years after radical groin dissection.[46]

## Malignant Melanoma

This is the most depressing of all anorectal malignancies. It contributes 1 to 3 per cent of all melanomas, with the anal canal being the third most common site, exceeded only by skin and eyes.[27] The sex distribution is about equal, the average age at presentation is 50 years.

They arise from the transitional zone of the anal canal and are mainly situated above the dentate line.[34] There are a few reports of these lesions arising and situated in the rectum.[2,20]

*Clinical Features.* Rectal bleeding is the most common symptom. Less frequent symptoms include anal pain, prolapse, loss of weight, anal irritation, and constipation.[34]

*Diagnosis.* Melanomas will be suspected when a deeply pigmented polypoid lesion on a short stalk is noted. However, unless ulceration with raised edges are present, this may be confused with thrombosed hemorrhoids. The majority of melanomas, however, are only lightly pigmented, or non-pigmented, and are often misdiagnosed as polyps or other neoplasms of the anal canal.[34] Microscopically, if melanin is seen, the diagnosis is simple. In the amelanotic melanoma, sheets of anaplastic cells can be misinterpreted as undifferentiated epidermoid carcinoma.

This malignancy is aggressive, with extensive local invasion and dissemination by both lymphatic and venous routes. Extensive invasion of the tissues around the anal canal was a feature of all cases in Morson and Volkstadts series.[34] Anal canal melanomas have a marked tendency to spread submucosally along the rectum, but rarely invade adjacent organs. Superior rectal node metastases accounted for 70 per cent of patients, while spread to inguinal lymph nodes is less common.[34] Widespread systemic metastases are early and rapid, most commonly to the liver, lung, and bone.[4,27]

*Treatment.* Melanomas of the anal canal are radioresistant and do not respond to chemotherapy or immunotherapy. The only chance for cure is early diagnosis followed by radical operation. Abdominoperineal resection with pelvic dissection represents the approach of choice, but the prognosis, nevertheless, remains poor. Of the 49 patients with malignant melanomas of the anorectum at Memorial Hospital, New York, only six patients lived five years following abdominoperineal resection.[41]

## REFERENCES

1. Ackerman, L. V., and Rosai, J.: Surgical Pathology. 491-492. St. Louis, C. V. Mosby, 1974.

2. Alexander, R. M., and Cone, L. A.: Malignant

melanoma of the rectal ampulla: Report of a case and review of the literature. Dis. Colon Rectum, *20:*53, 1977.

3. Arminski, T. C., and Pollard, R. J.: Paget's disease of the anus secondary to a malignant papillary adenoma of the rectum. Dis. Colon Rectum, *16:*46, 1973.

4. Beahrs, O. H., and Wilson, S. M.: Carcinoma of the anus. Ann. Surg., *184:*422, 1976.

5. Buroker, T. R., et al.: Combined therapy for cancer of the anal canal: A follow-up report. Dis. Colon Rectum, *20:*677, 1977.

6. Cabrera, A., Tsukada, Y., and Pickren, J. W.: Adenocarcinomas of the anal canal and perianal tissues. Ann. Surg., *164:*152, 1966.

7. Dillard, B. M., Spratt, J. S. Jr., Ackerman, L. V., and Butcher, H. R. Jr.: Epidermoid cancer of anal margin and canal. Arch. Surg., *86:*772, 1963.

8. Failes, D., and Morgan, B. P.: Squamous-cell carcinoma of the anus. Dis. Colon Rectum, *16:*397, 1973.

9. Fitzgibbons, R. J. Jr., Harkrider, W. W. Jr., and Cohn, I. Jr.: Review of abdominoperineal resection for cancer. Am. J. Surg., *134:*624, 1977.

10. Goligher, J. C.: Surgery of the Anus, Rectum and Colon. 3 ed. 222. Springfield, Charles C Thomas, 1975.

11. ———: Surgery of the Anus, Rectum and Colon. 3 ed. 824-825. Springfield, Charles C Thomas, 1975.

12. Gordon, P. H.: The chemically defined diet and anorectal procedures. Can. J. Surg., *19:*511, 1976.

13. Graham, J. H., and Helwig, E. B.: Bowen's disease and its relationship to systemic cancer. Arch. Dermatol., *83:*738, 1961.

14. ———: Bowen's disease and its relationship to systemic cancer. Arch. Dermatol., *80:*133, 1959.

15. Grinvalsky, H. T., and Helwig, E. G.: Carcinoma of the anorectal junction. Cancer, *9:*480, 1956.

16. Grodsky, L.: Uncommon non-keratinizing cancers of the anal canal and perianal region. NY State. J. Med., *65:*894, 1965.

17. ———: Extramammary Paget's disease of the perianal region. Dis. Colon Rectum, *3:*502, 1960.

18. ———: Bowen's disease of the anal region (squamous cell carcinoma in situ): Report of three cases. Am. J. Surg., *88:*710, 1954.

19. Hagihara, P., Vazquez, M. D., Parker, J. C. Jr.,

and Griffen, W. O. Jr.: Carcinoma of anal-ductal origin. Dis. Colon Rectum, *19:*694, 1976.

20. Hambrick, E., Abcarian, H., Smith, D., and Keller, F.: Malignant melanoma of the rectum in a negro man. Report of a case and review of the literature. Dis. Colon Rectum, *17:*360, 1974.

21. Hardcastle, J. D., and Bussey, H. J. R.: Results of surgical treatment of squamous cell carcinoma of the anal canal and anal margin. Proc. R. Soc. Med., *61:*623, 1968.

22. Helwig, E. G., and Graham, J. H.: Anogenital (extramammary) Paget's disease. A clinicopathological study. Cancer, *16:*387, 1963.

23. Holm, W. H., and Jackman, R. J.: Anorectal squamous-cell carcinoma: Conservative or radical treatment? JAMA, *188:*241, 1964.

24. Kline, R. J., Spencer, R. J., and Harrison, E. G. Jr.: Carcinoma associated with fistula-in-ano. Arch. Surg., *89:*989, 1964.

25. Klotz, R. G. Jr., Pamukcoglu, T., and Soniliard, D. H.: Transitional cloacogenic carcinoma of the anal canal. Cancer, *20:*1727, 1967.

26. Kuehn, P. G., Beckett, R., Eisenberg, H., and Reed, J. F.: Epidermoid carcinoma of the perianal skin and anal canal. N. Engl. J. Med., *270:*614, 1964.

27. Mason, J. K., and Helwig, E. B.: Anorectal melanoma. Cancer, *19:*39, 1966.

28. McConnell, E. M.: Squamous carcinoma of the anus—A review of 96 cases. Br. J. Surg., *57:*89, 1970.

29. Moller, C., and Saksela, E.: Cancer of the anus and anal canal. Acta Chir. Scand., *136:*340, 1970.

30. Morson, B. C.: Histologic typing of intestinal tumors. 62-65. Geneva, World Health Organization, 1976.

31. ———: The pathology and results of treatment of squamous cell carcinoma of the anal canal and anal margin. Proc. R. Soc. Med., *53:*416, 1960.

32. Morson, B. C., and Dawson, I. M. P.: Gastrointestinal Pathology. 624-625. Oxford, Blackwell Scientific Publications, 1972.

33. Morson, B. C., and Pang, L. S. C.: Pathology of anal cancer. Proc. R. Soc. Med., *61:*623, 1968.

34. Morson, B. C., and Volkstadt, H.: Malignant melanoma of the anal canal. J. Clin. Path., *16:*126, 1963.

35. ———: Muco-epidermoid tumors of the anal canal. J. Clin. Path., *16:*200, 1963.

36. Nielsen, O. V., and Koch, F.: Carcinomas of

# GRANOLA

½ Cup melted margarine
¼ Cup honey
3 Cups uncook oatmeal
1 Cup wheat germ
1 Cup slivered almonds (or sunflower seeds or walnuts
                        or a mixture)

Mix melted butter and honey. Add to oatmeal, wheat germ
and nuts; stir. Bake at 350° for 30 minutes. Stir after
15 minutes. Add 1 cup raisins if desired after baking.

the anorectal region of extramucosal origin with special reference to the anal ducts. Acta Chir. Scand., *139:*299, 1973.

37. Nigro, N. D., Vaitkevicius, V. K., and Considine, B. Jr.: Combined therapy for cancer of the anal canal: A preliminary report. Dis. Colon Rectum, *17:*354, 1974.

38. Pang, L. S., and Morson, B. C.: Basaloid carcinoma of the anal canal. J. Clin. Path., *20:*128, 1967.

39. Papillon, J.: Radiation therapy in the management of epidermoid carcinoma of the anal region. Dis. Colon Rectum, *17:*181, 1974.

40. Parks, T. G.: Mucus-secreting adenocarcinoma of anal canal origin. Br. J. Surg., *57:*434, 1970.

41. Quan, S. H. Q.: Anal and para-anal tumors. Surg. Clin. North Am., *58:*591, 1978.

42. Quan, S. H. Q., Magill, G. B., Leaming, R. H., and Hajdu, S. I.: Multidisciplinary preoperative approach to the management of epidermoid carcinoma of the anus and anorectum. Dis. Colon Rectum, *21:*89, 1978.

43. Raaf, J. H., Krown, S. E., Pinsky, C. M., Cunningham-Rundles, W., Safai, B. and Oettgen, H. F.: Treatment of Bowen's disease with topical Dinitrochlorabenzene and 5 Fluorouracil. Cancer, *37:*1633, 1976.

44. Sawyers, J. L.: Current management of carcinoma of the anus and perianus. Am. J. Surg., *43:*424, 1977.

45. Scoma, J. A., and Levy, E. I.: Bowen's disease of the anus: Report of two cases. Dis. Colon Rectum, *18:*137, 1975.

46. Stearns, M. W. Jr.: Abdominoperineal resection for carcinoma of the rectum. Dis. Colon Rectum, *17:*612, 1974.

47. Stearns, M. W. Jr., and Quan, S. H. Q.: Epidermoid carcinoma of the anorectum. Surg. Gynecol. Obstet., *131:*953, 1970.

48. Stout, A. P.: Malignant manifestations of Bowen's disease. NY State. J. Med., *39:*801, 1939.

49. Thompson, H. R.: Carcinoma of the anorectal region arising from the intramuscular and apocrine glands (two cases). Proc. R. Soc. Med., *49:*469, 1956.

50. Welch, J. P., and Malt, R. A.: Appraisal of the treatment of carcinoma of the anus and anal canal. Surg. Gynecol. Obstet., *145:*837, 1977.

51. Wolfe, H. R. I.: The management of metastatic inguinal adenitis in epidermoid cancer of the anus. Proc. R. Soc. Med., *61:*626, 1961.

52. Wolfe, H. R. I., and Bussey, H. J. R.: Squamous cell carcinoma of the anus. Br. J. Surg., *55:*295, 1968.

# 15

# Benign Neoplasms of the Rectum

## CLASSIFICATION OF COLORECTAL POLYPS

The most common benign condition of the large bowel are polyps, but the word "polyp" is a nonspecific clinical term which describes any projection from the surface of the intestinal mucosa regardless of its histologic nature or whether it is sessile or pedunculated. Many polyps are, in fact, not neoplastic but they are most conveniently considered here. There are four major subdivisions of colorectal polyps and, in each, polyps may be solitary or multiple. Only the neoplastic group has malignant potential.

## BENIGN EPITHELIAL NEOPLASMS

Although these lesions can be separated microscopically into distinct entities, they represent a spectrum of neoplastic change.[24] The macroscopic morphology of these neoplasms is non-specific, and does not necessarily correlate with the histological findings. It is the macroscopic appearance, however, which will determine the technique to be used to achieve total excisional biopsy, which is the treatment of choice when dealing with these lesions.

### Macroscopic Morphology

*Tubular Adenoma (Adenomatous Polyp).* This is a dark red, round to oval, lobulated,

With collaboration of William R. Johnson

solid neoplasm varying in size from less than 0.5 cm to greater than 2 cm in diameter.

*Tubulovillous Adenoma (mixed, papillary, villoglandular).* This is a convenient term for the description of those neoplasms which do not conform to the classical appearance of tubular adenomatous or villous growths. They may be sessile or pedunculated and have blunt, short, broad villous projections on their surface.

*Villous Adenoma (papilloma).* The typical villous adenoma is a broad based, sessile neoplasm with fine, finger-like projections on its surface.

### Histological Classification

Morson has categorized benign epithelial neoplastic polyps histologically regardless of the macroscopic appearance.[26] The relationship resulted from a study of 2500 polyps removed at St. Mark's Hospital, London. It is as follows: tubular adenoma, 75 per cent; tubulovillous adenoma, 15 per cent; villous adenoma, 10 per cent.

### Relationship to Carcinoma

*Polyps and Cancer.* It is well known that neoplastic polyps are found in association with carcinoma. Ekelund found that 22 per cent of 960 patients with large bowel malignancies had coexistent adenomatous polyps, either in proximity to the cancer or elsewhere in the colon.[10] This is a low figure since colonoscopy was not used in this study. The numbers were obtained from air contrast barium enemas, operative specimens, and a necropsy study of postopera-

TABLE **15-1.** Colorectal Polyps[29]

| TYPE | SOLITARY | MULTIPLE |
|------|----------|----------|
| *Neoplastic* | Tubular Adenoma<br>Villous Adenoma<br>Tubulovillous Adenoma | Familial Adenomatous Polyposis<br>Gardner's Syndrome |
| *Hamartomatous* | Juvenile<br>Peutz-Jeghers | Juvenile Polyposis<br>Peutz-Jeghers Syndrome |
| *Inflammatory* | Benign Lymphoid Polyp | Benign Lymphoid Polyposis<br>Inflammatory Polyposis in<br>Colitis |
| *Unclassified* | Metaplastic | Multiple Metaplastic Polyps |

tive patients. They established, however, that the polyps tended to be concentrated in the areas where the carcinoma was found. Of particular interest was the frequent association of polyps in the right and transverse colon when a carcinoma was found in these areas, and a correspondingly low incidence of polyps in the sigmoid colon and rectum of these patients.

*Adenoma-Carcinoma Sequence.* In his presidential address Morson described several aspects of polyp-cancer sequence.[27]

MORPHOLOGY OF THE POLYP-CANCER SEQUENCE. It is common to see tumors in the colon and rectum which are partly benign and partly malignant. In his large series of 1961 malignant tumors, 14 per cent had evidence of benign tumors, either adenomatous polyps or villous adenomas. He also found that the frequency of benign tumors varied with the extent of spread of the malignant component. If the carcinomas spread into the extramural tissues of the wall of the colon and rectum, benign tumors were found in 7 per cent. With spread in continuity limited to the wall of the bowel, it rose to 20 per cent, but if there was invasion of only submucosal tissues it was nearly 60 per cent. It is probable that as the cancers spread through the bowel wall, they tend to destroy the benign tumor cells.

MALIGNANT POTENTIAL OF TUBULAR ADENOMAS AND VILLOUS ADENOMAS. In the series of 2506 polyps 75 per cent were tubular adenomas, 10 per cent villous adenomas and 15 per cent intermediate type (villoglandular or tubulovillous). The general malignancy rate for tubular adenomas was 5 per cent, com-

pared to 40 per cent for villous adenomas, and 22 per cent for the intermediate type. The malignant potential of tubular adenomas and villous adenomas, including the intermediate type, is very low for a polyp under 1 cm in size. With diameter from 1 to 2 cm the malignancy rate increases to one in 10, but nearly half of all polyps with diameter over 2 cm contained evidence of invasive cancers. There is also a clear correlation of increasing epithelial dysplasia of the polyp with increasing malignant potential. When the grade of dysplasia in the polyp is mild the chance of malignancy is 6 per cent, compared to 18 per cent in the moderate, and 35 per cent in the severe dysplasia.

MULTIPLE BENIGN AND MALIGNANT TUMORS. There is abundant evidence that most cancers of the colon and rectum arise from previous benign tubular adenomas and villous adenomas. Out of 3002 patients at St. Mark's Hospital, London, 20 per cent had multiple synchronous tumors, either benign or malignant. In the same series 7 per cent developed a second or metachronous benign or malignant tumor during subsequent follow-up examination.

METACHRONOUS CARCINOMA OF THE COLON AND RECTUM. The cumulative risk of developing a second cancer increases with the length of follow-up, reaching about 5 per cent after 25 years. The risk varies according to whether tubular adenomas of villous adenomas were present in the first operative specimens. If they were present, then the risk of a second cancer rises steeply with time to reach 10 per cent at 25 years. If they were not present in the first operation, the curve flattens off to a metachronous cancer rate at 25 years of only about 4 per cent. This is evidence that there is an important relationship between polyp and cancer, and that the polyp-cancer sequence is probably a process which evolves over a period of many years.

LIFE HISTORY OF POLYP-CANCER SEQUENCE. It is rarely possible to make direct observation on the polyp-cancer sequence because polyps are usually removed by local excision at the time they are detected. In the few cases available for follow-up, carcinoma developed 5 to 12 years later.

THE POLYP-CANCER SEQUENCE IN FAMILIAL POLYPOSIS. A study of the life history of the polyp-cancer sequence in familial polyposis gives very useful information, which is relevant to the time it takes for cancer to evolve from isolated tubular adenomas or villous adenomas. The average age for diagnosis of polyposis without cancer is about 27 years, and for polyposis with carcinomas, 39 years. This gives a total time of approximately 12 years between the diagnosis of polyposis and the later development of cancers. More information about the time it takes for cancers to develop in patients with polyposis comes from the analysis of the age at onset of polyposis and cancers in patients who, for one reason or another, did not have any treatment for the disease. There were 59 such patients. The follow-up showed that at five years, 12 per cent developed cancers; at 10 years, 25 per cent; at 10 to 15 years, 30 per cent; at 15 to 20 years, over 50 per cent. These figures lend support to the concept that evolution of cancer of the colon and rectum, from tubular adenomas and villous adenomas, takes at least five years, and maybe more than 25 years, but on the average lies between 10 and 15 years. It must also be remembered that only very few cancers developed in polyposis, and that most benign tumors in this condition do not become malignant during a normal life span. As previously stated the malignancy rate for tubular adenoma is 5 per cent, and for villous adenomas approximately 40 per cent. This must mean that many tubular adenomas and villous adenomas never become malignant. Although the concept of adenoma-carcinoma sequence has gained increasing acceptance in recent years, much of the evidence in its favor

remains circumstantial, and falls short of direct scientific proof. There are others who believe that pure tubular adenomas do not become cancers, although villous adenomas and adenomas with villous component do.[34] Other investigators believe that most carcinomas of the large bowel derive de novo, and that if tubular adenomas do become invasive cancers they do so infrequently.[35] It appears that the controversy on adenoma-carcinoma sequence will continue.

*Significance of the Muscularis Mucosa.* The importance of the relationship of the lymphatic plexus to the mucous membrane is obvious when neoplastic spread is being considered. It has been assumed that the relationship of lymphatics to blood vessels in the gastrointestinal tract was on a one to one basis. It has now been shown by electron microscopy that the lymphatics do not enter the lamina propria, but ramify on and around the muscularis mucosa. There are some small lymphatic projections toward the base of the crypts but no lymphatic plexus is found within the lamina propria.[11] The muscularis mucosa, therefore, forms a demarcation zone, penetration of which is the basis for the diagnosis of malignant invasion. The diagrammatic representation of a pedunculated polyp is shown (Fig. 15-1). This simplifies the understanding of invasive and in situ carcinoma.[21] The same distinction exists with sessile adenomas.

The pathologist may call malignant change within the mucosa, above the muscularis mucosa, carcinoma in situ or severe dysplasia. The clinical relevance to the surgeon is that this lesion has no metastatic potential.[26] It is only when the muscularis mucosa is penetrated that a clinical diagnosis of carcinoma within a polyp should be made. Based on this information, and a review of the slides with the pathologist, the surgeon will be in a position to plan a therapeutic program. These considerations will be discussed in Chapter 16.

## Clinical Presentation

The symptoms produced by polyps (bleeding, diarrhea, prolapse, mucous discharge, and interference with defecation) are rarely severe, and in many cases absent, or unrecognized.

*Bleeding.* This is the most common finding either overt or occult. It is rarely severe. In

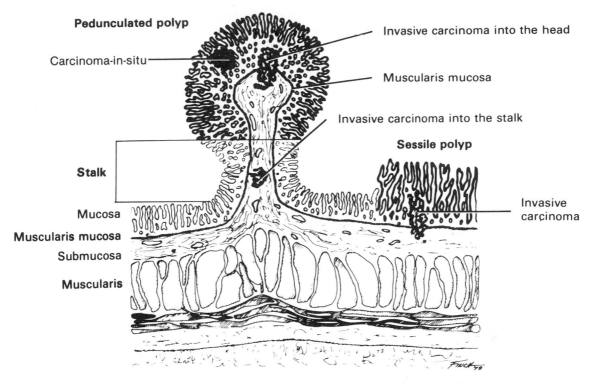

**Pedunculated polyp**

Carcinoma-in-situ

Invasive carcinoma into the head

Muscularis mucosa

Invasive carcinoma into the stalk

**Sessile polyp**

**Stalk**

Mucosa

**Muscularis mucosa**
**Submucosa**

**Muscularis**

Invasive carcinoma

FIGURE **15-1.** *The anatomic landmarks of the colon and rectal polyps.*

juvenile polyps, bleeding following autoamputation is common and may be brisk. Epithelial neoplasms tend to bleed intermittently. It is unusual for metaplastic polyps to bleed and, if this is the presentation and one of these the only lesion found, another cause should be sought. Gilbertsen has found that when Hemoccult tests are positive, 45 per cent of the patients have multiple pathology.[15]

*Diarrhea.* This is a common presentation of large villous adenomas, but can also occur with small pedunculated lesions. Duthie, in a study of the fluxes of sodium and water in relation to villous adenomas, found that there was a net loss into the lumen but that the surface of the villous lesion was absorptive.[9] It was the net loss of sodium and water which was predominantly responsible for the dehydration occurring in patients with large villous neoplasms. Potassium is in high concentration in the fluid lost from the villous lesion, and this explains the hypokalemia which may occur rather than any specific potassium secretory function. This secretory behavior is the exception rather than the rule.

*Prolapse.* Prolapse can occur as a result of intussusception with a polyp at the apex. In low villous lesions this can be mistaken for prolapsed hemorrhoids. Pedunculated polyps may prolapse and autoamputate.

*Mucous Discharge.* This may be noted during bowel movements or present as perianal soiling which the patient may describe as mild incontinence.

*Interference With Defecation.* Tendency to prolapse on straining, tenesmus, or a feeling of incomplete evacuation are common findings with low-lying benign rectal lesions.

**Management**

The primary aim in the management of rectal polyps is to achieve a histological diagnosis. Thus the treatment of choice is total excisional biopsy. If it were possible to distinguish among polyps macroscopically, then the removal of only the neoplastic ones would be required. Clearly, this is not always possible. Biopsy should be performed, unless this represents an unreasonable danger to the patient.

Because of the significance of the finding of neoplastic polyp in the rectum with regard to lesions elsewhere in the colon, the remainder of the colon should be examined thoroughly.[36]

In considering management, the rectum can be divided into thirds. Lesions in the lower two-thirds can usually be dealt with safely with a transanal approach. More care is required in excising lesions on the anterior wall in the middle third of the rectum because they are more likely to be intraperitoneal than an equivalent position on the posterior or lateral wall. Lesions in the upper one-third may be treated by a variety of techniques because the rectum is mobile and peritonealized, therefore access to it is more limited.

The valves of Houston do not include the longitudinal muscle layer of the rectum. Thus, great freedom exists in the depth of biopsy with less fear of perforation.

In the anal canal the dentate line is significant as an area of somatic sensation. It must be realized that this sensation can extend for 1 to 1.5 cm above this level, and local anesthetic may be required prior to excision.[32] Certainly, before any attempt at excision is made, a test of sensation should be performed. Before one decides to deal with a polyp the following questions should be answered: Is the lesion above or below the peritoneal reflection; Is the lesion sessile or pedunculated; How extensive is the lesion, particularly, where is the upper limit; What is the relationship of the lesion to the valves of Houston; Is the lesion on the anterior or posterior rectal wall; What is its relationship to the dentate line; Does the macroscopic appearance suggest malignancy?

We have already stated that total excisional biopsy is the treatment of choice. Small surface biopsies from a large neoplasm to assess the malignant status may be misleading. Not only are they deficient in achieving the primary goal, but also, they distort the surface of the tumor, thus removing the valuable criteria of texture from further consideration. However, if a lesion demonstrates an area which is hard or ulcerated, an appropriately selected biopsy may establish the diagnosis of invasive carcinoma, thereby allowing the surgeon to proceed with a definitive operation.

A host of methods are available to remove rectal lesions. The different methods are listed but details of their performance are described in the corresponding chapters.

---

*Techniques for Removal of Benign Anorectal Lesions*

Per anal approach (see Chapter 19)
  Prolapse, transfixion, excision
  Sigmoidoscopic technique
    Electrocautery snare
    Biopsy forceps excision
    Double scope technique
    Electrocoagulation
  Transanal excision
Posterior rectal approach (see Chapter 19)
  Transsphincteric (York-Mason)
  Transsacral (Kraske)
Sphincter-saving resections (see Chapter 16)
  Anterior resection, End to End Anastomosis (EEA) Stapler
  Pull-through operation

---

## Adenomatous Polyposis Syndrome

As study has progressed, it has become clear that there is a group of clinical diseases which have as their common denominator adenomatous polyposis of the colon and rectum. The gene responsible for adenomatous polyposis is an autosomal dominant with high penetrance. It appears that there are different loci on the gene where changes in an allele will determine the distribution of the adenomatous polyps, and the presence or lack of other associated neoplastic disease.[26] Both familial polyposis and Gardner's syndrome are precancerous conditions.

These two entities are within the spectrum of the adenomatous polyposis syndrome. It is best to think in terms of an adenomatous polyposis syndrome which may have extracolonic manifestations. These may be present at the time of initial diagnosis, or may develop many years later. Before a patient is classified, a full gastrointestinal work-up should be undertaken to document the presence of any associated lesions. At the time of laparotomy, careful examination of the remaining intestine should be performed to exclude the presence of extracolonic adenomatous polyps. We have not yet used the technique of small bowel endoscopy which has been used in some centers with a high degree of success.[31] Following these investigations the patient may be classified as either being in the "familial polyposis" group or in the group referred to as "Gardner's syndrome".

*How Many Polyps is Polyposis?* In the 150 colectomy specimens reviewed at St. Mark's Hospital, London, in no case were there fewer than 150 adenomas, and usually there were many more, the average being 1,000. An arbitrary minimum of 100 polyps is required for the diagnosis of familial polyposis. Patients with less than 100 are referred to as having multiple polyposis. This is thought to be transmitted by a recessive gene.[4] The polyps are distributed throughout the colon but there may be regional differences in density. Many of them are generally found in the rectum, which is always involved.

*Familial Polyposis.* This is a well-documented, hereditary disease of multiple adenomatous polyps of the large intestine, and occasionally other parts of the gastrointestinal tract. Transmission is by an autosomal dominant with a high degree of penetrance. In Bussey's series, 90 of 200 families had no history of any member other than the propositus having the disease.[2]

The risk of developing a carcinoma, if the disease is left untreated, approaches 100 per cent.[1,26] Of the patients presenting with symptoms, 50 to 70 per cent already have a carcinoma.[2,23] Clearly, the way to reduce the incidence of malignant transformation is to trace the family and operate early. Of the familial polyposis patients reviewed at St. Mark's Hospital, London, polyps rarely appeared before the age of ten, or caused symptoms before the age of fifteen.[3] It is suggested that examination should be initiated at fourteen years of age, and continued on a regular basis every two years. Parents should, however, be warned that polyps may appear earlier and any symptoms should be reported and examination performed at that time.

Although familial polyposis is considered to be a disease of youth, polyps have appeared at middle age. In the young patient, total abdominal colectomy should be timed so as not to interfere with school, but should be done before the age of 18. This is perhaps best related to the appearance of the polyps because reports of carcinoma in the young do exist, the youngest being a 14-year-old boy.[6] In general, if polyps are present at the first examination, the colon should be removed as soon thereafter as possible. When polyps develop later, the operation can be planned to fit with the patient's schedule, but should not be unduly delayed.

*Gardner's Syndrome.* Gardner and Richards described a clinical situation in which there is an association of adenomatous polyps of the large bowel, multiple osteomas of the skull and mandible, and multiple epidermoid cysts of the soft tissue of the skin.[12] Since then, the syndrome has been expanded to include abnormal dentition and postoperative desmoid tumors of the abdominal wall and abdominal cavity. In addition, carcinomas of the thyroid, ampulla of Vater, gallbladder and adrenal gland, as well as adenomas and carcinoids of the small intestine, skin pigmentation, and lymphoid polyps of the ileum have been reported.[3,28]

It must be emphasized that a patient classified as "familial polyposis" may later be reclassified as "Gardner's syndrome" because of the appearance of extracolonic manifestations. This shift can be expected to increase as the patient lives longer, and is a strong argument for considering all these patients under the single diagnosis of the "adenomatous polyposis syndrome."

The treatment of Gardner's syndrome is the treatment of adenomatous polyposis. Alm, et al, could find no clear-cut difference in the cancer risk between those patients with extracolonic manifestations of Gardner's syndrome and those without.[1] There are no additional follow-up measures required in patients with Gardner's syndrome, but it is clear that an awareness of the associated pathology will aid in early detection.

*Surgical Management of Multiple Adenomatous Polyposis.* Proctocolectomy assures freedom from the occurrence of colorectal cancer in this disease. The results reported by Moertel would support this operation.[25] His figures from the Mayo Clinic showed the incidence of carcinomatous transformation in the rectal stump to be 32 per cent in 178 cases available for follow-up. However, of those patients followed for more than 20 years, the incidence was 59 per cent in 17 patients. There was a rise, progressive with time, in the incidence of malignant conversion in the rectal stump.

On the other hand, at St. Mark's Hospital, London, the routine management of multiple polyposis is total colectomy and ileorectal anastomosis. Of 86 patients so managed, only two have developed cancer at two and seven years after colectomy. The study spans a 25 year period, with 11 patients cancer-free at between 20 and 25 years post colectomy. In both patients with cancer, the stage was Dukes' A. The follow-up practice is based upon a six-month review with electrocoagulation of rectal polyps, the aim being to keep the rectum clear of polyps.[26]

It is impossible to explain the reasons for such marked differences in the incidence of the development of carcinoma in the rectal stump. There are a few facts which may be helpful. The series reported by Moertel included patients who had invasive colonic cancers at the time of resection.[25] In addition, some patients with rectal cancer had this treated by electrocoagulation. The operation performed was ileorectosigmoidostomy, suggesting a longer portion of retained large bowel. No level of anastomosis is given, but it is significant that in those patients developing rectal cancer, the women outnumbered the men 2 : 1. Proctosigmoidoscopy, especially of the rectosigmoid region, is difficult in women. All but two patients were examined at six month intervals. The cancer at the time of diagnosis and treatment was advanced since only six of 25 patients survived five years; this would suggest that the cancer had been present for longer than six months. In addition, in a group of patients without polyps in the rectum, none developed rectal cancer.

The policy we, in general, recommend is total abdominal colectomy and ileorectal anastomosis. The site of the anastomosis must be such that the whole rectum is easily available for proctosigmoidoscopic evaluation. It is important to preserve the whole of the terminal ileum. The rectal stump is examined at two month intervals for the first year when the residual polyps are electrocoagulated. The patient is then followed at six month intervals. It is preferable that the management and followup be performed by one surgeon, or group of surgeons, experienced in the field of colon and rectal surgery.

The rectum is removed if, in the period of follow-up, it becomes carpeted with polyps, reducing the possibility of control, or if malignant or dysplastic change is found on biopsy. Proctocolectomy is performed if, at the time of diagnosis, malignant change is found in the rectum. It is strongly recommended for any patient who is unwilling or unable to comply with the rigid follow-up protocol. The question of the patient whose rectum is carpeted with polyps at initial presentation is more difficult. The situation is explained in detail to each patient, and then recommendation made. We encourage the patient to take part in the decision making process as much as possible as patient interest is essential to successful follow-up, which must continue as long as the rectum remains, hopefully for the life of the patient.

What about the patient who has 50 or 80 adenomatous polyps? Veale postulated that there are two genes which determine the presence of polyps.[37] One is a dominant gene giving rise to the adenomatous polyposis syndrome and the other a recessive gene responsible for, usually one or two, but perhaps as many as 80 to 90, adenomatous polyps. This genetic link to recessive adenomatous disease of the colon has not been proven but it remains an attractive theory, with evidence accumulating to support it.[23]

Few physicians today would suggest that, given a choice, adenomatous polyps should be left in situ. Colonoscopy provides a technique for the safe removal of colonic polyps.

The management of the patient with many scattered polyps is controversial. When multiple adenomas, distinct from polyposis are considered, 1 or 2 per cent develop more than five adenomas, and in this group 50 is rarely exceeded.[4] If colonoscopy can achieve and maintain a polyp-free colon without the use of unrealistically frequent follow-up examination then, for the patient who has multiple polyps, this is the method of choice. If an expert colonoscopist is unable to free the colon of polyps, the patient has numerous polyps scattered throughout the colon, and is an acceptable operative risk, a total colectomy and ileorectal anastomosis would seem more reasonable.

## BENIGN NON-EPITHELIAL NEOPLASMS

### Hemangioma

Rectal hemangioma is a rare condition. Jeffery, et al, reported only ten cases of diffuse rectal hemangioma treated at St. Mark's Hospital, London.[19] Head, et al, reviewed world literature, and could find only 120 reported cases of hemangioma involving the rectum and rectosigmoid.[18]

---

*Classification of Hemangiomas of the Gastrointestinal Tract*[14]

Capillary hemangioma
Mixed capillary cavernous hemangioma
Cavernous hemangioma
    Multiple phlebectasias (small cavernous)
    Simple polypoid (single cavernous)
    Diffuse expansive
        Single contiguous
        Multiple non-contiguous

---

*Clinical Presentation.* The great majority of patients present early in life with recurrent, painless, sometimes massive hemorrhage. The age of onset, type, frequency, and severity of bleeding are related to the size, number, and type of vascular malformation.

Capillary hemangiomas are characterized by slow, persistent bleeding producing dark stools and anemia. The diffuse cavernous hemangioma characteristically presents early with moderate to severe hemorrhage of a painless nature. At the time of definitive diagnosis, eight out of ten patients presenting at St. Mark's Hospital, London, had had at least one, and frequently many, surgical procedures performed on the mistaken diagnosis of a hemorrhoidal problem.[19] Patients in this series were all under 20 years of age, and bleeding had begun before ten years in all of them. In seven of the ten cases, bleeding had begun before five years of age, with the age range being three months to ten years.[19]

The incidence of bleeding in rectal hemangiomas approaches 90 per cent because of the trauma related to the passage of feces. Local rectal symptoms in addition to the hemorrhage are tenesmus, rectal urgency, and incomplete evacuation.

*Proctosigmoidoscopy.* If the hemangioma is visible as a bluish nodule or mass, the diagnosis may be relatively simple. Diffuse cavernous hemangiomas are sometimes diagnosed as mild proctitis, unless close examination is performed and the abnormal mucosal vessels recognized. It is important to determine the extent of the lesion when surgery is being considered, and to realize that the diffuse hemangioma tends to involve the whole bowel wall and to extend into the perirectal tissues.

Biopsy of hemangiomas, as a general rule, is contraindicated.

*Radiology.* Plain radiograph of the pelvis may be useful because of the frequent association of multiple phleboliths and hemangiomas. Barium enema may be helpful in indicating extrarectal involvement with the hemangioma. Angiographic studies add little additional information when the lesion has been identified and its upper limits defined.

*Treatment.* The treatment of rectal hemangiomas is surgery. If the lesion is small, electrocautery can be used to remove the tumor. Snare polypectomy with electrocautery can be used in some suitable cases. If the neoplasm is located in the rectosigmoid, anterior resection is the treatment of choice.

Diffuse cavernous hemangiomas present a significant problem. Gentry, et al, reviewed 30 such cases and found a 50 per cent intra- and perioperative mortality due to hemorrhage.[14] The problem is related to the extent of the angiomatous malformation, and thus makes abdominoperineal resection or any attempt to mobilize the rectum extremely hazardous. For this reason, Jeffery, et al, have proposed a sleeve resection of the rectal mucosa.[19] Obviously, this does not remove the hemangioma, and this is not the aim. However, with removal of the mucosal portion, which must be associated with meticulous hemostasis, the sigmoid colon is drawn down within the muscular rectal tube. In this way the residual hemangiomatous tissue, by interposition of the sigmoid colon, is protected from the trauma of fecal passage. They have achieved good results with this procedure.

The sleeve resection basically involves a combined approach to the lesion from above and below. Using a solution of 1 : 100,000 adrenalin in normal saline injected submucosally, complete mucosal excision of the rectum is performed and hemostasis of the muscular tube is achieved. From the abdominal approach the level of transection is decided upon, and the sigmoid colon is passed down within the muscular tube to be sutured 2 cm above the pectinate line. The only problem has been some early postoperative bleeding from the area of the suture line; otherwise, the operation has been remarkably free from complication. It can be seen that the problem of rectal mobilization is related to the extraperitoneal rectum; thus, the abdominal approach allows resection of any involved intraperitoneal rectum.

## Lipoma

Lipomas of the rectum are rare. There were five cases reported at Sloan Kettering-Memorial Hospital, New York over a 20 year period.[7] All rectal lipomas are submucosal lesions with an overlying intact mucosa. The lesions tend to be 2 cm or less in diameter and, although in most cases sessile, they can occur as pedunculated lesions. They are particularly innocent neoplasms and present only a point of differential diagnosis.

## Leiomyoma

Anorectal leiomyomas account for five per cent of the smooth muscle neoplasms of the gastrointestinal tract. The lesions may be pedunculated, present as sessile, submucosal, non-ulcerated masses, or as apparent extrarectal tumors, either in the abdomen or postrectal space, and attached by a stalk to the rectum.[30]

In the anal canal they may be found submucosally but are most commonly found in an intersphincteric position with a variable relationship to the sphincter muscles.[20] They are most commonly found in the age group of 50 to 59 years. Leiomyoma appears to be rare or absent in children, and there is a slight male predominance. The most common single finding is the presence of a mass. A small percentage of cases are totally asymptomatic and detected incidentally at proctosigmoidoscopic examination. Bleeding, constipation, and pain are the next most common group of presentations. There is frequently a long history of symptoms, possibly extending over years, and frequently tolerated by the patient because of their minor nature.

*Pathology.* Leiomyomas are commonly firm, rounded, sharply circumscribed neoplasms, but have no definite capsule. The differentiation between benign and malignant variants is controversial and unsatisfactory. It is the number of mitotic figures per high power field which most pathologists accept as the distinction between benign and malignant. Golden and colleagues proposed that if there are more than two mitoses seen per high power field the lesion is malignant.[17] The Broders classification is more complex but offers no advantage.

Local recurrence following excision is a common problem. This is related to the failure to appreciate the diagnosis, the fact that the neoplasm has no capsule but can be easily shelled out from a pseudocapsule, and the difficulty with reaching the diagnosis regarding malignancy.[20]

*Treatment.* Lesions less than 5 cm in diameter, and those that are pedunculated, can be treated by local excision. This should be wide; shelling out of the tumor should be avoided. When the tumor is greater than 5 cm in diameter a more aggressive approach is required. Some form of local resection will be the treatment of choice. Sphincter preservation should be attempted, but often this is impossible.

When recurrence develops, aggressive surgical correction is required. It is important to realize that the recurrence has a tendency to show less differentiation and frequently sarcomatous change occurs.[20] Following local resection 30 per cent of the patients can be expected to have a recurrence.

## HAMARTOMATOUS POLYPS

A hamartoma is a malformation, or inborn error of tissue development, characterized by an abnormal mixture of tissues endogenous to the part, with excess of one or more of these. It may show itself at birth or by extensive growth in the postnatal period.[28]

### Juvenile Polyps

Juvenile polyps are pink in color, with a glistening, smooth, round contour, unlike the lobulated appearance of an adenoma. They are usually pedunculated, and only rarely sessile. The cut surface has a cystic appearance; hence, the term "retention" polyp.

Histologically the lamina propria has a mesenchymal appearance and represents the hamartomatous portion of the polyp. The muscularis mucosa does not participate in the structure of the polyp. This is felt to be a reason for their tendency to autoamputate.

These polyps are found most commonly in children, but occasionally in adults. They are not precancerous and decrease in number with age. Cabrere, et al, recorded the findings in 32 pediatric patients.[5] These polyps were a frequent cause of minor colorectal complaints. Bleeding was the most common finding, but prolapse of the polyp, diarrhea, and crampy abdominal pain also occurred.

Brisk bleeding is felt to be related to the autoamputation of these polyps, a tendency which encourages a conservative approach when symptoms occur. If symptoms persist or become severe, in particular if anemia results from continued bleeding, then colonoscopic removal is required.[16] Colonoscopy in the young, particularly when a general anesthetic is required, may involve increased risks.

The syndrome of multiple juvenile polyposis is now recognized.[13] These polyps can be restricted to the colon, or distributed throughout the gastrointestinal tract. In the most severe form, symptoms of bleeding, prolapse, and malnutrition occur in the infant and, although only seven such cases have been reported, only one lived beyond infancy.[33] The St. Mark's Hospital Polyposis Register contains records of over 50 cases of juvenile polyposis encountered in 36 families. In three-fourths of these families there appeared to be only one affected member. The fact that about one-fourth of the investigated families contained two to five members with polyposis is suggestive of a genetic origin in this group. The more numerous solitary cases may result from environmental factors, or arise from new genetic mutations. Whether juvenile polyposis has malignant potential remains to be seen.[4]

### Peutz-Jegher's Syndrome

The Peutz-Jegher's syndrome is recognized as the combination of cutaneous pigmentation and gastrointestinal polyps.[24] The pigmentation is seen around the lips, on the hard palate, and on the dorsum of the fingers and toes. The pigmentation tends to fade, gradually, beyond the age of thirty so that parents may fail to exhibit this sign.[24]

Inheritance is by a single pleiotropic gene transmitted as a Mendelian dominant.[1] Neither gastrointestinal polyps nor pigmentation are found in all carriers of the gene.

These polyps are most commonly found in the small intestine and in only 50 per cent of cases are the colon and rectum involved, where the polyp tends to be solitary.

Histologically an overgrowth of the muscularis mucosa is the classical finding. The tree-like branching deformity reaches the periphery of the polyp and is covered by normal mucosa.

There is a slight, but definite, increase in the incidence of gastrointestinal cancer in these patients. Bussey reported four cases of gastrointestinal cancer and reviewed another ten from the literature.[3] The frequency of reports has been increasing but is still small. The cancer potential does not appear related to these polyps.

## INFLAMMATORY POLYPS
### Pseudopolyposis Coli

Pseudopolyposis can follow a severe attack of nonspecific ulcerative colitis, Crohn's disease, or one of the infective colitides. It results from incomplete mucosal sloughing. Two phases of the condition can be distinguished. In the acute situation, islands of edematous mucosa persist in a sea of ulceration, and appear as polypoid lesions. Histologically, there is an acute inflammatory infiltrate with marked mucosal and submucosal edema. When healing occurs there is a re-epithelialization of the ulcerated areas, together with varying degrees of fibrosis. This can result in the persistence of the mucosal projections which at this stage have, histologically, a chronic infiltration.

Radiologically, both the acute and chronic forms have a similar appearance. Distinction can be made with the proctosigmoidoscope but in the chronic stage biopsy may be necessary to distinguish the condition from familial polyposis. Inflammatory polyps are not, in their own right, precancerous, and their presence in no way influences the potential cancer status of the patient with ulcerative colitis, a development which remains related to the extent, age of onset, and duration of disease. That these are not precancerous in ulcerative colitis is a relative term; the potential cancer status of the pseudopolyp in this condition is no more or less than the adjacent mucosa.[29]

## UNCLASSIFIED
### Metaplastic (Hyperplastic Polyps)

These polyps are typical in appearance. They are commonly small (less than 0.5 cm in diameter), pale, sessile polyps found predominantly in the rectum. Occasionally they can be large (up to 2 cm), and a condition of metaplastic polyposis is recognized. Ekelund, et al, from a study of operative specimens and post-operative necropsy studies, found 84 per cent of metaplastic polyps in the rectum and sigmoid colon; the remainder were distributed evenly throughout the large bowel.[10]

Histologically, there is lengthening of the tubules which have a tendency to cystic dilation. The epithelium is serrated, with loss of the regular columnar pattern, and depletion of goblet cells. The lower half of the crypts shows a variable degree of epithelial hyperplasia.

These polyps do not cause symptoms, are not related to carcinoma, and would not require removal except for proof of their pathology.

## Benign Lymphoid Polyps

Benign lymphoid polyps are commonly found in the rectum, especially the lower third, and are also occasionally found in the terminal ileum. They are composed of normal lymphoid tissue and have the structure of lymph nodes with sinusoids. Benign lymphomatous polyposis is a rare variant.[22] In both cases biopsy is required to distinguish the condition from the malignant form.

The histologic criteria set out by Dawson, et al, for the diagnosis of benign lymphoid polyps are: the lymphoid tissue must be entirely within the mucosa and submucosa; there must be no invasion of the underlying muscle coat; at least two germinal centers must be present; and, if the rectal biopsy fails to include the muscle coat and no germinal centers are seen, then the diagnosis is inconclusive.[8]

## Cystic Pneumatosis

Cystica pneumatosis usually involves the small intestine, but may occasionally include the colon. Cyst-like spaces filled with gas are characteristic, and are found in the intestinal wall and mesentery. The condition may be related to trauma, but in most instances the etiology is obscure. Treatment is reserved for symptomatic patients who may develop obstruction secondary to the large, gas-filled cysts (see Chapter 30).

## REFERENCES

1. Alm, T., and Licznerski, G.: The intestinal polyposes. Clin. Gastroenterol., *2:*577, 1973.

2. Bussey, H. J. R.: Familial polyposis coli: Family studies, histopathology, differential diagnosis and results of treatment. 8. Baltimore, Johns Hopkins Univ Press, 1975.

3. ———: Gastrointestinal polyposis. Gut, *11:*970, 1970.

4. Bussey, H. J. R., Veale, A. M. O., and Morson, B. C.: Genetics of gastrointestinal polyposis. Gastroenterology, *74:*1325, 1978.

5. Cabrera, A., and Lega, J.: Polyps of the colon and rectum in children. Am. J. Surg., *100:*551, 1960.

6. Capps, W. F. Jr., Lewis, M. I., and Gazzaniga, D. A.: Carcinoma of the colon, ampulla of Vater and urinary bladder associated with familial multiple polyposis: A case report. Dis. Colon Rectum, *11:*298, 1968.

7. Castro, E. B., and Stearns, M. W.: Lipoma of the large intestine: A review of 45 cases. Dis. Colon Rectum, *15:*441, 1972.

8. Dawson, I. M. P., Cornes, J. S., and Morson, B. C.: Primary malignant lymphoid tumours of the intestinal tract: Report of 37 cases with a study of factors influencing prognosis. Br. J. Surg., *49:*80, 1961.

9. Duthie, H. L., and Atwell, J. D.: The absorption of water, sodium, and potassium in the large intestine with particular reference to the effects of villous papillomas. Gut, *4:*373, 1963.

10. Ekelund, G., and Lindstrom, C.: Histopathological analysis of benign polyps in patients with carcinoma of the colon and rectum. Gut, *15:*654, 1974.

11. Fenoglio, C. M., Kaye, G. I., and Lane, N.: Distribution of human colonic lymphatics in normal, hyperplastic, and adenomatous tissue; its relationship to metastasis from small carcinomas in pedunculated adenomas, with two case reports. Gastroenterology, *64:*51, 1973.

12. Gardner, E. J., and Richards, R. C.: Multiple cutaneous and subcutaneous lesions occurring simultaneously with hereditary polyposis and osteomatosis. Am. J. Hum. Genet., *5:*139, 1953.

13. Gathright, J. B. Jr., and Cofer, T. W.: Familial incidence of juvenile polyposis coli. Surg. Gynecol. Obstet., *138:*185, 1974.

14. Gentry, R. W., Dockerty, M. B., and Clagett, O. T.: Vascular malformations and vascular tumors of the gastrointestinal tract. International Abstracts of Surgery, *88:*281, 1949.

15. Gilbertsen, V. A.: Proctosigmoidoscopy and polypectomy in reducing the incidence of rectal cancer. Cancer, *34:*936, 1974.

16. Gleason, W. A. Jr., Goldstein, P. D., Shatz,

B. A., and Tedesco, F. J.: Colonoscopic removal of juvenile colonic polyps. J. Pediatr. Surg., *10:*519, 1975.

17. Golden, T., and Stout, A. P.: Smooth muscle tumors of the gastrointestinal tract and retroperitoneal tissues. Surg. Gynecol. Obstet., *73:*784, 1941.

18. Head, H. D., Baker, J. Q., and Muir, R. W.: Hemangioma of the colon. Am. J. Surg., *126:*691, 1973.

19. Jeffery, P. J., Hawley, P. R., and Parks, A. G.: Colo-anal sleeve anastomosis in the treatment of diffuse cavernous haemangioma involving the rectum. Br. J. Surg., *63:*678, 1976.

20. Kusminsky, R. E., and Bailey, W.: Leiomyomas of the rectum and anal canal: Report of six cases and review of the literature. Dis. Colon Rectum, *20:*580, 1977.

21. Lane, N.: The precursor tissue of ordinary large bowel cancer. Cancer. Res., *36:*2669, 1976.

22. Louw, J. H.: Polypoid lesions of the large bowel in children with particular reference to benign lymphoid polyposis. J. Pediatr. Surg., *3:*195, 1968.

23. Lovett, E.: Familial factors in the etiology of carcinoma of the large bowel. Proc. R. Soc. Med., *67:*751, 1974.

24. McConnell, R. B.: Genetic aspects of gastrointestinal cancer. Clin. Gastroenterol., *5:*483, 1976.

25. Moertel, C. G., Hill, J. R., and Adson, M. A.: Surgical management of multiple polyposis. Arch. Surg., *100:*521, 1970.

26. Morson, B. C.: Genesis of colorectal cancer. Clin. Gastroenterol., *5:*505, 1976.

27. ———: The polyp-cancer sequence in the large bowel. Proc. R. Soc. Med., *67:*451, 1974.

28. Morson, B. C., and Bussey, H. J. R.: Predisposing causes of intestinal cancer. Curr. Probl. Surg., *Feb.,* 1970.

29. Morson, B. C., and Dawson, I. M. P.: Gastrointestinal Pathology. 517-519. London, Blackwell Scientific Publication, 1972.

30. Nemer, F. D., Stoeckinger, J. M., and Evans, O. T.: Smooth-muscle rectal tumors: A therapeutic dilemma. Dis. Colon Rectum, *20:*405, 1977.

31. Ohsato, K., Yao, T., Watanabe, H., Iida, M., and Itoh, H.: Small-intestinal involvement in familial polyposis diagnosed by operative intestinal fiberscopy: Report of Four Cases. Dis. Colon Rectum, *20:*414, 1977.

32. Parks, A. G.: The surgical treatment of haemorrhoids. Br. J. Surg., *43:*337, 1956.

33. Sachatello, C. R., Hahn, I. S., and Carrington, C. B.: Juvenile gastrointestinal polyposis in a female infant: Report of a case and review of the literature of a recently recognized syndrome. Surgery, *75:*107, 1974.

34. Spjut, H. J., and Estrada, R. G.: The significance of epithelial polyps of the large bowel. Pathology Annual, 12. 147-170. New York, Appleton-Century-Crofts, 1977.

35. Spratt, J. S. Jr., and Ackerman, L. V.: Small primary adenocarcinomas of the colon and rectum. JAMA, *179:*337, 1962.

36. Theuerkauf, F. J. Jr.: Rectal and colonic polyp relationships via colonoscopy and fibersigmoidoscopy. Dis. Colon Rectum, *21:*2, 1978.

37. Veale, A. M. O.: Intestinal Polyposis. London, Cambridge University Press, 1965.

38. Wolff, W. I., and Shinya, H.: Definitive treatment of "malignant" polyps of the colon. Ann. Surg., *182:*516, 1975.

# 16

# Malignant Neoplasms of the Rectum

## CARCINOMA

It was estimated that in 1978 in the United States 100,200 new cases of carcinoma of the large bowel, including 31,000 carcinoma of the rectum, would occur.[13] Approximately 50 per cent of these patients will die from their disease.[115] Carcinoma of the rectum used to account for about 50 per cent of large bowel cancer.[31,113] More recent studies have shown a shift in the distribution of colorectal cancer toward the right side, with an increase in the right colon and a decrease in the rectum.[83,95] A study by Morgenstern of 1,009 consecutive cases of colorectal cancer from 1966 to 1977 inclusive, revealed the following distribution: rectum 15 per cent, rectosigmoid and sigmoid colon 38 per cent (Fig. 16-1).[83] The reason for this change in the distribution is not clear. One can only speculate that it may be the effect of more frequent proctosigmoidoscopy and eradication of rectal polyps. This important observation supports total evaluation of the large bowel whenever indicated with more frequent use of barium enemas and colonoscopy to detect more proximal lesions.

In recent years, increased research has been directed toward ascertaining the etiology of this disease; but it has been to little avail. Other efforts have been focused on improving the long-term survival with adjuvant therapy, but these, similarly, have been met with limited success. Operative therapy for carcinoma

of the rectum has also changed somewhat during the past several years. In carefully selected cases, carcinoma of the lower rectum has been successfully treated by local methods, and carcinoma of the middle third of the rectum has more often been treated by sphincter-saving operations. The most recent advance is the end-to-end anastomosis (EEA) stapler which has allowed surgeons to safely perform low anterior resections in a greater number of patients.

### Epidemiology

The etiology of rectal carcinoma is unknown. Hereditary factors have been implicated for some patients, but the overwhelming majority of cases appear to be related to extra-genetic factors.[72] The observations that the incidence of carcinoma of the large bowel is low in Japan but increases among Japanese immigrants to the United States, along with the high-prevalence of this disease among North Americans and Western Europeans, suggest that environmental factors are of etiological significance in the development of this disease.[118] A large-scale retrospective study by Wynder et al, aimed at uncovering the risk factors in patients with large bowel cancer, pointed to association of dietary factors.[119] Reddy and Wynder found that populations on a mixed Western diet, among whom the rate of large bowel cancer is high, degraded and excreted cholesterol and bile acid metabolites to a greater degree than those populations where the rate of colon cancer is comparatively low.[93] Hill found a significantly larger number of bacteroides in the stools of populations on

With collaboration of William R. Johnson

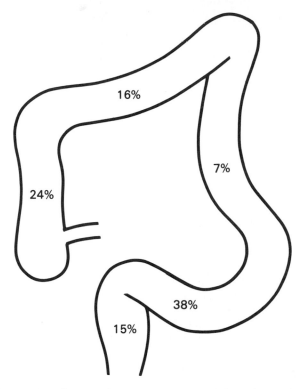

FIGURE **16-1.** *Distribution of 1009 carcinomas of the colon and rectum.*

Western diets than those on vegatarian diets.[56] Bacteroides are known to metabolize steroids more actively than the aerobes, and it is believed that a metabolite of bile acids by these bacteria is carcinogenic. With the available evidence, it has been suggested that a diet in which 30 to 45 per cent of the fat comes from meat is more likely to be associated with large bowel cancer.

Epidemiological studies by Burkitt suggested a relationship between a low fiber diet and the high incidence of large bowel cancer.[10] Relating this concept to the high fat, diet association, he postulated that the high fiber diet may decrease the incidence of large bowel cancer by decreasing the transit time, and thus, decrease the contact time of the carcinogen with the large bowel mucosa. Because of the increased bulk, and the consequent increased circumference of the bowel, the concentration of carcinogen is more diluted. The hypothesis that a high fiber diet has the ability to lower the incidence of carcinoma of the large bowel is supported by the experimental study of Chen et al.[16] They showed that a high fiber, bran diet had the ability to significantly lower the incidence of pathologic changes in the colon of mice receiving 1,2-dimethylhydrazine, a drug known for its specificity of causing carcinoma of the colon. One should remember that the etiology of colorectal cancer in humans is almost certainly multifactorial: diet alone is not likely the entire explanation.

**Premalignant Diseases of the Rectum**

*Adenomas.* At the present time there is overwhelming evidence suggesting the polyp-cancer sequence.[29,84] Indirect evidence supporting this concept is the fact that if rectal polyps are regularly destroyed, the incidence of rectal carcinoma is less than expected in a given population.[33] Much is still unknown regarding the average time for the malignant transformation, and what percentage, and which adenomas eventually become carcinoma in this polyp-cancer sequence.

*Familial Adenomatous Polyposis Syndrome*. This is a hereditary disease transmitted by an autosomal dominant gene. It is characterized by the development of at least 100 adenomatous polyps, and if left untreated, the subsequent development of adenocarcinoma of the large bowel, at an average age of 39 years old. The density of the polyps is greater in the left colon, and the rectum is invariably involved. The incidence of carcinoma developing in familial polyposis is highest in the rectum.[11]

*Chronic Ulcerative Colitis*. It is well-known that the incidence of carcinoma is higher in patients who have had a history of ulcerative colitis than in the normal population. This is especially true when the history includes: the presence of disease more than 10 years, total colonic involvement, and onset in childhood. Precarcinomatous change characterized by dysplasia, adenomatous, or villous change is a warning sign of the presence or future development of carcinoma somewhere in the colon or rectum.[67] The cancers in chronic ulcerative colitis are usually multiple, flat or plaque-like, often very aggressive, and develop at an earlier age than noncolitic cancers.[21]

*Irradiation Proctitis*. There have been sporadic reports of carcinoma of the rectum and colon developing years after irradiation for carcinoma of the cervix or uterus.[14] Over half of these carcinomas are mucin-producing, and the overall five-year survival is low. It is impossible to determine whether the relationship is one of cause and effect, or purely coincidental. Nevertheless, patients who are long term survivors of irradiation-treated carcinoma of the cervix and uterus should be followed for the late development of colorectal carcinoma.

*Schistosomiasis (Bilharziasis)*. In Egypt, carcinoma as a late complication of genitourinary schistosomiasis is well known.[87] Less clear is the relationship between carcinoma of the large bowel and intestinal schistosomiasis (Schistosoma mansoni, Schistosoma japonica).[101] A study by Wu and colleagues, in nonendemic and endemic areas of intestinal schistosomiasis in China, revealed that the incidence of carcinoma of the large bowel among infested patients is much higher, and occurs at an age about 10 years younger than patients without the disease.[117] They postulated that

repeated damage, with the consequent proliferation of bowel mucosa, provides a favorable condition for development of carcinoma in these individuals.

## Pathology

*Macroscopy*. The two most common macroscopic forms are the ulcerating type and the polypoid or fungating type. About 15 per cent display a bulky growth with a gelatinous appearance, and are referred to as colloid carcinomas.[109] In rare instances there is thickening of the rectal wall extending submucosally for at least 5 to 7 cm. This is the infiltrating carcinoma which is similar to linitis plastica of the stomach. The gross appearance of carcinoma may be of clinical importance. Greaney showed that ulcerated lesions, regardless of size, and polypoid or fungating lesions larger than 5 cm, are associated with a 50 per cent incidence of lymph node metastasis.[44] For polypoid carcinomas smaller than 5 cm, lymph node involvement is much less common.

*Microscopy*. Almost all carcinomas of the rectum are adenocarcinoma but their histologic appearances differ considerably. In 1925 Broder divided the microscopic features of carcinoma of the rectum into four grades according to the degree of differentiation.[9] Grinnell, in 1939, while trying to apply this grading to prognosis, found it more practical to grade large bowel carcinoma in relation to invasive tendency, glandular arrangement, nuclear polarity, and frequency of mitosis.[49] This grading system is used worldwide at the present time.

GRADE I. This variety displays a well-differentiated and compact glandular structure. The acini are lined with two to three layers of cells whose nuclei tend to remain close to the basal layer of the gland, leaving a clear zone near the luman. There is little tendency for individual cells or small groups of cells to extend into surrounding tissue. Mitoses are infrequent (Fig. 16-2).

GRADE II. The glandular arrangement is still preserved, but some glands appear to be loosely and irregularly arranged. The walls are thicker, and composed of cells in three or more layers with their nuclei scattered throughout the wall of the gland. The central zone in the cytoplasm of cells around the

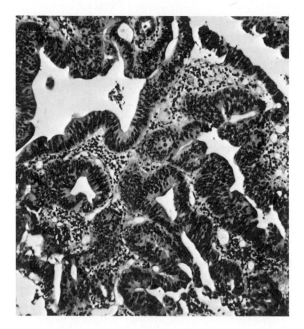

FIGURE **16-2.** *Grade I or well-differentiated adeno-carcinoma.*

lumen is largely lost. A tendency of the cells to stray off into adjacent tissue can be seen, especially at the deep, advancing edge of the lesion. Mitoses are more numerous (Fig. 16-3).

GRADE III. The glandular structure may be completely or nearly completely lost. At least parts of the growth may show neoplastic cells growing in solid masses, or cords with little or no tendency to arrange themselves around a central lumen. Nearly all the cells' polarity is lost. Mitoses are frequent (Fig. 16-4).

This grading system has been adopted by other as well differentiated (low grade), moderately differentiated (average grade), and poorly differentiated (high grade). In addition, about 15 per cent of colorectal carcinomas produce mucus and are called mucinous carcinoma (Fig. 16-5). This type of cancer has been found to have an adverse effect on the prognosis, although this is not universally agreed upon. The five-year survival is 18 per cent, compared to 49 per cent for the nonmucinous carcinoma in Symonds and Vickery series.[109]

*Relating Pathology to Prognosis.* GRADING. The relationship between the grade of the carcinoma and the incidence of lymph node metastases was studied by Grinnell, who found that the Grade III cases had a risk of lymph node metastases nine times greater than the Grade I cases (Table 16-1).[49] Grading has also proved to be of considerable value in rela-

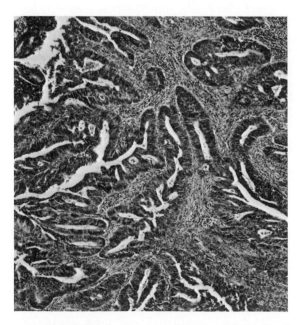

FIGURE **16-3.** *Grade II or moderately differentiated adenocarcinoma.*

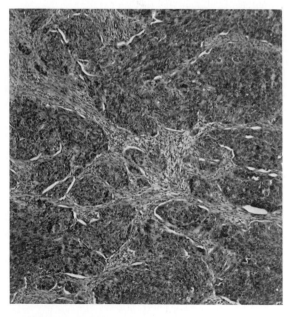

FIGURE **16-4.** *Grade III or poorly differentiated adenocarcinoma.*

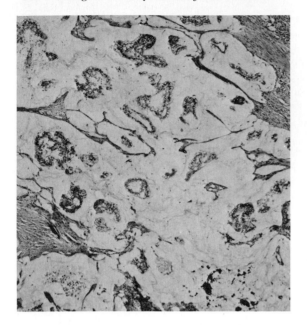

FIGURE **16-5.** *Mucinous adenocarcinoma.*

tion to prognosis as shown by Dukes and Bussey (Table 16-2).[27]

STAGING. Dukes divided carcinoma of the rectum into different stages, according to the depth of penetration by the carcinoma into the bowel wall and the presence or absence of lymph node metastases.[26,27] Thus, Stage A is when the invasion is into the muscularis propria but not through it and the lymph nodes are free from metastases. Stage B is the invasion through the full thickness of the bowel but the lymph nodes are free from metastases. Stage C, regardless of the depth of the invasion, lymph node metastases are present (Fig. 16-6). When the depth of invasion is limited to the muscularis propria the risk of lymph node metastases is about 12 per cent, whereas when invasion is full thickness, the risk of lymph node metastases is 50 per cent.[84] At the present time, this staging system is the best prognostic indicator. In their extensive experience

TABLE **16-1.** Risk of Lymph Node Metastasis

| GRADE | NO. OF CASES | PERCENT METASTASIS |
|---|---|---|
| *Low Grade* | 85 | 6 |
| *Average Grade* | 79 | 32 |
| *High Grade* | 52 | 54 |

TABLE **16-2.** Relationship of Grading to Survival

| GRADE | NO. OF CASES | CORRECTED 5-YEAR SURVIVAL (%) |
|---|---|---|
| *Low Grade* | 407 | 77 |
| *Average Grade* | 1266 | 61 |
| *High Grade* | 424 | 29 |

Dukes and Bussey found the five-year survivals of Stage A, B, and C carcinoma of the rectum (Table 16-3).[27]

Dukes further subdivided Stage C into $C_1$ and $C_2$.[37] Stage $C_1$ is when only adjacent regional lymph nodes contain metastases, whereas $C_2$ is when lymphatic spread involves the nodes at the point of ligature of the blood vessels (Fig. 16-7). The survival rates in these cases is also different (Table 16-4).[27]

The staging distribution is as follows: Stage A, 15 per cent; Stage B, 35 per cent; and Stage C, 50 per cent.[82] About two-thirds of Stage C cases correspond to the definition of $C_1$, and one-third to that of $C_2$. This distribution has not changed during the past thirty years.

NUMBER OF LYMPH NODE METASTASIS. To investigate the significance of the number of lymph node metastases, cases with lymphatic spread have been further subdivided into: one metastasis, two to five metastases, six to nine metastases, and 10 or more metastases.[27] Using these criteria, the five-year survivals are shown in Table 16-5.

## Mechanism of Spread in Carcinoma of Rectum

*Direct Spread.* Carcinoma of the rectum originates in the mucosa. As time goes by, it penetrates the thickness of the rectal wall rather than growing in the longitudinal axis. Untreated, it finally involves the full thickness of the rectum and invades adjacent tissues. It is unusual to find direct upward or downward spread greater than 1 cm beyond the visible borders of the lesion. This was substantiated by Quer, et al, and Grinnell.[48,91]

TABLE **16-3.** Relationship of Staging to Survival

| STAGE | NO. OF PATIENTS | CORRECTED 5-YEAR SURVIVAL (%) |
|---|---|---|
| *A* | 308 | 98 |
| *B* | 692 | 78 |
| *C* | 1037 | 32 |
| TOTAL | 2037 | 57.4 |

# THE DUKES' CLASSIFICATION

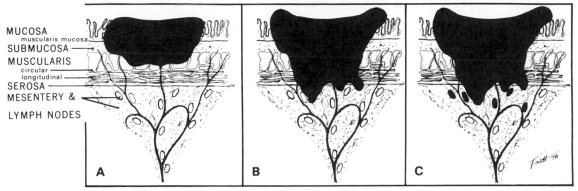

MUCOSA
muscularis mucosa
SUBMUCOSA
MUSCULARIS
circular
longitudinal
SEROSA
MESENTERY &
LYMPH NODES

**FIGURE 16-6.** *The Dukes' classification.*

*Transperitoneal Spread.* Peritoneal involvement of carcinoma of the rectum probably starts from local extension, continues through the peritoneum, and, subsequently, is disseminated within the peritoneal cavity. Once this occurs it is beyond hope for surgical cure.

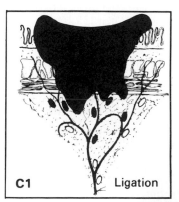

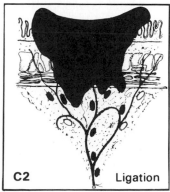

**FIGURE 16-7.** *The Dukes' classification.*

*Implantation.* It has been postulated that desquamated colonic or rectal cancer cells may implant on anal wounds after hemorrhoidectomy, fistulectomy, fissurectomy, and the cut ends of bowel.[38,61,68] Although this hypothesis has gained widespread acceptance, supporting evidence is predominantly circumstantial. The study by Rosenberg and colleagues failed to show the viability of exfoliated cells.[97] This finding would cast some doubt on this hypothesis. Such implantation may possibly be due to circulating cancer cells which are known to be increased during the induction of anesthesia and during operation.[45] Suture line recurrences of the rectum are usually caused by the extension of local pelvic recurrences.[114]

*Lymphatic Spread.* Ernest Miles believed that the lymphatic pathways of carcinoma of the rectum drained in three directions: upward along the superior rectal glands, laterally along the middle rectal nodes, and downward to the inguinal nodes.[79] This was based on an autopsy study where most patients died from advanced disease with proximal blockade of the lymph nodes. Later studies revealed that le-

**TABLE 16-4.** Prognosis of Dukes $C_1$ and $C_2$

| STAGE | NO. OF CASES | CORRECTED 5-YEAR SURVIVAL (%) |
|---|---|---|
| $C_1$ | 680 | 41 |
| $C_2$ | 282 | 14 |
| *unclassified* | 75 | 20 |
| TOTAL | 1037 | 32 |

TABLE **16-5.** Relationship of the Number of Lymph Node Metastases to Survival

| NO. OF LYMPH NODE METASTASES | NO. OF CASES | CORRECTED 5-YEAR SURVIVAL (%) |
|---|---|---|
| *1* | 125 | 64 |
| *2–5* | 249 | 31 |
| *6–10* | 138 | 22 |
| *more than 10* | 52 | 2 |

sions of the upper and middle thirds of the rectum drain upward along the superior rectal vessels; lesions in the lower third drain both upward along the superior mesenteric vessels, and laterally along the middle rectal vessels, and frequently along the internal iliac glands.[7] Retrograde drainage of carcinoma is unusual unless there is blockade of the proximal lymph nodes.[46] Spread to inguinal nodes generally does not occur unless the carcinoma has invaded the dentate line.

RETROGRADE INTRAMURAL METASTASES. With the present trend of performing a low anterior resection for carcinoma of the mid and upper rectum, the surgeon must select a site which compromises neither the adequacy of the resection nor the ability to perform a sphincter-saving procedure. It, therefore, becomes necessary to define an adequate distal margin. A comprehensive study of this subject was performed by Quer and colleagues in a prospective manner.[91] Examinations included 91 specimens which were obtained directly from the operating table. To obviate shrinkage, the specimens were stretched to conform with the preoperative or operative measurements of length, and were then immediately fixed for 48 hours in 10 per cent formalin. If the two patients who had clinically obvious metastatic deposits were excluded, only 1 of 89 patients had retrograde spread beyond 1.5 cm, and 86 had no retrograde intramural spread. To decrease the chance of error, they recommended a margin of 2.5 cm below the lowest, grossly palpable or visible edge of the carcinoma. This margin is adequate from the standpoint of retrograde intramural spread when the lesions were of low grade malignancy. For high grade malignancy they recommended not to perform low anterior resections unless a margin of 6 cm or more can be obtained.

A similar study was also carried out by Grinnell.[48] Sixty-seven of 76 patients with carcinoma of the rectum who had resection for cure had no retrograde intramural spread. Of the nine patients with retrograde spread, only three had spread beyond 1 cm from the lower margin of the carcinoma; two had a poorly differentiated carcinoma; while the other one had retrograde subserosal venous spread.

RETROGRADE EXTRAMURAL METASTASES. Spread of cancer cells in lymphatics is normally embolic from primary lesion to regional nodes, then from node to node, with occasional bypassing of a node or group of nodes. However, if lymph node metastases have developed, lymph flow may become blocked and be forced to seek alternate routes. As lymph pressure increases, lymphatic valves become incompetent, and retrograde flow and metastasis may occur. Metastases retrograde to pararectal nodes occurred in only 1.6 per cent of 309 cleared specimens of rectal carcinoma. All appeared to be the result of proximal lymphatic blockage from metastases.[46]

*Venous Spread.* The development of distant metastases from primary carcinoma can only result from dissemination of malignant cells into the blood stream. Circulating malignant cells are found infrequently in the peripheral blood of patients with carcinoma of the colon and rectum. However, the incidence rises during induction of anesthesia (28%), and such cells can be identified in the peripheral blood of 50 per cent of patients during the operation.[45] Surprisingly, follow-up studies of patients who had cancer cells in the peripheral blood during the operation have not shown any adverse affect on the ultimate prognosis.[45] Unfortunately, little is known about the factors which favor the implantation of circulating malignant cells and allow the subsequent formation of metastases. The incidence of hematologic spread correlates with the depth of invasion and histologic grade.[27] The most common site of distant metastases for carcinoma of the rectum is the liver, followed by the lungs.

LIVER METASTASIS. The incidence of liver metastases from carcinoma of the rectum, in patients who undergo curative or pilliative resection of the rectum, was found to be 14 per cent.[115] Goligher analyzed a series of 893 patient with carcinoma of the rectum undergoing laparotomy; by palpation 103 or 11.5 per cent were found to have metastases to the liver.[37] He further studied 31 patients whose livers were found to be free from metastases at operation, but who died in the immediate postoperative period. Necropsy revealed that one in six had a hidden metastasis not detected at laparotomy. Thus, the true incidence of liver metastases among patients undergoing operation was 26 per cent.

LUNG METASTASIS. Pulmonary metastases from colorectal carcinoma occur in 20 per cent of patients who die of their disease.[100] Of those patients who survive colorectal resection for cure, 15 per cent subsequently developed pulmonary metastases.

OTHER METASTASES. Metastases to other distant organs are much less common, but may include brain, bone, bone marrow, pancreas, thyroid, skin, adrenal glands, spleen, breast, ovary, penis, and nail bed.

*Spread Within Veins* (*Fixed Growth Within the Lumen of Veins*). A special search for evidence of this type of spread was made by Dukes and Bussey.[27] In 1795 operative specimens, the incidence was 11 per cent. The five-year survival in these patients was not as bad as might be expected. In the follow-up 197 cases in which venous spread was found, the overall five-year survival rate was 35 per cent, but increased to 64 per cent in the 52 cases with spread within the veins who had no lymphatic metastases. Thus, it appears that spread of cancer cells within the veins, per se, only slightly alters the prognosis; although, its presence may signify a late stage of the disease.

## Clinical Manifestations of Carcinoma of the Rectum

Initially, many carcinomas of the rectum produce no symptoms, and are discovered only as part of a routine proctosigmoidoscopy. Bleeding is the most common symptom of rectal cancer, and is, unfortunately, all too often, incorrectly attributed by the patients to hemorrhoids. Profuse bleeding is unusual, and anemia is found only in the late stage. Occasionally, there may be considerable mucus in the stool. As the disease progresses the patient will notice a change in caliber of the stool because of partial obstruction. Complete obstruction is rare with carcinoma of the rectum because of its large lumen and frequent slouging of the lesion. If it is located low in the rectum, there may be a feeling of incomplete evacuation after a bowel movement, or tenesmus. Mild abdominal symptoms such as bloating or cramps may occur. Severe pain in the rectum, or low back pain, occurs only when local fixation is extensive and the major nerve trunks are involved by pressure or invasion. If the carcinoma has invaded the bladder, signs of cystitis or fistula may become apparent.

## Physical Examination and Diagnostic Procedures

*Routine Procedures.* The general physical examination of the patient is important as a means of revealing the extent of the local disease, disclosing distant metastasis, and appraising the operative risk of the patient with regard to his nutritional, cardiovascular, pulmonary, and renal status.

Particular attention should be directed to the liver, inguinal and supraclavicular lymph nodes, and detection of jaundice. Digital rectal examination will detect about one-third of rectal carcinomas.[36] The size and extent of local disease can be determined. The status of the prostate gland should be noted. In women, pelvic examinations should be performed.

SIGMOIDOSCOPY is an essential part of the examination. It is of utmost importance to carefully record the size, distance of the lower margin from the anal verge, and the gross appearance of the lesion. Multiple biopsies should always be done to confirm the diagnosis and, hopefully, establish the grade of the carcinoma.

CHEST RADIOGRAPH is required for all patients with carcinoma of the rectum. It is the most practical and non-invasive method to detect pulmonary metastases. It is also a rough guide to evaluate pulmonary status.

*Special Procedures.* Unless patients with carcinoma of the rectum have a high grade obstruction, they should have a *barium enema,* perferably with air contrast, to rule out a more proximal carcinoma or polyps.

COLONOSCOPY should be done whenever there is any suspicious lesion on a good quality barium enema. Although it is controversial, some surgeons recommend routine colonoscopy on every patient with rectal carcinoma, while still others recommend colonoscopy on patients in lieu of a barium enema.

INTRAVENOUS PYELOGRAM should be done in all patients with carcinoma of the rectum in order to outline the anatomy of the ureters, to detect anomalies, to evaluate renal function, and to reveal any obstructive uropathy.

CYSTOSCOPY is indicated when there are bladder symptoms suspicious of invasion by the rectal carcinoma.

LIVER SCAN (RADIONUCLIDE IMAGING). Although liver scan is not completely accurate in the diagnosis of hepatic metastases, having both high false positive and false negative results, its major use today is as a baseline study during the followup period.[15,92] In addition, the presence of extensive metastases in an individual who would otherwise require radical extirpation of the rectum to remove the carcinoma, would direct the surgeon away from such a major operation if even palliation seemed hopeless.

COMPUTERIZED TOMOGRAM (CT SCAN). At the present time this has not proven to be superior to the less complicated liver scan or other less sophisticated clinical methods.

## Laboratory Studies

Laboratory studies to evaluate patients with carcinoma of the rectum are mandatory. These should include complete-blood-count, urinalysis, coagulation studies, liver and renal function tests, electrolytes, and carcinoembryonic antigen. Enough time should be allowed to correct any deficiencies, including the restoration of protein and blood volume.

## Preoperative Preparation

Patients should be admitted to the hospital in sufficient time to allow measures designed to establish their optimum physical and mental condition. In addition to the laboratory studies, electrocardiogram, especially in patients over 40 years old, should always be obtained, and pulmonary function tests performed if indicated.

It is generally agreed that a bowel preparation with vigorous mechanical cleansing and oral antibiotics results in a lower infection rate.[18,112] A popularly adopted method is that recommended by Condon and Nichols, and it is as follows: Day 1, Low residue diet, Bisacodyl, one capsule orally at 6:00 p.m.; Day 2, Continue low residue diet, Magnesium sulfate, 30 ml, 50 per cent solution (15 gm) orally at 10:00 a.m., 2:00 p.m. and 6:00 p.m., Saline enemas in the evening until return is clear; Day 3, Clear liquid diet, supplemental intravenous fluids as needed, magnesium sulfate, in dose above, at 10:00 and 2:00 p.m., no enemas, Neomycin 1 gm, orally at 1:00 p.m., 2:00 p.m. and 11:00 p.m., erythromycin base 1 gm orally at 1:00, 2:00 p.m. and 11:00 p.m., Day 4, Operation scheduled at 8:00 a.m.[20]

The potential complications, such as neurogenic bladder and impotence in men, should be fully discussed with the patients preoperatively. If abdominoperineal resection is anticipated, they should be visited by an enterostomal therapist who can discuss and give information regarding life as an ostomate. Successful stomal management usually begins with preoperative education, as does the adjustment to the colostomy, which is difficult for most patients. The ideal site for the colostomy is marked preoperatively.

*Prophylactic Antibiotics.* Current evidence indicates that the prophylactic administration of effective antibiotics has not been harmful to patients, and, in most instances, has been effective in decreasing of wound sepsis in colorectal procedures.[18]

SYSTEMIC ANTIBIOTICS. Prophylactic systemic antibiotics must be started prior to operation, allowing time for the drug to be present in the tissues before contamination takes place. Postoperative initiation of antibiotics has no benefit in decreasing wound infections.[107] The course of the drug should be brief, starting before the anesthesia, and continuing no longer than 24 hours. This brief course of antibiotics allows minimal opportunity for the bacteria to develop resistance to the antimicrobial agent.

Systemic antibiotics which have been found effective in sepsis prophylaxis for colorectal surgery conducted in controlled trails include: lincomycin and tobramycin, or lincomycin and gentamycin; cephaloridine; cefazolin; lincomycin; and doxycycline.[57,60,88,105,107] However, a Veterans Administration Cooperative study of preoperative prophylactic cephalothin, the most popular drug used by clinicians, failed to show a significant decrease in septic complications following colorectal operations.[20]

TOPICAL ANTIBIOTICS. Prophylactic antibiotics can also be applied topically to the wound. This can be done by mixing the antibiotic in a small amount of saline, or by sprinkling the antibiotic powder on the subcutaneous tissue. Reportedly effective antibiotics include: ampicillin, kanamycin, cephaloridine, and neosporin.[1,20,28,106]

## Operative Treatment of Carcinoma of the Rectum

*Basic Consideration.* For practical purposes, the rectum is conveniently divided into thirds (Fig. 16-8). The lower third is from the anorectal ring (3-4 cm from the anal verge) to 7 cm from the anal verge; The middle third is 7 to 11 cm from it; and, the upper third is 11 to 15 cm.

CARCINOMA OF THE LOWER AND UPPER THIRD OF THE RECTUM. With the present knowledge of the usual lymphatic pathway at different levels of the rectum, it is generally accepted that abdominoperineal resection is the treatment of choice for carcinoma of the lower third of the rectum, while anterior or low anterior resection is the treatment of choice for carcinoma of the upper third of the rectum.

CARCINOMA OF THE MIDDLE THIRD OF THE RECTUM. Controversy exists regarding the best curative resection for carcinoma of the middle third of the rectum. The technical

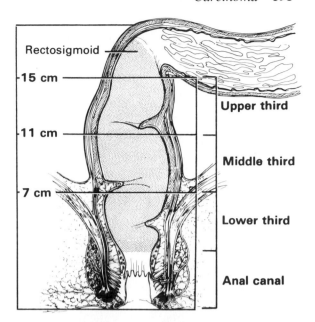

FIGURE **16-8.** *The three levels of the rectum.*

difficulties in performing the low anastomosis, and the high morbidity from anastomotic leaks and sepsis, are so well known that this level is frequently called "no-man's-land." Another concern to the surgeon is what constitutes an adequate distal margin for resection. Studies of operative specimens by many authors have shown that a distal margin of 2.5 cm from the lower border of the carcinoma is adequate to contain both intramural and retrograde lymphatic spread.[46,48,91] The exception to this generalization is the poorly differentiated carcinoma: one should obtain a distal margin of at least 6 cm from the lesions (see lymphatic spread). This observation is supported by the clinical studies by Wilson and Beahrs who noted no difference in suture line recurrence, pelvic recurrence, or five-year survival whether the distal margin was less than 2 cm or more than 5 cm from the lesion.[116] Localio has performed anastomoses as low as the levator ani muscle with complete maintenance of anal continence.[69]

That the proper selection of patients is the key to success has been well expressed in this statement by McGregor and Bacon, "The avoidance of a colostomy when indicated may jeopardize the patient's chance of cure, and this is an unfortunate mistake in surgical judgement. Equally tragic is the sacrifice of the patient's anal sphincter mechanism and all semblance of normality without his chance of survival."[77] The factors influencing the choice between a sphincter-saving operation and abdominoperineal resection for carcinoma of the middle third of the rectum include: build, obesity, local spread, perforation or abscess, size and fixation of the lesion, and histologic grade of the carcinoma (particularly undifferentiated carcinoma).

There have been numerous reports showing that sphincter-saving operations for carcinoma of the middle third of the rectum give comparable morbidity, mortality, and five-year survivals to abdominoperineal resection.[69,102,103] Although these reports were not controlled trials, and therefore not comparable, they do support the theory that in properly selected cases, a sphincter-saving operation is a good alternative method for carcinoma of the middle third of the rectum. Sphincter-saving procedures currently in use include low anterior resection, abdominosacral resection, and pull-through operation. Abdominosacral resection and pull-through operations are variants of low anterior resection in that the anastomosis is performed transsacrally in the former, and extraanally in the latter. In Localio's experience with 100 patients who underwent abdominosacral resection, the operative mortality was 2 per cent, compared to 1.7 per cent for low anterior resection and 2.3 per cent for abdominoperineal resection.[69] The five-year survivals and the pelvic recurrences were also comparable. The anastomotic leak rate was 12 per cent. Pull-through operations have never been popular, probably because of the high morbidity rate, especially due to sepsis and anal incontinence.[39] Success with this operation appears to be in the hands of a few experts who perform them regularly.[5,6,24,39,62] The recent introduction of the end-to-end anastomosis stapler may render the two procedures obsolete (see technique of EEA on p. 200)

*Other Considerations.* OVARIES AND TUBES. The incidence of occult ovarian metastases from carcinoma of the rectum and colon is approximately 6 per cent but can be as high as 16 per cent in Dukes' C carcinoma.[90] For this reason bilateral salpingo-oophorectomy should be considered, especially when the carcinoma is in the lower part of the rectum from where

direct communication by lymphatics to the ovaries and fallopian tubes exists (see lymphatic drainage in Chapter I). The risk of this added surgical procedure is small, and the benefit to the patient may be significant.[90] In addition, most of these patients have passed the menopause, so that they suffer no adverse physiological effects.

UTERUS. The lymphatic drainage from the lower part of the rectum also communicates with the uterus, cervix, and broad ligament (see lymphatic drainage in Chapter I). Theoretically, total hysterectomy should be performed along with abdominoperineal resection for carcinoma of the lower rectum. However, because this may add to the morbidity and mortality, such practice is usually limited to only those patients in whom associated pathology, such as direct extension of the carcinoma or large fibroids, exists.[3]

VAGINA. There is also a rich lymphatic communication between the lower rectum and the posterior vaginal wall. Excision of the posterior vaginal wall should, therefore, be included in abdominoperineal resection for carcinoma of the lower rectum. This should not add to the risk of the procedure.

SEMINAL VESICLES AND PROSTATE. These organs are not usually removed along with abdominoperineal resection unless there is direct extension of the carcinoma into them.

*The Assessment of Operability.* Cases classified as operable are those in which the surgeon considers the conditions favorable for extirpation of the disease by operation.

Inoperability is determined either by an unsatisfactory general condition which renders the patient unsuitable for a resection, or by an advanced state of the growth which places it beyond the hope for cure.[37] It is important to realize that in most cases it is only at exploratory laparotomy that an accurate assessment of the resectability of a rectal carcinoma can be made. Clinical examination alone gives no reliable information as to venous or lymphatic spread unless it is very extensive, or obvious distant metastases are present. Fixation of the primary growth, as determined by rectal examination, is unreliable in estimating the resectability. At laparotomy, the decision to resect is determined by the degree of fixation of the growth, presence and extent of hepatic metastases, and presence and extent of other metastases or peritoneal seedings.

*The Role of Palliative Resection in Rectal Carcinoma.* It is hard to justify a low anterior resection or abdominoperineal resection in patients who obviously have no chance for long term survival. On the other hand, most of these patients are symptomatic. If untreated, the symptoms invariably become worse by progression of the disease. The review by Bordos, et al of palliative abdominoperineal resections for carcinoma of the rectum sheds some light on this problem.[8] Thirty-four selected patients with carcinoma of the mid or lower part of the rectum who underwent palliative abdominoperineal resection were compared to 102 patients with a curative abdominoperineal resection. The operative mortality and the postoperative morbidity were similar. The perineal wound healed in all patients after palliative abdominoperineal resection. The significant result was that all the local symptoms disappeared after the palliative resection. Furthermore, a few patients survived five years. Among the 15 patients treated primarily by colostomy only, 11 patients continued to have varying amounts of pain, tenesmus, and bleeding. Lockhart-Mummery found the same gratifying result.[71] In 268 patients who had a palliative excision of the rectum for advanced carcinoma, the average survival time was 1.7 years; 24 lived more than five years. In light of these findings we tend to favor resection of the rectum, or a limited low anterior resection, unless the patient's general condition is considered too poor to withstand the operation or the malignant disease has disseminated extensively.

*The Place of the Hartmann Procedure.* Occasionally one encounters a situation where a carcinoma of the middle third of the rectum can be resected with an adequate lower margin of clearance but it is technically difficult to safely perform a low anastomosis, or, the likelihood of local recurrence is high. In such situations, closure of the distal rectal stump with establishment of an end sigmoid colostomy is another alternative to abdominoperineal resection. Likewise, in the presence of an obstructing carcinoma of the rectum where one is faced with poorly prepared bowel, a Hartmann's procedure might be considered. However, this procedure should be performed with caution since the complication of pelvic abscess as the principal cause of death is high (11 per cent).[41] If the pelvis is contaminated during the procedure, or bleeding can not be completely controlled, abdominoperineal resection should be considered rather than the Hartmann procedure.

*High Ligation of the Inferior Mesenteric Artery in Carcinoma of the Rectum.* In performing abdominoperineal resections for carcinoma of the rectum, Miles ligated the inferior mesenteric artery below the take-off of the left colic artery.[80] In a significant number of patients (7–11%) lymph node metastases, which would not have been removed unless a high ligation had been performed, were found at the origin of the inferior mesenteric artery. Based on this finding many surgeons advocated ligation of the inferior mesenteric artery at the origin of the aorta, hoping to improve long term survivals. In a study by Grinnell of 179 specimens with high ligation, 19, or 10.6 per cent, had lymph node metastases between the point of ligation of the artery at the aorta and the level of its left colic branch.[47] These were nodes which would not have been removed if ligation had been carried out at a point distal to the left colic artery. However, follow-up records of these 19 patients showed that none were salvaged by the radical procedure. This suggests that still higher aortocaval nodes were involved, and beyond the reach of surgery. A more recent study by Busuttil, et al, of treatment for carcinoma of sigmoid colon and upper rectum, also failed to show any benefit of ligating the inferior mesenteric artery at its origin.[12] Indeed, the complication rate after segmental colectomy was one-third as great as that for the radical left hemicolectomy. The hospital mortality was 1 per cent after the former, and 6.2 per cent after the latter; while five-year survival was 70.3 per cent after the former, and 56.3 per cent after the latter.

*The Place of Local Definitive Treatment for Carcinoma of the Rectum.* Before abdominoperineal resection was popularized by Miles, the standard treatment of carcinoma was perineal excision of the rectum through a posterior approach.[80] However, the recurrence was unacceptably high due to inadequate removal of nodes along the inferior mesenteric vessels. With the high morbidity of abdominoperineal resection, and low anterior resection, clinicians continued the search for a lesser procedure that was still adequate for long-term survival. Various methods of local treatment have been proposed. The goal is to identify patients with carcinoma which is still confined to the bowel wall without lymph node metastases (Dukes' A). This accounts for about 15 per cent of carcinoma of the rectum. Unfortunately, at the present time there is no reliable method to accurately identify these patients.

"Early rectal cancer" is defined by Morson and Bussey as invasive carcinoma that has not spread in direct continuity beyond the submucous layer, regardless of the presence of microscopic vascular or lymphatic invasion.[84] Of the 2,303 patients with rectal cancer admitted to St. Mark's Hospital, London, between 1948 and 1962 only 76 (3.3%) were in this category. A recent review by Morson of treatment in this group of patients showed that complete local excision was adequate for long-term survival in selected patients.[85] Most of the failures were those with a high grade malignancy, and those with an inadequate local excision.[70,85]

Many carcinomas of the lower and middle thirds of the rectum are treated locally for cure with electrocoagulation by some surgeons, and with endocavitary irradiation by others (see Chap. 18). The results have been encouraging.

*Technique of Abdominoperineal Resection.* For the abdominal part of the operation the patient is placed in the *supine position* in slight Trendelenberg for better exposure of pelvic structures and aid in venous return from the lower extremities. A number 16 Foley catheter is inserted into the bladder and the urine output is monitored continuously throughout the operation.

INCISION. We prefer a transverse incision at a level between the pubis and umbilicus, but a lower midline incision extending just above the umbilicus is also satisfactory (Fig. 16-9A).

MOBILIZATION OF SIGMOID COLON. The sigmoid colon is mobilized by incising the lateral peritoneal reflexion (white line of Toldt). This is carried cephalad to the distal descending colon, and caudad parallel to the rectum (Fig. 16-9B). The retroperitoneal areolar tissue is pushed aside with a stick sponge so that a fan-shaped flap of sigmoid mesentery is created. The left spermatic or left ovarian vein can be easily identified. At the level of the iliac crest, the ureter is just medial to this vein. The inferior mesenteric artery is identified and it is clamped, divided and doubly ligated just distal to the take-off of the left colic artery (Fig. 16-9C,D). The inferior mesenteric vein is ligated at the corresponding level. Next, the peritoneum on the right side of the sigmoid and rectum is incised, starting near the sigmoid vessels, and carried down to the pelvis. Unless there is invasion or inflammation in the pelvis the right ureter is not routinely identified.

POSTERIOR MOBILIZATION OF THE RECTUM. By drawing the rectum taut, a plane of areolar tissue behind the rectum, at the level just above the promontory of the sacrum, can be identified. Using blunt and sharp dissection the retrorectal space is entered easily, with minimal bleeding. At the $S_3$ or $S_4$ level the rectosacral fascia, which varies from a thin fibrous band to a thick ligament, is encountered. It is cut with a long heavy scissors (Fig. 16-9E,F). Failure to do so risks tearing the presacral venous plexus which may then bleed profusely and can be difficult to control. Once this fascia is cut, the coccyx is reached.

ANTERIOR MOBILIZATION OF THE RECTUM. The peritoneum at the rectovesical reflection is incised, and mobilization is continued in the plane between the seminal vesicles and Denonvillier's fascia. Dissection is extended distally until the rectum is separated from the seminal vesicles in men or vagina in women (Fig. 16-9G).

TAKING THE LATERAL LIGAMENTS (STALKS). At this stage the rectum has been mobilized posteriorly to the tip of the coccyx, and anteriorly to the level of the pubis. It is still attached laterally on each side by the pelvic fascia, called lateral ligaments (containing the accessory middle rectal vessels). The rectum is pulled taut with the left hand while the right hand is placed behind the rectum, and sweeps laterally on each side of the ligament, taking care to avoid the ureters. The ligaments are then clamped, divided, and ligated (Fig. 16-9H).

(*Text continues on p. 198*)

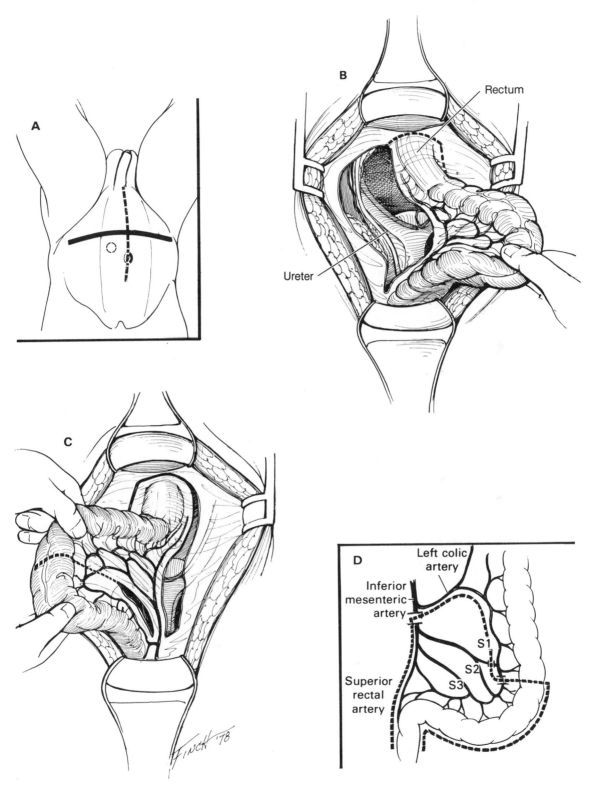

**FIGURE 16-9.** *Technique of abdominoperineal resection: abdominal part. (Continued on following pages)*

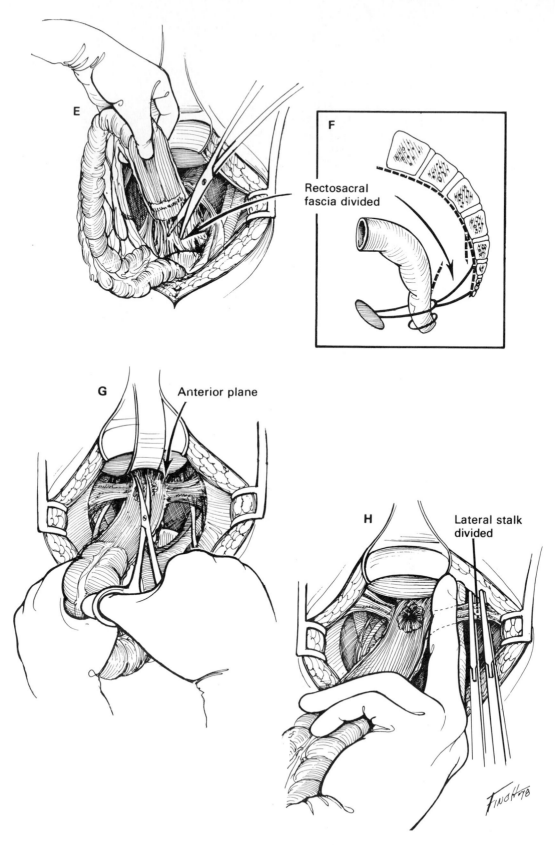

Rectosacral
fascia divided

Anterior plane

Lateral stalk
divided

FIGURE **16-9.** (*Continued*)

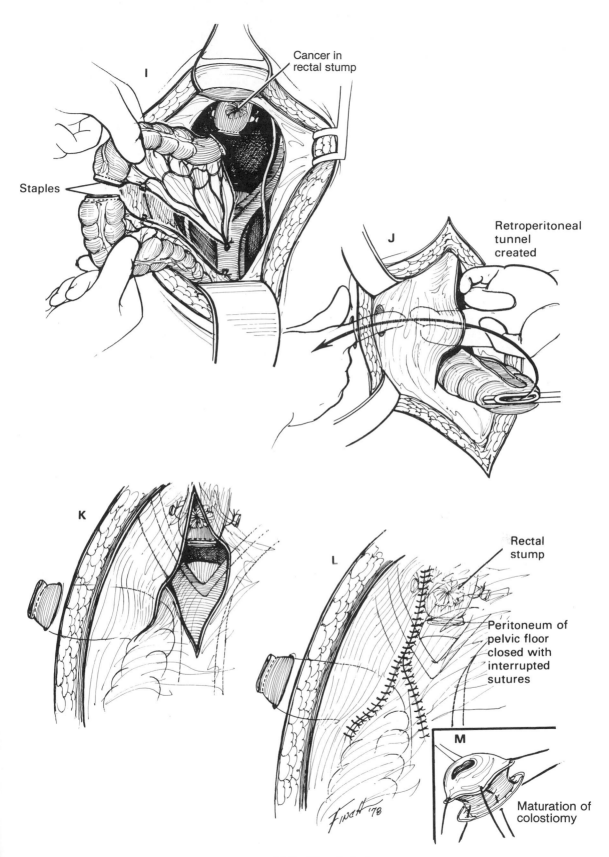

Cancer in rectal stump

Staples

J

Retroperitoneal tunnel created

K

L

Rectal stump

Peritoneum of pelvic floor closed with interrupted sutures

M

Maturation of colostiomy

FIGURE **16-9.** (*Conclusion*)

PREPARING THE COLOSTOMY AND RECONSTRUCTION OF PELVIC FLOOR. The site in the proximal sigmoid or distal descending colon chosen for the colostomy is cleaned and transected, an act easily accomplished with a stapler. The excess sigmoid and rectum are likewise transected above the carcinoma (Fig. 16-9I).

Using blunt finger dissection, an extraperitoneal tunnel is created, starting at the left flank and carried toward the site of the colostomy (Fig. 16-9J). A 2 cm disc of skin and subcutaneous tissue is excised at the premarked colostomy site. The anterior fascia is incised in a cruciate manner, the rectus muscle split, and the posterior fascia and peritoneum similarly incised in a cruciate manner. The opening should admit two fingers loosely. The colon is then brought through the extraperitoneal tunnel to the colostomy aperture (Fig. 16-9K). It should be matured at the completion of the abdominal part of the procedure.

With the stapled end of the rectal stump dropped into the pelvis, the pelvic peritoneum is closed with interrupted 4–0 silk (Fig. 16-9L). The abdominal cavity is irrigated with 2,000 to 3,000 ml of antibiotic solution. The abdominal cavity and the skin are then closed.

INTRAPERITONEAL COLOSTOMY. If the extraperitoneal colostomy cannot conveniently be performed, the colon is brought out through the colostomy aperture and the projecting limb is attached to the lateral abdominal wall using interrupted 4-0 silk to prevent herniation of the small bowel. Nevertheless the extraperitoneal technique is much preferred because of fewer complications related to peristomal herniation, prolapse, retractions and internal herniation.

MATURATION OF THE COLOSTOMY. The staples at the end of the colostomy are excised. The colostomy limb may be sutured to the anterior fascia. We prefer to evert the stoma 1 cm rather than making it flush with the skin. The stoma is immediately matured with interrupted 4-0 chromic catgut (Figure 16-9M). A temporary colostomy bag is then applied.

*Perineal Part of the Operation.* The patient is turned to the *prone position* with a 6″ roll under the pubis. The cheeks of the buttock are spread apart using 2″ tape (Fig. 16-10A). The perineal area is prepared and draped. A purse-string suture of #1 silk is placed around the anus to avoid fecal spillage. An elliptical incision is made around the anus, just lateral to the boundary of the external sphincter muscle (Fig. 16-10B). Bleeding points are electrocoagulated. The incision is deepened circumferentially. Posteriorly, the anococcygeal ligament and the anococcygeal raphe are incised close to the tip of the coccyx. Once this is completed the pelvic cavity is entered, and the rectal stump can be delivered (Fig. 16-10C). The levator ani muscles on each side of the rectum are clamped, cut, and tied. At this point the remaining rectum is attached only to the prostate in men or vagina in the women (Fig. 16-10D). An incision is made to include Denonvillier's fascia on the anterior wall of the rectum. Through this plane the rectum is sharply dissected from the prostate gland or vagina. Usually there is a moderate amount of bleeding over the prostatic capsule or vagina, requiring electrocoagulation or stick-tie.

CLOSURE OF THE PERINEAL SPACE. The perineal space is irrigated with an antibiotic solution. Meticulous hemostasis is obtained. One or more large, closed suction drains are placed in the perineal space and brought out through a small stab-wound more anteriorly so that the patient will not sit on them. The levator ani and the subcutaneous tissue are closed with interrupted absorbable sutures (Fig. 16-10E). The skin is closed. The drain is connected to continuous suction, and left in place until drainage is less than 25 ml per day, which usually takes about five days (Fig. 16-10F).

PACKING OF THE PERINEAL WOUND. Closure of the perineal space should not be done if there is continuous oozing of the wound, or if there has been fecal spillage. Instead, the wound should be packed with a rubber dam over Kerlex gauze. This should be removed in 48 hours. The rubber dam will permit removal without the gauze becoming adherent to adjacent tissue.

*Technique of Low Anterior Resection.* The term "low anterior resection" is applied when the rectosigmoid resection necessitates full mobilization of the rectum, and transection of both lateral ligaments. The anastomosis is performed below the anterior peritoneal reflection.

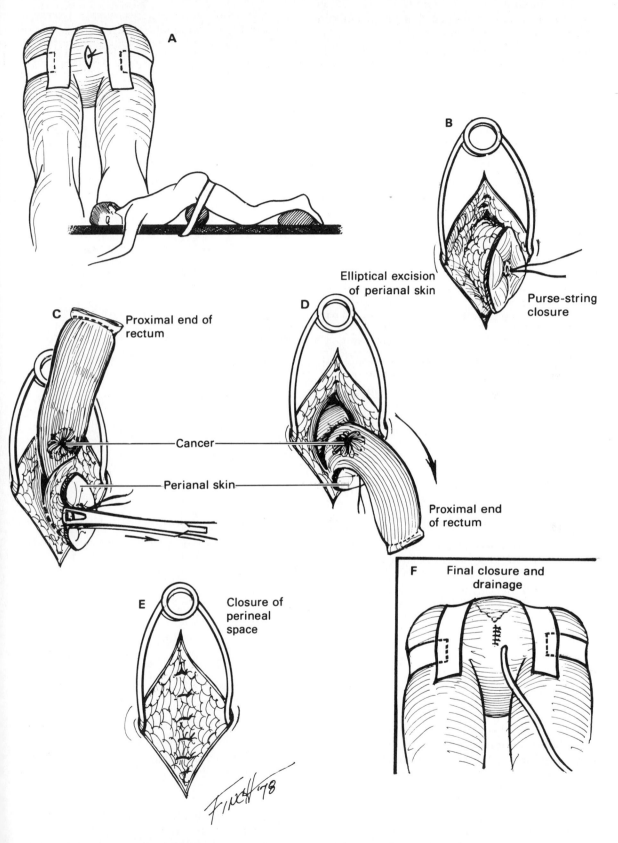

**A**

**B**

Elliptical excision
of perianal skin

Purse-string
closure

**C**

Proximal end of
rectum

**D**

Cancer

Perianal skin

Proximal end
of rectum

**E**

Closure of
perineal
space

**F** Final closure and
drainage

*Finch '78*

FIGURE **16-10.** *Technique of abdominoperineal resection: perineal part.*

Because of the lateral curves of the rectum, it is possible that a carcinoma at the 7 cm level may be at the 12 cm level after full rectal mobilization. This is especially true with a posterior lesion. The steps of the operation are exactly the same as the abdominal part of the abdominoperineal resection. The feasibility of low anterior resection is decided upon only after the rectum has been completely mobilized posteriorly, anteriorly, and laterally. If low anterior resection is to be done the distal clearance should be at least 2.5 cm from the lower margin of the carcinoma. The splenic flexure must be taken down if there is any question of tension at the anastomosis. At the completion of the anastomosis the pelvic peritoneum is left open so that the hollow of the sacrum is communicating freely with the peritoneal cavity to allow drainage of the accumulated fluid. Closed suction drainage may be used in selected patients when the pelvis is not completely dry, or in patients with narrow and deep pelves, which are more common in men. Proximal colostomy is rarely performed, but in those circumstances where the surgeon is not entirely satisfied with the integrity of the anastomosis, he should not hesitate to perform a complementary transverse colostomy.

SINGLE-LAYER ANASTOMOSIS. We adopt the open technique with no clamps applied on the bowel ends. A popularly used suture is 4–0 polypropylene with four square-knots tied on each suture, or 4–0 polyglycolic acid or polyglactin.

The colonic end lies in a convenient location within the abdominal cavity for closure of the posterior wall. Sutures are tied after they have all been placed (Fig. 16-11A). Vertical mattress sutures are used: the first bite is full thickness on each side, but on the return bite only mucosa and submucosa are included (Fig. 16-11B,C). All knots are tied inside the lumen.

An interrupted, full thickness with only mucosal inversion as described by Gambee is used on the anterior wall (Fig. 16-11D,E).[32]

TWO-LAYER ANASTOMOSIS. Many surgeons prefer a two-layer anastomosis: an outer seromuscular layer of 4–0 nonabsorbable suture, and a continuous inner layer of 4–0 absorbable suture.

ANASTOMOSIS USING END-TO-END ANASTOMOSIS (EEA) STAPLER. The recently introduced EEA stapler has extended the limits of the low anterior resection by enabling surgeons to perform a highly reliable anastomosis at a lower level than was technically possible utilizing a traditional hand-sewn anastomosis. The initial steps of the operative procedure are identical to those utilized in the performance of a low anterior resection (as described above), except that the position of the patient is modified. The patient is placed supine on the operating table, and the sacrum is raised slightly on a pad at the end of the table (Fig. 16-12A). The legs are placed in the padded Lloyd-Davies leg supports, and abducted at the hips with no more than 10 to 15° of flexion at the hips and knees. This provides excellent exposure for both the abdominal and perineal operators.

Having determined that a low anterior resection with EEA anastomosis is feasible, one proceeds as follows.

In the preparation of the proximal bowel, the mesentery is cleared for a 2.0 to 3.0 cm distance from the proposed proximal resection margin. The bowel is transected between clamps, and a 2–0 Prolene, full-thickness pursestring suture is placed approximately 2 to 3 mm from the cut edge, with each bite taken 4 to 5 mm apart. This pursestring suture is more conveniently applied using the specially designed fenestrated clamp (Fig. 16-13).

To prepare the rectum the mesentery is cleared for a 2.0 to 3.0 cm distance from the proposed distal resection margin. The rectum is transected, preferably between clamps. The rectosigmoid is resected, leaving in the pelvis a short rectal stump. A 2–0 Prolene, full-thickness pursestring suture is placed on the rectum 2 to 3 mm from cut edge with each bite taken 4 to 5 mm apart. Unfortunately for the extremely low anastomosis, the width of the pelvis is not adequate to permit the application of the instrument and the Keeth needle needed to insert the suture.

Before the insertion of the instrument the perineal operator confirms that the EEA stapler is properly assembled and that the safety is in the locked position. The appropriate sized stapler cartridge is slipped over the center rod and locked in position. The anvil is slipped on the center rod and the screw tightened. The lubricated stapler is inserted in a closed position, with the handle up (Fig. 16-12B). The abdominal operator loosens the rectal pursestring and, with a hand posterior to

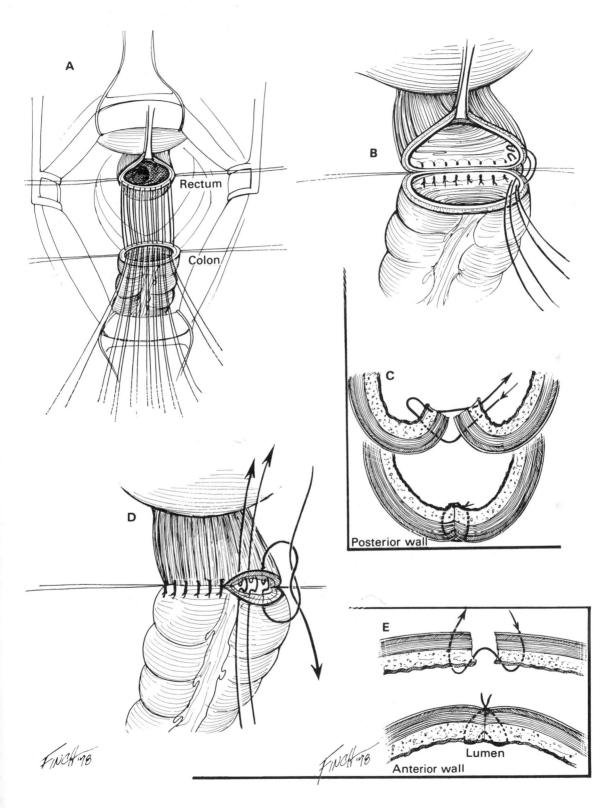

Labels within figure:
Rectum
Colon
A
B
C
Posterior wall
D
E
Lumen
Anterior wall

FIGURE **16-11.** *Technique of single-layer anastomosis.*

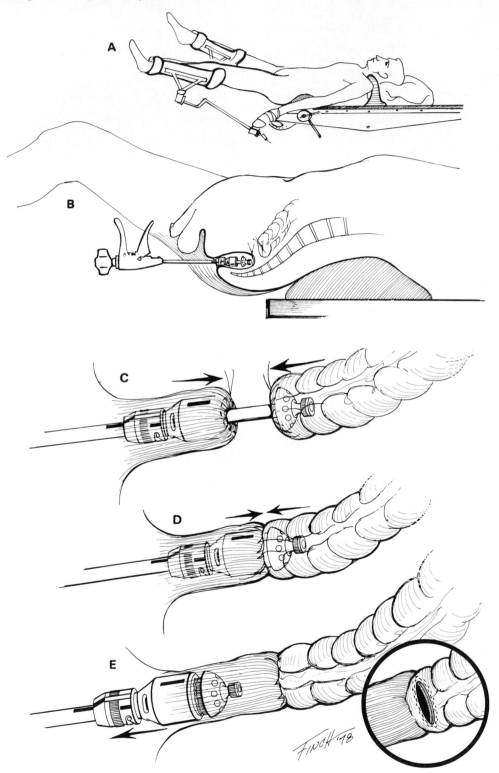

FIGURE **16-12.** *Technique of EEA stapler.*

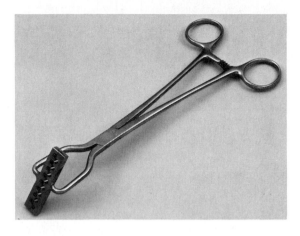

FIGURE **16-13.** *Fenestrated clamp for purse-string suture.*

the rectal stump, directs the perineal operator in advancing the instrument until the tip of the anvil protrudes through the rectal lumen.

In securing bowel on the stapler the perineal operator opens it fully by turning the wing nut counterclockwise. The proximal bowel is dilated, and the proximal colon advanced over the stapler anvil. The proximal and distal pursestring sutures are tied, thus securing the bowel around the center rod of the stapler (Fig. 16-12C).

Next, the stapler is closed fully by turning the wing nut clockwise as the abdominal operator keeps the "gap" free of mesentery, bladder, and other tissues. When the stapler is closed, the abdominal operator checks the proposed anastomosis to be certain it contains no excess tissue, and that during closure the rectal wall and colon wall have not extruded outside the diameter of the cartridge. The safety is released and the stapler fired by squeezing the handle firmly (Fig. 16-12D). This places a double, staggered, circular row of stainless steel staples to join the two ends of bowel while a circular knife simultaneously cuts two rings of tissue inside the staple line, thus creating an inverted end-to-end anastomosis.

To remove the instrument the safety is returned to the locked position, and the stapler is opened by turning the wing nut counterclockwise three complete turns as the abdominal operator gently steadies the anastomosis. The stapler, which should move independently of the bowel, is rotated and

rocked gently, and slowly withdrawn (Fig. 16-12E).

The abdominal operator checks the completed anastomosis visually and by palpation. The perineal operator removes the anvil and cartridge, confirms that all staples have fired, and that the proximal and distal margins of resection consist of intact rings of full-thickness bowel. The perineal operator inserts a proctoscope and insufflates air into the distal rectum after the abdominal operator has covered the anastomosis with saline. As air is insufflated, the abdominal operator checks for bubbles arising from the anastomosis. The anastomosis must be airtight (Fig. 16-12F).

Of our first 50 operations using the EEA stapler, 27 patients had low anterior resections and 23 patients had anterior resections or left colectomies. There was one clinical anastomotic leak in a patient with low anterior resection, and one patient died of a pulmonary embolus on the day of discharge from the hospital. There were also a few technical problems (Table 16-6).

Whether the EEA stapler is more secure than hand-sewn anastomoses for the low an-

TABLE **16-6.** Technical Problems in 50 Patients Using EEA Stapler

| PROBLEM | NO. OF PATIENTS | MANAGEMENT |
|---|---|---|
| *Incomplete excised rectal ring* | 9 | Transverse loop colostomy  −6 No further treatment  −2 Anastomosis redone  −1 |
| *Incomplete excised proximal ring* | 2 | Suture reinforcement |
| *Rectal tear (extraperitoneum)* | 1 | Perineal drain |
| *Anterior serosal tear* | 1 | Suture reinforcement |
| *Staple fired but knife blade failed to cut* | 1 | Anastomosis redone |
| *Massive hemorrhage from sacral veins* | 1 | Transfusion, packing, drain |
| *Marked discrepancy between anvil & proximal bowel* | 1 | Additional 10 cm resected |

terior resection remains to be seen. There is no question that lower level anastomoses can be achieved by using the EEA stapler than by hand-sewn anastomoses (Fig. 16-14). Encouraging results are also reported by Goligher, et al.[40]

*Technique of Local Excision.* The patient is placed in the prone or supine position, depending upon the location of the lesion. A full-thickness excision is made around the lesion with a rim of normal rectal wall of 1 cm. The wound is closed with full-thickness mattress sutures of 4–0 polyglycolic acid or polyglactin (Fig. 16-15).

### Adjuvant Therapy for Carcinoma of Rectum

*Irradiation Therapy.* PREOPERATIVE IRRADIATION. Although the resectability rate of carcinoma of the rectum has remarkably increased during the past decades, the five-year survival rate has not improved.[115] The search for additional modalities of treatment to employ in conjunction with surgical excision has been widespread during the past two decades. It has long been known that carcinoma of the rectum is relatively sensitive to irradiation.[42,108] Since the publication of Stearns, et al, in 1959, reporting the increase in five-year survivals in Dukes' C carcinoma of the rectum there has been a number of studies using preoperative irradiation for carcinoma of the rectum.[104] Interpretation of the results in the literature is difficult. Most of the reports were

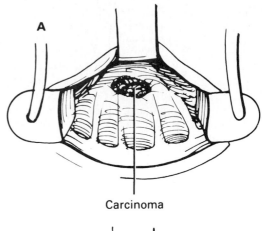

Carcinoma

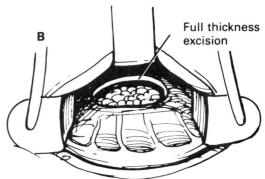

Full thickness excision

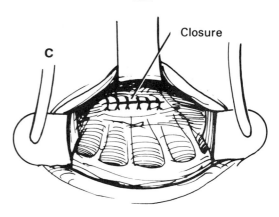

Closure

FIGURE **16-15.** *Local excision of the rectal carcinoma. (After Parks, A., G., Local excision of rectal carcinoma, in Operative Surgery, Ed. Rob, C., and Smith, R., p. 163. London, Butterworth and Co., 1977)*

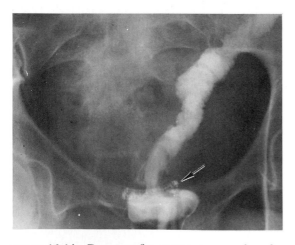

FIGURE **16-14.** *Gastrografin enema two weeks after the operation showing the metal ring of anastomosis* (arrow) *about 3 to 4 cm. from the anal verge.*

not controlled trials, the modes of treatment were different, and the dosage varied widely, from a mere single dose of 500 rads in the immediate preoperative period to multiple doses totalling 5000 rads.[30,96] These reports showed no increase in morbidity and mortality as the result of the preoperative irradiation in patients undergoing abdominoperineal resection.

The most comprehensive study is the controlled clinical trial from the *Veterans Administration Cooperative group*.[54] In this study 2000 rads were delivered to the mid-plane, employing 10 daily fractions of 200 rads each over a two-week period. When the carcinoma was located within 8 cm of the anal verge, an additional dose of 500 rads (10 daily, fractions of 50 rads each) was delivered through a perineal portal. Randomization of 700 patients was well balanced for age, resectability, and type of resection. Of the 453 patients in whom resection was considered to be clinically "curative", five-year survival in the irradiation group was 48.5 per cent compared with 38.8 per cent for surgery alone. Although this data suggests a possible treatment benefit, the difference is not considered statistically significant.

Further examination of the data showed that the difference in favor of those receiving the combined therapy was largely confined to patients on whom abdominoperineal resection was performed, that is, those patients with lesions below 8 cms. Of the 305 patients having abdominoperineal resection for cure, the five-year survival in the combined therapy group was 47 per cent, compared with 34 per cent in the surgery alone group. This apparent improvement in survival was explained by the facts that 500 rads were added to the perineal port, and that the low lying carcinoma permitted the radiotherapist to center the beam in the region of the carcinoma more easily than if it were at a higher level.[54]

Positive lymph nodes were found in 28 per cent of the specimens resected in patients who received preoperative irradiation, as compared to 41 per cent in the control group. This difference was more pronounced in patients having low lying carcinomas requiring abdominoperineal resection (26% vs. 44%). Despite these observations, it might be questioned whether this dosage of irradiation, and the time interval used, could destroy malignant cells in the adjacent lymph nodes. As well, there was no histologic evidence of dying or ghost neoplastic cells in the lymph nodes, or any other evidence to suggest the destruction of malignant cells in the nodes.[54] In the ongoing Veterans Administration II study, only abdominoperineal resections are included, and the lymph node data from the first 117 specimens was quite similar to that reported in the first study. When combined, this evidence is highly suggestive that preoperative irradiation can destroy foci of cancer cells in the lymph nodes adjacent to the carcinoma, with conversion to a more favorable stage of disease.[54] Whether this will be translated into five-year survivals of Dukes' A or B instead of Dukes' C remains to be seen.

From follow-up of the 305 patients who underwent "curative" abdominoperineal resection, it was apparent that there was no appreciable difference between the treated and the control group during the first three postoperative years. However, among 171 patients who were still living beyond three years, 93 per cent of the treated group survived to the fourth year compared with 75 per cent of the control group; and 88 per cent and 83 per cent, respectively, survived the fifth postoperative year. Thus, the apparent benefit in survival in the treated group appeared to occur predominantly between the third and fifth postoperative years (83 per cent vs. 62 per cent). This was logically explained by the alteration of cancer cells by the irradiation so that they are less apt to become implanted distally if disloged, and spread at the time of the operation. Thus, the benefit would not become apparent until enough time had elapsed for implants to develop to lethal size, that is 3 to 5 years.[54]

Of the 461 patients who had microscopically "curative" resection but who died during the five-year postoperative period, complete autopsy information was available on 180. An effort was made to determine whether death was attributable to recurrent or metastatic carcinoma. There was a consistently smaller number of patients having cancer at autopsy in those receiving preoperative irradiation than in the control group. This strongly suggests that preoperative irradiation exerts a long-term beneficial effect on postoperative recurrence.[54]

With the information available at the present time, the effect of preoperative irradiation in carcinoma of the rectum can be summarized as follows: the resectability may be improved; cancer cells in the regional lymph nodes may be destroyed, and thus may convert the disease to a more favorable stage; local seeding of cancer cells, as well as distant dissemination, may be decreased by altering the viability of shedded cancer cells. At the present time however, there is no unanimous agreement in the dose of radiation to be delivered.

POSTOPERATIVE IRRADIATION. Since most recurrent carcinoma of the rectum is localized in the pelvis, and usually occurs in those patients with Dukes' B or C lesions, it was thought it might be more appropriate to use postoperative irradiation, when details of the pathologic staging have been established. The advantages of postoperative irradiation are: (*1*) The total extent of the carcinoma is known and thus eliminates unnecessary irradiation particularly to those patients with Dukes' A lesions; (*2*) Postoperative irradiation could be used in patients with either anterior resection or abdominoperineal resection and, therefore, would potentially benefit a larger number of patients.[53] The theoretical disadvantages of postoperative irradiation are: (*1*) Postoperative irradiation has no effect on cells which may be spread at the time of operation; (*2*) Residual malignant cells in tissues rendered hypoxic as a result of operation may be more resistant to ionizing irradiation than those in a normal oxygenated environment; (*3*) A long delay in initiating postoperative irradiation could ensue if there are any postoperative complications, or if there is a delay in the healing of the perineal wound.[53]

There have been only a few institutions undertaking postoperative irradiation.[52,78] Gunderson reported a series of 36 patients with colorectal carcinoma, treated with operation and postoperative irradiation, in a prospective but nonrandomized study.[52] Only patients with carcinomas extending through the bowel wall or those with positive lymph nodes were included. The dose ranged from 4500 rads in five weeks, to 5100 rads in six weeks. When the lesion extended through the bowel wall or to a nodal capsule 5500 rads were given in 6 to 6½ weeks. Six thousand to 7000 rads were given in seven to eight weeks if there was residual or recurrent carcinoma after the operation. Of the 31 patients who had resection for cure only one (3%) was considered a local failure. Of five patients who had palliative resection with residual carcinoma, two (40%) had local failure. Although this result of the postoperative irradiation is encouraging, because of the small number of patients and short period of follow-up no conclusions can be drawn.

PREOPERATIVE COMBINED WITH POSTOPERATIVE IRRADIATION. Further searches have continued with the aim to improve the survival in carcinoma of the rectum, and to reduce morbidity and unnecessary treatment. The positive results from the Toronto trial, using 500 rads preoperatively, is an attractive one since this amount of irradiation does not interfere with wound healing.[96] The most recent adjuvant radiation treatment is the "sandwich technique" which uses a single dose of 500 rads preoperatively, and 4500 rads in five weeks postoperatively.[81] In an initial pilot study using this combination of pre- and postoperative irradiation, 18 of 19 patients with rectal carcinoma underwent radical resection. Eleven patients with full thickness involvement, or with positive lymph nodes were given postoperative irradiation. All patients tolerated the treatment well, with no undue side effects. The follow-up was too short to evaluate, but this attractive modality deserves further attention.

*Adjuvant chemotherapy* is the postoperative use of cancerocidal drugs to eradicate microfoci of cancer cells. The most useful single agents for colorectal cancer have been 5-fluorouracil (5-FU) and 5-fluorodeoxiuridine (5-FUDR). Most investigators use 5-FU because its effectiveness is identical to 5-FUDR while being much less expensive. 5-FU blocks the formation of thymidylic acid and, therefore, the biosynthesis of DNA.[59]

To study the possible effects of adjuvant 5-FU in conjunction with operative resection, cooperative trials conducted by the Veterans Administration group and the Central Oncology Group showed improvement in survival, but it was not statistically significant.[43,55] For its ongoing trial the Veterans Administration Surgical Adjuvant Group is using a combination of methyl-CCNU and 5-FU for colonic cancer.[55] The National Surgical Adjuvant Project for Breast and Bowel Cancers (NSABP) is using 5-FU, Methyl-CCNU and vincristine.

An alternate route of administering chemotherapy is by injecting 5-FU directly into the bowel lumen at the time of operation. The rationale of this approach is the modification or control of cancer spread by injuring or destroying malignant cells within the isolated area of bowel, and also permitting absorption of the drug into the mesenteric vein, lymphatics, and nodes.[55] A controlled study conducted by Lawrence, et al, showed no significant benefit from the treatment, whereas, Grossi, et al, noted improvement in the five-year survival rate in the group with Dukes' C rectal carcinoma.[51,66] However, the number of patients was too small for statistical analysis.

*Immunotherapy.* Cancer cells have repeatedly been found in the systemic venous blood in a high percentage of patients undergoing colonic or rectal excision for carcinoma.[45] Their presence or absence in the peripheral blood during the operation in no way correlates with survival, suggesting that host factors are important in preventing the growth of these circulating cancer cells.[58] Many other observations support the premise of a close relationship between immunologic competency and the growth of human cancer.[58]

The rationale of using immunotherapy for cancer assumes that there is potential antitumor immunity present in patients which is either blocked or at a low level, but which can be effectively stimulated to destroy malignant cells.[73]

A variety of modalities have been used to increase immunocompetence. Specific methods include the use of living carrier cells, neuraminidase, and purified tumor antigen.[74] Nonspecific immunologic adjuvants have been shown to be effective in eliciting an immune response against a wide range of tumor types, including colorectal cancer. The most widely used immunoadjuvants are bacillus Calmette-Guerin (BCG), Corynebacterium parvum (C-parvum), and Methanol Extracted Residue of BCG (MER). Only nonspecific adjuvants have been used in colorectal cancer.

Another current approach is combination immunotherapy and chemotherapy. Chemo-immunotherapy aims at combining the "debulking" capacity of chemotherapy with the potential for control of microscopic disease by immunotherapy and, therefore, producing long term disease-free survival.

Reed, et al, noted that the immunotherapeutic group of patients using C-parvum had less immunosuppression secondary to chemotherapy than the control group, and were able to receive chemotherapy twice as frequently. It may be that C-parvum exhibited no immunotherapeutic value in these patients but merely allowed the more aggressive utilization of chemotherapy.

Immunotherapy is most effective when the bulk of the cancer is small, either surgically removed, or in response to chemotherapy or irradiation therapy.[99] Immunotherapy can only be effective in an immunocompetent host. Immunocompetence in a patient can be judged by his ability to express delayed cutaneous hypersensitivity to antigens such as tuberculin purified derivative (TPD) and 2–4 dinitrochlorobenzene.[58]

Most of the current immunotherapeutic trials in bowel cancer are in a very early stage with small numbers of patients, and short follow-ups, and therefore, without evaluable data. There has never been any documentation that adjuvant immunotherapy of any form increased long term survival in patients with resected colorectal cancer. The immunotherapy by M. D. Anderson Hospital Group, using BCG, showed improvement in survival.[76] Unfortunately the results were not compared to a control group, making interpretation difficult. In the NSABP study, BCG is being used.

Immunotherapy is still in its infancy. It has shown a good potential to delay or prevent recurrence in colorectal cancer. Patients with Dukes' B and Dukes' C colorectal cancer would make excellent candidates for adjuvant immunotherapy, and are currently being entered into the NSABP study.

## CARCINOIDS

Rectal carcinoids account for 17 per cent of all gastrointestinal carcinoids. When the embryologically derived divisions of foregut, midgut, and hindgut are considered, the carcinoid neoplasm arising in each area has a characteristic chemicopathological manifestation.[110] Hindgut carcinoids, which include rectal carcinoids, do not produce serotonin or any other hormonal agent, rarely metastasize, and are not considered to give rise to the carcinoid syndrome.[86] There has been one reported exception to this involving a patient who failed to show elevation in 5HIAA when symptoms of flushing were maximum, except for a mild elevation on the day of her death three years after hepatic metastases.[98] It is possible the 5HIAA was the wrong marker, and that this neoplasm may have been secreting another hormonal agent.

## Clinical Presentation

There is no sex predominance, and carcinoids are most commonly found in the sixth and seventh decades of life. The typical finding at rectal examination is a solitary, mobile submucosal nodule with an intact overlying mucosa. Its color varies from yellow-grey to tan-pink. The size is usually 1 to 1.5 cm. In only 2 to 4 per cent are they multiple. In 32 per cent of the cases reported by Orloff the patient was asymptomatic, and in 20 per cent the symptoms were related to other pathology.[86] When symptoms were caused by the neoplasm, they were usually bleeding or constipation and only rarely did obstruction occur.

Malignancy has been reported in 39 per cent of cases, and in these the significant findings related to a size greater than 2 cm in diameter with invasion into the muscularis propria. The malignant variety is frequently ulcerated, with bleeding being part of the clinical presentation. Bates related size to malignancy and found that 1.7 per cent of carcinoids less than 1 cm, 10 per cent of carcinoids between 1 and 2 cm, and 82 per cent of carcinoids greater than 2 cm, were malignant.[4]

## Pathogenesis

Carcinoids are a member of the amine precursor uptake decarboxylation (APUD) group of neoplasms. These cells have the ability to secrete small polypeptide hormones. The two ultrastructural characteristics of enterochromaffin cells are secretory granules and lysosomes; hence, all are potentially secretory. Serotonin is responsible for the manifestations of the carcinoid syndrome, but proteases such as kallikrein may have a role and have also been extracted from metastatic carcinoids.

## Histochemical Characteristics

The histochemical staining reaction of carcinoids depends upon whether they are of foregut, midgut, or hindgut origin. All have an affinity for chromate salts; hence, the term "chromaffin tumors". However, the terms "argentaffin" and "argyrophil" are more specific. Argentaffin refers to tissues which re-

duce silver salts to black metallic silver in the absence of other reducing agents. This property depends upon the presence of serotonin. Carcinoids of the midgut are typically argentaffin. Argyrophil refers to tissues which have an affinity to silver, but these tissues do not reduce the salt to the black metal unless an additional reducing agent is present. Carcinoids of the foregut tend to be argyrophil, but not argentaffin. These histochemical properties have clinical significance, since carcinoids arising from foregut tend to produce typical variants of the carcinoid syndrome. Carcinoids of the hindgut tend to be negative for both the argentaffin and argyrophil reactions, and thus it is extremely rare for metastatic carcinoids from the rectum to produce any manifestations of the carcinoid syndrome.[110]

## Pathology

Macroscopically carcinoids may have a yellow appearance, but in most cases this is not a striking feature. Microscopically, they consist of rozettes, ribbons, or masses of uniform small, round, or polygonal cells with prominant nuclei and acidophillic cytoplasmic granules.

No absolute histologic difference exists between benign and malignant rectal carcinoids. Size and histologic evidence of invasion into the muscularis propria are helpful in distinguishing benign from malignant lesions. In Orloff's series of 15 carcinoids that were greater than 2 cm in diameter, 13 had invasion, 12 had metastasized to local lymph nodes, and six to distal organs.[86] When the lesion was larger than 2 cm, only 7 per cent were benign, whereas, when the lesion was smaller than 2 cm, only 4 per cent were malignant.

## Treatment

From the pathological data of these neoplasms it will be seen that those greater than 2 cm in diameter should, in general, be treated by abdominoperineal resection. For smaller lesions, an absolute essential for treatment is total excisional biopsy, which will be necessary to make a distinction.

## LEIOMYOSARCOMA

Leiomyosarcoma of the rectum occurs at all ages and in both sexes, but it is more common beyond the sixth decade of life. Bleeding, constipation, and rectal pain are the most common symptoms. In addition, the patient may complain of a pressure sensation, dysuria, or difficult defecation.[63] The majority of lesions are palpable on digital examination. They may be large, predominantly endorectal lesions, and in the more malignant forms have extensive perirectal invasion.[64] The surface may be ulcerated but generally has a rubbery feel. As with other sarcomas, the primary pathways of spread are by direct invasion and the hematogenous route. Lymph node metastases are not common even in advanced disease with pulmonary and hepatic metastases.

## Microscopy

The criterion of malignancy is simple in the high grade forms. It is based upon the number of mitoses per high power field. Golden and Stout state that two or more mitoses per high power field are required for a diagnosis of malignancy.[34] The Broder's classification of malignancy for sarcomas is also based upon the number of mitoses per high power field. It appears to offer little advantage over that of Golden and Stout which is the most useful criterion presently available. It is upon this definition that the decision for more definitive surgery is based.

## Treatment

There have been attempts to modify the treatment according to the histological classification of the neoplasm. It will be seen that because of the difficulty in deciding upon malignancy there is a high recurrence rate among supposedly benign lesions treated by local excision.[63] When local recurrence develops, and in those lesions that are diagnosed primarily as malignant, the treatment of choice is wide local excision rather than lymphatic clearance, but abdominoperineal resection may be necessary. Leiomyosarcoma of the rectum is radioresistant.

# MALIGNANT LYMPHOMA

These lesions are less common than the rectal carcinoid. The disease is more common in women (2 : 1), and is usually seen beyond the age of 50.

## Clinical Presentation

The presentation is usually because of rectal bleeding or alteration in bowel habits. However, a significant proportion may present with nothing more than generalized malaise and vague abdominal pain.

The lesion is usually detected on rectal examination and sigmoidoscopy. The macroscopic appearance bears no relationship to the histological structure. The growth patterns seen in the rectum are variable. They may be bulky, protuberant growth with ulceration; annular or plaque-like thickenings of the bowel wall; multiple malignant lymphomatous polyposis.[22]

## Microscopy

The criteria of malignancy depend upon invasion of the muscularis propria and the absence of a follicular pattern.[25] It should be stressed that a biopsy must include the muscle layer. Clearly, advanced lesions do not need this, but it is particularly important in the lymphomatous polyp group. The predominant pattern is that of a lymphosarcoma and thus, the pattern commonly seen is that of a reticulum cell sarcoma.

The growth tends to be rapid, with early involvement of lymph nodes. Dawson and associates found, however, that the presence of enlarged nodes at surgery did not, invariably, indicate involvement: this determination should be left to the pathologist.[25]

## Treatment

Surgical resection should be attempted wherever possible. Radiotherapy has a limited place in the primary treatment of rectal lymphoma, and is not a substitute for surgery.[25] Radiotherapy is useful in the palliation of inoperable cases and as an adjunct to surgery when resection is considered incomplete, either in relation to the primary lesion or the associated lymph node metastases. Adjuvant chemotherapy has an important role in the treatment of these malignancies.

Five-year survivals are few. Goligher had only two cases; neither of them survived five years.[36] It appears that a ten-year survival indicates a cure, and that despite a five year disease-free period, recurrences have been recorded in the five to ten year gap. It is important to realize that long term survivors have been reported following incomplete removal of gastrointestinal malignant lymphomas, including those with lymph node involvement. With advances in cytotoxic drug therapy and, to a lesser extent, in radiotherapy, surgical resection has a prominent place even when the surgeon feels doubtful as to the completeness of his resection and, thus, ultimate success.

Lymphosarcoma has been reported in association with chronic ulcerative colitis.[23,111] Caution is emphasized with these patients when reviewing rectal biopsies for staging of colitis because in some of the cases confusion has arisen between chronic inflammatory infiltrate and lymphosarcoma. In such cases radical excision of the colon is clearly required.

## SECONDARY CARCINOMA

It is unusual for the rectum to be invaded secondarily by carcinoma. The most common malignancies to do so are large bowel cancers, usually of the sigmoid colon, which may involve pelvic structures, including the rectum. It is rare for prostatic cancers to invade Denonvillier's fascia and present as a rectal neoplasm. It is more common for prostatic cancer to grow in a circumferential fashion around the rectum giving the appearance of an annular carcinoma without a break in mucosal continuity. This has the appearance of a bulky, infiltrating, rectal carcinoma. The diagnosis can only be made following a biopsy.[65]

The pouch of Douglas is a common site for metastatic implantation following transperitoneal spread from carcinoma of any of the intraabdominal organs. The most common sites of origin are the stomach and ovary. Any metastatic neoplasm can present in this site; breast is a typical example of such a malignancy. Carcinoma of the cervix rarely involves the rectum.[17]

## REFERENCES

1. Andersen, B., Korner, B., and Ostergaard, A. H.: Topical ampicillin against wound infection after colorectal surgery. Ann. Surg., *176:*129, 1972.

2. Bacon, H. E., Dirbas, F., Myers, T. B., and Ponce DeLeon, F.: Extensive lymphadenectomy and high ligation of the inferior mesenteric artery for carcinoma of the left colon and rectum. Dis. Colon Rectum, *1:*457, 1958.

3. Bacon, H. E., and Zuber, W. F.: Panhysterectomy concomitant with bowel resection for carcinoma: 75 cases. Surgery, *57:*370, 1965.

4. Bates, H. R. Jr.: Carcinoid tumors of the rectum. Dis. Colon Rectum, *5:*270, 1962.

5. Bennett, R. C., Hughes, E. S. R., and Cuthbertson, A. M.: Long-term review of function following pull-through operations of the rectum. Br. J. Surg., *59:*723, 1972.

6. Black, B. M., and Walls, J. T.: Combined abdominoendorectal resection: Reappraisal of a pull-through procedure. Surg. Clin. North Am., *47:*977, 1967.

7. Block, I. R., and Enquist, I. F.: Lymphatic studies pertaining to local spread of carcinoma of the rectum in female. Surg. Gynecol. Obstet., *112:*41, 1961.

8. Bordos, D. C., Baker, R. R., and Cameron, J. L.: An evaluation of palliative abdominoperineal resection for carcinoma of the rectum. Surg. Gynecol. Obstet., *139:*731, 1974.

9. Broders, A. C.: The grading of carcinoma. Minn. Med., *8:*726, 1925.

10. Burkitt, D. P.: An epidemiologic approach to cancer of the large intestine: the significance of disease relationship. Dis. Colon Rectum, *17:*456, 1974.

11. Bussey, H. J. R.: Familial Polyposis Coli. Baltimore, The Johns Hopkins University Press, 1975.

12. Busuttil, R. W., Foglia, R. P., and Longmire, W. P., Jr.: Treatment of carcinoma of the sigmoid colon and upper rectum. Arch. Surg., *112:*920, 1977.

13. Cancer Statistics. American Cancer Society, Inc., 24, 1978.

14. Castro, E. B., Rosen, P. P., and Quan, S. H. Q.: Carcinoma of large intestine in patients irradiated for carcinoma of cervix and uterus. Cancer, *31:*45, 1973.

15. Cedermark, B. J., Schultz, S. S., Bakslu, S., Parthasarathy, K. L., Mittelman, A. and Evans, J. T.: The value of liver scan in the follow-up study of patients with adenocarcinoma of the colon and rectum. Surg. Gynecol. Obstet., *144:*745, 1977.

16. Chen, W. F., Patchefsky, A. S., and Goldsmith, H. S.: Colonic protection from dimethylhydrazine by a high fiber diet. Surg. Gynecol. Obstet., *147:*503, 1978.

17. Christodoulopoulos, J. B., Papainnou, A. N.,

Drakopoulou, E. P., Kantos, E. K., and Razis, D. V.: Carcinoma of the cervix presenting with rectal symptomatology: Report of three cases. Dis. Colon Rectum, *15:*373, 1972.

18. Condon, R. E.: Rational use of prophylactic antibiotics in gastrointestinal surgery. Surg. Clin. North Am., *55:*1309, 1975.

19. Condon, R. E., Bartlett, J. G., Nichols, R. L., Schulte, W. J., Gorbach, S. L. and Ochi, S.: Preoperative prophylactic cephalothin fails to control septic complications of colorectal operations: Results of controlled clinical trial. A Veterans Administration Cooperative Study. Am. J. Surg., *137:*68, 1979.

20. Condon, R. E., and Nichols, R. L.: The present position of the Neomycin-Erythromycin bowel prep. Surg. Clin. North Am., *55:*1331, 1975.

21. Cook, M. G., and Goligher, J. C.: Carcinoma and epithelial dysplasia complicating ulcerative colitis. Gastroenterology, *68:*1128, 1975.

22. Cornes, J. S.: Multiple lymphomatous polyposis of the gastrointestinal tract. Cancer, *14:*249, 1961.

23. Cornes, J. S., and Smith, J. C.: Lymphosarcoma in chronic ulcerative colitis. Br. J. Surg., *49:*50, 1961.

24. Cutait, D. E., and Figliolini, F. J.: A new method of colorectal anastomosis in abdominoperineal resection. Dis. Colon Rectum, *4:*335, 1961.

25. Dawson, I. M. P., Cornes, J. S., and Morson, B. C.: Primary malignant lymphoid tumors of the intestinal tract. Report of 37 cases with study of factors influencing prognosis. Br. J. Surg., *49:*80, 1961.

26. Dukes, C. E.: The classification of cancer of the rectum. J. Pathol. Bacteriol., *35:*1, 1932.

27. Dukes, C. E., and Bussey, H. J. R.: The spread of rectal cancer and its effect on prognosis. Br. J. Cancer., *12:*309, 1958.

28. Evans, C., Pollock, A. V., and Rosenberg, I. L.: The reduction of surgical wound infection by topical cephaloridine: A controlled clinical trial. Br. J. Surg., *61:*133, 1974.

29. Fenoglio, C. M., and Lane, N.: The anatomic precursor of colorectal carcinoma. JAMA, *231:*640, 1975.

30. Fletcher, W. S., Allen, C. V., and Dunphy, J. E.: Preoperative irradiation for carcinoma of the colon and rectum. Am. J. Surg., *109:*76, 1965.

31. Floyd, C. E., Stirling, C. T., and Cohn, I. Jr.: Cancer of the colon, rectum and anus. Review of 1687 cases. Ann. Surg., *163:*829, 1966.

32. Gambee, L. P.: A single-layer open intestinal anastomosis applicable to the small as well as the large intestine. West J. Surg. Obstet. Gynecol, *59:*1, 1951.

33. Gilbertsen, V. A., and Nelms, J. M.: The prevention of invasive cancer of the rectum. Cancer, *41:*1137, 1978.

34. Golden, T., and Stout, A. P.: Smooth muscle tumors of the gastrointestinal tract and retroperitoneal tissues. Surg. Gynecol. Obstet., *73:*784, 1941.

35. Goligher, J. C.: The Dukes' A, B and C categorization of the extent of spread of carcinomas of the rectum. Surg. Gynecol. Obstet., *143:*793, 1976.

36. ———: Surgery of the Anus, Rectum and Colon. 3 ed. 483-484, 836. Springfield, Charles C Thomas, 1975.

37. ———: The operability of carcinoma of the rectum. Br. Med. J., *2:*393, 1941.

38. Goligher, J. C., Dukes, C. E., and Bussey, H. J. R.: Local recurrences after sphincter-saving excisions for carcinoma of the rectum and rectosigmoid. Br. J. Surg., *39:*199, 1951.

39. Goligher, J. C., Duthie, H. L., DeDombal, F. T., and Watts, J. M.: Abdomino-anal pull-through excision for tumors of the mid-third of the rectum. Br. J. Surg., *52:*323, 1965.

40. Goligher, J. C., Lee, P. W. R., Macfie, J., Simpkins, K. C., and Lintot, D. J.: Experience with the Russian model 249 suture gun for anastomosis of the rectum. Surg. Gynecol. Obstet., *148:*517, 1979.

41. Gongaware, R. D., and Slanetz, C. A. Jr.: Hartmann procedure for carcinoma of the sigmoid and rectum. Am. J. Surg., *178:*28, 1973.

42. Gordon-Watson, C.: The treatment of carcinoma of the rectum with radium. Br. J. Surg., *17:*643, 1930.

43. Grage, T. E., et al: Adjuvant chemotherapy with 5-FU after resection of colorectal carcinoma—A preliminary report. Am. J. Surg., *133:*59, 1977.

44. Greaney, M. G., and Irvin, T. T.: Criteria for the selection of rectal cancers for local treatment: A clinicopathologic study of low rectal tumors. Dis. Colon Rectum, *20:*463, 1977.

45. Griffiths, J. D., McKinna, J. A., Rowbotham, H. D., Tsolakidis, P., and Salsbury, A. J.: Carcinoma of the colon and rectum: Circulating malignant cells and five-year survival. Cancer, *31:*226, 1973.

46. Grinnell, R. S.: Lymphatic block with atypical and retrograde lymphatic metastasis and

spread in carcinoma of the colon and rectum. Ann. Surg., *163:*272, 1966.

47. ———: Results of ligation of inferior mesenteric artery at the aorta in resections of carcinoma of the descending and sigmoid colon and rectum. Surg. Gynecol. Obstet., *120:*1031, 1965.

48. ———: Distal intramural spread of carcinoma of the rectum and rectosigmoid. Surg. Gynecol. Obstet., *99:*421, 1954.

49. ———: The grading and prognosis of carcinoma of the colon and rectum. Ann. Surg., *109:*500, 1939.

50. Grinnell, R. S., and Hiatt, R. B.: Ligation of the inferior mesenteric artery at the aorta in resections for carcinoma of the sigmoid and rectum. Surg. Gynecol. Obstet., *94:*526, 1952.

51. Grossi, C. E., et al: Intraluminal fluorouracil chemotherapy adjunct to surgical procedures for resectional carcinoma of the colon and rectum. Surg. Gynecol. Obstet., *145:*549, 1977.

52. Gunderson, L. L.: Combined irradiation and surgery for rectal and sigmoid carcinoma. Curr. Probl. Cancer, *1:*40, 1976.

53. Gunderson, L. L., and Sosin, H.: Areas of failure found at reoperation (second or symptomatic look) following "curative surgery" for adenocarcinoma of the rectum. Cancer, *34:*1278, 1974.

54. Higgins, G. A. Jr.: The pros and cons of irradiation treatment of colorectal cancer. *In* Nehus, L. M., (ed.) Surgery Annual. New York, Appleton-Century-Crofts, 1978.

55. Higgins, G. A. Jr.: Chemotherapy, adjuvant to surgery, for gastrointestinal cancer. Clin. Gastroenterol., *5:*795, 1976.

56. Hill, M. J., et al: Bacteria and aetiology of cancer of large bowel. Lancet, *1:*95, 1971.

57. Hojer, H., and Wetterfors, J.: Systemic prophylaxis with Doxycycline in surgery of the colon and rectum. Ann. Surg., *187:*362, 1978.

58. Homes, E. C., Eilber, F. R., and Morton, D. L.: Immunotherapy of malignancy in humans. Current status. JAMA, *232:*1052, 1975.

59. Humphrey, E. W.: Cancer chemotherapy. Curr. Probl. Surg., 16, Sept. 1966

60. Keighley, M. R. B., Crapp, A. R., Burdon, D. W., Cooke, W. T., and Williams, J. A.: Prophylaxis against anaerobic sepsis in bowel surgery. Br. J. Surg., *63:*538, 1976.

61. Killingback, M., Wilson, E., and Hughes, E. S. R.: Anal metastasis from carcinoma of the rectum and colon. Aust. NZ. J. Surg., *34:*178, 1965.

62. Kirwan, W. O., Turnbull, R. B. Jr., Fazio, V. W., and Weakley, F. L.: Pull-through operation with delayed anastomosis for rectal cancer. Br. J. Surg., *65:*695, 1978.

63. Kusminsky, R. E., and Bailey, W.: Leiomyomas of the rectum and anal canal: Report of six cases and review of the literature. Dis. Colon Rectum, *20:*580, 1977.

64. Labow, S. B., and Hoexter, B.: Leiomyosarcoma of the rectum: Radical VS conservative therapy and report of three cases. Dis. Colon Rectum, *20:*603, 1977.

65. Lasser, A.: Adenocarcinoma of the prostate involving the rectum. Dis. Colon Rectum, *21:*23, 1978.

66. Lawrence, W. Jr., Terz, J. J., Horsley, S. III, Donaldson, M., Lovett, W. L., Brown, P. W., Ruffner, B. W. and Regelson, W.: Chemotherapy as an adjunct to surgery for colorectal cancer. Ann. Surg., *181:*616, 1975.

67. Lennard-Jones, J. E., Morson, B. C., Ritchie, J. K., Shove, D. C., and Williams, C. B.: Cancer in colitis: Assessment of the individual risk by clinical and histological criteria. Gastroenterology, *73:*1280, 1977.

68. LeQuesne, L. P., and Thompson, A. D.: Implantation recurrence of carcinoma of the rectum and colon. N. Engl. J. Med., *258:*578, 1958.

69. Localio, S. A., Eng, K., Gouge, T. H., and Ranson, J. H. C.: Abdominosacral resection for carcinoma of the mid rectum: Ten years experience. Ann. Surg., *188:*475, 1978.

70. Lock, M. R., Cairns, D. W., Ritchie, J. K., and Lockhart-Mummery, H. E.: The treatment of early colorectal cancer by local excision. Br. J. Surg., *65:*346, 1978.

71. Lockhart-Mummery, H. E.: Surgery in patients with advanced carcinoma of the colon and rectum. Dis. Colon Rectum, *2:*36, 1959.

72. Lynch, H. T., and Krush, A. J.: Heredity and adenocarcinoma of the colon. Gastroenterology, *53:*517, 1967.

73. MacDonald, J. S.: The immunobiology of colorectal cancer. Semin. Oncol., *3:*421, 1976.

74. Martin, D.: The necessity for combined modalities in cancer therapy. Hosp. Pract., 129, Jan. 1973.

75. Mathe, G., et al: Active immunotherapy for acute lymphoblastic leukemia. Lancet, *1:*697, 1969.

76. Mavligit, G. M., Gutterman, J. V., Burgess, M. A., Khankhanian, N., Seibert, B., Speer, J. F., Reed, R. C., Jubert, A. V., McBride, C. M., Copeland, E. M., Gehan, E. A. and

Hersh, E. M.: Adjuvant immunotherapy and chemoimmunotherapy in colorectal cancer of the Dukes' C classification: Preliminary clinical results. Cancer, *36* (suppl): 2421, 1975.

77. McGregor, J. K., and Bacon, H. E.: The surgical management of carcinoma of the mid and upper rectum. Abdominoperineal proctosigmoidectomy without abdominal colostomy and with sphincter muscle preservation: A critical analysis of 699 cases. Arch. Surg., *85:*807, 1962.

78. Mendiondo, O. A., Wang, C. C., Welch, J. P., and Donaldson, G. A.: Postoperative radiotherapy in carcinomas of the rectum and distal sigmoid colon. Radiology, *119:*673, 1976.

79. Miles, W. E.: Pathology of spread of cancer of rectum and its bearing upon surgery of cancerous rectum. Surg. Gynecol. Obstet., *52:*350, 1931.

80. ———: A method of performing abdominoperineal excision for carcinoma of the rectum and of the terminal portion of the pelvic colon. Lancet, *2:*1812, 1908.

81. Mohinddin, M., and Kramer, S.: Adjuvant radiotherapy—preoperative, postoperative, or both: A proposal for a new approach. Cancer Clinical Trials, *1:*93, 1978.

82. Morgan, C. N.: Treatment of cancer of the rectum. Am. J. Surg., *115:*442, 1968.

83. Morgenstern, L., and Lee, S. E.: Spatial distribution of colonic carcinoma. Arch. Surg., *113:*1142, 1978.

84. Morson, B. C., and Bussey, H. J.: Predisposing causes of intestinal cancer. Curr. Probl. Surg. 23-24 (Feb), 1970.

85. Morson, B. C., Bussey, H. J. R., and Samoorian, S.: Policy of local excision for early cancer of the colorectum. Gut, *18:*1045, 1977.

86. Orloff, M. J.: Carcinoid tumors of the rectum. Cancer, *28:*175, 1971.

87. Plorde, J. J.: Harrison's Principles of Internal Medicine. 8 ed. 1106-1110. Thorn, Adams, Braunwald, Isselbacher, Petersdorf, (eds.) New York: McGraw-Hill Book Co., 1977.

88. Polk, H. C. Jr., and Lopez-Mayor, J. F.: Postoperative wound infection: A prospective study of determinant factors and prevention. Surgery, *66:*97, 1969.

89. Pollock, A. V., Leaper, D. J., and Evans, M.: Single dose intra-incisional antibiotic prophylaxis of surgical wound sepsis: A controlled trial of cephaloridine and ampicillin. Br. J. Surg., *64:*322, 1977.

90. Quan, S. H. Q., and Sehdev, M. H.: Pelvic surgery concomitant with bowel resection for carcinoma. Surg. Clin. North Am., *54:*881, 1974.

91. Quer, E. A., Dahlin, D. C., and Mayo, C. W.: Retrograde intramural spread of carcinoma of the rectum and rectosigmoid. Surg. Gynecol. Obstet., *96:*24, 1953.

92. Read, D. R., Hambrick, E., Abcarian, H., and Levine, H.: The preoperative diagnosis of hepatic metastasis in cases of colorectal carcinoma. Dis. Colon Rectum, *20:*101, 1977.

93. Reddy, B. S., and Wynder, E. L.: Large bowel carcinogenesis: Fecal constituents of populations with diverse incidence rates of colon cancer. J Natl Cancer Inst, *50:*1437, 1973.

94. Reed, R. C., Gutterman, J. W., Mavligit, G. M., and Hersh, E. M.: Phase I trial of intravenous and subcutaneous Corynebacterium parvum. Proc. Am. Assoc. Can. Res., Am. S. Clin. Onc., *16:*228, 1975.

95. Rhodes, J. B., Holmes, F. F., and Clark, G. M.: Changing distribution of primary cancers in the large bowel. JAMA, *238:*1641, 1977.

96. Rider, W. D., Palmer, J. A., Mahoney, L. J., and Robertson, C. T.: Preoperative irradiation in operable cancer of the rectum—the report of the Toronto trial. Ontario Cancer Institute. Can. J. Surg., *20:*335, 1977.

97. Rosenberg, I. L., Russell, C. W., and Giles, G. R.: Cell viability studies on the exfoliated colonic cancer cell. Br. J. Surg., *65:*188, 1978.

98. Salgesser, F., and Gross, M.: Carcinoid syndrome and carcinoid tumors of the rectum. Amer. J. Proct., *20:*27, 1969.

99. Schabel, F. M., Skipper, H. E., Lester, W. R. Jr., Trader, M. W., and Thompson, S. A.: Experimental evaluation of potential anticancer agents XX. Development of immunity to leukemia L1210 in BDF$_1$, mice and effects of therapy. Cancer Chemother. Rep., *50:*55, 1966.

100. Schulten, M. F., Heiskell, C. A., and Shields, T. W.: The incidence of solitary pulmonary metastasis from carcinoma of the large intestine. Surg. Gynecol. Obstet., *143:*727, 1976.

101. Shindo, K.: Significance of schistosoma japonicum in the development of cancer of the large intestine: Report of a case and review of the literature. Dis. Colon Rectum, *19:*460, 1976.

102. Slanetz, C. A., Herter, F. P., and Grinnell, R. S.: Anterior resection versus abdominoperineal resection for cancer of the rectum and rectosigmoid. Am. J. Surg., *123:*110, 1972.

103. Stearns, M. W. Jr.: The choice among anterior resection, the pull-through and abdomino-perineal resection of the rectum. Cancer, *34:*969, 1974.

104. Stearns, M. W. Jr., Deddish, M. R., and Quan, S. H. Q.: Preoperative roentgen therapy for cancer of the rectum. Surg. Gynecol. Obstet., *109:*225, 1959.

105. Stokes, E. J., Waterworth, P. M., Franks, V., Watson, B., and Clark, C. G.: Short term routine antibiotics prophylaxis in surgery. Br. J. Surg., *61:*739, 1974.

106. Stone, H. H., and Hester, T. R. Jr.: Topical antibiotic and delayed primary closure in the management of contaminated surgical incisions. J. Surg. Res., *12:*70, 1972.

107. Stone, H. H., Hooper, C. A., Kolb, L. D., Geheber, C. E., and Dawkins, E. J.: Antibiotic prophylaxis in gastric, biliary and colonic surgery. Ann. Surg., *184:*443, 1976.

108. Symonds, C. J.: Cancer of the rectum: Excision after application of radium. Proc. R. Soc. Med., *7:*153, 1914.

109. Symonds, D. A., and Vickery, A. L. Jr.: Mucinous carcinoma of the colon and rectum. Cancer, *37:*1891, 1976.

110. Tilson, M. D.: Carcinoid syndrome. Surg. Clin. North Am., *54:*409, 1974.

111. Vieta, J. O., and Delgado, G. E.: Chronic ulcerative colitis complicated by colonic lymphoma: Report of a case. Dis. Colon Rectum, *19:*56, 1976.

112. Washington, J. A. II, Dearing, W. H., Judd, E. S., and Elveback, L. R.: Effect of preoperative antibiotic regimen on development of infection after intestinal surgery: Prospective, randomized, double-blind study. Ann. Surg., *180:*567, 1974.

113. Welch, C. E., and Giddings, W. P.: Carcinoma of colon and rectum. Observations on Massachusetts General Hospital cases 1937–1948. N. Engl. J. Med., *244:*860, 1951.

114. Welch, J. P., and Donaldson, G. A.: Detection and treatment of recurrent cancer of the colon and rectum. Am. J. Surg., *135:*505, 1978.

115. Whittaker, M., and Goligher, J. C.: The prognosis after surgical treatment for carcinoma of the rectum. Br. J. Surg., *63:*384, 1976.

116. Wilson, S. M., and Beahrs, O. H.: The curative treatment of carcinoma of the sigmoid, rectosigmoid, and rectum. Ann. Surg., *183:*556, 1976.

117. Wu, T. T., Ch'en, T. H. and Ch'i, C.: The relationship of schistosomiasis to carcinoma of large intestine. Chin. Med. J., *80:*231, 1960.

118. Wynder, E. L., and Reddy, B.: The epidemiology of cancer of the large bowel. Digestive Diseases, *19:*937, 1974.

119. Wynder, E. L., and Shigematsu, T.: Environmental factors of cancer of the colon and rectum. Cancer, *20:*1520, 1967.

# 17

# Retrorectal Tumors

Located in the presacral region is a heterogeneous group of neoplasms and cysts which comprise what has been categorized as retrorectal tumors. In addition to the usual tissues from which neoplasms may arise, this is an area of embryological fusion and remodelling, and thus, the common site for the persistence of embryological remnants from which neoplasms may also arise. The following is an account of these rare but interesting lesions. The anatomy of the region will first be reviewed.

The retrorectal space lies between the upper two-thirds of the rectum and the sacrum, above the retrorectal fascia. It is limited anteriorly by the fascia propria covering the rectum, posteriorly by the presacral fascia, and laterally by the lateral ligaments of the rectum (stalks). Superiorly, it communicates with the retroperitoneal space, and inferiorly is limited by the rectosacral fascia which passes forward from the $S_4$ vertebra to the rectum 3 to 5 cm proximal to the anorectal junction. Below the rectosacral fascia is the supralevator space, a horseshoe-shaped potential space limited anteriorly by the Denonvilliers fascia, and below by the levator ani (Fig. 17-1).

The retrorectal space contains loose connective tissue. The presacral fascia protects the presacral vessels which lie deep to it. The presacral vessels are part of the extensive vertebral plexus, and are responsible for the major bleeding problems encountered in this area during surgery.

With collaboration of William R. Johnson

## CLASSIFICATION

Lovelady and Dockerty proposed a classification which has formed the basis for the more expanded versions we now have.[14] Uhlig and colleagues, aided by the composite classification of Freier and associates, proposed the following classification.[3,25]

---

*DIFFERENTIAL DIAGNOSIS OF*
*RETRORECTAL TUMORS AND CYSTS*

Congenital
  Developmental cysts (epidermoid, dermoid and mucus-secreting cysts and teratoma)
  Chordoma
  Teratocarcinoma
  Adrenal rest tumor
  Anterior sacral meningocele
  Duplication of rectum
Inflammatory
  Foreign-body granuloma
  Perineal abscess
  Internal fistula
  Pelvirectal abscess
  Chronic infectious granuloma
Neurogenic
  Neurofibroma and sarcoma
  Neurilemmoma
  Ependymoma
  Ganglioneuroma
  Neurofibrosarcoma
Osseous
  Osteoma
  Osteogenic sarcoma
  Simple bone cyst, sacrum
  Ewing's tumor

Chondromyxosarcoma
Aneurysmal bone cyst
Giant-cell tumor
Miscellaneous
  Metastatic carcinoma
  Liposarcoma
  Hemangioendothelial sarcoma
  Lymphangioma
  Extra-abdominal desmoid tumor
  Plasma-cell myeloma
  Lipoma
  Fibroma
  Fibrosarcoma
  Leiomyoma
  Leiomyosarcoma
  Hemangioma
  Pericytoma
  Endothelioma

## INCIDENCE

These lesions are rare. Uhlig and associates reviewed all the cases presenting to local hospitals in Portland, Oregon, and found a total of 63 cases over a thirty year period.[25]

Mayo and colleagues, in 1958, reviewed 161 tumors, and in 1962 Spencer and Jackman reviewed 38 precoccygeal cysts presenting in the preceding five years.[16,24] McColl, in 1963, presented 23 cases of presarcal tumors seen at St. Mark's Hospital, London.[17] Most reviews are restricted to the adult population and do not include the pediatric group. Sacrococcygeal teratomas, which form the majority seen in the pediatric group, are estimated to have occurred once in every 40,000 births.[19]

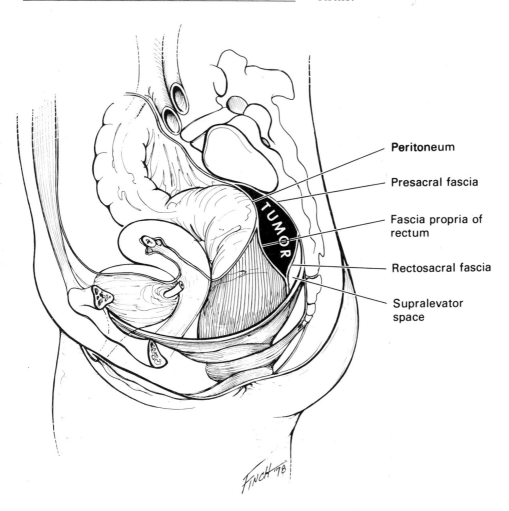

Peritoneum

Presacral fascia

Fascia propria of rectum

Rectosacral fascia

Supralevator space

**FIGURE 17-1.** *The retrorectal space.*

## PATHOLOGY

It is not proposed to give an exhaustive review of pathology of this area. Many of the tumors are universal in presentation and the reader is referred to any standard pathology text. The tumors and cysts chosen for emphasis are those typical of the retrorectal area.

### Developmental Cysts

As indicated in Table 17-1, developmental cysts may arise from any of the germ layers.

*Epidermoid and Dermoid Cysts.* There is general agreement that these result from defects of closure of the ectodermal tube with heterotopic inclusions of skin and sometimes with accessory skin appendages.

THE EPIDERMOID CYST is lined by stratified squamous epithelium with keratohyaline granules and intracellular bridges. There are no skin appendages within the epithelium.

DERMOID CYSTS. In addition to the stratified squamous epithelium seen in the epidermoid cysts, these have either sweat glands, hair follicles, sebaceous glands or all three. These appendages characterize dermoid cysts.

Both epidermoid and dermoid cysts tend to be rounded, and circumscribed with a thin connective tissue outer-layer, and contain viscid green/yellow material. These cysts can communicate with the skin surface, where they appear as a postanal dimple. The cysts are more common in women than in men and

have a high rate of infection (30–40 per cent).[7] In the infected state they may appear as a retrorectal abscess or perirectal suppuration. When the postanal dimple communicates with an infected cyst a mistaken diagnosis of a fistula-in-ano is commonly made.

*Enterogenous Cysts.* The current belief is that enterogenous cysts result from sequestration of the developing hindgut. It is interesting that, on occasion, layers of either squamous or transitional epithelium may be found within the lining of an otherwise mucus-secreting cyst. This is not surprising when the embryology of the area is considered, since the terminal hindgut, or cloaca, gives rise to rectal and urogenital structures.

Generally these are thin-walled cysts lined by mucus-secreting columnar epithelium. They tend to be multilocular, usually with one dominant cyst and a series of minor or daughter cysts. In the uninfected state they are filled with a clear to green mucoid material.

These cysts are more common in women and, as with the epidermoid/dermoid cysts, have a tendency to become infected. In the majority of cases, however, they remain asymptomatic. Frequency of developmental cyst of female to male occurrence is 5 : 1. The majority are asymptomatic and, because the tension in the cyst is low, they may be easily missed on rectal examination. Of all the cysts presenting at the Mayo Clinic, only 45 per cent were symptomatic and, of these, 70 per cent of the symptoms were related to the presence of infection in the cyst.[24] The average age of pre-

TABLE **17-1.** Germ Layer Origin of Developmental Cysts

|  | EPIDERMOID | DERMOID | ENTEROGENOUS | TERATOMATOUS |
|---|---|---|---|---|
| *Tissue of Origin* | Ectoderm | Ectoderm | Endoderm | All three germ cell layers represented |
| *Histological Characteristics* | Stratified Squamous | Stratified squamous with skin appendages (sweat glands, sebaceous glands, hair follicles) | Columnar or cuboidal lining ± secretory function | Varying degrees of differentiation between cysts and germ cell layers of single cyst |
| *General State* | Benign* | Benign* | Benign | Benign or Malignant |

\* Malignant variant rare

sentation of these cysts is in the fourth decade. The duration of symptoms, if they exist, is frequently measured in years.

### Teratoma and Teratocarcinoma

These are true neoplasms arising from totipotential cells. They classically have representative tissue from each germ cell layer, although the degree of differentiation may vary among the elements. Malignancy, when it occurs, tends to arise from one of the germ cells; however, in the anaplastic variety, it may be impossible to distinguish the tissue of origin. The more mature the tissue appears, the more benign the neoplasm tends to be, but all should be viewed as potentially malignant.[26]

Of the 32 germ cell neoplasms reviewed by Conklin and colleagues, all but four occurred in children, the oldest being two years.[2] Of this group, 23 had lesions visible at birth, and only one of these recurred, metastasized, and caused death of the infant following surgical treatment.

Malignancy is rare beyond the second decade; however, the neonatal malignancy rate is 4 per cent.[19] Of those neoplasms present at birth and not treated immediately, 7 per cent can be expected to be malignant by the fourth month.[22] Hunt reported that between the fourth month and the fifteenth year, this figure increases to 42 per cent.[11] Beyond the twentieth year, malignancy is less common, as indeed, are retrorectal teratomas. Killen, et al, reviewed the literature and found 35 reported cases to which they added two of their own.[12] Of these 37 cases of adult teratoma (beyond 20 years), 76 per cent occurred in women, and only 5 of 37 were malignant.[12] Thus, the potential for malignant conversion is the greatest during the period of growth, in particular during the early years of life.[5] It significantly decreases, but is still present, in the adult. Hence, there is a need for adequate, early surgical removal.

The sacrococcygeal teratoma presents most commonly as an obvious external mass in the perineal area of the neonate. Occasionally the dominant mass is toward the peritoneal cavity. These neoplasms can vary in size from a small retrorectal mass to one weighing more than the infant and is, thus, capable of causing pelvic obstruction during labor. In children there is a 2 : 1 female to male ratio. In the adult, the lesions present most commonly as a retrorectal mass; however, they may be seen externally as pedunculated or protuberant tumors in the sacrococcygeal area.

### Chordoma

The chordoma is a malignant tumor arising from the remnants of the fetal notochord. The notochord is the primitive flexible vertebral column extending from the basilar portion of the occipital bone to the caudal limit of the embryo.

In the adult, the only notochordal remnant is found in the nucleus pulposus of the intervertebral disc. The chordoma does not appear to arise from the nucleus pulposus but from the vertebral bodies. Although it can occur anywhere from the hypophysis cerebri to the coccyx, the sacrococcygeal area is the most common site.

The persistence of aberrant buds of notochordal tissue in the sacrococcygeal region was described by Horwitz.[10] There is little doubt that remnants of these are the source of sacro-coccygeal chordomas.[26]

The neoplasms may arise in either sex at any age, but are more frequent in men, in the fifth decade of life. The preponderance of men is more marked in the sacral than in the cranial group. Harvey and Dawson, reviewing 220 cases, found a sex distribution of 144 men and 76 women.[6]

Macroscopically, the chordoma is typically a slow growing, lobulated, well-defined structure composed of soft gelatinous tissue, often with areas of hemorrhage. It invades, distends, and destroys the neighboring bone and extends into adjacent regions.

Microscopically, they are said to resemble the various stages of notochordal development. The cells are usually aggregated in irregular groups, separated by stromal tissue. Peripheral cells contain mucus droplets in the cytoplasm. As these cells mature, the droplets coalesce so that in older cells, single, large vacuoles exist giving the characteristic physaliphorous cell typical of chordoma. Toward the center of the neoplasms, cords of cells appear to float in mucus, cell boundaries are indistinct, and the appearance is that of a syncytium.

### Neurogenic Tumors

Neurogenic lesions in this location are the typical neoplasms of peripheral nerves, and arise along the nerve. Evidence of motor and sensory dysfunction are usually confined to a single peripheral nerve. In this region, however, because of the cauda equina, a neoplasm arising from a nerve root within the spinal canal may have devastating effects on all the local nerves, even resulting in paraplegia. These lesions usually reach a significant size before detection. They are related to the lateral wall of the pelvis, are slow growing, and good results are obtained with surgical removal. It is rare for a malignant variant to be found here.

In a Uhlig, et al, series, the average age of presentation was 33 years, and except in the case of one patient with an ependymoma who was paraplegic but stable, the group had good results.[25] It must be remembered that the prognosis for life is good with most peripheral nerve neoplasms, but the morbidity can be significant.

### Osseous Lesions

Primary bone neoplasms in this region, as elsewhere, are far less common than metastatic neoplasms. In spite of this, virtually all possible types of bone lesions, both benign and malignant, have been found in this area. Persistent skeletal pain frequently calls attention to these neoplasms which are usually well-advanced when detected. Malignant sarcomas, either of cartilaginous or osseous origin, and other lesions such as Ewings sarcoma, have a disastrous prognosis when they occur. When found they are usually inoperable and widespread.

Benign neoplasms, apart from bone cysts and osteomas, present the problem of recurrence. If feasible, a block resection is the treatment of choice. Unfortunately, because of the site, the neoplasm is often advanced, requiring extensive surgery which is frequently incomplete. Every attempt must be made to achieve primary resection.

### Miscellaneous Tumors

Other connective tissue sarcomas have been reported in this area (e.g., liposarcoma, fibrosarcoma, hemangiosarcoma). These are, fortunately, rare and the prognosis is, as with bone sarcoma, poor. In Uhlig's series, nine patients had recurrent or metastatic carcinoma in the presacral area.[25] This should always be kept in mind when the history is being taken.

## THE RISK OF MALIGNANCY IN THE RETRORECTAL TUMOR

The incidence of malignancy in teratoma has been given. In general, the chance that a presacral tumor in an adult will be malignant is 33 per cent. In other words, two-thirds of presacral tumors in adults will be benign. The male to female incidence of malignancy is equal. This finding is interesting when the usual female predominance of these lesions is considered. This reflects the fact that malignancies always, eventually present clinically, whereas benign lesions may remain asymptomatic. This is significant when it is considered that many of the lesions in women are found during the reproductive years of life when pelvic examinations are more frequent. Thus, the female predominance may to some extent be artificial.

## CLINICAL PRESENTATION

### Symptoms

The symptoms caused by these tumors are related to their site, size and, in the case of retrorectal cysts, the presence or lack of infection.

*Pain.* This is a common finding with the neoplastic group, and with the infected cysts. It is generally poorly localized as low back or perianal pain, a rectal ache, or deep rectal pain. If the sacral plexus is involved, referred pain into the legs or buttocks may be experienced. It is unusual for the pain to be accompanied by paralysis in the early stages.

Characteristically, the pain experience in retrorectal neoplasms is frequently postural. The patient will relate it to sitting or standing, and often the onset of pain will be related to some local trauma such as a fall on the sacrum or coccyx.

*Infection.* This may be an isolated event with fever, chills, rigors, and pain, or manifest as recurrent episodes of perianal suppuration, frequently with a history of recurrent surgical attempts at treatment. This latter history in a female should always precipitate a careful search to exclude a retrorectal cyst.

*Interference with the Pelvic Outlet.* CONSTIPATION. Large tumors may interfere with the passage of stool or give the feeling of unsatisfied defecation. Straining may result in the appearance of hemorrhoids, sometimes with rectal bleeding, but the tumors as a rule do not bleed.

INCONTINENCE. Whether from paradoxical diarrhea secondary to obstruction or to interference with sphincter nerve supply, incontinence is an occasional presentation. In its early stages, gross perianal soiling may be the only manifestation of an early loss of fecal control.

OBSTRUCTED LABOR. Many of the solid tumors first come to light during pregnancy. Occasionally a missed retrorectal tumor presents for the first time as a cause of obstructed labor.

*Urinary Symptoms.* Disturbances in bladder function are not uncommon and may be due to interference with the pelvic parasympathetic supply, to direct pressure on the bladder or urethra, or to obstruction of the pelvic ureters.

*Central Nervous System Manifestations.* Although rare, anterior sacral meningoceles may present as central nervous system problems. Headache and recurrent episodes of meningitis have been reported to result from recurrent infections of an adult meningocele.[18] The meningomyelocele is a gross disorder of sacral neurogenic and osseous formation, and presents with varying degrees of neurogenic disorder in the infant.

### Associated Pathology

Although not included in this group as retrorectal tumors, two conditions are occasionally manifest as retrorectal pathology. The first is a complication of diverticulitis with extension of suppuration into the retrorectal space, occasionally presenting as a suppurating mass. The second situation is seen in patients with Crohn's disease, in whom sinus formation and possible fistulization may present as retrorectal induration.

### Previous Surgery

A history of recurrent local surgery for perianal suppuration is important in the context of the retrorectal cysts. In addition, a history of surgery for malignant neoplasms of the genitourinary or gastrointestinal tract, in particular, bladder, prostate, or rectum, is highly significant from the point of recurrence. The retrorectal space is a common site for metastatic spread.

### Examination of Retrorectal Tumors

Rectal examination allows a decision to be made of potential operability and the surgical approach required in the individual patient.

Examination begins with inspection of the perianal area. The presence of soiling and a pouting anus may suggest interference with the nerve supply to the anal sphincters. Laxity of the anal sphincters on rectal examination and the presence of saddle anesthesia of the perineum further support involvement of coccygeal nerves.

As the finger passes into the rectum a solid retrorectal mass should be obvious. High retrorectal tumors may escape detection unless careful assessment of the sacral curve is made, a sudden anterior angulation being the first indication. Location of the mass should be recorded as well as whether it is lobulated or solitary, and whether it is possible to define its upper limits. In particular, a clear assessment must be made of its relationship to the sacrum and the coccyx. This assessment is important, as the location will determine the operative approach to the problem (Fig. 17-2).

Cystic neoplasms may be more difficult since, if flaccid, they tend to feel like mucosal folds. However, if the finger is swept across the posterior mucosal surface, fluid within the cyst will be pushed before the finger into the lateral aspect of the cyst which will become tense and distended, thus allowing clear delineation. With tense cysts it is sometimes difficult to distinguish between a supralevator abscess or a deep posterior space infection. Associated features such as a postanal dimple should be sought in these cases.

An anterior meningocele can be mistaken for a simple cyst. In an infant, pressure over the cysts can cause a rise in fontanelle pressure which can be palpated. Once the fontanelle has closed, the use of the valsalva maneuver can be used to demonstrate spinal canal cyst continuity.

Sigmoidoscopy should be performed to determine whether the rectal wall is involved. A note should be made of the state of the overlying rectal mucosa, in particular, whether there is any evidence of submucosal edema which may indicate underlying infection. Frequently, the mucosa will be totally normal.

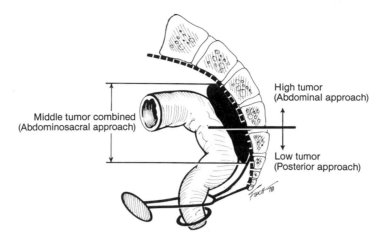

High tumor
(Abdominal approach)

Middle tumor combined
(Abdominosacral approach)

Low tumor
(Posterior approach)

FIGURE **17-2.** *Location of retrorectal tumors and the operative approaches to their treatment.*

## DIAGNOSTIC MEASURES
### Radiology

*Plain Films.* The solid tumors which arise from, compress, invade, or displace the sacrum and coccyx make a plain radiograph of the pelvis one of the most useful diagnostic procedures. Anterior sacral meningocele have a characteristic, 'scimitar' sacrum caused by the presence of a unilateral sacral defect with increased ossification of the smooth, rounded outer border with no associated bony destruction.[18] Destruction of the bones in the area may indicate the presence of a malignancy. Osteoblastic metastases from prostatic carcinoma are frequently found in this area, and have a characteristic radiographic appearance. Such an appearance must not be confused with Paget's disease of the pelvic bones. With teratomas, the presence of bone, or even teeth, have been reported as a radiographic finding.

*Fistulography.* When a chronic fistula is present, particularly following repeated surgery, a fistulogram may be extremely useful in defining the presence of a retrorectal cyst, and its ramifications which may not have been appreciated previously.

*Computerized Tomography (CT) Scan.* Although this method has not been fully evaluated for use with these lesions, it appears to be useful in defining the surface of the tumor in relationship to the sacrum, in particular, giving an indication of invasion or destruction of that structure. It also allows a clearer definition of the extent of the lesion, which will aid in deciding upon the surgical approach.

*Ultrasonography.* Although very successful in gynecological work, its usefulness in presacral tumors is limited because of the site of the lesion. Because it lies deep in the pelvis, with overlying bowel, and, in women, the genital structures, access by use of ultrasonography is limited.

*Angiography.* This has provided information regarding vascularity of these neoplasms, therefore, when this information is required, clearly this modality has a place. However, it is fair to say that it is infrequent that angiography will alter the decision to operate or add to the decision regarding the surgical approach.

### Biopsy of Retrorectal Tumors

Preoperative biopsy of a lesion considered to be operable has no place. In this situation, the best biopsy is total surgical excision. When the lesion is considered to be inoperable, then it is necessary to obtain a tissue diagnosis so that adjuvant therapy can be planned. When doubt as to the diagnosis exists, and it is clear that surgical excision cannot be undertaken without significant risk to the patient, a preoperative diagnosis is necessary to prevent inappropriate surgery.

There are two routes by which biopsy can be achieved. The first is a direct approach through the posterior wall of the rectum; this is simple, direct, and does not appear to be associated with any morbidity. The second technique is that of an extrarectal, presacral approach, with the finger in the rectum being used to direct the needle to the site of biopsy. The latter technique is successful in all but a few retrorectal tumors. Our preference is for the extrarectal biopsy technique.

## SURGERY FOR RETRORECTAL TUMORS

### Abdominal Approach

Indications for an abdominal approach include the high retrorectal tumors where safe access is not possible from below. This approach is also indicated for extraspinal, neurogenic tumors. The abdomen is entered through a transverse incision. The sigmoid colon is mobilized, and the rectum placed on stretch so that the pelvis can be examined and the relationship of the tumor to the rectum appreciated (Fig. 17-3). The presacral sympathetics are identified, and the retrorectal space entered through a plane anterior to these structures. In this way the rectum is displaced forward and the tumor defined with a minimum of hemorrhage. The middle sacral vessels are often significantly enlarged in the case of solid retrorectal tumors and these should be sought and ligated before mobilization is attempted.[23] The presacral veins produce the most difficult hemorrhage to control because they retract when cut and are, thus, difficult to isolate. Careful dissection with particular attention to hemostasis is essential, and protection of all nervous structures should be attempted at all times.

By slow, meticulous dissection the tumor is mobilized; hemoclips are useful in this procedure. The tumor is then removed. This simplified description should in no way down-play the difficulties encountered during this dissection. With persistance, provided the tumor is high and the sacrum uninvolved, this procedure can be accomplished.

### Posterior Approach

The posterior approach is useful for low-lying lesions as well as infected cysts. It is not suited for high lesions or ones with high exten-sions. A vigorous mechanical bowel preparation, in conjunction with antibiotics as would be used for any large bowel surgery, is obtained.

The patient is placed in the prone jackknife position. A midline, curvilinear, or horizontal incision is made and deepened to define the sacrum, coccyx, and the anococcygeal ligament. This is detached from the coccyx and displaced, revealing the levator ani with the central decussating fibers passing from the rectum to the coccyx. This is divided and the supralevator space entered. The coccyx is disarticulated from the $S_5$ vertebra allowing entrance into the supralevator space. Varying amounts of levator ani muscle are incised in order to gain adequate access. At this point a decision whether the distal one or two sacral segments require excision is made. This will depend upon the size of the lesion, its relationship to the sacrum, and the exposure required. If this is necessary, the gluteus maximus muscle can be detached from each side and a portion of the sacroiliac ligaments may be incised. The sacral nerves related to the lowest two sacral vertebrae can be divided without fear of any significant neurological deficit. In addition, there is no problem with sacral instability. Bleeding is frequently a problem until the bone has been completely removed. To some extent this bleeding is reduced if the jackknife position is chosen as the means of positioning the patient. Removal of a portion of the sacrum will be necessary to achieve a block excision of any neoplasm arising from that bone, or to achieve greater access to the retrorectal space. Caution, however, must be taken in the presence of a high extension, because the vascular supply tends to come from above, and an uncontrolled vessel in a deep, inaccessible hole will prove troublesome. It must be remembered, however, that in all cases of retrorectal tumors and cysts the coccyx must always be sacrificed, not only to achieve a better exposure but because the commonest associated feature of recurrence was failure to remove this bone.[24] All of the cystic lesions in this area should be assumed to take origin in the coccyx; hence, its removal is mandatory (Fig. 17-4).

The posterior approach is best suited for the removal of cystic lesions, especially precoccygeal cysts. It can be seen that this approach is ideal for all low tumors, and many tumors

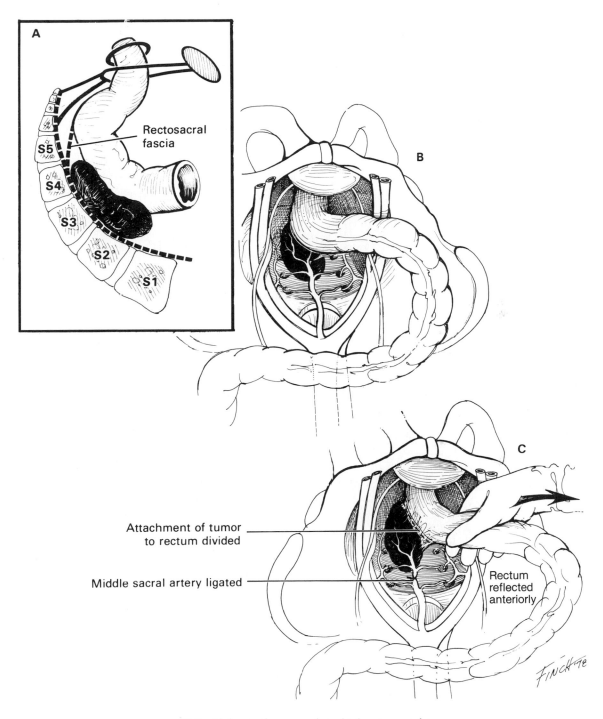

Rectosacral
fascia

**A**

**S5**
**S4**
**S3**
**S2**
**S1**

**B**

**C**

Attachment of tumor
to rectum divided

Middle sacral artery ligated

Rectum
reflected
anteriorly

FINCH 78

FIGURE **17-3.** *Abdominal approach to high retrorectal tumor.*

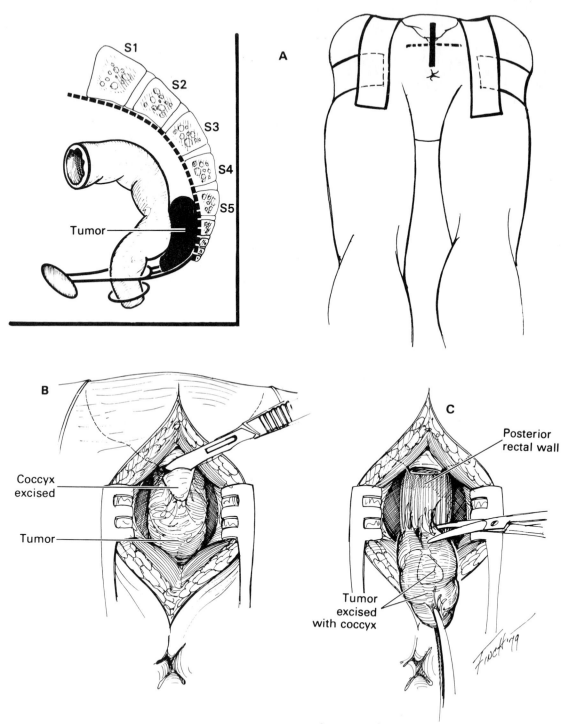

Labels in figure:

S1
S2
S3
S4
S5
Tumor

A

B

Coccyx
excised

Tumor

C

Posterior
rectal wall

Tumor
excised
with coccyx

FIGURE 17-4. *Posterior excision of retrorectal tumor.*

below the sacral promontory can be removed by this route. Preoperative examination is obviously important since a mistake in assessing the upward extent of the lesion can be very difficult to retrieve in the operating room. Maneuverability through this incision is limited. Should significant, uncontrolled hemorrhage occur from deep within the wound, pressure packs should be applied. It hemostasis still cannot be achieved, the patient should be repositioned and the abdominal approach used. Having removed the tumor, closure of the wound is performed in layers around suction catheters. These catheters ensure elimination of the dead space which is left when the tumor is removed.

*Management of Infected Cysts.* Unless the cyst has ruptured into the rectum at the time of presentation the surgical approach should be by an extrarectal posterior route. If, however, rupture into the rectum has occurred, the posterior approach is clearly contraindicated. In this situation adequate transrectal drainage should be assured, curettage of the cavity performed, and expectant treatment adopted with regular follow-up examination. If the cyst is acutely inflamed it may be necessary to perform a staged procedure with drainage as the first step. Once inflammation has settled, excision of the cyst and the coccyx will be necessary.

When the chronic sinus tracts are associated with an infected cyst these tracts should be laid open, the cyst excised, and this excision must include the coccyx. In this situation the wound should be left open to heal by secondary intention.

## Abdominosacral Approach

This approach has been used successfully by Localio, et al, and MacCarty, et al, for removing large retrorectal chordomas in adults.[13,15] Pediatric surgeons have found it a useful approach for large retrorectal teratomas with abdominal extension.

Localio, et al, advocate a combined approach. The abdominal dissection is completed as previously described, peritoneum closed, the patient placed into a jackknife position, and the sacral approach performed for definitive removal. These approaches do not differ from those performed as isolated operations. The main advantages of the abdominal approach are to achieve ligation of the middle sacral vessels, which can be so significant in these tumors, and at the same time to achieve mobilization down to a level which makes lower resection a simpler procedure.

In the case of chordoma, block resection of the tumor and sacral segment is necessary to achieve an adequate resection. With the large teratomas having abdominal extension, some surgeons have advocated partial removal by the abdominal route, with completion of removal by the sacral approach.[1] This depends upon the size of the tumor and is usually unnecessary.[8]

In the case of chordoma where many surgical disciplines are involved, MacCarty has stressed the team approach, with a combination of specialty surgeons.[15] His aim is complete block excision with the preservation of the nerve structures as an essential part of the procedure. Localio has gone as high as transection of the sacrum at the level of $S_2$, making no attempt at preservation of the nervous structures and has had excellent postoperative results with regard to bladder and sphincter function.[13] In addition, he has found no problems with spinal column stability. Freier agrees with this approach, and supports the results.[3] This is at variance with other investigators.[4,15]

When preservation of nervous structures compromises the otherwise successful removal of a tumor, the nerves should be sacrificed, and the consequences accepted as a price for cure (Fig. 17-5).

## Transrectal Approach

This has been advocated for the removal of retrorectal cysts.[1] We do not use this approach unless the cyst has ruptured at the time of presentation.

## Intersphincteric Approach

A rarely recognized approach to the removal of presacral lesions is through the intersphincteric plane. Access is gained posteriorly, between the internal and external sphincter, until the retrorectal space is reached. The technique is similar to that described by Parks for his postanal repair.[20] In this way, small lesions can be adequately removed.

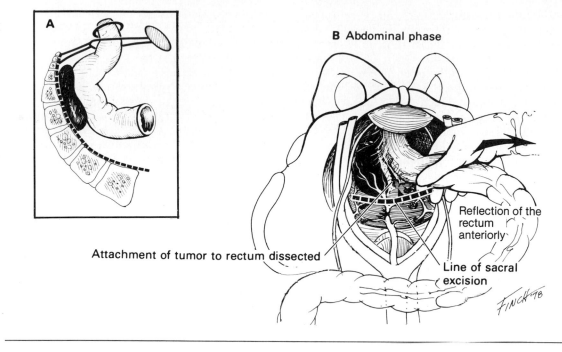

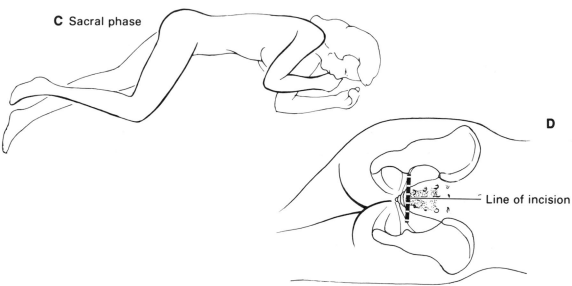

FIGURE **17-5.** *Abdominosacral approach to retrorectal tumor. (After Localio, S., A., et al. Ann Surg 166:394, 1967)*

## ADJUVANT THERAPY IN RETRORECTAL NEOPLASMS

### Radiotherapy

In the case of inoperable malignancies, this is the only modality which can provide adequate palliation. This is particularly true in the case of soft tissue sarcomas since these characteristically present in an advanced stage.

In the case of chordoma, despite the fact that these are relatively radioresistant tumors, high dose radiotherapy can provide palliation.

Pearlman and Friedman recommend giving doses up to and in excess of 7000 rads by supervoltage techniques with the avoidance of vital structures.[21] They have achieved significant palliation in slightly over 50 per cent of cases so treated. As a result, they recommend this form of therapy in either inoperable chordomas, or following inadequate surgical excision. This regime means that virtually all postoperative chordomas receive radiotherapy; when long-term surgical results are assessed, adequate excision is achieved in only a small number. The recommendation of this group is primary excision followed by radiotherapy. If there is recurrence, they recommend repeated excision rather than repeated radiotherapy since the problems of radiation damage become significant following such large doses.

Complications related to radiotherapy may be significant. These can manifest as severe skin reactions in the perineal area, severe proctitis, and radiation cystitis. All these conditions are troublesome but can be minimized with modern techniques of radiotherapy.

### Chemotherapy

There are few tumors in this area that respond satisfactorily to cytotoxic therapy and this is not, so far, a popular method of therapy. We have been unable to find a satisfactory regime that can be recommended.

### RESULTS

The results of treatment of retrorectal neoplasms and cysts reflect the nature of the tumor and the adequacy of resection. Malignant tumors in this area have a poor prognosis: few patients survive five years with either soft tissue sarcomas or teratocarcinomas.

In the case of the chordoma despite a low grade of malignancy, Gray reported a 10 per cent incidence of metastases.[4] The five year survival rates are difficult to interpret because of the slow growth. In the past, virtually all have recurred, and the 10 year survival rate was 15 to 20 per cent in the series reported by Pearlman and Friedman.[21] At Sloan-Kettering Memorial Hospital, New York, the five year survival, free of disease, was reported as 10 per cent, and metastases had occurred in 43 per cent of the patients seen.[9]

Localio and associates could find only four long term survivors from 198 surgically treated patients with chordoma.[13] These figures are depressing; however, with the modern therapeutic approach combining surgery and radiotherapy improvement can be expected.

Benign tumors and congenital cysts can be adequately treated by surgical excision. It is only when the cysts are not recognized or are inadequately treated or, in the case of benign neoplasms, inadequately removed, that recurrent problems arise. This is an area where access is limited and, therefore, it is essential that the primary procedure be adequate.

### REFERENCES

1. Caropreso, P. R., Wengert, P. A. Jr., and Milford, H. E.: Tailgut cyst—a rare retrorectal tumor: Report of a case and review. Dis. Colon Rectum, *18:*597, 1975.

2. Conklin, J., and Abell, M. R.: Germ cell neoplasms of the sacrococcygeal region. Cancer, *20:*2105, 1967.

3. Freier, D. T., Stanley, J. C., and Thompson, N. W.: Retrorectal tumors in adults. Surg. Gynecol. Obstet., *132:*681, 1971.

4. Gray, S. W., Singhabhandhu, B., Smith, R. A., and Skandalakis, J. E.: Sacrococcygeal chordoma: Report of a case and review of the literature. Surgery, *78:*573, 1975.

5. Gross, R., Clatworthy, H., and Meeker, I.: Sacrococcygeal teratomas in infants and children: A report of 40 cases. Surg. Gynecol. Obstet., *92:*341, 1951.

6. Harvey, W. F., and Dawson, E. K.: Chordoma. Edinb. Med. J., *48:*713, 1941.

7. Hawkins, W. J., and Jackman, R. J.: Developmental cysts as a source of perianal abscesses, sinuses and fistulas. Am. J. Surg., *86:*678, 1953.

8. Hendren, W. H., and Henderson, B. M.: The surgical management of sacrococcygeal teratomas with intrapelvic extension. Ann. Surg., *171:*77, 1970.

9. Higinbotham, N. L., Phillips, R. F., Farr, H. W., and Hustu, H. O.: "Chordoma"—Thirty-five year study at Memorial Hospital. Cancer, *20:*1841, 1967.

10. Horwitz, T.: Chordal ectopia and its possible relation to chordoma. Arch. Pathol., *31:*354, 1941.

11. Hunt, P., VanLeeuwen, G., Bingham, H., and Sights, W.: Sacrococcygeal teratomas—A report

of three cases and survey of present knowledge. Clin. Pediatr., *7:*165, 1968.

12. Killen, D. A., and Jackson, L. M.: Sacrococcygeal teratoma in the adult. Arch. Surg., *88:*425, 1964.

13. Localio, S. A., Francis, K. C., and Rossano, P. G.: Abdominosacral resection of sacrococcygeal chordoma. Ann. Surg., *166:*394, 1967.

14. Lovelady, S. B., and Dockerty, M. B.: Extragenital pelvic tumors in women. Am. J. Obstet. Gynecol., *58:*215, 1949.

15. MacCarty, C. S., Waugh, J. M., Coventry, M. B., and O'Sullivan, D. C.: Sacrococcygeal chordomas. Surg. Gynecol. Obstet., *113:*551, 1961.

16. Mayo, C. W., Baker, G. S., and Smith, L. R.: Presacral tumors: Differential diagnosis and report of case. Mayo Clin. Proc., *28:*616, 1953.

17. McColl, I.: The classification of presacral cysts and tumors. Proc. R. Soc. Med., *56:*797, 1963.

18. Oren, M., Bennett, L., Lee, S. H., Truex, R. C. Jr., and Gennaro, A. R.: Anterior sacral meningocele: Report of five cases and review of the literature. Dis. Colon Rectum, *20:*492, 1977.

19. Pantoja, E., and Rodriguez-Ibānez, I.: Sacrococcygeal dermoids and teratomas: Historical review. Am. J. Surg., *132:*337, 1976.

20. Parks, A. G.: Anorectal incontinence. Proc. R. Soc. Med., *68:*681, 1975.

21. Pearlman, A. W., and Friedman, M.: Radical radiation therapy of chordoma. Am. J. Roentgenol., *108:*333, 1970.

22. Scobie, W. G.: Malignant sacrococcygeal teratoma—A problem in diagnosis. Arch. Dis. Child., *46:*216, 1971.

23. Smith, B., Passaro, E., and Clatworthy, H. W. Jr.: The vascular anatomy of sacrococcygeal teratomas: Its significance in surgical management. Surgery, *49:*534, 1961.

24. Spencer, R. J., and Jackman, R. J.: Surgical management of precoccygeal cysts. Surg. Gynecol. Obstet., *115:*449, 1962.

25. Uhlig, B. E., and Johnson, R. L.: Presacral tumors and cysts in adults. Dis. Colon Rectum, *18:*581, 1975.

26. Willis, R. A.: Pathology of Tumours. 4 ed. 938. London, Butterworth and Co., 1967.

# 18

# The Basic Application of Electrosurgery

The application of diathermy and electrosurgery is based on the fact that with a radio-frequency current above 10,000 cycles per second, stimulation of muscle and nerve does not occur.[4] When two large (over 100 cm²) electrodes of near-equal size are used, the current is evenly dispersed within the intervening tissue and only warm heat is produced (Diathermy) (Fig. 18-1A).[8] On the other hand, when one electrode is large and the other small, the current is concentrated in the smaller electrode. It produces a high concentration of heat and causes destruction of cells (Electrosurgery) (Fig. 18-1B).[8]

## CLINICAL USAGE

Electrosurgery in clinical use, at the present time, consists of electrocutting, electrocoagulation, and fulguration. Electrocutting is the severing of tissue by a blade electrode energized from a high frequency electrosurgical unit. Electrocoagulation is the heating, desiccation, and destruction of tissue at the point of contact using needle tip, ball tip, or blade electrode (Fig. 18-2A).[3] Fulguration is a method of coagulation wherein the active electrode is held some distance (e.g., 1 to 10 mm) away from the tissue and the energy is dissipated in the area by means of sparking (Fig. 18-2B). Thus, fulguration, by its nature, requires a relatively high voltage applied in order to ionize the gas between the electrode and the tissue. Fulguration has greater depth of penetration,

and greater dehydration of the tissue, than the effect of electrocoagulation.[8]

The mode of operation, cutting or coagulation, or a combined effect (blended), depends on the waveform of the current. It has been found that an undamped, continuous sinusoidal waveform is best for strictly cutting tissue. A series of damped, sinusoidal waves has been found best to achieve coagulation, but has very limited or no cutting capability. For cutting with simultaneous coagulating, a waveform of interrupted sinusoids has been found to be effective (Fig. 18-3). The exact reasons why some waveforms cut and others coagulate have not yet been explained.[4]

### Current Density and Volume of Tissue

The current density or the total heat generated by electrosurgery is directly related to the surface area of the tissue in contact with the active electrode.[3] For example, assuming that a given current passing through a cross section of 1 mm² results in a temperature rise of 100° C, the same current through 2 mm² gives a rise of 25° C. If the area is increased to 1 cm², the temperature rise is only 0.1° C (Fig. 18-4). The two electrodes normally used are a large area patient-plate and a small area active electrode (Fig. 18-1B). The patient-plate, in good contact with a large area of the skin, assures a low current density and makes the temperature rise at that electrode negligible.

Resistance of tissue varies. Fat has greater electrical resistance than does muscle. Wet tissue increases the area of contact and reduces the current density. Hence, it requires a

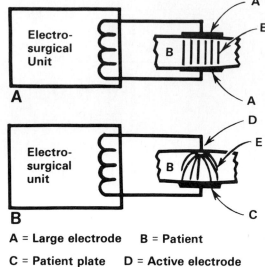

A = **Large electrode**   B = **Patient**

C = **Patient plate**   D = **Active electrode**

E = **Current flow pattern**

FIGURE **18-1.** *Principles of operation of* (A) *diathermy, and* (B) *electrosurgery.* (*After Sittner, W. R. et al.:* In *Endoscopy. Berci, G.* (*ed.*) p. 215. *New York, Appleton-Century-Croft, 1976*)

higher coagulating setting. Total heat production is also related to the power delivered and duration of the application. A power of 50 watts for one second gives the same total heating as a power of 5 watts for 10 seconds, but the distribution of the heat is different. At a lower power and longer duration, the temperature is lower near the active electrode, but more heat is generated deeper in the tissue.[3]

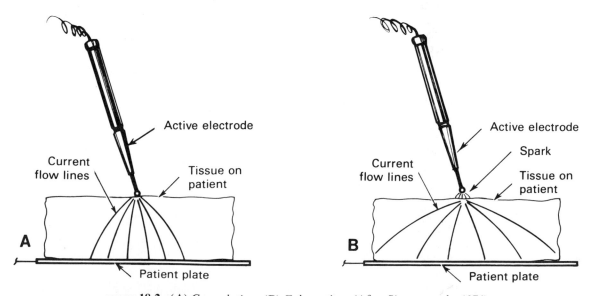

FIGURE **18-2.** (A) *Coagulation.* (B) *Fulguration.* (*After Sittner et al., 1976*)

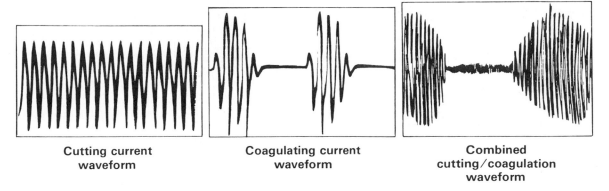

| **Cutting current waveform** | **Coagulating current waveform** | **Combined cutting/coagulation waveform** |

FIGURE **18-3.** *Different waveforms of current.*

## Hazards

*Excessive Application of Heat.* The dial calibration on each electrosurgery unit is arbitrary and varies widely (Fig. 18-5). When the equipment is unfamiliar, one should always start at a lower setting and gradually increase. Short bursts of power are also desirable in order to minimize the depth of the heat.

*Electrical Burns.* Skin burns can occur if the patient-plate is in poor contact with the patient, or if the conductive paste dries out during a long procedure. Another burn location is the site of alternate current paths, such as the points of attachment of the electrocardiogram monitor.[4]

*Explosion.* The wide spread use of non-flammable, non-explosive anesthetic gases today safely allows the use of electrosurgery. A more important hazard is explosion due to bowel gas. It has been shown that the explosive gases of the bowel are methane and hydrogen which are liberated by bacteria in the colon.[1] When the large bowel is well prepared, such as is done for colonoscopy, this hazard is negligible.[1,7] However, if poorly prepared, serious explosions can occur with other procedures such as electrocoagulation or snaring of rectal polyps by way of the sigmoidoscope.[2] This problem can be eliminated by adequate aspiration of gases from the rectum before each application of the electric current.

*Electrical shock.* Shock hazards usually involve leakage or faulty currents which flow along conductive paths from a power line-connected, electrical device to the ground-line, or between two such devices. Among such devices are the light source, electrosurgical unit, and cardiac monitoring machine. A preferred arrangement for minimizing shock

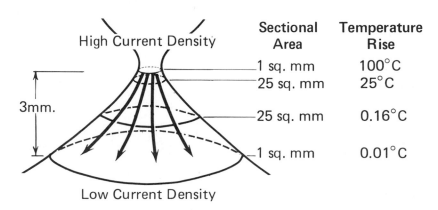

| | Sectional Area | Temperature Rise |
|---|---|---|
| High Current Density | 1 sq. mm | 100°C |
| | 25 sq. mm | 25°C |
| | 25 sq. mm | 0.16°C |
| | 1 sq. mm | 0.01°C |
| Low Current Density | | |

3mm.

FIGURE **18-4.** *The current density, and volume of tissue. (After Curtis, L. E.: Gastrointest. Endosc., 20:10, 1973)*

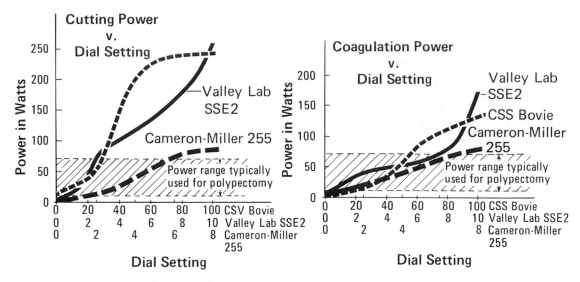

FIGURE **18-5.** *Relationship between power and dial setting in different electrosurgical units.* (*After Curtis, L. E.: Gastrointest. Endosc., 20:11, 1973*)

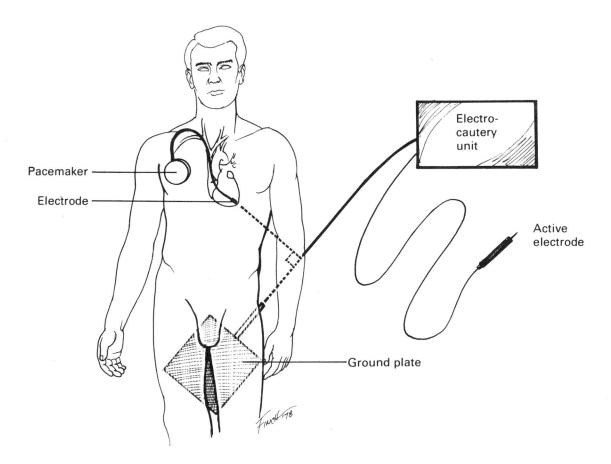

FIGURE **18-6.** *Active electrode and ground plate are connected perpendicular to the pacemaker electrode.*

hazard is to ground the exterior conductive surfaces of all power line-connected equipment to a common point, and to isolate all conductors contacting the patient. Since a faulty connection may render supposedly grounded equipment even more hazardous than ungrounded equipment, the hospital engineer should periodically check the ground integrity of all power line-connected equipment.[3] Improper function of electrosurgical equipment has also been reported to cause ventricular fibrillation or other arrhythmias.[6]

*Interference With the Function of Cardiac Pacemakers.* Earlier cardiac pacemakers were susceptible to deactivation by external radiofrequency waves, especially electrosurgery which may cause cardiac arrhythmias.[5] Most recently implanted pacemakers are protected by shielding and filtering layers to reduce the effects of external interference. Nevertheless, precautions should be taken to minimize the possibility of such interference. Green and Merideth give the following useful safety guides when electrosurgery is used in patients with cardiac pacemakers: (*1*) the patient-plate is best placed beneath the patient's buttocks, keeping the radio-frequency small; (*2*) the wires connecting the active electrode and the patient-plate to the electrosurgical unit should be perpendicular to the wires of the pacemaker electrodes, because parallel wires serve as a better receiving antenna for radio-frequency fields; (*3*) if an external battery pacemaker is used, the pack should be as far removed as possible from the electrosurgical field; and, (*4*) monitor the patient's heart rhythm with an electrocardiograph, and have defibrillation-resuscitation equipment available (Fig. 18-6).

## REFERENCES

1. Bond, J. H., and Levitt, M. D.: Factors affecting the concentration of combustible gases in the colon during colonoscopy. Gastroent., *68:*1445, 1975.
2. Bond, J. H., Levy, M., and Levitt, M. D.: Explosion of hydrogen gas in the colon during proctosigmoidoscopy. Gastrointest. Endos., *23:*41, 1976.
3. Curtiss, L. E.: High frequency currents in endoscopy: A review of principles and precautions. Gastrointest. Endos., *20:*9, 1973.
4. Glover, J. L., Bendick, P. J., and Luik, W. J.: The use of thermal knives in surgery: Electrosurgery, lasers, plasma scalpel. Curr. Prob. Surg., 15:26, 1978.
5. Greene, L. F., and Merideth, J.: Transurethral operations employing high frequency electric currents in patients with demand cardiac pacemakers. J. Urol., *108:*446, 1972.
6. Hugenbuchler, R. F., Swope, J. P., and Reeves, J. G.: Ventricular fibrillation associated with use of the electrocautery. JAMA, *230:*432, 1974.
7. Ragins, H., Shinya, H., and Wolff, W. I.: The explosive potential of colonic gas during colonoscopic electrosurgical polypectomy. Surg. Gynecol. Obstet., *138:*554, 1974.
8. Sittner, W. R., and Fitzgerald, J. K.: High-frequency electrosurgery. *In* Berci, G. (ed.): Endoscopy. New York, Appleton-Century-Crofts, 1976.

# 19

# Techniques of Endorectal and Transrectal Procedures

Procedures such as rectal biopsy, electrocoagulation, and snaring of rectal polyps are usually performed in the office or outpatient clinic. It is important that the office or clinic be well equipped with essential instruments and spare parts. The clinician should be proficient in the use of these instruments. Sedation or anesthesia is rarely, if ever, necessary. If a barium enema study is indicated, it should be done a few days before or three to four weeks after the procedure in order to avoid the risk of perforation. However, if a carcinoma is biopsied, a barium enema can be safely performed anytime thereafter.

In many normal people the colon contains a variable amount of hydrogen and methane.[15] The frequently used, packaged phosphosoda enema is not adequate to eliminate these gases, and explosions from electrocoagulation or snaring can occur, although it is rare.[1,2] This can be prevented by the frequent use of suctioning to evacuate the gases prior to applying the electric current.

The patients are usually sent home immediately following the procedure. No dietary restrictions are recommended, but patients are advised to take a bulk-forming agent as a stool softener for a week to 10 days. Following removal of larger sessile lesions, a liquid diet for 24 to 48 hours may be in order. The patients are forwarned to report any profuse rectal bleeding, persistent abdominal or shoulder pain, or fever. When in doubt, a flat plate, upright of the abdomen, and lateral decubitus films should be performed.

## RECTAL BIOPSY

Many local and systemic disorders can be diagnosed by rectal biopsy. Conditions in which rectal biopsy is essential, or useful for diagnosis or management include: malignant and benign neoplasms of the rectum, chronic ulcerative colitis, Crohn's colitis, ischemic colitis, pseudomembranous colitis, radiation proctitis, amebiasis, schistosomiasis, bacillary dysentery, pneumatosis cystoides intestinalis, amyloidosis, solitary ulcer of the rectum, Hirschsprung's disease, and colitis cystica profunda.[8,9,21]

The biopsy specimens are inevitably small; they are rarely larger than 8 mm. However, with an adequate biopsy and proper orientation of the specimen, an accurate interpretation can be achieved.

### Technique

We use the 1.5 × 25 cm sigmoidoscope, and prefer the inverted semiprone position. A cup-shaped, or alligator biopsy forceps is suitable (Fig. 19-1).

*Biopsy of Rectal Carcinoma.* The best area from which to take a biopsy is the junction between the carcinoma and the normal mucosa. Multiple areas should be sampled. Bleeding is usually minimal but may require coagulation.

*Biopsy of the Rectal Mucosa.* The lower valve of Houston is frequently the ideal loca-

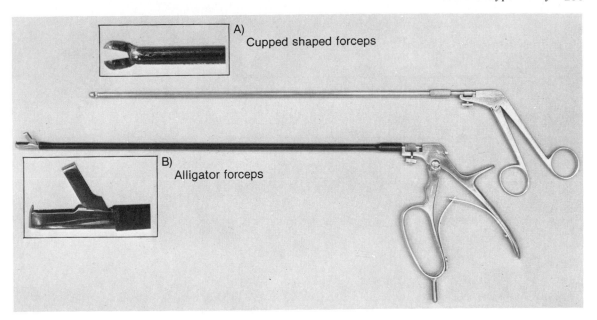

A) Cupped shaped forceps

B) Alligator forceps

FIGURE **19-1.** *Biopsy forceps.*

tion for biopsy. Other surgeons believe the best location for biopsy is the posterior part of the middle valve of Houston. At this location, if bleeding occurs, the sigmoidoscope can be pressed against the sacrum to constrict the blood vessels, and electrocoagulation can be accurately applied in a bloodless field. A small piece of frosted glass, nylon mesh, or filter paper is lightly applied to the submucosal surface of the specimen, which will adhere to it by the specimen's own stickiness.[21] The mounted specimen is then dropped into the fixative.

## ELECTROCOAGULATION OF RECTAL POLYPS

During a routine sigmoidoscopy it is common to find small polyps, ranging in size from 1 to 5 mm, in the rectum. The majority of them are metaplastic (hyperplastic) polyps or lymphoid hyperplasia, which have no malignant potential.

Small adenomatous polyps of 1 to 5 mm in size have an extremely low incidence of carcinoma. However, because of the minimal risks of the complications during a properly performed excisional biopsy, all such polyps

within the reach of the sigmoidoscope should be biopsied so that the histologic morphology is known. Where several polyps are present, the rest may be electrocoagulated.

### Technique

Either an inverted semiprone position, or a Simm's position can be used, and a 1.5 × 25 cm. or a 1 × 25 cm sigmoidoscope is suitable. A ball-tip or a suction-coagulation electrode is used, connected to the electrocoagulation unit which is set at approximately 30 per cent of the maximal power (Fig. 19-2). Following biopsy the electrode is placed either 1 to 2 mm from the polyp and the spark is used to fulgurate it, or the electrode is placed directly in contact with the polyp to coagulate it. The duration of each burning should not be more than three seconds, but this can be repeated until the entire polyp becomes white. A "pop" noise may be heard. This is from the explosion of the cells from the pressure of steam generated within them.

### SNARE POLYPECTOMY

Both inverted semiprone or Simm's position can be used, and a 1.5 × 25 cm sigmoidoscope is preferred. Different commercial snar-

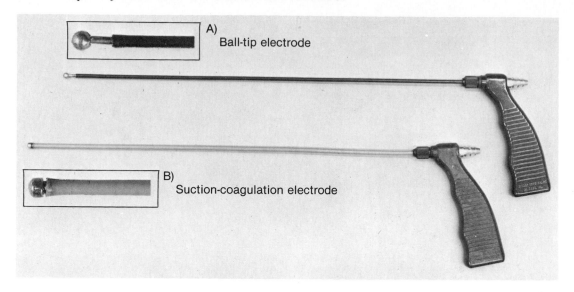

FIGURE **19-2.** *Electrocoagulation electrodes.*

ing devices are available (Fig. 19-3). These are connected to the coagulator which is set between 30 and 40 per cent of the maximal power, depending upon the size of the polyp. Prior to transection of a polyp, it is important to have the stalk or the base fully visualized in order to avoid drawing the bowel wall into the snare. If the polyp is at the limit of sigmoidoscopic visualization, and the base not adequately visualized, then it may be safer to perform a colonoscopic polypectomy.

*Pedunculated Polyp.* The snare wire is looped around the polyp, and is positioned onto the stalk a few millimeters from the bowel wall. Once the loop is in a satisfactory position, the snare is pushed caphalad so that the base of the wire loop touches the stalk (Fig. 19-4A). This will fix the snare wire in the proper position for closing the loop. One must always check that there is no mucosal fold inadvertently caught in the snare (Fig. 19-4B). Before applying the coagulation, the polyp is manipulated toward the center of the rectal lumen to avert the polyp from resting on the rectal wall. This maneuver will avoid the possibility of burning the mucosa of the opposite wall, since the current is transmitted through

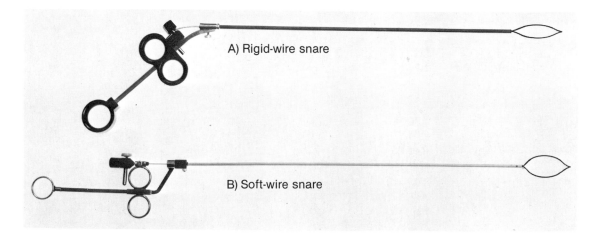

FIGURE **19-3.** *Electrocautery snares.*

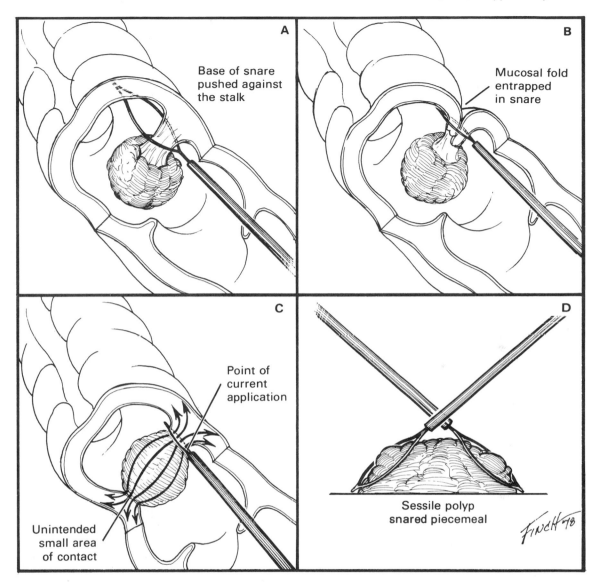

**A** Base of snare pushed against the stalk

**B** Mucosal fold entrapped in snare

**C** Point of current application / Unintended small area of contact

**D** Sessile polyp snared piecemeal

FIGURE **19-4.** *Technique of snare polypectomy.*

the polyp (Fig. 19-4C).[5] Coagulation is applied no longer than three seconds. The snare is gently tightened while applying the electric current. If the polyp is not cut, wait for approximately 10 to 15 seconds to allow the tissue to cool, and then repeat the coagulation and tightening of the snare until the stalk of the polyp is completely transected. The polyp can easily be retrieved by the use of suction, or with a polyp grasper or biopsy forceps. The polyp site should be checked for bleeding or perforation.

*Sessile Polyp.* A small sessile polyp can be snared in the same way as a pedunculated polyp by including a small part of the underlying mucosa tented up as a pseudopedicle. A sessile polyp larger than 2 cm should be removed piecemeal. The snare wire is cut through the substance of the polyp to divide it into multiple pieces of 1 to 1.5 cm in size (Fig. 19-4D). The residual polyp at the base can be electrocoagulated. It may be necessary to remove a large sessile polyp in more than one session. The patient should return after four to six weeks for examination and removal of any residual polyp.

## PER ANAL EXCISION OF LARGE SESSILE VILLOUS ADENOMAS OF THE RECTUM

Villous adenoma is a premalignant neoplasm: it comprises approximately 8 per cent of all polyps of the colon and rectum.[24,32] The most common location is the rectum, and 43 per cent of these rectal villous lesions are in the distal half.[12,32,37] Because of the frequency of multifocal areas of malignancy, a standard punch biopsy sample is not sufficient for reliable diagnosis. Livstone and co-workers found that a 2 mm spherical specimen contains only 1/8,000 of the volume of a 4 cm polyp; therefore, the entire lesion should be excised and submitted for histological examination.[16]

Most villous neoplasms of the lower rectum, and many of those of the middle part of the rectum, can be removed per anally.[25,31,36] Indurated or ulcerated areas are signs of an invasive carcinoma, therefore it is useful to biopsy these areas. Lesions which are entirely soft do not require biopsy as this may increase the difficulty of excision and confuse the histologic evaluation. All patients who have rectal villous lesions should be thoroughly investigated with barium enema and/or colonoscopy to rule out another more proximal lesion.

### Technique

The bowel is thoroughly prepared mechanically in the same manner as it is for colon resection. In addition, 250 ml of a one per cent neomycin solution is given per rectum, and the patient is asked to retain it overnight. Two units of blood should be available. Preferably under general anesthesia, the patient is placed in the semi-prone position with a roll under the pubis. A Pratt or Park's speculum is inserted to obtain exposure. Prior to dissection of the neoplasm, a saline solution containing 1 : 200,000 epinephrine is infiltrated beneath the lesion in the submucosal plane to reduce bleeding (Fig. 19-5). Dissection is started at the distal end of the lesion with a 5 mm rim of normal mucosa and submucosa. The sequence of the excision is as follows:

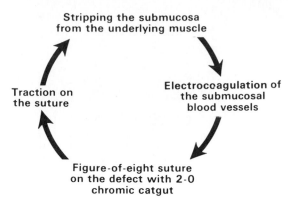

Stripping the submucosa from the underlying muscle → Electrocoagulation of the submucosal blood vessels → Figure-of-eight suture on the defect with 2-0 chromic catgut → Traction on the suture →

If the procedure is feasible, the neoplasm should be removed in a lateral direction so that the defect created can be closed in a transverse manner. As traction is placed on the sutures the neoplasm prolapses, thereby masking the underlying mucosa. To overcome this handicap, a dinner fork can be placed under the lesion to lift the submucosa and displace the neoplasm proximally (Fig. 19-6). This tool is ideal for exposing the underlying submucosa during the repeated sequences of excision.[26] It is customary to leave several of the chromic catgut sutures long so that traction can be used to prolapse the suture line into the lower part of the rectum in the event of postoperative bleeding. Sigmoidoscopic examination is performed at the completion of the procedure to make sure that the lumen is patent. The excised specimen is pinned out flat on a piece of cardboard, and then placed in a fixative solution (Fig. 19-7). By properly orienting the specimen, the pathologist can do accurate serial sections for histological examination.

Postoperatively, the patient should be on a clear liquid diet for two days, to make sure that perforation did not occur. Once the patient is on a regular diet, a bulk-producer should also be added. The first postoperative check should be in six weeks. Any residual tumor can be electrocoagulated in the clinic or office. Thereafter, sigmoidoscopy at three month intervals for the first year and then annually is desirable.

## POSTERIOR APPROACH TO THE RECTUM

Large villous or sessile adenomas of the mid-rectum, not accessible to the per anal tech-

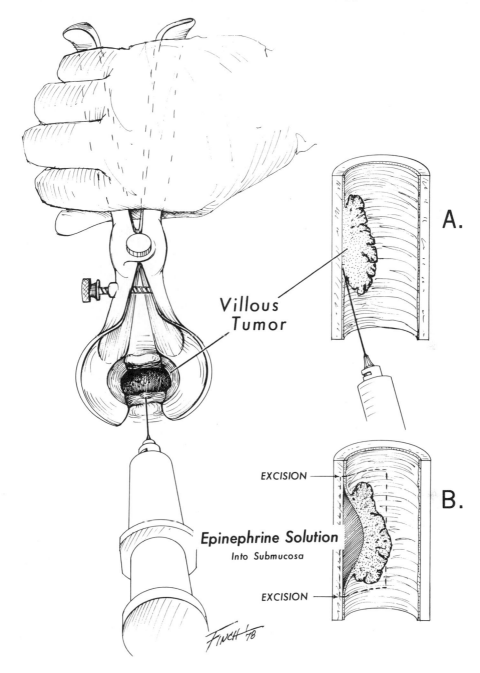

Villous Tumor

A.

Epinephrine Solution

Into Submucosa

EXCISION

EXCISION

B.

**FIGURE 19-5.** *Local infiltration of villous tumor. (After Nivatvongs, S., et al.: Dis. Colon Rectum. 16:510, 1972)*

nique, can be removed through a posterior proctotomy. A neoplasm in the upper part of the rectum should be removed by anterior resection. Posterior proctotomy has a rather high incidence of wound infection and fecal fistulae, although most of these heal spontaneously. A thorough preoperative mechanical bowel preparation and oral antibiotics should

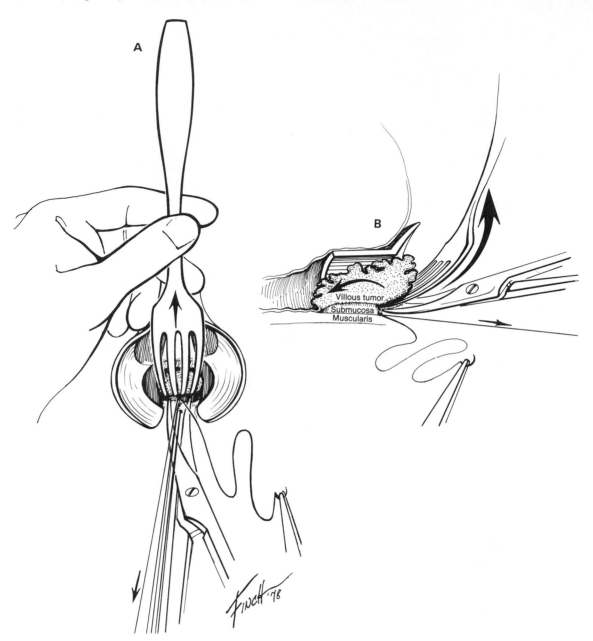

**FIGURE 19-6.** *The use of dinner fork as a retractor. (After Nivatvongs, S., et al.: Dis. Colon Rectum. 21:534, 1978)*

be used. Suction drainage is employed in the retrorectal space. A clear liquid diet is given for two or three days postoperatively.

**The Kraske Approach**

In 1885 Kraske described a method of excising carcinoma of the rectum through the pos-

terior approach.[14] Because of the high incidence of recurrence of the malignancy and the high rate of fecal fistulization, this method was abandoned after the introduction, by Miles in 1906, of abdominoperineal resection. More recently, this Kraske approach has been revived for the excision of benign rectal neoplasms.[4,27,38]

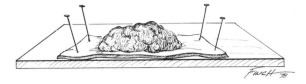

FIGURE **19-7.** *The specimen pinned on cardboard.*

*Technique.* The patient is placed in the semi-prone position with a roll under the pubis and the buttocks taped apart (Fig. 19-8A). A transverse or midline incision is made from the sacrococcygeal joint to a point just proximal to the anus. The anococcygeal ligament is detached from the coccyx, and the coccyx is then excised. The middle sacral artery is tied or electrocoagulated. The incision is deepened to expose the levator ani muscle which is incised in the midline to expose the posterior rectal wall (Fig. 19-8B). The rectum is opened through the posterior wall and the lesion is excised submucosally (Fig. 19-8C,D). The defect is approximated, if possible, using 4—0 chromic catgut. The posterior proctotomy wound is closed transversally with a one-layer interrupted suture of 4—0 polypropylene. A two layer closure may be performed if desired. Hemostasis is obtained, and the entire wound is irrigated with an antibiotic solution. The levator ani muscle is approximated with interrupted 2—0 chromic catgut, and the anococcygeal ligament is sutured to the gluteus muscle with 2—0 chromic catgut (Fig. 19-8E). A small suction drain is placed in the retrorectal space. The skin is closed with 4—0 polypropylene suture.

### The York-Mason Transsphincteric Approach

In order to provide better exposure of the interior of the rectum, York-Mason popularized the complete division of the sphincter muscles.[20] This approach also gives an ideal exposure for the repair of a prostatorectal or rectovaginal fistula.[20] In his extensive experience with more than 180 patients using this method, none has suffered loss of anal continence.[19] He strongly emphasizes the accurate suturing of the divided sphincters with restoration of the anatomical layers.

*Technique.* The position of the patient is the same as in Kraske's approach. The skin incision is made from a point just to the left of the sacrococcygeal junction passing obliquely downward to the anal verge in the midline (Fig. 19-9A). With this incision it is not necessary to remove the coccyx, and the incision can be enlarged by incising the lower part of the gluteus muscle. The incision is deepened to expose the external sphincter complex, puborectalis, and levator ani muscle. These are divided along the lines of incision, tagging the divided edges step by step. The nerve supply to these muscles lies lateral to the incision and is, therefore, safe from injury. It is important to accurately mark each layer and component of the muscles with stay sutures for correct identification when the time comes to reapproximate them (Fig. 19-9B). Next, the internal sphincter is divided with proximal extension through the thinner muscle wall of the rectum. The submucosa and mucosa are then incised to expose the interior of the rectum and the anal canal (Fig. 19-9C). The lesion is excised, and the wound is closed in layers (Fig. 19-9D). The mucosa and submucosa are closed with continuous 4—0 chromic catgut; the internal sphincter is closed with interrupted 3—0 chromic catgut; and, the external sphincter and the levator ani are closed with interrupted 2—0 chromic catgut (Fig. 19-9E). Each layer of the wound is washed with an antibiotic solution. A suction drain, placed in the ischiorectal space, is used. The skin is closed with 4—0 polypropylene.

## ELECTROCOAGULATION OF CARCINOMA OF THE RECTUM

Since the report by Strauss in 1935 of the excellent results with electrocoagulation of carcinoma of the rectum, there have been sporadic reports of this approach.[35] It was generally reserved for palliative treatment of rectal carcinoma, or for poor surgical risk patients. Madden and Kandalaft, in 1967, reported a small series of patients with carcinoma of the rectum treated by electrocoagulation as the primary and preferred method.[18] Other investigators also reported favorable results in more selected cases.[3,13,33] This method of treatment was stimulated by the poor long term survival and the high morbidity and mortality, especially in the elderly, from abdominoperineal resection.

The obvious advantages of electrocoagulation for carcinoma of the lower part of the rec-

(*Text continues on p. 244*)

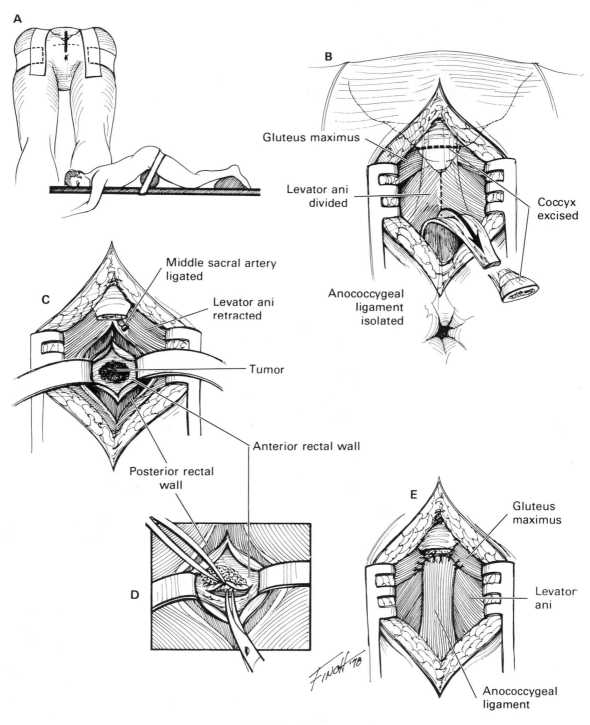

**A**

**B**

Gluteus maximus

Levator ani divided

Coccyx excised

Anococcygeal ligament isolated

**C**

Middle sacral artery ligated

Levator ani retracted

Tumor

Anterior rectal wall

Posterior rectal wall

**D**

**E**

Gluteus maximus

Levator ani

Anococcygeal ligament

FIGURE **19-8.** *Kraske's approach.*

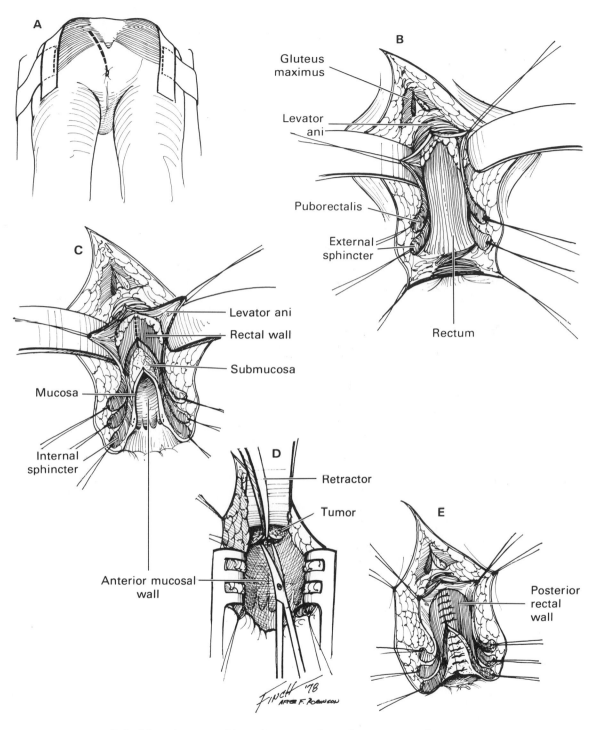

FIGURE **19-9.** *Mason's transsphincteric approach to the rectum. (After Mason, A., Y. In Surgical Technique Illustrated. Malt, R. A.(ed.), p. 75–77. Boston, Little, Brown Co. 1977)*

tum are the 0 per cent mortality from the procedure, and the avoidance of the permanent colostomy.[17] The disadvantages are: (*1*) Electrocoagulation may fail to eradicate the primary malignancy; (*2*) Electrocoagulation certainly fails to cure patients who have lymph node metastasis.

The carcinoma which is fixed or has penetrated the bowel wall gave a poor result and should not be treated by electrocoagulation with hope for cure. The entire lesion has to be accessible to the procedure. Generally, it should not be higher than 10 cm from the anal verge.[17]

At the present time the main objection to electrocoagulation is the lack of knowledge of the presence or absence of metastatic lymph nodes. Digital examination of the rectum may detect pararectal nodes at the level of, or just above the carcinoma. In addition, certain factors may provide indirect evidence in predicting the probability of lymph node metastases. It is well known that an undifferentiated adenocarcinoma of the rectum and rectal carcinoma with full thickness involvement have a high incidence of lymph node metastases.[6] Studies by Greaney showed that an ulcerating carcinoma, regardless of size, and a polypoid, non-ulcerated carcinoma larger than 5 cm are associated with a high incidence of lymph node metastases.[11] With polypoid, non-ulcerated carcinomas smaller than 5 cm, lymph node involvement is a much less common feature (11 per cent). Unfortunately, favorable lesions account for only 8 per cent of the carcinomas of the rectum.[11] The surgeon must weigh the risks of lymph node metastases in a given patient against the risks of a radical operation.

### Preparation

Electrocoagulation of rectal carcinoma is not an office procedure. All patients are hospitalized, and have the bowel prepared in the same manner as for colon resection. Spinal or general anesthetics are required, and the operative time may range from one to three hours.[18]

### Technique

The semi-prone position is used for carcinomas located anteriorly, while the lithotomy position is used for posterior ones. A Pratt speculum is used to visualize low lying lesions, while an operating proctoscope is used for higher ones. Exposure is the key to success: the entire lesion must be seen. A needle-point electrode is employed in preference to the ball-tip type because of its greater heat production and deeper penetration. The coagulator is set between 40 and 55 per cent of the maximal power. The needle is embedded into the carcinoma, the depth depending upon the extent of penetration into the wall. The coagulation is applied repeatedly, in an orderly manner, until the entire carcinoma becomes flat and soft. Suction is used frequently to evacuate the smoke and the possible explosive gases. A uterine currette or a biopsy forceps can be used to remove the coagulum. Carcinomas located in the posterior or lateral quadrant of the lower and middle portion of the rectum can be coagulated vigorously since they are extraperitoneal, whereas lesions located in the anterior wall of the mid-rectum must be treated more cautiously because of their intraperitoneal location. In women, anterior wall carcinomas may require coagulation in multiple stages in order to avoid the development of a rectovaginal fistula.

### Postoperative Management and Follow-up

Patients usually have no significant amount of pain. Fever from the reaction of the coagulation may last for several days, and should be treated symptomatically only. Only clear liquids are allowed for the first two days until it is certain that no perforation has occurred. When advanced to a regular diet, a bulk-producing agent is prescribed. Postoperative bleeding is the most common complication, and occurred in 19 per cent of Madden and Kandalaft's latest series of 131 patients.[17] In half of these patients, the bleeding stopped spontaneously. The frequency of perforation and rectovaginal fistulae is surprisingly low (1.5 and 2.5%, respectively).[17] Patients should be re-examined in the clinic one month after the coagulation. Any ulcerated or exophytic area should be biopsied and, if proven to be malignant, the patient must be re-admitted and a repeat coagulation is performed. It may be necessary to repeat the coagulation several times for complete eradication of the malignancy.

### Failure of Electrocoagulation

It is frequently necessary to readmit patients for repeat coagulations because of residual or recurrent carcinoma. One should establish a time limit with each patient for unsuccessful coagulation, and proceed with the appropriate radical operation if the patient's condition permits. Three to six months is acceptable. In a poor risk patient, one might have no choice but to continue the electrocoagulation therapy.

## Results

In Madden and Kandalaft's series, the five year survival for the 41 patients who were clinically suitable for abdominoperineal resection was 78 per cent. The five year survival in the clinically inoperable patients (22 patients) was 32 per cent. The overall five year survival in their series was 62 per cent.[17]

Electrocoagulation of carcinoma of the lower and middle part of the rectum as primary treatment is highly successful in a limited number of patients. The most important key to success is the proper selection of patients.[3,13] Preferably, the lesions should be within 10 cm of the anal verge, on the posterior rectal wall, mobile, polypoid, nonulcerated, smaller than 5 cm, and well differentiated. Of course, all these criteria do not have to be met, but they are the ideal. Electrocoagulation is also useful for the palliative treatment of poor risk patients.

## INTRACAVITARY IRRADIATION OF CARCINOMA OF THE RECTUM

In 1973 Papillon of France introduced a local form of treatment for highly selected cases of carcinoma of the rectum, using contact irradiation.[30] The apparatus consists of a portable Philips contact machine with 50 kilovolts power. The treatment distance is 4 cm from the focal spot. A special proctoscope 3 cm in diameter, equipped with a fiberoptic light is placed directly over the carcinoma (Fig. 19-10). The treatment is performed as an outpatient, requires no anesthetic, and is, generally, well tolerated by elderly patients. The usual dose is 3000 to 4000 rads administered within three minutes, given every seven to 10 days, for a total dose of 9000 to 15,000 rads. Total elapsed time for the treatment is 4 to 6 weeks.[29] The advantage of intracavitary irradiation over external irradiation is its mas-

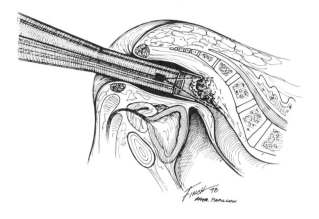

FIGURE **19-10.** *Endocavitary irradiation.* (*Papillon, J.: Dis. Colon Rectum.* 17:*173, 1974*)

sive dose delivered to a small area, compared to the much smaller dose delivered to a much wider area with external irradiation.

### Interstitial Curie Therapy

After completion of the contact irradiation, intracavitary radium implants are employed as complementary irradiation to the bed of the carcinoma, using a dose of 2,000 to 3,000 rads over two to three days.[28] Admission to the hospital is necessary but anesthesia is not indicated. This form of therapy is used for residual carcinomas.

### Selection of Patients

This technique should be applied to carcinomas that are within 10 cm from the anal verge, and not larger than 3 × 5 cm Polypoid, non-ulcerated, mobile, and well-differentiated adenocarcinomas are the most suitable for contact irradiation.[28,34]

### Results

In Papillon's series of 186 patients, of the 133 patients followed more than 5 years, 104 were alive and well, a 5 year survival of 78 per cent.[28] Three treatment failures underwent radical surgery, and one died postoperatively. There were 16 deaths from intercurrent disease, while 12 patients died from metastases. Failure to control local disease in the first 18 month period was observed in 14 per cent. In the group of patients with polypoid cancers, failure occurred in 9.5 per cent, while in patients with ulcerative lesions failure occurred in 26 per cent. Some of these patients were saved by radical surgery so that the overall rate of local or regional failure was 7.5 per cent.

## REFERENCES

1. Bond, J. H., Levy, M., and Levitt, M. D.: Explosion of hydrogen gas in the colon during proctosigmoidoscopy. Gastrointest. Endosc., *23:*41, 1976.

2. Carter, H. G.: Explosion in the colon during electrodesiccation of polyps. Am. J. Surg., *84:*514, 1952.

3. Crile, G. Jr., and Turnbull, R. B.: The role of electrocoagulation in the treatment of carcinoma of the rectum. Surg. Gynecol. Obstet., *135:*391, 1972.

4. Crowley, R. T., and Davis, D. A.: A procedure for total biopsy of doubtful polypoid growths of the lowest large bowel segment. Surg. Gynecol. Obstet., *93:*23, 1951.

5. Curtiss, L. E.: High frequency currents in endoscopy: A review of principles and precautions. Gastrointest. Endosc., *20:*9, 1973.

6. Dukes, C. E., and Bussey, H. J. R.: The spread of rectal cancer and its effect on prognosis. Br. J. Cancer, *12:*309, 1958.

7. Fenoglio, C. M., and Lane, N.: The anatomical precursor of colorectal carcinoma. Cancer, *34:*819, 1974 suppl.

8. Gabriel, W. B., Dukes, C. E., and Bussey, H. J. R.: Biopsy of the rectum. Br. J. Surg., *38:*401, 1951.

9. Gear, E. V. Jr., and Dobbins, W. O.: Rectal biopsy: A review of its diagnostic usefulness. Gastroenterology, *55:*522, 1968.

10. Gilbertsen, V. A., and Nelms, J. M.: The prevention of invasive cancer of the rectum. Cancer, *41:*1137, 1978.

11. Greaney, M. G., and Irvin, T. T.: Criteria for the selection of rectal cancers for local treatment: A clinicopathologic study of low rectal tumors. Dis. Colon Rectum, *20:*463, 1977.

12. Hanley, P. H., Hines, M. O., and Ray, J. E.: Villous tumors: Experience with 217 patients. Am. Surg., *37:*190, 1971.

13. Jackman, R. J.: Conservative management of selected patients with carcinoma of the rectum. Dis. Colon Rectum, *4:*429, 1961.

14. Kraske, P.: Zur Exstirpation Hochsitzender Mastdarmkrebse. Verhandl. Deutsch. Gellesch. Chir., *14:*464, 1885.

15. Levitt, M. D.: Volume and composition of human intestinal gas determined by means of an intestinal washout technic. N. Engl. J. Med., *284:*1394, 1971.

16. Livstone, E. M., Troncale, F. J., and Sheahan, D. G.: Value of a single forceps biopsy of colonic polyps. Gastroenterology, *73:*1296, 1977.

17. Madden, J. L., and Kandalaft, S.: Electrocoagulation in the treatment of cancer of the rectum. *In* Nehus, L. M. (ed.): Surgery Annual 6. 195-212. New York, Appleton Century Croft, 1974.

18. ———: Electrocoagulation. A primary and preferred method of treatment for cancer of the rectum. Ann. Surg., *166:*413, 1967.

19. Mason, A. Y.: Transphincteric approach to rectal lesions. *In* Nehus, L. M. (ed.): Surgery Annual. 6. 171-194. New York, Appleton Century Croft, 1974.

20. ———: Transphincteric exposure of the rectum. Ann. R. Coll. Surg. Engl., *51:*320, 1972 suppl.

21. Morson, B. C.: Rectal and colonic biopsy in inflammatory bowel disease. Am. J. Gastroent., *67:*417, 1977.

22. ———: Evolution of cancer of the colon and rectum. Cancer, *34:*845, 1974 suppl.

23. Morson, B. C., Bussey, H. J. R., and Samoorian, S.: Policy of local excision for early cancer of the colorectum. Gut, *18:*1045, 1977.

24. Nicoloff, D. M., Ellis, C. M., and Humphrey, E. W.: Management of villous adenomas of the colon and rectum. Arch. Surg., *97:*254, 1968.

25. Nivatvongs, S., Balcos, E. G., Schottler, J. L., and Goldberg, S. M.: Surgical management of large villous tumors of the rectum. Dis. Colon Rectum, *16:*508, 1973.

26. Nivatvongs, S., and Goldberg, S. M.: Use of a dinner fork as a retractor during transanal excision of large rectal villous adenomas. Dis. Colon Rectum, *21:*534, 1978.

27. O'Brien, P. H.: Kraske's posterior approach to the rectum. Surg. Gynecol. Obstet., *142:*413, 1976.

28. Papillon, J.: Intracavitary irradiation of early rectal cancer for cure. A series of 186 cases. Cancer, *36:*696, 1975.

29. ———: Endocavitary irradiation in the curative treatment of early rectal cancers. Dis. Colon Rectum, *17:*172, 1974.

30. ———: Endocavitary irradiation of early rectal cancers for cure. A series of 123 cases. Proc. R. Soc. Med., *66:*1179, 1973.

31. Parks, A. G., and Stuart, A. E.: The manage-

ment of villous tumours of the large bowel. Br. J. Surg., *60:*688, 1973.

32. Quan, S. H. Q., and Castro, E. B.: Papillary adenomas (villous tumors): A review of 215 cases. Dis. Colon Rectum, *14:*267, 1971.

33. Salvati, E. P., and Rubin, R. J.: Electrocoagulation as primary therapy for rectal carcinoma. Am. J. Surg., *132:*583, 1976.

34. Sischy, B., and Remington, J. H.: Treatment of carcinoma of the rectum by intracavitary irradiation. Surg. Gynecol. Obstet., *141:*562, 1975.

35. Strauss, A. A., Strauss, S. F., Crawford, R. A., and Strauss, H. A.: Surgical diathermy of carcinoma of the rectum; its clinical end results. JAMA, *104:*1480, 1935.

36. Thomson, J. P. S.: Treatment of sessile villous and tubulovillous adenomas of the rectum: Experience of St. Mark's Hospital, 1963-1972. Dis. Colon Rectum, *20:*467, 1977.

37. Welch, J. P., and Welch, C. E.: Villous adenomas of the colorectum. Am. J. Surg., *131:*185, 1976.

38. Wilson, S. E., and Gordon, H. E.: Excision of rectal lesions by the Kraske approach. Am. J. Surg., *118:*213, 1969.

# 20

# Rectal Prolapse

Rectal procidentia may be defined as the protrusion of the entire thickness of the rectal wall through the anal sphincter. It was one of the earliest surgical problems recognized by the medical profession, yet many facets of this condition remain controversial.

## GENERAL PRINCIPLES

### Etiology

There are two theories concerning the etiology of rectal procidentia. The first of these was proposed by Moschcowitz in 1912.[29] He conceived the idea that a rectal procidentia was a sliding hernia through a defect in the pelvic fascia. This idea was based on the observation that an abnormally deep rectovaginal or rectovesical pouch was a striking and constant feature in most patients with complete rectal prolapse (Fig. 20-1).

The second theory was proposed more recently by Broden and Snellman who demonstrated by cineradiography that the initial step in the genesis of prolapse was circumferential intussusception of the rectum with its starting point about three inches from the anal verge (Fig. 20-2).[6] They believed that they disproved conclusively the theory that herniation of the pouch of Douglas into the rectal lumen is the primary process in the formation of a complete prolapse of the rectum. Studies by Theuerkauf, and associates support this view.[43]

It is possible that either one or the other of these abnormalities is present in different patients, a concept that appears to have been the basis of Altemeier's classification of the condition into three types of rectal prolapse.[2] Type I is a protrusion of the redundant mucosal layer (labelled as a false prolapse, and usually associated with hemorrhoids). Type II is an intussusception without an associated cul-de-sac sliding hernia. Type III is a sliding hernia of the cul-de-sac which he believes occurs in the vast majority of cases.

Without trying to degrade the excellent thought processes involved in describing this condition as a sliding hernia, nor trying to take credit away from the beautiful radiological studies demonstrating intussuscepting bowel, it is not difficult to realize that these two processes are really one and the same. The invagination of the anterior rectal wall classically described as a sliding hernia might just as well be described as an intussusception which has not yet involved the total circumference of the bowel. On the other hand, during operative correction on patients in whom the total circumference is involved, herniation of other viscera has been seen. Of greater value than arguing about names would be to pursue studies aimed at better understanding of the pelvic musculature. For example, there is already good electromyographic evidence that demonstrates an abnormality which might explain more rationally the underlying defect that leads to prolapse. Porter found that the reflex suppression of the resting activity of the external sphincter and levator muscles that occurs normally on distention of the rectum with a balloon is more profound and prolonged in cases of complete rectal prolapse.[36] However, the importance of some subtle disorder

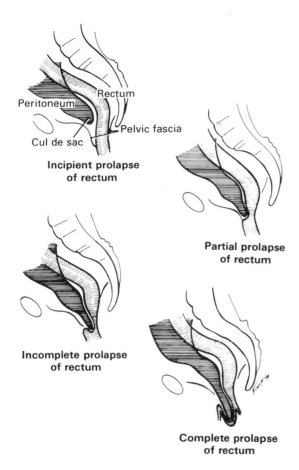

**Incipient prolapse of rectum**

**Partial prolapse of rectum**

**Incomplete prolapse of rectum**

**Complete prolapse of rectum**

FIGURE **20-1.** *Rectal procidentia as conceived by Moschowitz. (After Goldberg, S. M., et al.: Clin. Gastroenterol., 4:490, 1975)*

of the sphincteric mechanism as the primary etiological factor is diminished by the fact that cineradiographically, the prolapse starts well above the pelvic floor, and thus, laxity of the pelvic musculature cannot be a primary factor in the causation of this condition.

**Predisposing Factors**

In reviewing 536 cases of rectal prolapse treated at St. Mark's Hospital, London, in the years 1948 to 1960, Mann reported that 52 per cent of the patients gave a clear history of straining associated with intractable constipation, while another 15 per cent of the patients experienced diarrhea. He listed additional factors which were considered contributory causes of anatomical or neuromuscular deficit: pregnancy, previous operations, and neurological disease.

More recently Parks has suggested that the pelvic floor weakness is secondary to nerve entrapment or nerve stretching which leads to a muscular deficiency, and hence, complete procidentia.[33]

**Pathologic Anatomy**

The anatomic defects that have been described as occurring with prolapse of the rectum include: a defect in the pelvic floor with diastasis of the levatores ani and a weakened endopelvic fascia; loss of the normal horizontal position of the rectum due to its loose attachment to the sacrum and pelvic walls; an abnormally deep cul-de-sac of Douglas; a redundant rectosigmoid colon; and a patulous weak anal sphincter. Those who believe that rectal prolapse is primarily an intussusception feel that these anatomic changes are secondary to the recurring prolapse (Fig. 20-3).

**Clinical Features**

*Sex.* Women predominate in the proportion of 6:1. This was shown in the above men-

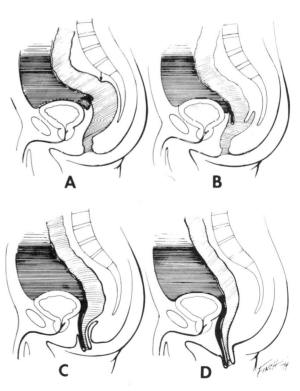

FIGURE **20-2.** *Intussusception drawing analogous to Broden and Snellman's idea. (After Goldberg, S. M., et al.: Clin Gastroentrol., 4:491, 1975)*

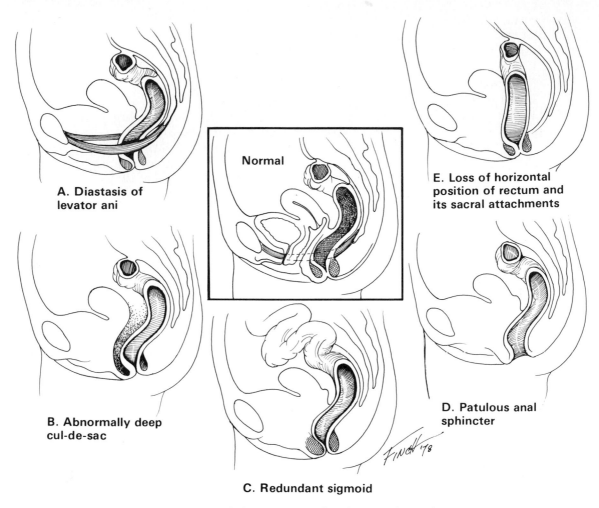

A. Diastasis of levator ani

Normal

E. Loss of horizontal position of rectum and its sacral attachments

B. Abnormally deep cul-de-sac

D. Patulous anal sphincter

C. Redundant sigmoid

FIGURE **20-3.** *Pathologic anatomy found in rectal procidentia.*

tioned St. Mark's study as well as by Kupfer and Goligher.[22]

*Age.* In women the incidence is maximal in the fifth and subsequent decades, but in men it is evenly distributed throughout the age range.[22] Mann reported that in men the rate of incidence falls off after the age of 40, whereas in women it climbs steadily to reach its maximum incidence in the seventh decade.[25]

*Symptoms.* The presenting complaints may be related to the prolapse itself, or to the disturbance of anal continence which frequently coexists. Initially, the mass may extrude only with defecation, but in a more advanced form, occurs with any slight exertion, such as cough-

ing or sneezing. In its early stage, symptoms may include difficulty in bowel regulation, discomfort, the sensation of incomplete evacuation, and tenesmus. In its florid form, this very disabling condition is characterized by a permanently extruded rectum which is excoriated and ulcerated. This leads to mucous discharge and bleeding which causes soiling of the underclothes. Fecal incontinence is almost always a symptom. Constipation with straining is frequently associated. Impairment of anorectal sensation, due to the persistently extruded mass, contributes to the incontinence. In some individuals, associated urinary incontinence may occur. This may or may not be seen in conjunction with uterine prolapse. The psychological trauma is formidable and, because of embarrassment, many of these patients avoid all social contact.

## Physical Examination

*Inspection.* In its florid form, rectal procidentia with its protruding, large, red mass is quite unmistakable for anything else. At the initial examination, however, the prolapse is frequently reduced. However, in many cases, the anal orifice may be quite patulous. If the patient is asked to bear down, the full thickness of the rectal wall will prolapse and the concentric folds are readily noted (Fig. 20-4). Not infrequently, the mucosa shows superficial ulceration due to repeated trauma.

*Palpation.* Digital examination usually demonstrates a diminished tone of the sphincter muscle. Voluntary contraction of this muscle upon the examining finger is either deficient or absent. Another feature is the lack of discomfort experienced by the patient for such an examination. Bi-digital palpation of the prolapsing tissue will make it apparent that the entire bowel wall thickness is involved.

*Sigmoidoscopy.* The first 8 to 10 cm on the anterior wall of the rectum may appear red and inflamed, even to the point of being mistaken for inflammatory bowel disease. On rare occasions, granuloma formation may occur. This may be the early, telltale sign of the so-called hidden or occult rectal procidentia.

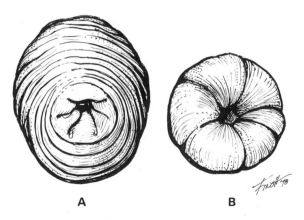

**FIGURE 20-4.** (A) *Concentric folds of rectal procidentia vs.* (B) *radial folds in prolapsing internal hemorrhoids.*

## Differential Diagnosis

In the situation where the mucosa appears hesitatingly at the anal orifice, the distinction of a mucosal prolapse or prolapsing internal hemorrhoids from a complete rectal procidentia may cause some difficulty. Helpful points in differentiating the two conditions include the facts that with complete procidentia the furrows are in a concentric ring, while with mucosal prolapse they are radial; with complete procidentia, the anus is in a normal anatomical position, while with the mucosal prolapse it is everted; with the complete prolapse there is a sulcus between the anus and the protruding bowel, while no sulcus is present with only a mucosal prolapse.

Occasionally a large polypoid tumor of the rectum or colon may emerge through the anal orifice giving the impression of a prolapse. However, associated symptoms, sigmoidoscopy, and a barium enema will confirm this diagnosis.

## INVESTIGATIONS
### Radiological

*A barium enema* should be performed in order to assess the possible association of another disease process such as a neoplasm, inflammatory bowel disease, or diverticular disease. The presence of another disease process may modify the treatment recommended.

*Spine.* Radiographs of the lumbar spine and pelvis may be a clue to frank neurological disease (e.g., spina bifida occulta). If clinically warranted, neurological consultation might prove in order. Such radiographs would not be indicated in all situations.

*Intravenous Pyelogram.* It has been recommended that an intravenous pyelogram be performed for the purpose of demonstrating the course of the ureters.[25] When the pelvic floor descends, the ureters may also descend, being pulled along with the rectum. They are therefore at risk in an operation upon the rectum.

*Cineradiography.* In the case where the diagnosis of procidentia is suspected, but cannot be demonstrated, cineradiography may demonstrate the prolapse.

## Anorectal Manometry

As pointed out in the chapter on physiology, patients with rectal procidentia have specific detectable abnormalities. Such studies may help in the earlier diagnosis of this condition (see Chap. 2).

## Electromyographic Studies

Studies have demonstrated electromyographical abnormalities in patients with rectal prolapse. These are also discussed in the chapter on physiology (see Chap. 2).

## OPERATIVE TREATMENT

Among the more contentious arguments are those concerned with the best operative procedure that has the fewest problems. A discussion of the operative management naturally centers around the presumed etiological factors, and the pathological anatomy. It is upon the concept of these underlying features that the great multitude of widely different procedures have been based. Classification of many of these procedures has been previously outlined.[13]

When trying to decide upon the operative procedure for complete prolapse of the rectum, a surgeon must consider the mortality and morbidity rate, the chance of recurrence, and the probability of restoration or maintenance of continence to be expected from each particular operation. The general health of the patient must also be considered.

The extensive number of procedures which have been proposed all have their disadvantages. The following discussion will present the more popular techniques in current use. This discussion does not apply to the treatment of mucosal prolapse, because this is a relatively minor problem and its management is dealt with in chapter six.

### Abdominal Approaches

*Ripstein Procedure.* In the United States, one of the more commonly used techniques for the correction of rectal procidentia is that described by Ripstein.[39] He suggests that massive procidentia is an intussusception that only occurs when the rectum loses its attachment and becomes a straight tube. The pelvic floor defects, he believes, are secondary and not primary in this condition. Therefore, he postulated that if one can prevent the straightening of the rectum by keeping it fixed to the hollow of the sacrum, intussusception, and hence, procidentia would not occur. With the pressures which are exerted by defecation, the forces acting on the long axis of the tube create an intussusception which begins at the rectosigmoid junction, and finally protrudes through the anus. The aim of his operation, then, is to restore the posterior curve of the rectum, and maintain it during the act of straining. He feels there is no reason to remove the peritoneal sac or repair the pelvic floor. The only requirement of the operation is to produce a sling which firmly fixes the rectum to the sacrum. The first material he used which proved to be effective was fascia lata, but in order to avoid an extra incision, a Teflon mesh was later substituted. More recently Marlex mesh has been utilized.[5]

The technique involves mobilization of the rectum down to the tip of the coccyx by opening the lateral peritoneal folds, and bluntly freeing the bowel from the sacrum. A 5 cm band of Teflon or Marlex mesh is then placed around the rectum at the level of the peritoneal reflection, and the free ends are sutured firmly to the presacral fascia and periosteum 5 cm below the promontory. Nonabsorbable sutures are placed about 1 cm from the midline, carefully avoiding presacral blood vessels. The opposite edge of the synthetic material is then sutured to the presacral fascia, 1 cm from the midline on the opposite side. The rectum is pulled upward and rendered taught. The upper and lower borders of the sling, as well as an apron-like projection, if desired, are sutured to the rectum with nonabsorbable sutures in order to prevent the sling from sliding up and down on the bowel. The sling must be loose enough to allow one or two fingers to pass between the bowel and the sacral fascia. If it is too snug, it may cause problems ranging from mild constipation to fecal impaction. If angulation of the rectum by the sling is apparent, a "hitch" suture can be placed between the anterior surface of the lumbosacral disc and the mesorectum. The peritoneal defect can then be closed with a running catgut suture (Fig. 20-5).

The largest series in which this technique was used has been reported by Ripstein.[38] He has operated on 289 patients with only one

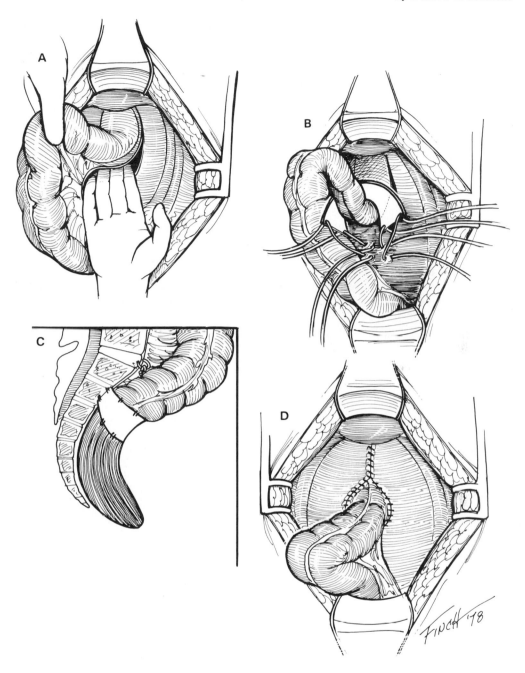

FIGURE **20-5.** *Technique of Ripstein repair. (After Britten-Jones, R.: In Operative Surgery. Todd, I. P. (ed.), p. 228. London, Butterworths, 1977)*

death, this being due to pulmonary embolus. Only 3 per cent of patients required resection of the redundant rectosigmoid. He claims that his morbidity is minimal, and that problems such as pulmonary atelectasis, phlebitis, wound infection, and related problems have not been unduely frequent. Results of other authors are summarized in Table 20-1.

COMPLICATIONS. In order to augment the incomplete information available regarding the results of this procedure, Gordon and Hoexter

TABLE **20-1.** Results of Ripstein Procedure

| AUTHOR | | NO. OF PATIENTS | % RECURRENCES Complete | Mucosal | % MORTALITY |
|---|---|---|---|---|---|
| Ripstein | 1972[37] | 289 | 0 | ? | 0.3 |
| Romero-Torres | 1972[40] | 6 | 0 | 0 | 0 |
| Jurgeleit, et al | 1975[21] | 55 | 7.3 | ? | 0 |
| Morgan | 1975[26] | 42 | 0 | 7.1 | 2.4 |
| Bomar, et al | 1977[3] | 36 | 0 | ? | 0 |

polled the members of the American Society of Colon and Rectal Surgeons.[15] Information on a total of 1,111 procedures was obtained (Table 20-2). This review revealed a recurrence rate of 2.3 per cent, while complications which were directly related to placement of the sling occurred in 16.5 per cent. The overall reoperation rate was 4.1 per cent. Indications for reoperation included fecal impaction, small bowel obstruction, stricture, pelvic abscess, rectal erosion, and hemorrhage. Reoperations for mucosal prolapses and recurrences were not included in this calculation.

The complication of fecal impaction was not easy to evaluate. Some respondents described severe constipation which was worse than in the preoperative phase. Other patients gladly substituted intermittent enemas for prolapse, and failed to report them. However, included in this group were only those patients with fecal impaction who were treated with repeated enemas, disimpaction, or reoperation for release of the fecal impaction.

Presacral bleeding ranged from mild to severe. However, only those cases requiring transfusion were included.

Strictures were common, but only those that required further operation, either division or removal of the sling, or resection of the segment of the bowel, were included. Excluded

TABLE **20-2.** Results of 1,111 Ripstein Procedures

| CONDITION | NO. OF PATIENTS | % RECURRENCE |
|---|---|---|
| Recurrences | 26 | 2.3% |
| Complications | 183 | 16.5% |
| Fecal impaction | 74 | 6.7% |
| Presacral hemorrhage | 29 | 2.6% |
| Stricture | 20 | 1.8% |
| Pelvic abscess | 17 | 1.5% |
| Small bowel obstruction | 15 | 1.4% |
| Impotence | 9 | 0.8% |
| Fistula | 4 | 0.4% |
| Misc. | 15 | 1.4% |

were cases of documented narrowing of the rectum with barium enema for whom no operative intervention was yet performed.

Sepsis referred to the presence of an abscess in the pelvis. Pelvic abscesses and sepsis were usually relieved by removal of the sling and drainage but some required diverting colostomies.

Small bowel obstruction was described as developing due to adhesions of the bowel to the site of the placement of the sling.

The exact incidence of impotence was impossible to evaluate, especially since the distribution of men and women was not determined, and because many of the patients who underwent the procedure were elderly. However, despite meticulous dissection, young, male patients were reported to have become impotent.

The fistulae were due to piercing the bowel, or, possibly, due to erosion of the sling.

Some very unusual complications related to the placement of the sling included erosion through the rectum by the sling. This appears to have been the result of excessive tension placed around the rectum which resulted in ischemia. The late occurrence of this complication may be due to the repeated pressure exerted upon the bowel wall by stool as it passes through the sling. One of the most unusual complications was an erosion of the sling into the urinary bladder.

In regard to the recurrence rate, this operation is a good one with a recurrence rate of only 2.3 per cent. The reported complication rate of 16.5 per cent is related to the specific placement of the sling and, if to this, one adds non-specific complications such as urinary problems, pulmonary problems, and wound infections, which were reported to be approximately 13 per cent by the Lahey Clinic, then an overall complication rate may approximate 30 per cent.

An alternative is to place the sling posteriorly. If one were to place the sling posteriorly to the rectum, leaving the anterior one-fourth to one-third of the circumference of the rectum free to expand, the complication rate might be reduced by half.[47] This speculation would seem to be borne out by the reports of Morgan and associates, and Penfold and associate in using the Ivalon sponge repair, where fecal impaction was not a noted postoperative problem.[28,35]

*The Ivalon sponge wrap operation,* first described by Wells, has become increasingly popular.[46,47] In the United Kingdom it is becoming established as the treatment of choice in most cases of complete rectal prolapse. Minor variations of surgical detail occur, but all surgeons using this technique insist that the rectum is, initially, fully mobilized down to the anorectal ring posteriorly. Part (often the upper one-third) of the lateral ligament is divided to permit adequate posterior mobilization. Hemostasis must be meticulous, as subsequent hematoma formation might predispose to an infected sponge. A rectangular sheet of Ivalon (polyvinyl alcohol) sponge is then sutured to the periosteum of the concave surface of the sacrum by means of nonabsorbable stitches (silk, nylon or linen). The mobilized rectum is then drawn upward from the pelvic floor, and placed onto the front of this sheet, the lateral extremities of which are folded around so as to just fail to meet anteriorly. A certain portion (2–3 cm) of the anterior circumference of the rectum must remain uncovered to prevent constriction of the lumen. A further series of sutures are then used to fasten the anterior aspect of the sponge to the rectal wall. Finally, the pelvic peritoneum is sutured over the fixed rectum. Penfold and Hawley pointed out that care must be taken to ensure that the base of the sigmoid mesocolon is not shortened as this would predispose to sigmoid volvulus (Fig. 20-6).[35]

Morgan and Wells suggested that this technique provided a very effective method of controlling rectal prolapse, and that it also contributed toward the management of the notoriously difficult functional bowel problems that beset these patients.[27] Fifty per cent of their patients became continent postoperatively and, as a result of this, were able to manage their difficult bowel habits more easily.

COMPLICATIONS. In the series of Morgan, Porter, and Klugman, the mortality and morbidity of this operation were each 2.6 per cent.[28] They felt this constituted a reasonable safety level for major pelvic surgery in the advanced age group. The other criterion of effectiveness is the cure rate of 96 per cent. Three of their patients developed a recurrent prolapse, and it was noted that these all occurred within three years of the operation. Prolapse of the mucosa through the anal canal, considered by some patients as trivial compared to the complaints of the previous complete prolapse, occurred in 8.6 per cent of patients. Half of those with mucosal prolapse failed to respond to submucosal injections of 5 per cent phenol in almond oil, and required operative excision. There is no doubt that mucosal prolapse causing leakage of fecal-stained mucus results in pruritus and discomfort. Control of mucosal prolapse will improve the patients continence, and, therefore, their attitudes toward the use of aperients or suppositories in the management of their bowel habits. The results published by other authors are summarized in Table 20-3.

Pelvic sepsis developed in 2.6 per cent of Morgan's series.[28] If the bowel is opened or injured during dissection, the Ivalon sponge implant method should be abandoned. It is clear that, should sepsis occur, an expectant policy

TABLE **20-3.** Results of Ivalon Sponge Operation

| AUTHOR | NO. OF PATIENTS | % RECURRENCES | | % MORTALITY |
| | | *Complete* | *Mucosal* | |
| --- | --- | --- | --- | --- |
| *Theuerkauf, et al 1970*[43] (review of literature) | 109 | 1.8 | ? | 3.7 |
| *Stewart 1972*[42] | 41 | 7.3 | 24.4 | 0 |
| *Penfold, et al 1972*[35] | 101 | 3.0 | 30.7 | 0 |
| *Morgan, et al 1972*[28] | 150 | 3.2 | 5.3 | 2.6 |
| *Boutsis, et al 1974*[4] | 26 | 11.5 | 34.6 | 3.8 |

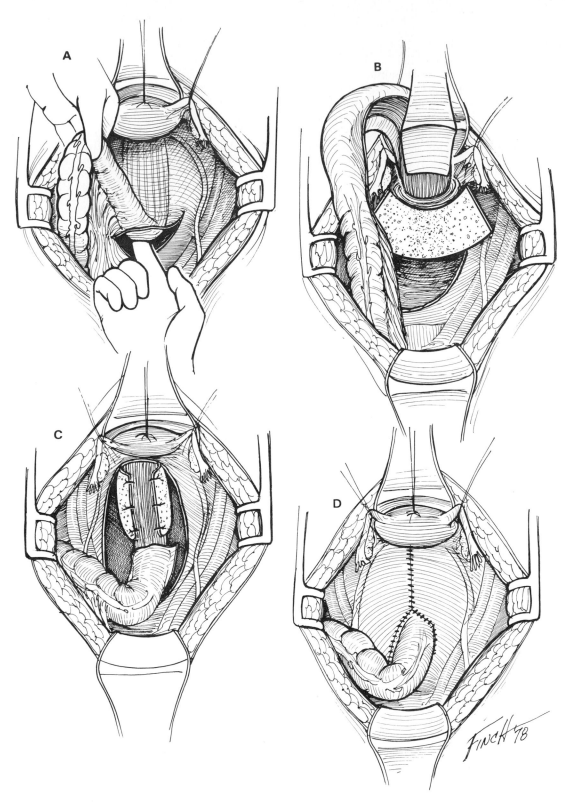

FIGURE **20-6.** *Technique of Ivalon sponge repair.* (*After Porter, N. H.: In Operative Surgery, Todd, I. P. (ed.), pp. 222–224 London, Butterworths, 1977)*

is not justified, and the sponge should be removed as a matter of urgency. If an abscess points into the vagina or rectum, removal of the sponge through the wall of either viscus is possible, and complete resolution can be expected. Kupfer and Goligher found a pelvic sepsis rate of 16 per cent.[22]

In rats, polyvinyl alcohol sponge has been shown to produce sarcomas. However, there is no evidence yet that it predisposes to malignancy in humans. Ivalon has been found to be present in human tissues for 5 years, producing a foreign body reaction with only moderate fibrosis. Reoperation on patients with previously implanted Ivalon has been surprisingly straightforward. It is felt that the minimal amount of fibrous tissue between the sacrum and the rectum suggests that the success of the operation in controlling prolapse is not due to fixation of the rectum to the sacrum, but rather, to a stiffening of the rectum itself, thus preventing rectal intussusception.[35]

*Abdominal proctopexy and sigmoid resection*, a technique, originally described by Frykman in 1955, is a composite surgical procedure using selected techniques designed to eliminate the abnormal factors that contribute to the formation of rectal procidentia.[9] The entire procedure is performed through a transverse abdominal incision, and as described by him, consists of four essential steps (Fig. 20-7). (*1.*) Mobilization of the rectum by the abdominal route. The dissection of the rectum is carried out exactly as in the abdominal phase of a Miles abdominoperineal resection, except for preserving the blood supply to the rectum, and keeping the lateral stalks intact. (*2.*) Elevation of the rectum as high as possible, and fixation of the lateral stalks by suturing them to the periosteum of the sacrum. Here the rectum is completely mobilized down to the levator muscles. The freed rectum is drawn up into the abdomen, which makes the lateral stalks stand out prominently. These are then sutured to the periosteum of the sacrum with silk to hold the organ firmly in this elevated position. Care must be taken not to narrow the bowel by placement of the fixation sutures, as this may lead to an obstruction. The cavity created posterior to the rectum by the dissection and elevation fills in with scar tissue as described by Pemberton and Stalker, achieving firm fixation of the posterior rectal wall.[34] (*3.*) Suture of the endopelvic fascia anteriorly to the rectum in order to obliterate the cul-de-sac. The excess peritoneum of the cul-de-sac is excised, and the new peritoneal floor is sutured snuggly

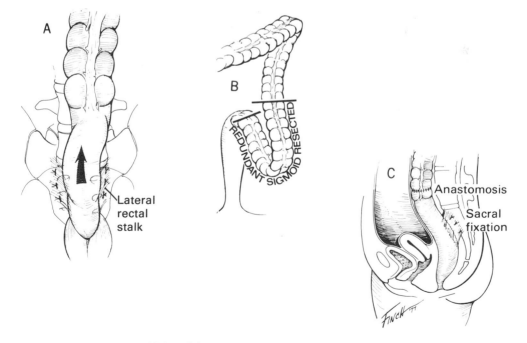

FIGURE **20-7.** *Abdominoproctopexy and sigmoid resection.*

about the elevated intestine with interrupted silk sutures. No attempt is made to approximate the levator muscles anterior to the rectum. (*4.*) Segmental resection of all the excess sigmoid colon with an end-to-end anastomosis. The peritoneum lateral to the descending colon is incised up to the splenic flexure, and the entire left colon is mobilized from the retroperitoneal structures. A wedge resection of the colon is then done with preservation of the major blood vessels. The redundant colon is resected so that the anastomosis can be accomplished without tension. Any convenient site may be selected for the anastomosis. The raw surfaces are reperitonealized except for the left gutter.

Over the 25 year period from 1952 to 1977, 103 patients underwent this operative procedure by Goldberg and associates.[11] There was one death. There were no known complete recurrences, although nine patients returned with mucosal prolapses. Initially these were treated with phenol in oil injections, but in recent years rubber band ligatures have been applied with good results.

COMPLICATIONS. There were 12 major complications, for a rate slightly under 12 per cent. There were three colonic obstructions and one anastomotic leak, each requiring temporary colostomy. Following the closure of one of these colostomies, a fecal fistula developed which closed spontaneously. There was one case of severe presacral bleeding which required six units of blood, and one patient had a wound dehiscence. There were three small bowel obstructions, two requiring operative intervention, and one patient had a cardiac arrest from which she was successfully resuscitated. In addition, there is one case of acute pancreatitis, and one acute incarceration of a hiatal hernia.

The ever present problem of continence plagued this group of surgeons in a similar fashion in which it has bothered others. Problems of sphincteric control were encountered in at least one-half of the patients. In addition, it was impossible to determine the degree of proper rectal function in many of the mentally defective patients. It was of interest that none of the men had problems with persistent incontinence; this was probably due to the fact that the sphincter is better developed in the male.[10]

IS COLONIC RESECTION REALLY NECESSARY? A very pertinent question which should be asked at this juncture relates to whether a colonic resection is a necessary component in the correction of rectal procidentia. Advocates of this procedure believe that maximal resection of the left colon is an essential step in the treatment of rectal procidentia. It is argued that shortening of the left colon should permanently prevent recurrence, irrespective of the type or the multiplicity of etiological factors that may be involved, since the straight left colon firmly supported proximally by the phrenocolic ligament has little mobility and cannot slide. Of all the weaknesses or abnormalities required to produce rectal prolapse, the only factor that can be controlled with any degree of certainty is the length of the colon. Stress and strain may break down the rebuilt rectal support and, again, deepen the cul-de-sac, but the configuration of the straight, short left colon will not change. Without slack and mobility in the left colon, the rectum cannot descend, and rectal prolapse cannot recur.

The low anterior resection as recommended by Muir has the decided advantage in that it is an operation familiar to all surgeons because of its use in carcinoma of the rectum.[30] However, the low end-to-end anastomosis between the dilated rectum and a smaller proximal sigmoid makes the procedure technically difficult. The difficulties predispose to the problems inherent in a low anastomosis, notably a leak and its subsequent complications. A resection at any convenient level seems to make much more sense than a low resection. Another aspect not previously considered is that removal of a large, redundant sigmoid will result in smoother bowel function. With less constipation there would be less straining, thus decreasing the chance of an anatomical recurrence.[12]

Theuerkauf and colleagues reported the surgical experience at the Mayo Clinic with 124 cases of rectal prolapse treated over 16 years.[43] Various techniques were used, and it was found that with the Pemberton suspension-fixation operation there was a recurrence rate of 32.4 per cent, with the Altemeier proctosigmoidectomy procedure it was 38.5 per cent, and with anterior resection, 3.7 per cent. Combining a review of the literature with their own results they came to the conclusion that anterior resection, with or without a suspension procedure, should be recommended for good risk patients of all ages. The Thiersch operation was recommended for the older, debilitated, poor risk patients, while the Pemberton procedure with suture of the rectal stalks to the sacral fascia may be used in the intermediate risk group. While fixation of the rectum is taking place, some type of temporary suspension is wise, but not necessary. They feel that pelvic floor repair is unnecessary in any operation for prolapse.

The recurrence rate reported by Loygue and co-workers for patients treated by rectopexy alone is 3.6 per cent after follow-up intervals of up to 15 years.[24] There were only two postoperative deaths in 140 procedures. Intervertebral disc infection was found in two cases. Of 44 patients in whom incontinence was due solely to loss of tone in the anal sphincter, 41 recovered completely.

Although resection of the excess bowel increases the magnitude of the procedure, it provides a greater potential for permanent cure, hence, may be worthwhile. This procedure, of course, is primarily designed for use in those individuals whose general physical condition justifies an aggressive approach.

### Perineal or Sacral Procedures

*Thiersch Operation.* A very simple palliative procedure for prolapse, first described by Thiersch, is the encirclement of the anal orifice with a silver wire.[44] It was initially imagined that such circumanal wiring would be beneficial in two ways: by mechanically supporting and containing the prolapse; and by provoking a reaction in the tissues of the anal region leading to a ring of fibrosis reinforcing the atonic sphincters. However, the wire is nonirritating, and does not stimulate a significant tissue reaction (Fig. 20-8).

Virtues of the procedure are that it causes a minimal degree of surgical trauma, and can be performed easily under local anesthesia. Also,

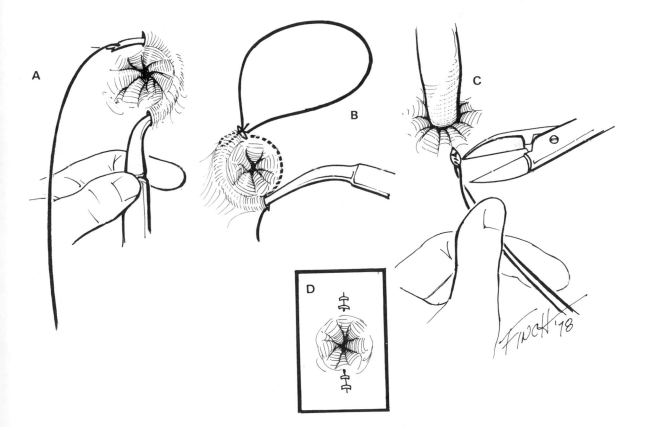

FIGURE **20-8.** *The Thiersch operation. (After Golingher, J. C.: Anus, Rectum and Colon. 330. Springfield, Ill., Charles C Thomas, 1975)*

if it is not satisfactory, the wire can be easily withdrawn and re-introduced on two or three successive occasions. The disadvantages of this procedure are that it is only palliative, does not cure the prolapse, and does not restore continence, but carries with it a high degree of recurrence. In Goligher's series, there was a 56 per cent recurrence rate. Complications of this procedure include fecal impaction, infection, breakage or sloughing of the circumanal band, and mucosal prolapse. In addition, rectovaginal fistulae secondary to erosion of the wire have been seen.

Over the years, there have been numerous modifications of this encirclement procedure. Such materials as silk, fascia, tendon, muscle, crimped Teflon, rigid steel wire, nylon tapes, and, most recently, a folded half inch mesh of Marlex have been advocated.

Some of the problems of this procedure may be obviated by the insertion of a silicone rubber perianal suture described by Hopkinson and Hardman.[17] This elastic material can expand and contract to allow normal defecation, and yet control continence and prolapse. With use of this soft, elastic material, one hopes to achieve gentle support of the sphincter muscle without the complications of fracture, cutting out, or fecal impaction.

A modification currently enjoying some popularity is the use of a polypropylene mesh (Marlex) described by Lomas and Cooperman.[23] With the patient under regional or local anesthesia in the prone jackknife position, perianal radical incisions 2 cm long are made in the left posterior and right anterior quadrants, starting about 1 cm from the anal border. Each incision is made 2.5 cm deep. A curved hemostat is inserted through the left posterior incision, emerging through the right anterior incision outside the external sphincter. The previously prepared mesh which consists of a four-ply piece of Marlex 1.5 cm wide and 20 cm long which had sutures placed at 1 cm intervals is then drawn through half the circumference of the anus. The hemostat is reintroduced, and the mesh is delivered around the other half of the circumference. Care must be taken not to break through the posterior vaginal wall or the anterior rectal mucosa. The mesh is drawn tightly over the index finger in the anal canal, and four to six sutures of Marlex are used to fix the overlapping mesh. Excess mesh is cut off, and the wound irrigated.

The original authors recommend a solution of Kanamycin for irrigation. The wounds are closed in two layers using 3-0 chromic for the fibroadipose tissue and 4-0 nylon for the skin (Fig. 20-9). Postoperatively, stool softeners are administered.

Lomas and Cooperman have performed 50 such repairs with excellent results in 47 patients. Postoperative fecal impactions were rare, and infected wounds were drained without requiring the removal of the mesh.[23]

*The transsacral repair* of rectal prolapse was described by Davidian and Thomas.[7] The procedure, conducted through a posterior approach, consists primarily of resection of the coccyx and distal sacrum, repair of the lax levatores ani and endopelvic fascia by anterior approximation of the structures with fine wire sutures, and excision of the redundant peritoneal cul-de-sac. This repair serves the dual role of securing the rectum posteriorly in a horizontal position, as well as contributing to the strength of the pelvic floor. When necessary, a resection of redundant rectosigmoid can be accompanied without disturbing the existing anorectal reflexes, thus maintaining sphincteric reservoir continence. Thomas claims excellent results in 44 patients operated on in this fashion with no mortality or recurrence.[45] Resection was performed in eight of the 44 patients. A morbidity of 38 per cent was encountered, primarily a consequence of wound infection (20 per cent). Anastomotic leaks occurred in two patients. Two cases of fecal fistulae were encountered: one necessitated a temporary, and the other a permanent colostomy. A stricture that could be handled only by dilatation was also seen.

The operation is of modest magnitude, and associated with maintenance of or improvement in fecal continence. Although this procedure requires an unfamiliar approach and may be technically difficult, nevertheless, it may be used in debilitated patients, and those with a deformed or a narrow pelvis.

*Perineal rectosigmoidectomy* was first described by Mikulicz in 1889, powerfully advocated by Miles in 1933, and for some time remained the favorite method of treatment in Great Britain. In the United States, this procedure was championed by Altemeier and colleagues.[2] Hughes (1949) reported on the follow-up studies of 150 consecutive patients who

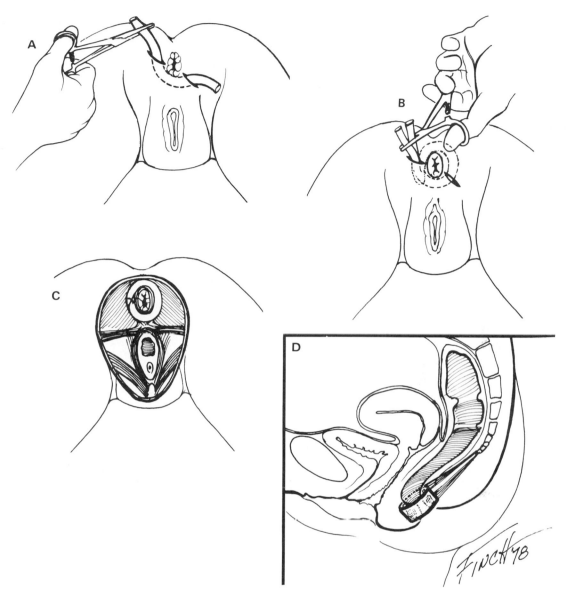

FIGURE **20-9.** *Lomas and Coopermam modification of Thiersch. (After Lomas, M. I., and Cooperman, H.: Dis. Colon Rectum, 15:416, 1972)*

underwent perineal rectosigmoidectomy at St. Mark's Hospital in London, and discovered an ultimate recurrence rate of over 60 per cent with more than half of these patients being incontinent.[19] Porter (1962) subsequently reported 110 additional patients who underwent rectosigmoidectomy from 1949 to 1960 at St. Mark's Hospital, many of whom also underwent perineal suture of the puborectalis muscle as part of the operation.[36] The results were improved very little by the perineal suturing of the levator ani muscle, and recurrences developed in 58 per cent of patients. Consequently, this has led many to believe that the approximation of puborectalis muscle is not of prime importance in the repair of the procidentia. Altemeier, et al reported excellent results with the one stage perineal operation of rectosigmoidectomy, having only three recurrences after 106 operations.[2] However,

*(Text continues on p. 264)*

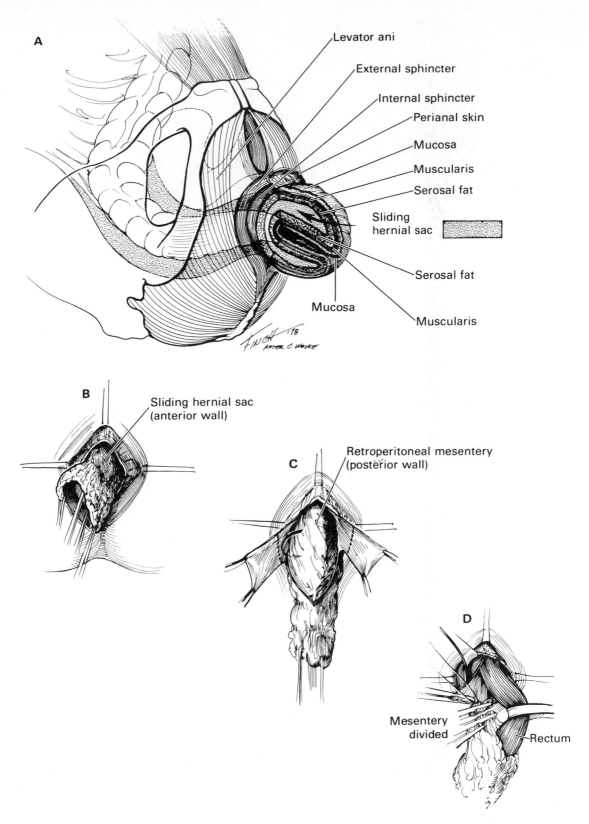

Levator ani

External sphincter

Internal sphincter

Perianal skin

Mucosa

Muscularis

Serosal fat

Sliding
hernial sac

Serosal fat

Mucosa

Muscularis

**B** Sliding hernial sac
(anterior wall)

**C** Retroperitoneal mesentery
(posterior wall)

**D**

Mesentery
divided

Rectum

FIGURE **20-10.** *Altemeier perineal rectosigmoidectomy. (After Altemeier, W. A., Hosp Pract. 7:102, 1972) (Continued opposite page)*

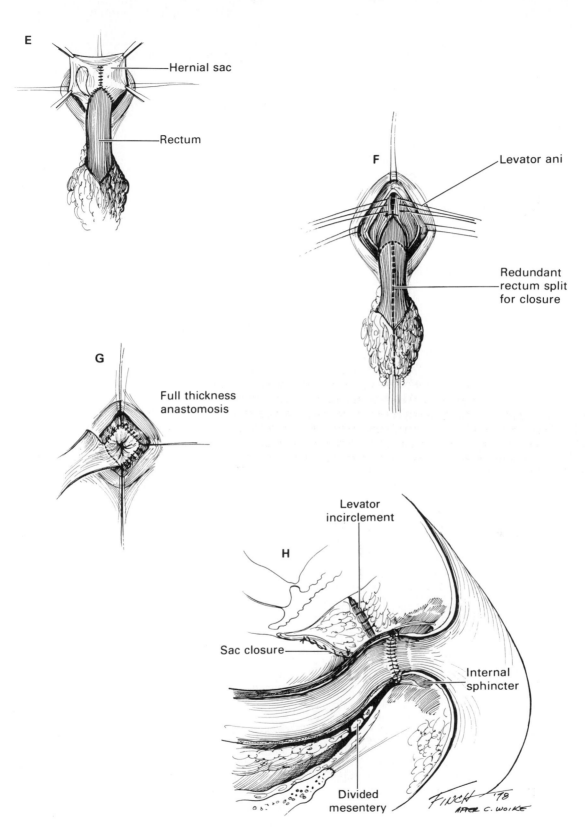

**E**

Hernial sac

Rectum

**F**

Levator ani

Redundant
rectum split
for closure

**G**

Full thickness
anastomosis

Levator
incirclement

**H**

Sac closure

Internal
sphincter

Divided
mesentery

FINCH '78
AFTER C. WOIKE

FIGURE **20-10.** (*Conclusion*)

these good results cannot be matched by other surgeons. The technique of perineal sigmoidectomy may also induce further damage to the already altered anatomy and physiology. Our feeling is that perineal rectosigmoidectomy should probably be considered as a palliative procedure, and relegated to use in the poor risk patient who is confined to a nursing home; amputation of the massive prolapse would unquestionably facilitate the care of these patients.

As advocated by Altemeier, the one stage perineal procedure includes obliteration of the hernial sac by high ligation, approximation of the levator ani muscles to repair the defect in the pelvic diaphragm through which the hernia protruded, and resection of the prolapsing and redundant bowel with primary end-to-end anastomosis.[1] The procedure also involves the reduction of the distended anus to a normal size.

TECHNIQUE. Under general anesthesia, the patient is placed in the lithotomy position with slight trendelenburg in order to minimize distention of the hemorrhoidal vessels so as to reduce operative bleeding and to allow the small intestine to retract into the peritoneal cavity (Fig. 20-10). The four quadrants are marked for traction and orientation. A circumferential incision through all layers of the rectum is made 3 mm proximal to the pectinate line. This length is adequate for establishing the anastomosis, yet short enough to prevent postoperative protrusion. The anterior wall of the hernial sac is thus exposed, and the outer cuff of the prolapse is peeled down to reveal the sliding hernia. The sac is opened to determine the full extent, and the excess peritoneal reflections are trimmed away. The mesentery to the redundant bowel is then divided and ligated. The pouch of Douglas is obliterated by a continuous suture of 2-0 chromic catgut, which produces an inverted Y-suture.

Next, the medial borders of the retracted levator ani muscles are grasped anteriorly to the rectum, and approximated with approximately four interrupted sutures. As the defect in the pelvic diaphragm is eliminated, a sacral curve is imparted to the bowel, increasing the effectiveness of the puborectalis. The defect in the pelvic diaphragm is narrowed down to fit snugly around the surgeon's finger.

The redundant bowel is divided into halves by anterior and posterior incisions carried to the level of the proposed resection. The anterior and posterior angles of the bowel are anchored to the mucocutaneous border, alignment with the original quadrant traction sutures is made, and the bowel is then transected progressively in quadrants. This completes the anastomosis of all layers of the bowel wall to the anal ring. The everted anastomosis is then reduced.

Complications encountered with this procedure include abscesses secondary to leaking anastomoses, rectal stricture, and nonspecific complications.

## SUBSEQUENT MANAGEMENT
### Postoperative Management

It is of paramount importance, that regardless which operative procedure is utilized, the patient understands that the bowels must move on a regular basis without any straining.

### Management of Residual Incontinence

An all-important consideration to be mentioned is that of continence. The greatest weakness of the present day operative treatment for rectal prolapse is its limited capacity to restore in all patients normal anorectal function despite the excellent anatomical results. In Goligher's series of 91 cases, using the abdominal repair as the method of choice, some 40 per cent of patients failed to show any improvement in anal continence.[22] One-half of Altemeier's patients had return of function of the external sphincters within the six month to one year period following operation.[2] In addition, his patients regularly had incontinence for 20 to 30 days following the operation after which time some control was acquired. Penfold and Hawley state that 40 per cent of patients do not have satisfactory continence after the Ivalon sponge operation.

Because of the difficult, if not impossible, task of attempting to classify degrees of incontinence, and because individual interpretations are subjective rather than objective, reports of different authors cannot be compared precisely. Morgan and associates defined incontinence as the uncontrolled leak of solid or loose stools, and found 80.6 per cent of patients incontinent preoperatively.[28] Almost all their patients had a variable degree of urgency at defecation, and some of them restrained the act only with difficulty. In their series, 38.8 per cent were incontinent postoperatively; further operative procedures for incontinence were performed in 7.5 per cent.

The return of continence may take as long as six to twelve months, consequently, one should resist demands for further operative treatment for incontinence until a year has passed. Improvement in continence appears to be due to three factors. First, the patients learn to adjust their aperient regimen better after operation. In this respect the most useful is a bulk-forming agent. The second factor is that operation narrows the rectum by surrounding fibrosis, which is appreciable on digital examination, for at least 18 months postoperatively. This often leads to the passage of frequent, pellet-like stools. The third important factor is the absence of continuing dilatation of the anal canal by a large complete prolapse, so that there is reduction in the diameter of the anal canal. However, after operation, one is unable to detect any clear quantitative improvement in pelvic electromyograms. Nevertheless, there is no doubt that elimination of complete rectal prolapse allows the patient to practice sphincter exercises more effectively, and the use of faradism appears to reeducate the proprioceptive reflexes and improve the patients' consciousness of when their sphincters are contracting. Unfortunately, pelvic faradism has not been shown to produce an objective improvement.

Morgan and associates published the results of 150 patients who were operated on using the Ivalon sponge method.[28] A number of these patients were investigated preoperatively and postoperatively by means of cineradiography during defecation. Postoperative studies showed good fixation of the rectum in the sacral hallow, and improvement in the position of the levator muscular shelf on which the distal portion of the rectum lay. Preoperative and postoperative electromyographic studies of the pelvic floor were also performed in some patients. In all these patients there was a gross disturbance of the normal postural pelvic floor reflexes preoperatively, and only two of the patients who were followed-up postoperatively (both were young) showed any significant recovery in the pelvic muscle function. This indicates that whatever the cause of the prolapse may be (and they believe it is due to a large extent to abnormal habits of defecation), these etiological factors produce muscle failure in the pelvic floor before prolapse occurs, and this defect is not cured by fixing the rectum in the sacral hallow. These observations are in keeping with those of Parks and associates on the "descending perineum" syndrome.[33] They also contribute toward explaining the fact that correction of the rectal prolapse alone does not entirely solve the functional problems of continence and abnormal bowel habits.

The anal stimulator described by Hopkinson and Lightwood was introduced in the hope of controlling both the prolapse and incontinence.[18] However, at St. Mark's Hospital, London, little, if any, improvement has been noted with the aid of the stimulator.[16] It is difficult to imagine such a stimulator curing a patient with a massive prolapse of the rectum because they almost certainly need definitive repair. However, the electrical stimulator might prove to be an aid in those patients with residual incontinence, thus improving the ultimate success rate.

For patients with residual incontinence following a successful anatomical repair, Parks has described a method of treatment whereby the levator ani is repaired from below by introducing a lattice of nylon floss through an approach through the intersphincteric plane.[32] In addition, this operation restores the anal canal to a narrow tube, and creates a prominent anorectal angle. Provided the patient does not bear down or strain in any way after the operation, the results of the procedure appear satisfactory (chap. 22). In Morgan's series, four patients with residual incontinence were operated on using this nylon floss repair, and three subsequently regained full continence.

## COMPLICATIONS OF RECTAL PROCIDENTIA
### Strangulation and Gangrene

Very rarely, a rectal prolapse may become incarcerated. In circumstances where it is irreducible, and there is doubt as to the viability of the bowel, an emergency rectosigmoidectomy would appear to be the treatment of choice.

### Ulceration and Hemorrhage

Minor ulceration of the exposed mucosa may cause minimal bleeding, but more extensive ulcerations, on very rare occasions, may cause a severe hemorrhage.

### Rupture of the Prolapse

This exceedingly rare complication would obviously require urgent operation, and is probably best handled through an abdominal approach.

## PROLAPSE IN CHILDREN

In children, the incidence is highest in the first two years of life and declines thereafter.[14] Boys are affected slightly more frequently than girls. The condition is usually the mucosal type. Predisposing factors that are generally held to be important in the development of the prolapse include the absence of the sacral curve so that in the sitting or standing position, the rectum and anal canal form an almost vertical straight tube. Excitement causes comprise conditions leading to excessive straining at stool, such as diarrhea, overpurgation, and constipation. Mucoviscidosis may also be associated with rectal prolapse.

The mother complains that when the child defecates the rectum projects from the anus. This may be associated with a slight discharge of mucus or blood. Upon examination, the ring of prolapsing mucosa may be noted to project 2 to 4 cm beyond the anal orifice. Palpation of the prolapsing tissue reveals that only two layers of mucosa are present. Rarely, a complete rectal procidentia may occur.

The differential diagnosis includes a prolapsed rectal polyp or the apex of an intussusception protruding through the anus.

It is important to realize that in children, prolapsing rectal mucosa is a self-limiting disease. Consequently, treatment should be directed at the correction of constipation and the institution of proper habits of defecation. Strapping of the buttocks has been advocated but this is probably only buying time until the self-limiting disease resolves. In nonresponding cases, submucosal injection of a sclerosing agent such as phenol in almond oil has proven effective.[14] Stephens has recommended the insertion of a subcutaneous stitch of catgut, which, in fact, is a temporary Thiersch operation.[41] For a complete rectal prolapse, perirectal injections of alcohol have been advocated in order to stimulate a periproctitis and fix the rectum to the sacrum.[8]

Actual surgical resection for prolapse in children is a very rare necessity, but Goligher has had to perform emergency rectosigmoidectomies for large, irreducible prolapses in children.

## "HIDDEN" PROLAPSE (INTERNAL PROCIDENTIA)

This refers to the earliest stage of procidentia when the intussuscepting rectum occupies the rectal ampulla but has not yet continued through the anal canal. The most common complaint is difficulty in bowel emptying, often described as a sensation of incomplete evacuation or obstruction. The second most common symptom is incontinence. Other symptoms include pain, bleeding, mucous discharge, pruritus, and diarrhea.[20] Sigmoidoscopic findings have included a solitary ulcer or reddening of the mucosa 6 to 8 cm from the anus, in addition to a bulging edematous mucosa.

Follow-up by Irhe of 40 patients who underwent a Ripstein repair revealed that 25 patients were subjectively improved, 10 had unchanged symptoms, and four were worse.[20] One death occurred in that series, a patient developed a rectovaginal fistula; and two strictures requiring operation for removal of the sling occurred. The procedure restored continence in 75 per cent of patients. When indications for surgery were pain or a sensation of obstruction, the results were poor. Therefore, in patients who are continent, it is recommended to avoid operation. In patients with incontinence early operation is justified. Ripstein operated upon 12 such patients with relief of symptoms in 11 patients.[37]

## SUMMARY

In this chapter an attempt has been made to present the current information available on the more popularly used techniques in the repair of complete rectal procidentia. No one procedure has been recommended as the treatment of choice, as we recognize that each procedure has advantages and disadvantages. The particular method of repair used by a surgeon will depend upon his previous training, and exposure to a certain technique modified by his own personal experience. At the present time we would usually favor a pelvic fixation procedure in which the rectum is not completely surrounded anteriorly by a synthetic material. However, in an individual who has symptomatic diverticular disease or suffers from severe constipation in association with a very redundant colon, a resection might be recommended instead of one of the fixation procedures. Certainly, one would hesitate to insert a foreign body into the pelvis in association with a resection. An abdominal approach is favored but, in poor risk patients, a perineal rectosigmoidectomy or some encirclement procedure may prove satisfactory.

## REFERENCES

1. Altemeier, W. A.: One-stage perineal surgery for complete rectal prolapse. Hosp. Pract., *7:*102, 1972.

2. Altemeier, W. A., Cutbertson, W. R., Schowengerdt, C. J., and Hunt, J.: Nineteen years' experience with the one stage perineal repair of rectal prolapse. Ann. Surg., *173:*993, 1971.

3. Bomar, R. L., and Sawyers, J. L.: Transabdominal proctopexy (Ripstein procedure) for massive rectal prolapse. Am. Surg., *43:*97, 1977.

4. Boutsis, C., and Ellis, H.: The Ivalon-sponge-wrap operation for rectal prolapse: An experience with 26 patients. Dis. Colon Rectum, *17:*21, 1974.

5. Britten-Jones, R.: Complete rectal prolapse: Ripstein operation in operative surgery. *In* Rob, C., Smith, R. (eds.): Colon, Rectum and Anus., London, Butterworths, 1977.

6. Broden, B., and Snellman, B.: Procidentia of the rectum studied with cineradiography: A contribution to the discussion of causative mechanism. Dis. Colon Rectum, *11:*330, 1968.

7. Davidian, V. A. Jr., and Thomas, C. G.: Transsacral repair of rectal prolapse. Am. J. Surg., *123:*231, 1972.

8. Findlay, L., and Galbraith, J. B. D.: Injection of alcohol in the treatment of prolapse of the rectum in infancy and childhood. Lancet, *1:*76, 1923.

9. Frykman, H. M.: Abdominal proctopexy and primary sigmoid resection for rectal procidentia. Am. J. Surg., *90:*780, 1955.

10. Frykman, H. M., and Goldberg, S. M.: The surgical treatment of rectal procidentia. Surg. Gynecol. Obstet., *129:*1225, 1969.

11. Goldberg, S. M.: unpublished, 1977.

12. Goldberg, S. M., and Gordon, P. H.: Treatment of rectal prolapse. Clin. Gastroenterol., *4:*489, 1975.

13. Goldberg, S. M., and Gordon, P. H.: Operative treatment of complete prolapse of the rectum. In Najarian, J. S., and Delaney, J. P. (eds.) Surgery of the Gastrointestinal Tract. New York, Intercontinental Medical Book Corporation, 1974.

14. Goligher, J. C.: Surgery of the Anus, Rectum and Colon. 3 ed. 292. Charles C Thomas, Springfield, Ill., 1975.

15. Gordon, P. H., and Hoexter, B.: Complications of Ripstein procedure. Dis. Colon Rectum, *21:*277, 1978.

16. Hawley, P. R.: Personal communication, 1974.

17. Hopkinson, B. R., and Hardman, J.: Silicone rubber perianal suture for rectal prolapse. Proc. R. Soc. Med., *66:*1095, 1973.

18. Hopkinson, B. R., and Lightwood, R.: Electrical treatment of anal incontinence. Lancet, *1:*297, 1966.

19. Hughes, E. S. R.: In discussion on rectal prolapse. Proc. R. Soc. Med., *42:*1007, 1949.

20. Ihre, T., and Seligson, U.: Intussusception of the rectum—internal procidentia: Treatment and results in 90 patients. Dis. Colon Rectum, *18:*391, 1975.

21. Jurgeleit, H. C., Corman, M. L. Coller, J. A., and Veidenheimer, M. C.: Procidentia of the rectum: Teflon sling repair of rectal prolapse, Lahey Clinic experience. Dis. Colon Rectum, *6:*464, 1975.

22. Kupfer, C. A., and Goligher, J. C.: One hundred consecutive cases of complete prolapse of the rectum treated by operation. Br. J. Surg., *57:*34, 1970.

23. Lomas, M. I., and Cooperman, H.: Correction of rectal procidentia by use of Polypropylene mesh (Marlex). Dis. Colon Rectum, *15:*416, 1972.

24. Loygue, J., Hugier, M., Malafosse, M., and Biotois, H.: Complete prolapse of the

rectum—A report on 140 cases treated by rectopexy. Br. J. Surg., *58:*847, 1971.

25. Mann, C. V.: Rectal prolapse in Diseases of the Colon, Rectum and Anus. 238. London, Medical Books Ltd., 1969.

26. Morgan, B.: Procidentia of the rectum; the Ripstein operation. Dis. Colon Rectum, *18:*468, 1975.

27. Morgan, C., and Wells, C.: The use of the Ivalon sponge. Proc. R. Soc. Med., *55:*1084, 1962.

28. Morgan, C. N., Porter, N. H., and Klugman, D. J.: Ivalon (polyvinyl alcohol) sponge in the repair of complete rectal prolapse. Br. J. Surg., *59:*841, 1972.

29. Moschcowitz, A. V.: The pathogenesis, anatomy and cure of prolapse of the rectum. Surg. Gynecol. Obstet., *15:*7, 1912.

30. Muir, E. G.: Post-anal perineorrhaphy for rectal prolapse. Proc. R. Soc. Med., *48:*33, 1955.

31. Nay, H. R., and Blair, C. R.: Perineal surgical repair of rectal prolapse. Am. J. Surg., *123:*557, 1972.

32. Parks, A. G.: Post-anal perineorrhaphy for rectal prolapse. Proc. R. Soc. Med., *60:*920, 1967.

33. Parks, A. G., Porter, N. H., and Hardcastle, J. D.: The syndrome of the descending perineum. Proc. R. Soc. Med., *59:*477, 1966.

34. Pemberton, J. de J., and Stalker, L. K.: Surgical treatment of complete rectal prolapse. Ann. Surg., *109:*799, 1939.

35. Penfold, J. C. B., and Hawley, P. R.: Experiences of Ivalon-sponge implant for complete rectal prolapse at St. Mark's Hospital 1960–1970. Br. J. Surg., *59:*846, 1972.

36. Porter, N. H.: A physiological study of the pelvic floor in rectal prolapse. Ann. R. Coll. Surg., *31:*379, 1962.

37. Ripstein, C. B.: Procidentia of the rectum: Internal intussusception of the rectum (Stage I rectal prolapse). Dis. Colon Rectum, *18:*458, 1975.

38. Ripstein, C. B.: Definitive corrective surgery. Dis. Colon Rectum, *15:*334, 1972.

39. Ripstein, C. B., and Lanter, B.: Etiology and surgical therapy of massive prolapse of the rectum. Ann. Surg., *157:*259, 1963.

40. Romero-Torres, R.: Sacrofixation with marlex in total prolapse of the rectum. Am. J. Surg., *124:*381, 1972.

41. Stephens, F. D.: Minor surgical conditions of the anus and perineum (in pediatrics). Med. J. Aust., *1:*244, 1958.

42. Stewart, R.: Long-term results of Ivalon wrap operation for complete rectal prolapse. Proc. R. Soc. Med., *65:*777, 1972.

43. Theuerkauf, F. J. Jr., Beahrs, O. H., and Hill, J. R.: Rectal prolapse: causation and surgical treatment. Ann. Surg., *171:*819, 1970.

44. Thiersch. *Quoted by* Carrasco, A. B.: Contribution à l'Etude du Prolapsus du rectum. Paris, Masson, 1934.

45. Thomas, C. G.: Procidentia of rectum: Transsacral repair. Dis. Colon Rectum, *18:*473, 1975.

46. Wells, C.: Rectal prolapse. Nurs. Times., *67:*345, 1971.

47. Wells, C.: New operation for rectal prolapse. Proc. R. Soc. Med., *52:*602, 1959.

# 21

# Constipation

Devoting an entire chapter to a single symptom might, at the outset, appear unwarranted. Nevertheless, the magnitude of the problem in patients who have sustained a long-standing history of constipation of "idiopathic" origin is great. The pharmacology of the various medications used in the treatment of constipation is, frequently, poorly understood. In addition, newer modalities of investigation, which have included transit studies and manometric studies of the anorectal mechanism, have suggested that there may, indeed, be a sound indication for a surgical approach to the problem of constipation in many patients. One realizes, of course, that any suggestion of the use of an operation for the treatment of constipation will undoubtedly be the most controversial topic discussed in this textbook. Nonetheless, patients, often young women, incurr distressing days, and even weeks, before having a bowel movement. The use of a great variety of different laxatives, and/or suppositories, followed by combinations of these with or without the regular use of enemas, becomes the rule in many of these troubled patients. Consequently, a review of the etiology, the pharmacological treatment and the potential use of surgery in the treatment of constipation is appropriate.

## GENERAL PRINCIPLES

### Definition

The word *constipation* has different meanings to different patients, therefore, one must determine what is meant by a complaint of

constipation. The term may imply that stools are too small, too hard, too difficult to expel, or that there is the sensation of incomplete evacuation. These parameters are unreliable or difficult to evaluate. One is, therefore, left with stool frequency as a clinical guide.

In a review of 1,055 presumed normal people working in three factories, and among 400 patients attending a general practitioner's office, Connell and associates found that over 98 per cent of subjects fell within the frequency limits of three bowel actions weekly to three bowel actions daily.[9] There was no correlation with the age of the subjects, but all the subjects with two or fewer bowel actions weekly were women. Therefore, constipation in terms of frequency alone might be defined as fewer than three bowel actions weekly.

Devroede feels that with the available information a patient should be considered constipated if the stool weight is less than 35 grams per day, if fewer than three stools for women, and five for men, per week are passed while following a high residue diet (14.4 grams crude fiber); or if more than three days pass without a bowel movement.[11]

### Etiology

Any attempt at listing the numerous causes of constipation is met immediately with frustration. The causes are numerous and diversified, and, therefore, attempts at classification become either oversimplified or excessively detailed. Numerous classifications have been described (Devroede[11], Jones and Godding[21], Hinton and Lennard-Jones[20], Darlington[10],

Benson[5], French's differential diagnosis[13]). The classification presented in the list below, although not exhaustive, is fairly comprehensive.

---

### CLASSIFICATION OF CAUSES OF CONSTIPATION

FAULTY DIET AND HABITS
  Inadequate bulk (fiber)
  Excessive ingestion of foods which harden stools, (e.g. cheese)
  Lack of exercise
  Ignoring the call to stool
  Environmental changes (hospitalization, vacation)
  Laxative abuse
SPECIFIC DISORDERS OF BOWEL STRUCTURE
  Anal—fissures, hemorrhoids, stenosis, fistulous abscess
  Obstructions—neoplasms (intrinsic or extrinsic), volvulus, hernia, intussusception, inflammations (diverticulitis, ischemic colitis, amoeboma, tuberculosis, syphilis, lymphogranuloma venereum), anastomotic stricture, endometriosis
  Rectocele
  Rectal procidentia
  Descending perineum syndrome
DISORDERS OF MOTILITY
  Idiopathic slow transit
  Irritable bowel syndrome
  Diverticular disease
  Idiopathic megacolon and/or megarectum
PSYCHIATRIC DISORDERS
  Depression
  Psychoses
  Anorexia nervosa
IATROGENIC
  Medication especially codeine, antidepressants and other psychoactive drugs, iron, anticholinergic drugs
  Immobilization
NEUROLOGICAL
  Aganglionosis (Hirschsprung's disease, Chagas' disease)
  Defective innervation (resection of nervi erigentes)
  Spinal cord—neoplasm, lumbosacral cord trauma, multiple sclerosis, paraplegics
  Cerebral—neoplasm, Parkinson's disease
ENDOCRINE AND METABOLIC
  hypothyroidism
  hypercalcemia
  pregnancy
  diabetes mellitus
  dehydration
  hypokalemia
  uremia
  pheochromocytoma
  hypopituitarism
  lead poisoning
  porphyria

---

## FAULTY DIET AND HABIT

A recent advance of outstanding importance is the epidemiological studies of Painter, Burkitt, Walker and others which have shown that the fiber content of our foodstuffs is the prime factor which determines the rate of transit through the colon.[8,30,44] Inadequate dietary fiber, as occurs in the usual western diet, produces sparse inspissated stools; whereas, populations with a high fiber diet may have a normal bowel habit of two or three large, soft motions per day.[44] Since peristaltic movements are stimulated by distention of the intestine they tend to be sluggish when the food bulk is insufficient to cause a normal amount of distention. Excessive ingestion of foods which harden stools, such as processed cheese, will be a contributing factor. Lack of exercise will also decrease colonic activity.

Repeatedly ignoring the call to stool will result in insensitivity of the reflex initiated by a fecal mass in the rectum. This results in adaptation of the sensory mechanism so that arrival of further propulsive waves fails to produce an adequate call to stool. Ultimately all natural periodic urges disappear.

One of the imagined causes of constipation is the belief that a daily stool is necessary for good health. This leads to the chronic abuse of harsh laxatives. After the bowel has been completely emptied by a purgative, it generally takes two days for fecal material to accumulate in sufficient quantity to stimulate the desire for a bowel action. While this may seem self evident, it often increases the distress of a patient whose attention is focussed on his bowel function. Further purgation (because of the failure to have a bowel movement the very next day), will unnecessarily abuse the intestine, and ultimately lead to a complete loss of natural bowel habits (cathartic colon).

Environmental circumstances such as un-favorable working conditions, travel, and admission to the hospital may all cause the patient to ignore the call to stool. Some of these are obviously only temporary problems.

## SPECIFIC DISORDERS OF BOWEL STRUCTURE

Constipation may be only one of several symptoms with which a patient with disorders of bowel structure will present. In association with other symptoms, the examining physician will be led to the appropriate diagnosis, often with the aid of certain investigative modalities. Clearly, obstructive lesions will explain constipation, but these patients may have both an alternating constipation and diarrhea. Similarly, individuals with painful anal lesions will suppress the call to stool because of the fear of the pain of defecation. This, of course, only aggravates the problem as the stool becomes harder and more difficult to pass. A detailed discussion of each cause in this group is out of the scope of this book.

## DISORDERS OF MOTILITY

Using radiopaque markers, a slow transit rate, particularly along the transverse, descending, and sigmoid colon, may be demonstrated. The exact cause is unclear. Patients with idiopathic megabowel have a dilated rectum or distal colon, but ganglion cells are present. Transit studies may also show abnormalities. Patients with irritable bowel syndrome have the dominant complaint of abdominal pain. Constipation is only an associated finding. Constipation is not an uncommon symptom associated with diverticular disease and may result from the tendency of the colon to form closed high pressure segments.

## PSYCHIATRIC DISORDERS

Psychiatric disturbances are often associated with constipation. One must remember, however, that the medications used in the treatment of psychiatric illnesses very frequently contribute to or cause constipation in their own right. Some patients may become obsessed with their bowel function or lack thereof, and resort to excessive laxative abuse. One must also remember that certain psychiatric patients will deny bowel actions while, in fact, their bowels are moving. Such patients can be detected with the use of radiopaque markers.

## IATROGENIC

A host of medications may contribute to constipation (frequent offenders are listed above). One might add that bedpans are uncomfortable, and should be replaced by bedside commodes whenever feasible.

## NEUROLOGICAL

Aganglionosis, as it occurs congenitally with Hirschsprung's disease or is acquired due to the neurotoxin of Trypanosoma cruzi, will cause constipation. Defects of innervation such as those following surgery, as well as diseases of the spinal cord and brain, will be contributing factors.

## ENDOCRINE AND METABOLIC

Various endocrine abnormalities with their characteristic clinical patterns may cause constipation. Also included in this group are those who are pregnant.

## INVESTIGATIONS
### History

One must first confirm the diagnosis of constipation because the patient's presenting symptoms may be more imagined than real. Next, one must determine the onset of the symptoms because onset in childhood may point to a congenital cause such as Hirschsprung's disease, while a more recent onset might pont to one of the specific disorders of bowel structure. Specific questions regarding laxative ingestion and other associated symptoms, bowel, and dietary habits, may lead one to the correct diagnosis. A recent onset in adults is more commonly associated with significant colorectal pathology.

## Physical Examination

In most patients with constipation, abdominal findings will be unremarkable. One might palpate a stool-filled colon. Rarely, one may find a mass suggestive of a carcinoma, or hepatomegaly suggestive of metastases.

The anal region should be carefully inspected for such findings as fissures, hemorrhoids, fistulae, and abscesses. Digital examination of the rectum might reveal a mass suggestive of a carcinoma or, possibly, a rock hard fecaloma.

Almy has pointed out that the absence of stool in the rectum suggests that the difficulty lies above the rectum, and makes a disorder of defecation unlikely.[1] This observation is not valid if the patient is using laxatives, enemas or suppositories.

Anal sensitivity and reflexes should be checked next. Deficient sensation may represent a neurogenic disorder and cutaneosphincteric reflexes may be absent. Characteristically, in Hirschsprung's disease, after rectal examination a profuse fecal discharge occurs.

## Stool Examination

The gross examination of the stool might reveal a large hard mass, or pellet-like stools that are characteristically seen in patients with diverticular disease and also in the irritable bowel syndrome, possibly related conditions. Stool should then be examined for occult blood, and positive findings further investigated.

## Proctosigmoidoscopy

Endoscopic examination is mandatory to rule out the presence of a neoplasm. On occasion, one might find a distal proctitis. Nevertheless, in the vast majority of patients presenting with constipation, proctosigmoidoscopic examination is within normal limits. Not infrequently, patients with long standing laxative abuse, mainly of the anthracene family, will demonstrate melanosis coli, a discoloration of the mucosa which may range from light brown to black.

## Barium Enema

Although plain films of the abdomen occasionally show the extent of fecal accumulation, the main diagnostic tool to demonstrate structural abnormalities in the colon is the barium enema. Certainly, in constipation of recent origin, a barium enema is mandatory. Sometimes an unusually redundant colon is noted, while other times an unusually dilated rectum and/or colon are found.

## Biopsy

When mucosal abnormalities are detected endoscopically, a biopsy is definitely indicated.

When Hirschsprung's disease is suspected, a biopsy is indicated, as classically, aganglionosis is diagnostic of Hirschsprung's disease. However, Devroede has pointed out several difficulties in the histopathological interpretation which prevent him from relying too heavily upon the histology.[11] He is pleased if the neuropathologist finds an abnormality, but disregards the report of a normal biopsy if transit studies and anorectal manometry are abnormal. There are several difficulties in relying too heavily on histology. First, the distal segment of bowel does not contain neurons for up to 25 mm. from the distal edge of the internal sphincter and the normal value for adults is unknown. Second, the severity of the clinical course correlates poorly with the length of the aganglionic segment. A third problem of the histopathological interpretation lies in the potential existence of "skip" lesions. A fourth problem concerns the qualitative appearance of the nervous plexuses. And, finally, quantitatively, hypoganglionosis causes constipation but it is not known what the normal range is.[45] For all these reasons the value of histopathological diagnosis of constipation of local neurogenic origin is, at present, not clearly defined.

## Transit Studies

The next major step in the evaluation of constipation is the measurement of colonic transit time. A technique for measuring gastrointestinal transit time by the use of radiopaque barium-impregnated polythene pellets has recently been described by Hinton.[19] The technique may establish an abnormality, but also may demonstrate a normal transit time in a patient with a bowel neurosis or in the occasional patient who denies having bowel actions. To use this method, the patient stops all laxatives for at least 48 hours prior to and during the investigation. On the first day 20 opaque markers are given before breakfast. On day four and day six plain abdominal radiographs are taken and the number of markers on each film are counted. If all 20 markers are still present on day four, or more than four markers remain on day six, transit is slower than normal. Further films may be taken on subsequent days until all markers are passed to give an indication of the extent of abnormality.

Martelli and colleagues have described a somewhat different technique whereby the patient ingests 20 radiopaque markers which, in fact, are 1 to 2 mm thick rings cut from a radiopaque Levin tube.[27] The patient consumes a high residue diet and refrains from laxatives, enemas, and all other non-essential medications. To distinguish among the different types of constipation, the progression of these markers is followed by daily films of the abdomen until complete expulsion of the markers occurs, but for a maximum of seven days after ingestion. Normal values were obtained by them under controlled conditions. By following the stools daily, one may distinguish the patients suffering from outlet obstruction where the markers proceed quickly along the colon but accumulate in the rectum, from those suffering from colorectal inertia where at the end of the test, markers are distributed throughout the large bowel from the cecum to the rectum. In situations where only a portion of the colon demonstrates inertia, the markers may collect in either the right or left colon.

### Anorectal Manometry

The study of anorectal pressures and reflexes might enable the attending physician to select patients who may be candidates for operative treatment for their constipation problem. For instance, in patients with Hirschsprung's disease, rectal distention does not induce internal sphincter relaxation. In addition, one should realize that there are many other demonstrable pressure abnormalities that can be detected by anorectal manometry in patients with idiopathic constipation.[26] The reflex may be normal, or the amplitude of relaxation may be less than in normal controls, or the reflex may be totally absent. The resting pressure of the anal canal may be greater than expected, and occasionally, this is accompanied by a rectoanal inhib-

itory reflex whose amplitude is greater than normal. Finally, at rest, wide variations of pressure may be demonstrated, far exceeding normal spontaneous oscillations. This may or may not be accompanied by a superimposed rectoanal inhibitory reflex. Several probes have been used to study anorectal pressure profiles and reflexes. (Lawson[24], Shuster[33], Arhan[4])

## WHY TREAT CONSTIPATION?
### Dispel Myths

Patients must first be reassured that there is a wide variation of normality in regard to the frequency of bowel movements. The folklore and mythology associated with the need for daily evacuation must be dispelled. Advertising encourages self purgation by making people feel "guilty" about constipation, and by portraying daily bowel movements as the secret to a healthy and happy life. Erroneous concepts such as the belief that toxic substances may be absorbed into the body without a daily bowel movement must be cast aside.

### Associated Symptoms and Daily Activity

Martelli and colleagues noted that constipation is not without associated symptoms and complications.[26] They noted the disappearance of a multitude of symptoms after successful surgical care of constipation.

Symptoms described included hard stools, stools difficult to evacuate, abdominal distention and bloating, and anorexia. Signs included fecalomas, abdominal masses, and abdominal tenderness. To this list Thompson added foul breath, furred tongue, flatulence, headache and irritability.[41]

Regardless of the cause of constipation, absence of the numerous associated symptoms should allow the patient to function better in his usual daily activity.

### Potential Disease

The latest food fad encourages a diet containing large amounts of unprocessed bran. While the immediate adverse effect of low fiber diets is constipation, the long-term adverse effects may include diverticular disease and malignancy. This is based upon studies that link the low-fiber content of the usual

Western diet with an increased risk of colonic cancer and diverticulosis.[30]

Three studies establish the link between cancer and constipation.[7,18,46] More women with cancer of the colon had antecedent constipation than a comparable group of unconstipated controls. More men with cancer of the rectum had a history of constipation. In Wynder's study, having three stools per week for a long period of time was considered a risk factor.[46]

There are no available data to substantiate the claim that volvulus of the large bowel is frequently preceeded by long standing constipation. In many cases, hard stools with straining are the initiating factors in the development of fissures and hemorrhoids.

### Economic Consideration

Constipation creates an economic problem of staggering proportions. Well over 200 million dollars is spent annually for non-prescription laxatives.[10] A common misconception is that non-prescription medication is totally safe and without adverse effect. If a bowel movement is induced by a laxative, it may be several days before enough stool is present for another bowel movement. Therefore, when an individual attempts to maintain a daily bowel movement with the prolonged use of laxatives, a viscious cycle may develop in which either more of the same laxative or a more potent one must be used. A "cathartic colon" may then develop. This long standing use of laxatives creates a varying degree of financial burden upon a given patient.

### TREATMENT

Almy described the aims in the treatment of a patient with chronic constipation to be the restoration of normal frequency and consistency of stools, freedom from the discomforts ordinarily associated with constipation, the maintenance of reasonably regular elimination without artificial aids, and the relief of any generalized illness of which constipation may be a symptom.[1,2] Although these are the ideal goals, one should nevertheless seek to achieve them if at all possible.

### Correction of Faulty Diet and Habits

Since the commonest cause of constipation is faulty diet and habits management often re-

quires no more than a careful examination and reassurance, together with simple guidance. Patients should be advised not to ignore the call to stool, as neglect only disrupts the normal adaptive relaxation mechanism of the rectum yielding fecal stasis. Simple exercise should be encouraged: some patients, with nothing more than a regular walk in the morning or evening, claim an easier and more satisfactory bowel action. Environmental factors such as working conditions, are often difficult to change. If the history reveals excessive ingestion of foods which cause hardened stools such as processed cheese, then such foods might be eliminated, or at least reduced in quantity.

Fiber-containing foodstuffs have hydrophilic properties which soften the stool. The increased volume of feces favors the stimulation of a natural peristaltic reflex. Cereals, especially bran, are good agents in this regard. The most inexpensive, and highest concentration of crude fiber, is unprocessed bran or Miller's bran.[28] This easily obtainable material has been found to be effective in lowering intraluminal pressure, and decreasing transit time in patients with constipation and diverticular disease. Coarser bran is more beneficial because of its greater water-holding capacity.[22] In addition, the diet should contain generous portions of vegetables and fruits. Foods with fat (not excessive) are of value. Patients who are unable to achieve adequate intake of fiber-containing foods should supplement their diets with hydrophilic preparations such as psyllium seed extracts which act in a similar fashion.

In his diet trial Devroede recommends that patients have an average intake of 14.4 gm. of crude fiber per day.[11] Sample diets are shown in Appendix B. Patients are instructed to record each bowel movement. They are also instructed to stop taking drugs, if not essential, particularly laxatives, and not to resort to enemas. This treatment is continued for a month. Patients who fail to respond to a change in diet, (men should have more than five and women more than three stools per week) may require further studies, such as colonic transit time and manometry.

### Medical Treatment

Obviously specific metabolic and endocrinological problems such as hypothyroidism must be treated on their own merits. A favorite recommendation is for the patient to sit on the toilet at regular intervals, and for prolonged periods of time, regardless whether there is an urge to defecate or not. However, the value of such a ritual is open to debate. Antispasmodics may relieve cramping in individuals with the irritable bowel syndrome. Nevertheless, constipation remains a common and sometimes formidable challenge.

*Laxatives.* Laxatives are compounds that facilitate the passage and elimination of feces from the colon and rectum. In addition to the treatment of constipation, valid indications for the use of laxatives include preparation for gastrointestinal investigations, and surgery.

With the almost countless number of laxatives available on the market today classification of such drugs becomes extremely important, but correspondingly difficult. Darlington reported that there are more than 700 proprietary laxative preparations available in almost every dosage form.[10] The classification presented is a modification of the ones presented by Goodman and Gilman and Steinberg.[15,38] This classification is based on the mechanism of action of the drug.

---

### CLASSIFICATION OF LAXATIVES
STIMULANTS
    Anthracene (emodium, anthraquinone)
        cascara sagrada
        senna (Senokot)
        danthron
        rhubarb
    Castor Oil
    Diphenylmethane Cathartics
        bisacodyl (Dulcolax)
        phenolphthalein
        oxyphenisatin acetate
MECHANICAL
    Saline Laxatives
        magnesium sulphate (epsom salts), Milk of Magnesia, magnesium citrate, magnesium carbonate, sodium sulphate (Glauber's salt), sodium phosphate, potassium sodium tartrate (Rochelle salt)
    Bulk-Forming Agents
        psyllium seed preparations (Plantago) Metamucil, Konsyl, LA Formula, Hydrocil, Mucilose, Siblin
        synthetic mucilloids (Methylcellulose, sodium carboxymethylcellulose
        agar

---

        tragacanth
        karaya gum
        bran
    Mineral Oil
    Surface-Active Agents
        dioctyl sodium sulfosuccinate (Colace, doxinate, Bulax, DOSS)
        dioctyl calcium sulfosuccinate (Surfak)
        Poloxalkol
MISCELLANEOUS
    Lactulose
OBSOLETE CATHARTICS
    calomel, aloe, podophyllum, jalap, colocynth, elaterin, ipomea, gambage, croton oil, sulfur

---

One must also remember that all cathartics are contraindicated in a patient with abdominal cramps, colic, nausea, vomiting, or any undiagnosed abdominal pain.

The drugs in each group act similarly and will hence be described in groups.

STIMULANT LAXATIVES. This group chemically stimulates the intestinal wall to increased peristaltic activity, and hence causes gripping, intestinal cramps, increased mucus secretion, and excessively rapid evacuation in some patients. The mechanism of action is by irritation of the intestinal mucosa, or selective action upon the intramural nervous plexus or intestinal smooth muscle. Increased water and electrolyte excretion is attributed to more rapid transit of feces through the intestine. The initiation of the irritant activity may be in either the small intestine or the large bowel. Although it might be expected that the colon must always be the site of laxative irritant activity, this is not the case. Any agent that increases the propulsive activity of the small intestine necessarily accelerates large bowel peristalsis.

These agents are useful in the treatment of acute constipation as well as constipation due to prolonged bed rest or hospitalization, and preparation for radiological examinations. Abuse, however, may lead to "cathartic colon": a poorly functioning large intestine and, hence, prolonged use should be discouraged.

MECHANICAL CLEANSING. This group increases propulsive activity by either increasing the bulk of the stool or changing the consistency of the stool. Traditional teaching dictates that hypertonic salts attract and retain a large volume of isotonic fluid in the gastrointestinal tract, thus stimulating peristalsis in the small intestine, reducing transit time, and causing the passage of a watery stool. Recent findings suggest that saline cathartics stimulate the release of cholecystokinin, stimulating small bowel motility, and inhibiting absorption of fluid and electrolytes from the jejunum and ileum.[17] These laxatives should be given with adequate amounts of water for two reasons: first, the holdover in the stomach is shortened; and second, the patient suffers less dehydration. Upon oral administration, laxation occurs in three to six hours.

The laxative effect of bulk-forming agents is due to the absorption and retention of large amounts of water. Mechanical distention caused by this increased residue of unabsorbed material promotes peristalsis, and facilitates passage of stool. The laxative effect is usually seen within 24 hours of ingestion but may take up to three days. Side effects are relatively rare. Minor adverse effects include frequent flatulence and borborygmi. Esophageal, gastric, small intestinal, and colonic obstructions, as well as fecal impactions have been reported. Therefore, this group of agents should be taken with generous amounts of fluids in order to avoid such problems.

Liquid petrolatum retards the absorption of water from the stool, and thus softens fecal material. The onset of action is approximately six to eight hours. It can be administered orally or as an enema. The usual dose is 15 to 45 ml. Mineral oil should not be taken at bedtime because of the dangers of aspiration. It is best taken between meals to obviate any tendency for interference with absorption of fat soluble-vitamins. It should not be used in the presence of dysphagia because of the threat of lipoid pneumonia. Pruritus ani and anal leakage are minor annoying side effects.

Dioctyl sulfosuccinates in their sodium or calcium salt lower surface tension at the oil-water interface of the stool, thereby softening the stool by permitting a greater penetration of feces by water and fat. More recently, it has been suggested that dioctyl sulfosuccinate stimulates fluid and electrolyte secretion as well.[12] The usual daily dose is 100 to 200 mg. They act within 24 to 48 hours.

Lactulose is a synthetic disaccharide not digested by small intestinal or pancreatic enzymes. In the colon it is metabolized by microflora with resultant acidification of the stool and release of gas. It is effective in treating constipation, and changes the nature of the colon flora. The resultant anions may cause osmotic catharsis, and for this reason, the agent might be classified with the saline laxatives. However, it is too costly for routine administration, and, with long term use, there is the risk of superinfection.[41]

SUPPOSITORIES are useful for evacuating the lower bowel, and have been advocated when considering an enema. They are probably not as effective as an enema but are more aesthetically acceptable to patient and nurse. The insertion of an inert cylinder such as a glycerine suppository often initiates a defecation response, usually within 30 minutes. This appears to be a reflex act. Other suppositories contain bisacodyl, dioctyl sodium sulfosuccinate, senna, or carbon dioxide.

ENEMAS. Clinical indications for enemas include preparation for endoscopic examination, surgery or childbirth, removal of fecal impaction and barium, and certain cases of acute constipation. Warm tap water or warm saline enemas are preferred. Soapsuds and hydrogen peroxide enemas are quite irritating to the colonic mucosa, and should be avoided. As well, hypertonic phosphate salts are quite irritating to the colonic mucosa, and tend to stimulate the rectum to produce a large amount of mucus which may interfere with an evaluation of the state of the mucosa. They work within approximately five minutes, and act by causing distention and by osmotic activity. They may give rise to sodium retention. However, the practical advantage of the packaged enemas recommends their use in a busy office practice. Enemas should be administered with the patient lying on his left side or prone and the enema bag 2 feet above the level of the rectum. Material should be introduced slowly with as many temporary interruptions as are necessary to prevent cramps. Repositioning the patient on his right side might help assure adequate distribution of the enema fluid.

Certain dangers are involved with enemas including electrolyte depletion, water intoxication, colonic perforation, and even psychologic dependence.

There are several potential adverse effects that may result from the overconsumption of laxatives. The ill-effects of laxative abuse may be greater than those of constipation. They include: (*1.*) dehydration and electrolyte disturbance, (*2.*) hypokalemia, (*3.*) hypermagnesemia, (*4.*) nausea, vomiting and abdominal distress, (*5.*) malabsorption, (*6.*) parafinomas, (*7.*) lipoid pneumonia, (*8.*) intestinal obstruction, (*9.*) specific toxic effect, (*10.*) anal stenosis, (*11.*) dependence, and (*12.*) colonic structural injury.

### Surgery

The indications for surgery in constipation of recent origin are relatively clear, and are related to the underlying cause of the constipation such as cancer or diverticular disease. Patients suffering from Hirschsprung's disease are usually operated on during childhood, but some reach adulthood before the problem is recognized.[15] In short segment, Hirschsprung's disease, anorectal myotomy may suffice to cure the patient.[6,25,26,29,34,36,39]

On the other hand, the indications for surgery in chronic constipation are poorly defined and controversial, at best. Martelli, et al, in a radically different approach to constipation, reported that good results in this group could be achieved through adequate selection and choice of treatment.[26] The high cost of treating constipation, and the uncontrolled utilization of laxatives with their complications would seem to support the contention that no patient should need to resort to a life long consumption of laxatives and administration of enemas, if another solution is available.

Devroede has classified patients with constipation of unknown origin in terms of the segment of bowel which has the disordered function.[11] He described three groups: outlet obstruction is when the anorectal junction does not relax properly; hind-gut dysfunction is when the right colon empties very well, but markers accumulate in the left, sigmoid colon, and rectum; and, colonic inertia is when the entire large bowel fails to propel contents. Although this classification leaves the physician with the task of uncovering the cause of each type of constipation, it has the advantage of permitting a rational surgical approach to the problem.

Preliminary results with anorectal myectomy appear promising with regard to outlet obstruction, and can be achieved without mortality and with little morbidity. Indications for surgery are based on colonic function, taking into account an abnormally low frequency of defecation, delayed transit time of radiopaque markers, and/or abnormalities detected with anorectal manometry. These abnormalities include an absent rectoanal inhibitory reflex, anal contraction instead of relaxation when the rectum is distended, spontaneous variations of pressure in the rectum and anal canal, a hypertonic anal canal, abnormalities of the rectoanal inhibitory reflex with sometimes lesser and other times greater amplitudes of relaxation, and pressure exceeding predistension values before returning to the resting level (overshoot).

The technique consists of a submucosal resection of a 1 cm wide strip of muscle posteriorly. It includes the full thickness of the internal sphincter, and both muscular layers of the rectal wall up to 6 cm above the dentate line (Fig. 21-1).

Anorectal myectomy was performed in 62 patients: 62 per cent of the 50 patients with fewer than three stools per week had more than three per week one year after myectomy.[26] The six patients who were operated on because of the abnormal transit of radiopaque markers, and the six patients for abnormal manometric findings were all asymptomatic. Of the 26 per cent of patients who were incontinent preoperatively, two-thirds became continent postoperatively. However, 16 per cent of the patients who were continent preoperatively became incontinent post-operatively. The degree of incontinence experienced was similar to that following sphincterotomy for anal fissure. Shandling, et al performed poste-

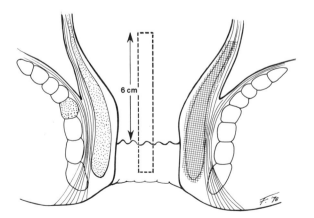

**FIGURE 21-1.** *Posterior anorectal myectomy.*

rior internal sphincterotomy in children with constipation and reported good results.[34]

Theory based on rather extensive experience with lateral internal sphincterotomy in the treatment of fissure-in-ano would suggest that a lateral internal sphincterotomy would result in fewer problems than a posterior sphincterotomy. In addition, a sphincterotomy would probably also suffice rather than a myectomy. But these opinions are only conjecture at the present time.

Aminev and associates have recommended operative management for constipation in certain selected cases.[3] Thompson recommends colectomy and ileorectal anastomosis for patients with severe constipation and megacolon secondary to laxative abuse which, because of long standing usage, has destroyed the colon's power of propulsion.[40]

Patients who suffer from colonic inertia may also occasionally be cured by surgery. Should the inertia involve only a portion of the colon, such as the right colon, then, possibly, a right hemicolectomy might overcome the constipation problem. If the transit studies demonstrate inertia of the left colon then a left hemicolectomy might correct the problem. Patients with total colonic inertia should have a total abdominal colectomy and ileorectal anastomosis. Very seldom, if the patients also complain of fecal incontinence, a proctocolectomy and ileostomy can be performed. Devroede recommends a Soave procedure in patients who have undergone an anorectal myectomy with no success, and in whom markers have demonstrated a delayed transit time in the descending and sigmoid colon.[11]

## SPECIAL PROBLEMS
### Prevention of Constipation

There are certain clinical circumstances in which straining at stool presents an added hazard to the patient. Patients who have had a myocardial infarction, patients with cerebral and cardiovascular disease and thromboembolic disease are at special risk. These patients should be placed on bulk-forming agents, either in natural foodstuffs or with a psyllium seed preparation.

### Fecal Impaction

Fecal impaction is a serious crisis which may constitute an intestinal obstruction. Ninety-eight per cent of fecal impactions occur in the rectum. Fecal impaction in an undistressed individual can be evacuated with oral laxatives, such as Senokot, in doses of six tablets twice daily. More likely, administration of enemas will be required, and tap water enemas will prove effective. Mineral oil and dioctyl sodium sulfosuccinate have been advocated, although their effectiveness is probably due to the fluid volume. In an acutely distressed individual, digital evacuation can be achieved with moderate sedation.

Recurrent fecal impaction should be prevented by reviewing the background factors which have led to the impaction, and eliminating or avoiding them in the future. Dietary management as previously mentioned, as well as suppositories, and senna preparations may have to be given. Lactulose in a dose of 10 ml twice a day is useful, especially in the unusual cases where fecalomas pack the large bowel all the way to the cecum.

### Psychiatric States

As noted above, various psychiatric states are associated with constipation. The clinician should also remember that various antidepressent drugs are constipating. Constipation due to the latter cause is amenable to the stimuant laxatives. One must be careful not to overlook an organic cause of constipation in this group of patients.

### Idiopathic Megarectum and Megacolon

Among the many adult patients who complain of chronic constipation, there will be a few who have adult megacolon. In some of these, the myenteric plexus may be damaged. Abnormalities of motor function remain incompletely understood, and consequently, present considerable frustration to patient and clinician alike. The role of surgery in their management is still controversial and often disappointing. Resection may appear drastic but as Dyer and colleagues pointed out, it is the treatment of choice since local procedures in the sphincter may not be of permanent benefit, and bypass operations may not prove adequate because of their failure to produce progressive movements in the intestine.[14]

Todd pointed out that while a megabowel may result from recognized neurological, toxic, mechanical, and degenerative pathology such as Hirschsprung's disease, Chagas' disease, volvulus and systemic sclerosis, there is a type of dilatation where the muscle layers of the intestine and their intrinsic and extrinsic innervations appear to be normal.[42] This is called idiopathic megabowel. Large amounts of feces accumulate without initiating defecation. He feels that the treatment of pathological megabowel is mainly surgical, but that of idiopathic megabowel is mostly medical. Treatment consists of keeping the rectum empty without waiting for an urge to defecate. The untreated patients with gross distention may require repeated oil enemas followed by evacuatant enemas and sometimes digital manipulation. Senokot usually proves to be very helpful to these patients. Most of them will need to use a glycerine or Dulcolax suppository. Optimum treatment is probably Senokot tablets in a dosage sufficient to have the desired effect of keeping the stools soft, together with a suppository as required. However, using Devroede's criteria, some of these patients might, in fact, be surgical candidates.

### Spinal Cord Injuries

About the third or fourth night after injury, a laxative is given, followed, if necessary, by a suppository the next morning. This is continued until a regular bowel habit is achieved. Digital removal, and one or two enemas may be required in the first week or two. One should aim at bowel evacuation every other day. Diet should contain plentiful amounts of fiber-containing foods. A chemical stimulant such as Senokot or Dulcolax should be administered on alternate nights. Stimulation to initiate defecation might include body movement, eating, drinking, massage of the abdomen, anal digital stimulation, or insertion of a suppository.

### Constipation in the Geriatric Population

Delay in transit time, incomplete emptying, diminished awareness, and neglect of the call to stool are the four most commonly occurring causes of constipation in the elderly.[19] Because they are physically inactive individuals, often immobile in bed, a loss of tone in the musculature of the elderly makes it difficult to empty the bowel completely without the consequent necessity of straining at stool.

Jones and Godding pointed out that there are several complications of constipation which are more prone to occur in the elderly.[21]

These include: cardiovascular changes, gastrointestinal effects (including pain simulating angina pectoris), and fecal impaction. As a consequence of fecal impaction, fecal incontinence may occur, and if unrecognized may cause a patient to be institutionalized unnecessarily. Other consequences of impaction include intestinal obstruction, restlessness and confusioned states, rectal hemorrhage due to stercoral ulceration, and urinary retention.

Therapeutic measures have emphasized reassurance with retraining the bowels; encouragement of physical activity, in-take of adequate fluids, and dietary alterations; avoidance of constipation; and treatment of known underlying diseases, especially hypothyroidism. Such recommendations infer a readily curable problem, but when the patient is elderly, such hope is unrealistic.[31] These patients usually require laxatives: the agents of choice are stimulant laxatives such as Senokot or Dulcolax. Saline purgatives may disturb water and electrolyte balance, while the hazards of liquid paraffin are well recognized. Bulk-forming agents must be accompanied by adequate amounts of fluids, but are contraindicated where fecal accumulations are already present. Stool "softeners" may be inappropriate if the stool is already soft, but rather the neuromuscular responses in the colon need stimulation. Successful therapy turns out to be an individual trial and error proposition.

For the nursing home patient who is debilitated and unable to promptly heed the call to stool an acceptable routine for management includes the regular use of enemas. Tap water enemas administered every three to five days will effectively keep the colon empty, and the patient comfortable.

### Constipation in Obstetrical Patients

Multiple etiological factors are implicated in the occurrence of constipation during pregnancy. Decreased physical activity, changes in hormonal concentration (possibly contributing to atony of the gut muscle), decreased bulk in the diet, and the use of drugs such as iron, may all contribute. During pregnancy the aim should be prevention of constipation, and this is best accomplished with adequate dietary fiber augmented by bulk-forming agents if necessary. Laxatives are best avoided, but if necessary, the choice lies between Bisocodyl and

Senna. Senna is safe for both mother and baby with no known adverse effects on nutrition or lactation.[35] Soft stools passed without straining may help prevent the problems of hemorrhoids and anal fissures so frequently associated with pregnancy. In the puerperium, results have shown that a simple safe, and inexpensive method of preventing constipation has been established by the use of Senokot.

## Terminally Ill Patients

Lamberton has reported that patients who are dying, especially from carcinomatosis, present an often neglected problem.[23] Their constipation, frequently aggravated by the universal administration of an opiate analgesic, leads to the distressing symptoms of abdominal distention, and excessive gas with added pain and even vomiting. He feels that these patients may benefit by an enema, and greater attention should be paid to make their dying days more comfortable and peaceful. They should prophylactically receive a laxative with the opiate analgesic.

## REFERENCES

1. Almy, T. P.: Constipation. *In* Sleisenger, M. H., and Fordtran, J. S. (ed.): Gastrointestinal Disease. Philadelphia, W. B. Saunders, 1973.

2. Almy, T. P.: Management of chronic constipation. *In* Turell, R. (ed.): Diseases of the Colon and Anorectum. Philadelphia, W. B. Saunders, 1969.

3. Aminev, A. M., Golovachev, V. L., and Veretenkov, V. I.: The surgical management of intestinal stasis. Am. J. Proct., *27:*37, 1976.

4. Arhan, P., Faverdin, C., and Thouvenot, J.: Anorectal motility in sick children. Scand. J. Gastroenterol., *7:*309, 1972.

5. Benson, J. A.: Simple chronic constipation pathophysiology and management. Postgrad. Med., *57:*1:55, 1975.

6. Bentley, J. F. R.: Posterior excisional anorectal myotomy in management of chronic fecal accumulation. Arch. Dis. Childhood, *41:*144, 1966.

7. Bjelke, E.: Epidemologic studies of cancer of the stomach, colon and rectum. Scand. J. Gastroenterol. [Suppl], *9:*31, 1974.

8. Burkitt, D. P.: Epidemiology of the cancer of the colon and the rectum. Cancer, *28:*3, 1971.

9. Connell, A. M., Hilton, C., Irvine, G.,

10. Darlington, R. C.: *In* Griffenhagen, G. B. and Hawkins, L. L. (eds.): Handbook of Non-Prescription Drugs. 4 ed. 66-76. Washington, D.C., American Pharmaceutical Association, 1973.

11. Devroede, G.: Constipation: Mechanisms and management. *In* M. H. Sleisenger, and Fordtran, J. S. (eds.): Gastrointestinal Disease. 2 ed. Philadelphia, W. B. Saunders, 1978.

12. Donowitz, M., and Binder, H. J.: Effect of Dioctyl sodium sulfosuccinate on colonic fluid and electrolyte movement. Gastroenterol., *69:*941, 1975.

13. Douthwaite, A. H., (Ed.): French's Index of Differential Diagnosis, 9 ed. 185, Chicago, John Wright and Sons, 1967.

14. Dyer, N. H., Dawson, A. M., Smith, B. F., and Todd, I. P.: Obstruction of bowel due to lesion in the myenteric plexus. Br. Med. J., *1:*686, 1969.

15. Fairgrieve, J.: Hirschsprung's disease in the adult. Br. J. Surg., *50:*506, 1962.

16. Goodman, L. S., and Gilman, A. (eds.): The Pharmacological Basis of Therapeutics. 5 ed. New York, Macmillan Publishing, 1975.

17. Harvey, R. F., and Read, A. E.: Mode of action of the saline purgatives. Am. Heart J., *89:*810, 1975.

18. Higginson, J.: Etiological factors in gastrointestinal cancer in man. J. Nat. Cancer Instit., *37:*527, 1966.

19. Hinton, J. M.: Studies with drugs and hormones on the human colon. Proc. Roy. Soc. Med., *60:*215, 1967.

20. Hinton, J. M., and Lennard-Jones, J. E.: Constipation: definition and classification. Postgrad. Med. J., *44:*720, 1968.

21. Jones, F. A., and Godding, E. W.: Management of Constipation. London, Blackwell Scientific Publications, 1972.

22. Kirwan, W. O., Smith, A. N., McConnell, A. A., Mitchell, M. D., and Eastwood, M. A.: Action of different bran preparations on colonic function. Br. Med. J., *4:*187, 1974.

23. Lamerton, R.: Resurrected by an enema. Nursing Times, *72:*1653, 1976.

24. Lawson, J. O. N., and Nixon, H. H.: Anal canal pressures in the diagnosis of Hirschsprung's disease. J. Ped. Surg., *2:*544:1967.

25. Lynn, H. B.: Rectal myectomy for aganglionic megacolon. Mayo Clin. Proc., *41:*289, 1966.

Lennard-Jones, J. E., and Misiewicz, J. J.: Variation of bowel habit in two population samples. Proc. Roy. Soc. Med., *59:*11, 1966.

26. Martelli, H., Devroede, G., Arhan, P., and Duguay, C. Mechanisms of idiopathic constipation: outlet obstruction. Gastroenterol., *75:*623, 1978.

27. Martelli, H., et al: Some parameters of large bowel function in normal man. Gastroenterol., *75:*612, 1978.

28. Medical Letter, *15:*98, 1973.

29. Nissan, S., and Bar-Maor, J. A.: Further experience in the diagnosis and surgical treatment of short segment Hirschsprung's disease and idiopathic megacolon. J. Ped. Surg., *6:*738, 1971.

30. Painter, N. S., and Burkitt, D. P.: Diverticular disease of the colon: a deficiency disease of Western civilizations. Br. Med. J., *2:*450, 1971.

31. Palmer, E. D.: "Presbycolon" problems in the nursing home. JAMA., *235:*1150, 1976.

32. Pietrusko, R. G.: Use and abuse of laxatives. Am. J. Hosp. Pharm., *34:*291, 1977.

33. Schuster, M. M., Hookman, P., Hendrix, T. R., and Mendeloff, A. I.: Simultaneous manometric recording of internal and external anal sphincter reflexes. Bull. Johns Hopkins Hosp., *116:*79, 1965.

34. Shandling, B., and Desjardins, J. G.: Anal myomectomy for constipation. J. Ped. Surg., *4:*115, 1969.

35. Shelton, M. G. *cited by* Jones, F. A., and Godding, E. W.: Management of Constipation. London, Blackwell Scientific Publications, 1972.

36. Shermeta, D. W., and Nilprabhassorn, P.: Posterior myectomy for primary and secondary short segment aganglionosis. Am. J. Surg., *133:*39, 1977.

37. Smith, B.: Pathologic changes in the colon produced by anthraquinone purgatives. Dis. Colon Rectum, *16:*455, 1973.

38. Steinberg, H.: *In* Turell, R. (ed.): ?. Applied pharmacology related to the colon. *In* Diseases of the colon and Anorectum. Philadelphia, W. B. Saunders, 1969.

39. Thomas, C. G., Bream, C. A., and DeConnick, P.: Posterior sphincterotomy and rectal myotomy in the management of Hirschsprung's disease. Ann. Surg., *171:*796, 1970.

40. Thompson, H. R.: Colectomy for colitis and constipation. Transactions of the Medical Society of London, *80:*107, 1964.

41. Thompson, W. G.: Constipation and catharsis. Can. Med. Assoc. J., *114:*927, 1976.

42. Todd, I.: Some aspects of adult megacolon. Proc. Roy. Soc. Med., *64:*561, 1971.

43. Travell, J.: Pharmacology of stimulant laxatives. Ann. NY Acad. Sci., *58:*416, 1954.

44. Walker, A. R. P., Walker, B. F., and Richardson, B. D.: Bowel transit times in Bantu populations. Br. Med. J., *3:*48, 1970.

45. Weinberg, A. G.: The anorectal myenteric plexus: its relation to hypoganglionosis of the colon. Am. J. Clin. Path., *54:*637, 1970.

46. Wynder, E. L., and Shigematsu, T.: Environmental factors of cancer of the colon and rectum. Cancer, *20:*1520, 1967.

# 22

# Anal Incontinence

Anal continence is dependent on a complex series of learned and reflex responses to colonic and rectal stimuli. There is also considerable individual variation in bowel habits that make clear distinction of derangement of continence difficult. The patient who has lost complete control of solid feces has complete incontinence. The patient who complains of inadvertent soiling or escape of liquid or gas has partial incontinence. Less fastidious individuals may not offer complaints of partial incontinence, and therefore, careful questioning may be necessary. Therapeutic recommendations for incontinence can best be made with a better understanding of the anatomy and physiology of the anorectal region. The reader is thus referred to those chapters for review.

## ETIOLOGY
### Previous Surgical Procedures

*Internal Sphincterotomy.* In performing an internal sphincterotomy for treatment of fissure-in-ano, various amounts of the internal sphincter are incised. This may lead to partial incontinence of liquid or gas due to inadequate closure of the anal canal by the internal sphincter. This is usually temporary, but may be permanent.

*Fistula surgery* is the anorectal procedure most commonly followed by postoperative incontinence. Gross incontinence of feces may be avoided if the anorectal ring is preserved. However, minor defects in continence may

With collaboration of John D. Nicholson

follow if even a small amount of sphincter muscle is severed. This complication may be reduced by avoiding wide retraction of the severed ends of the sphincter mechanism. This may be accomplished by either placing a seton or "coring out" the fistulous tract, with subsequent sparing of the sphincter mechanism (see Chap. 8).

*Hemorrhoidectomy.* In modern surgery for hemorrhoids, incontinence is a rare complication. However, if the sphincter mass is inadvertently injured as in blind clamping techniques where the internal sphincter is grasped by a clamp, incontinence may result. It has been suggested that minor alterations in continence may be due to the removal of the hemorrhoidal tissue: a tissue described as possibly functioning as a corpus cavernosum of the anus.[16] When incorrectly performed, the Whitehead operation leads to eversion of the rectal mucosa onto the anoderm. This results in incontinence by destruction of the normal sensory mechanism, and mucosal leak from the exposed mucosal surface onto the perineum. Rarely, a circumferential scar will form following hemorrhoidectomy. This may lead to improper closure of the anal canal causing partial incontinence.

*Sphincter Saving Operations.* In the usual anterior resection normal continence for gas, liquid, or solid feces is generally maintained. However, when the anastomosis is performed in the distal third of the rectum, impairment of normal continence is not infrequent. Incontinence to liquid or gas often follows, and the patient may be unaware of a sudden bolus of stool. These problems are frequent in the early postoperative period, but subside within six months in the great majority of patients. The lower limit of an anastomosis without interfering with gross mechanism of incontinence is at the uppermost level of the anal canal at the top of the anorectal ring which is approximately 4 cm from the anal verge in most individuals.

Abdomino-anal pull-through resection of the rectum has a high incidence of partial incontinence. In a review of his results with this procedure, Hughes found that only 29 per cent of the patients were classified as having normal function postoperatively; 23 per cent were classified as having severe incontinence; and the remaining 48 per cent admitted to minor incontinence.[9]

Parks describes a colo-anal sleeve anastomosis for treatment of rectal mucosal lesions. In a limited series of five patients reported in 1976, all had an alteration in continence. They were continent for solid feces, and none had to wear a pad to prevent soiling despite some difficulty with loose stools or flatus.[8]

The abdomino-transsacral approach popularized by Localio for resection of mid rectal neoplasms preserves the sphincter mechanism. He reported on 100 patients in 1978 who were all continent for fluid, flatus, and feces postoperatively.[10] In this procedure, as with low anterior resection, it is the extent of the distal dissection that is the prime determinant of sphincter function.

Utilizing new mechanical devices for performing end-to-end anastomoses (EEA Stapler), it is now technically possible to perform extremely low rectal anastomoses. However, if the anorectal ring is disturbed, partial or total incontinence may be observed. The severity and duration of the dysfunction is not predictable. Goligher recently reported on 62 patients in which a low anterior anastomosis was performed using the Russian Model 249 stapling device. In all 50 patients with the anastomoses 7 cm or greater from the anal verge, continence was complete. In the 12 patients with the anastomosis less than 7 cm from the anal verge, all initially had less than perfect continence. With time, however, five have subsequently developed perfect continence, three have nearly perfect continence, and four are still imperfect.[5]

## Obstetrical Lacerations

Vaginal delivery and its complications are among the most common causes of surgically correctable incontinence seen in practice today. During vaginal delivery, tears of the perineum are common. To prevent this complication, obstetricians have devised various controlled incisions to facilitate delivery. One popular method is a median epistiotomy. This usually heals well, and without complication following primary suture repair. However, if there is a breakdown of the repair, or if infection occurs, the patient may become incontinent.

## Aging

A very common cause of anal incontinence is old age and general debilitation. With better investigative equipment becoming available, future research may reveal a specific abnormality; but currently, elderly individuals frequently suffer from incontinence without one of the other underlying or precipitating factors described in this section being present.

## Procidentia

In the case of procidentia or complete rectal prolapse, the internal and external sphincter mechanisms may be chronically impaired. This is associated with incontinence in over 50 per cent of cases.[12] Repair of the procidentia generally does little to change the status of the sphincter mechanism. Various treatments have been applied in the past including waiting and hoping the sphincter tone would return, electrical stimulation of the sphincter mechanisms, and various plicating operations.[1,2] None of these methods meet with uniform success, although the Parks post anal repair described below has proven useful. Therefore, the problem of procidentia with incontinence would best be treated by preventative means, correcting the prolapse before incontinence occurs. (see Chap. 20)

## Trauma

In the case of impalement injuries, the sphincter mechanism is often disrupted. Depending upon the extent of the injury, primary repair may be achieved without a protective colostomy. However, if the tissues are badly destroyed, and there has been a delay in recognition, protective colostomy with later definitive repair is preferable.

## Irradiation

With the treatment of cervical and uterine cancers by extracavitary and intracavitary irradiation, varying degrees of destruction of the muscular components of the rectum and anal canal occur, resulting in various degrees of irradiation proctitis. Although no treatment of irradiation-induced incontinence is uniformly rewarding, two or three daily cleansing enemas are generally recommended, along with a high bulk diet. If the condition becomes intolerable, colostomy is the last recourse, and if severe bleeding remains a problem, proctectomy may be advised.

## Neurogenic

In cases of myelomeningocele, the nerve supply, both sensory and motor, is disturbed in a variety of ways leading to various forms of incontinence. Any form of trauma, neoplasm, vascular accident, infection, or demyelinating disease to the central nervous system or spinal cord may interfere with normal sensation or motor function leading to incontinence.

## Imperforate Anus

The various operative procedures designed for imperforate anus depend upon the type of deformity. The ultimate goal is to establish a perineal opening with adequate sensory and motor control. Rarely are sensory mechanisms preserved, therefore, some defect in continence usually results. Gross incontinence can usually be avoided by careful placement of the colon or rectum through residual sphincter mechanisms (i.e. the puborectalis sling).

## Miscellaneous

Overflow secondary to fecal impaction is a frequent cause of incontinence. This problem is often missed because the patient complains of profuse diarrhea. Digital examination usually reveals a rectum full of stool. This problem generally occurs in elderly debilitated patients, or patients and young children recovering from surgical procedures, usually anorectal. Thus, physicians must be aware of this potential problem, and routinely institute early preventative measures. In general, hospital patients should be on a bulk-forming stool softener of a psyllium seed derivative. If impaction should occur, gentle enemas with a combination of tap water, phosphate soda, and hydrogen peroxide may be used. If these measures fail, disimpaction, with or without anesthesia, is the treatment of choice.

Large prolapsing third or fourth degree hemorrhoids may cause partial incontinence by interfering with the normal closure mechanism of the internal sphincter. This may result in either the escape of gas or liquid feces, or mucosal irritation.

Chronic inflammatory processes of the anorectal region as seen in ulcerative colitis, amoebic colitis, or lymphogranuloma venereum infections may result in local sensory derangement, interference of the sphincter mechanism, and/or mucosal irritability resulting in a loss of the rectal reservoir function.

Carcinoma of the anal canal may also present with incontinence either because of infiltration into the sphincter mechanism, or by preventing adequate closure of the anal canal.

# DIAGNOSIS

## History

As in the investigation of any pathological condition, a careful history is necessary. Particular attention must be paid to the characteristics of incontinence. Complete incontinence may be defined as the uncontrolled passage of solid feces, whereas partial incontinence may be defined as the uncontrolled passage of liquid or gas. This condition must also be distinguished from urgency, where the patient's diet or own individual bowel habits lead to a frequent passage of liquid stool accompanied by a great sense of urgency. In these cases simple dietary change may be all that is necessary.

Congenital abnormalities such as Hirschsprung's disease generally present with some form of constipation and megacolon. An accurate history is necessary to distinguish the condition from acquired megacolon in the adolescent and adult age group. In acquired megacolon, there is often soiling of the perineum by the overflow incontinence secondary to fecal impaction. In Hirschsprung's disease, there is rarely any incontinence of liquid or gas due to the constantly closed internal sphincter.

It is important to note if the patient had any previous anorectal operations or low colon anastomosis since these procedures may lead to anal incontinence. Also, dietary factors such as coffee or beer may lead to frequent loose bowel movements. Any history of remote or recent trauma to the anorectal area may also aid in establishing the cause of incontinence.

### Physical Examination

In patients with incontinence it is important to note if incontinence is a manifestation of a generalized disease or neurologic disorder, or if it is a local phenomenon. Inspection of the perineum is important. By simple retraction of the gluteal muscles, a large patulous anus, that is seen with rectal procidentia, can be easily recognized. Also, any large prolapsing hemorrhoids or evidence of pruritus may point to the fact that local anatomic factors may be responsible for the minor soiling by liquid or gas. Previous surgical scars may also be identified.

Palpation will point out any "keyhole deformity" of the anal canal which might lead to soiling which may be misinterpreted as partial incontinence. The assessment of anal tone is, at best, a very indistinct barometer of sphincter function. The ability to assess strength of voluntary sphincter contraction is, at best, subjective. The patient's complaints should provide a more reliable index of incontinence.

Anoscopic and proctosigmoidoscopic examinations will reveal any inflammatory process of neoplasm contributing to the patient's complaint.

### Special Investigations

The ability to retain a disposable enema is a very useful clinical guide in the assessment of incontinence. If the patient is able to retain a 100 cc, water enema, thoughts of any surgical correction or prolonged treatment plan are unnecessary. Reassurance that there is not a more serious problem is all that is indicated for such a patient.

Electromyography may be a useful test in evaluating the patient with anal incontinence secondary to disruption of the external sphincter mechanism. Its primary benefit is in locating the severed ends of the sphincter muscle. It is fortunate that a denervated external sphincter, as opposed to other skeletal muscles, retains its muscle mass. However, if extensive injury or perineal infection destroy the majority of responsive muscle tissue, any primary sphincter repair would be ill-advised.

Various manometric devices have been utilized for measurement of rectal sensation and sphincter activity.[14,17] At best, the method and materials are somewhat cumbersome, and more suitable for the laboratory.

Henriksen has devised a method for which sphincter strength can be quantitated.[6] A metal ball, 2 cm in diameter, is inserted into the rectum. A string is attached to one end of the ball, passed over a small wheel, and affixed on the other end to a scale pan. Weights are then placed on the scale pan for a two second duration, 50 gms at a time. The sphincter is allowed to relax between the placement of each weight on the pan. In studying incontinent patients, the highest value recorded for which patients could retain the ball was 175 gms; whereas, in the normal group, the lowest value recorded was 450 grams. This is a wide variation between normal and abnormal, and allows for objective evaluation of relative sphincter strength.

## TREATMENT
### Operative Procedures Available

*Sphincteroplasty* (Fig. 22-1). The technique of sphincteroplasty, as applied by Slade, et al, provides good to excellent results in most patients who have adequate residual muscle mass.[15] The technique of surgery involves preparing the patient by evacuation of the large bowel with enemas and laxatives. At the time of operation an indwelling urethral catheter is placed and maintained until decreased pain permits voluntary voiding.

The operation is performed with the patient in the prone position with the buttocks elevated over a 6″ roll. Anesthesia may be regional or general, but the entire operative site is infiltrated with local anesthetic and 1:200,000 epinephrine in order to relax the muscles and improve hemostasis. The first step is mobilization of the anoderm from the underlying sphincter mechanism and scar. The incision is curvilinear, and parallels the outer edge of the external sphincter. This incision should extend for at least 200 to 240 degrees of arc, depending upon the amount of scar tissue present. Cephalad mobilization should extend approximately to the distal edge of the anorectal ring. The entire sphincter mechanism is then widely dissected free from its bed. Care must be taken to preserve the branches of the

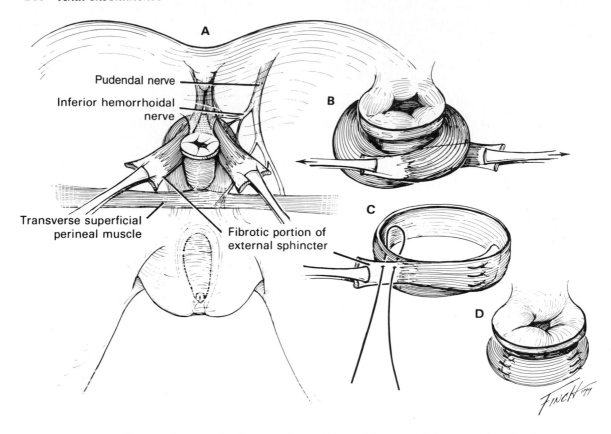

FIGURE 22-1. *Technique of sphincteroplasty. (A) Mobilization of the severed ends of sphincter muscle. (B) Muscle ends are overlapped. (C) Mattress sutures applied. It is important to leave the scar at each end of the muscle, to hold the sutures. (D) At completion, the anal canal should admit 1 finger snugly. The wound is packed open.*

pudendal nerves as they enter into the muscle posterolaterally. Wide dissection permits approximation without tension. Two-thirds of the circumference should be adequate in most instances. It is often easiest to begin at the normal muscle and advance to the scarred area once a proper plane has been established. The entire sphincter mechanism is sectioned transversely through the middle of the scar tissue preserving this for suture placement. The muscle ends are overlapped to decrease the anal aperature until it fits snugly over the index finger. Six to nine mattress sutures are carefully placed to maintain the desired aperture. The material used is generally a 2—0 synthetic absorbable suture. The tendency of the sphincter ends to pull apart must be minimal, as this is a sign of inadequate mobilization of the muscle from its bed, and will predispose to the separation at the suture line.

When all sutures are placed they may be pulled up tight, and the orifice is checked again to insure proper placement of the sutures, which are then tied. The anoderm is then carefully sutured over the sphincter with interrupted sutures, the horseshoe-shaped defect outside the muscle is partially closed, and the remainder is packed open with a fine gauze.

Patients are given a low residue diet for the first week, and opiates are given to decrease pain and frequency of bowel movements. A colostomy is not required, and postoperative therapy with antibiotics is unnecessary. Patients usually leave the hospital in 10 to 14 days.

We have recently reviewed 47 cases of acquired anal incontinence that were treated by sphincteroplasty as described above from 1953 to 1978. The etiology of the incontinence was obstetrical or gynecological in 22 patients

(47%), anorectal pathology in 21 (45%), and trauma in 4 (8%). The patients had antecedent symptoms for an average of 9.4 years (the range was from three weeks to more than 30 years). Thirty-six were women and 11 men, with a mean age of 44 years. Four (8.5%) had existing colostomies at the time of sphincteroplasty, but none of these were specifically performed to "protect" the repair. Twelve (25%) had had one or more previously attempted repairs at other institutions.

The total complication rate was 8.5%: there was one immediate postoperative death secondary to a myocardial infarction; one patient had a postoperative hemorrhage; and two developed abscesses. Results, as evaluated by an independent examiner, were excellent in 24 cases (52%), good in 17 (37%), fair in 4 (9%) and poor in one (2%). The poor results were in a patient who had had symptoms for over 30 years, and had had two previous sphincteroplasties elsewhere.

*Post Anal Repair.* The posterior sphincteroplasty and suture of the puborectalis as devised by Parks is another method of treatment.[12] Again, adequate muscle mass must be present for this operation to be successful. Essential parts of this operation are restoration of the anorectal angulation, as well as increase of the length of the anal canal. As Parks describes the operation, a posterior angular incision is made through the anoderm and proceeds through the intersphincteric plane between the external and internal sphincter (Fig. 22-2A,B). This intersphincteric plane is pursued upward until the puborectalis is reached (Fig. 22-2C). The pelvic cavity is entered, by dividing the recto-sacral fascia, and the perirectal fat is swept off the levator ani muscles (Fig. 22-2D,E,F). At this point most of the levator ani muscle can be seen, therefore, sutures can be placed from one side of the pelvis to the other incorporating the levator ani muscle on each side. These muscles will not meet: the sutures only form a lattice (Fig. 22-2G). A 2—0 propylpropylene suture is used. Next, a row of sutures is placed to oppose the two limbs of the puborectalis which further buttress the anorectal angle (Fig. 22-2H). This also makes the pull of the puborectalis more efficient. Plicating sutures are also placed in the external sphincter muscles to narrow their arc of action (Fig. 22-2I).

By placing a finger in the anal canal one can feel if the whole area is somewhat stenosed, a state essential for a successful result to be obtained. The wound is closed over a suction drain (Fig. 22-2J) and systemic antibiotics are given. Although Parks recommends purging the patient for a 10 day period with Magnesium Sulfate to ensure liquid stools, we would suggest the use of an elemental diet, and Loperamide HCl (Imodium) to quiet the bowel, and codeine as an analgesic. Parks reports 83 per cent successful outcome of the operation.[12]

*Thiersch operation* for incontinence is a procedure devised to narrow the anal ring by a foregin body implant either of wire, teflon, or silastic.[4] This is a static barrier to the passage of rectal contents, and offers nothing in the way of voluntary control and the maintenance of continence. This procedure may offer some control of solid feces but offers little in the control of liquid or gas. Often these foreign bodies will later extrude and become secondarily infected.

*Gracilis Muscle Transposition.* This procedure is reserved for situations in which massive trauma or infection in the perineum has destroyed the bulk of the patient's sphincter mechanism. A procedure described by Pickrell and associates is to use a sling of gracilis muscle still attached to one end of the pubis to encircle the anus, and reattach the severed end to the opposite ischial tuberosity.[13] We feel that this can be summarized as a "living Thiersch procedure" because of the inability of the gracilis muscle, or any other skeletal muscle other than the external sphincter mechanism, to maintain both the tonic and phasic contraction necessary for continence. We have no direct personal experience with this procedure, but there have been scattered successful reports.[11]

*Colostomy.* As a last resort for patients with anal incontinence so severe that they are disabled by their problem and unable to control their pattern by conventional means such as medication, diet, and enemas, colostomy may become necessary. This is especially appropriate in patients with irradiation destruction of the rectum. It is important to perform the colostomy outside of the irradiated field to prevent subsequent breakdown or problems

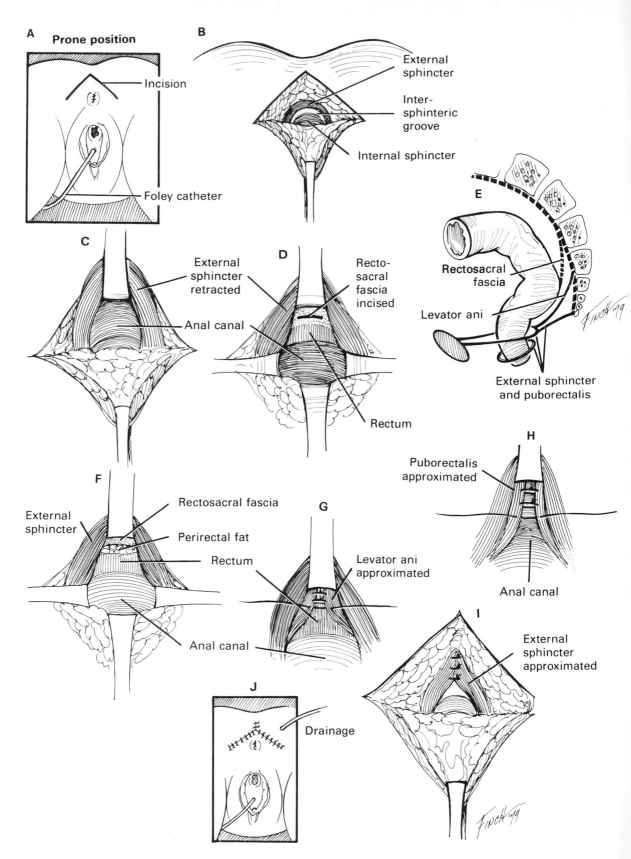

**A** Prone position

Incision

Foley catheter

**B** External sphincter

Inter-sphinteric groove

Internal sphincter

**C** External sphincter retracted

Anal canal

**D** Recto-sacral fascia incised

Rectum

**E** Rectosacral fascia

Levator ani

External sphincter and puborectalis

**F** External sphincter

Rectosacral fascia

Perirectal fat

Rectum

Anal canal

**G** Levator ani approximated

Anal canal

**H** Puborectalis approximated

Anal canal

**I** External sphincter approximated

**J** Drainage

FIGURE 22-2. *Technique of postanal pelvic floor repair.*

with the colostomy. Whether the rectum should be left in situ or removed is a question that can only be answered in discussion with the patient, and by considering the degree of the chance of morbidity that continued rectal discharge might cause. This must be balanced with the increased morbidity which accompanies proctectomy.

### Nonoperative Procedures

Electrical control of sphincteric dysfunction can be provided by direct electrical implants to the muscle tissue, or by externally activated "plugs".[7] The electrical implants have the inherent problem of infection and dislodgement, and the continued contraction of these sphincter mechanisms can only be sustained for 40 to 60 sec. Often this is inadequate to maintain continence. The anal stimulator plug is a more complex apparatus but it has the advantage of being a noninvasive technique. By gradually decreasing the size of the anal plugs, normal anal tone is gradually returned. There are only scattered reports mentioning the success of this procedure. Most trials are discouraging, perhaps again attributable to the inability of the sphincter mechanism to maintain tonic contraction for any prolonged period of time.

Another nonsurgical method popularized by Schuster consists of operant conditioning of rectosphincteric response.[3] This is achieved by screening patients for incontinence, and selecting well motivated, alert patients for a three-phase instruction of voluntary control mechanisms. The method involves placing a balloon in the rectum and connecting pressure transducers to a graph in order to give the patient visual feedback corresponding to his sphincteric responses to command. Gradually, the visual feedback is eliminated but checked by a trained observer to see if the patient can respond to rectal sensations of varying amounts. Engel studied seven patients and was able to get subjective improvement in all but one using this technique.[3] One major disadvantage is the time involved. Each session takes at least two hours, and involves a significant amount of sophisticated physiologic monitoring apparatus. However, this technique does appear promising, and perhaps with further refinement may attain a role in the treatment of congenital or acquired anal incontinence.

## SELECTION OF APPROPRIATE OPERATIVE PROCEDURE

In patients incontinent secondary to injury to the external sphincter, we prefer to perform a sphincteroplasty, as described above, when there is intact innervation to at least one-half of the sphincter. However, if the sphincter is intact and incontinence is secondary to a stretching of the puborectalis, with subsequent loss of the normal 80° angle between the axis of the rectum and anal canal, as may occur with aging or rectal procidentia, the Park's post anal repair is used.

In cases in which the sphincteric mechanism is denervated, procedures such as a gracilis muscle transplant or a Thiersch operation might be considered. As a last resort, a colostomy may be the only reasonable alternative.

The results of nonsurgical methods such as "conditioning" or electrical implants are inconclusive as of this writing, and bear further investigation. We personally have no experience with these methods.

## "KEYHOLE" DEFORMITY

With the advent of the lateral internal sphincterotomy the "keyhole" deformity will, fortunately, become increasingly uncommon. For the patient already afflicted with the problem, instruction in personal hygiene to include careful cleansing, with special attention to cleaning the partially everted anus, should be given. The patient should be counselled to keep the stool formed because liquid stools will be associated with more leakage. A wisp of cotton placed at the anal verge may help prevent skin irritation. Operative correction will probably not be helpful and may even prove meddlesome.

### REFERENCES

1. Caldwell, K. P. S.: The electrical control of sphincter incompetence. Lancet, 7:174, 1963.
2. Castro, A. F., and Pittman, R.: Repair of the incontinent sphincter. Dis. Colon Rectum, 21:183, 1978.
3. Engel, B. T., Mikoomanesh, P., and Schuster,

M. M.: Operant conditioning of recto-sphincteric responses in the treatment of fecal incontinence. N. Engl. J. Med., *290:*646, 1974.

4. Goligher, J. C.: Surgery of the Anus, Rectum and Colon, 3 ed. 329-330. Springfield, Charles C Thomas, 1975.

5. Goligher, J. C., Lee, P. W. R., MacFie, J., Simpkins, K. C., and Lintott, D. J.: Experience with the Russian Model 249 suture gun for anastomoses of the rectum. Surg. Gynecol. Obstet., *148:*517, 1979.

6. Henriksen, F. W., and Huthouisen, B.: Measurement of the anal sphincter strength by a simple method suitable for routine use. Scand. J. Gastroent., *7:*555, 1972.

7. Hopkinson, B. R., and Lightwood, R.: Electrical treatment of anal incontinence. Lancet, *2:*297, 1966.

8. Jeffery, P. J., Hawley, P. R., and Parks, A. G.: Colo-anal sleeve anastomoses in the treatment of diffuse cavernous haemangioma involving the rectum. Br. J. Surg., *63:*678, 1976.

9. Kennedy, J. T., McOmish, D., Bennett, R. C., Hughes, E. S. R., and Cuthbertson, A. M.: Abdomino-anal pull-through resection of the rectum. Br. J. Surg., *57:*589, 1970.

10. Localio, S. A., Eng, K., Gouge, T., and Ranson, J. H. C.: Abdominosacral resection for carcinoma of the midrectum: Ten years experience. Ann. Surg., *188:*475, 1978.

11. Nieves, P. M., Valles, T. G., Aranguren, G., and Maldonado, D.: Gracilis muscle transplant for correction of traumatic anal incontinence. Dis. Colon Rectum, *18:*349, 1975.

12. Parks, A. G.: Anorectal incontinence. Proc. R. Soc. Med., *68:*681, 1975.

13. Pickrell, K. L., Broadbent, T. R., Masters, F. W., and Metzger, J. T.: Construction of a rectal sphincter and restoration of anal continence by transplanting the gracilis muscle. Ann. Surg., *135:*853, 1952.

14. Schuster, M. M.: Diagnostic value of anal sphincter pressure measurements. Hospital Practice, 115, 1976.

15. Slade, M. S., Goldberg, S. M., Schottler, J. L., Balcos, E. G., and Christenson, C. E.: Sphincteroplasty for acquired anal incontinence. Dis. Colon Rectum, *20:*33, 1977.

16. Stelzner, F.: The morphological principles of anorectal continence. Prog. Pediatr. Surg., *9:*1, 1976.

17. Varma, F. K., Hunt, T. W., and Stephens, F. D.: The anomanometer: Its use in the assessment of continence and in the diagnosis of Hirschsprung's disease. Aust. NZ J. Surg., *42:*185, 1972.

# 23

# Injuries to the Anus and Rectum

Trauma to the lower bowel, particularly the colon, rectum, and anus, is not rare. Injuries occur through "normal" living, and by events that are related to purposeful or accidental manipulation of these organs for one reason or another. The natural injuries that result from ingested particles that pass in the feces, and from parturition are extremely uncommon compared to the "man-related" events that pertain to diagnostic or operative procedures, criminal, civilian, and military injuries, and to acts perpetrated by one human upon another. While the greatest discussion and disagreement pertaining to these injuries centers around specific procedures required to repair the damage, there is little disagreement that expeditious evaluation, an organized approach, and mature surgical judgment will all contribute to a successful outcome in these injuries.

## ETIOLOGY
### Operative Procedures

Intraoperative injuries, during procedures on the anorectum or the urogenital organs, do occur. While anorectal complications or injuries that occur will be discussed in a separate section, suffice it to say that any operation on the anal canal or rectum, particularly for hemorrhoids, fistulae, or fissures, as well as anal canal injuries can cause anal stenosis, ectropion, sphincteric muscle injury or soft tissue perineal injuries.

Injuries to the rectum and anus can occur during operations on adjacent organs. Dilatation and curettage of the uterus has been associated with uterine perforation, and subsequent perforation of the rectum or rectosigmoid. Injuries to the rectum and rectosigmoid may occur during any complicated pelvic or abdominal procedure. Commonly performed procedures such as total abdominal hysterectomy, vaginal hysterectomy, perineal or suprapubic prostatectomy, radical cystectomy, and transurethral resection of the prostate can cause injury to the rectum, although this occurence is infrequent. The rare rectoprostatic fistula is another example. McLaughlin recommends the use of anal stretching (dilatation) without proximal colostomy, and a primary repair of the inadvertent rectal laceration incurred during perineal prostatectomy.[40] The stretch (another form of rectal trauma) "decompresses" the rectum by temporary anal sphincter atony, thus preventing development of high pressure and subsequent "blow out" of the rectal repair. However, we would recommend exercising great caution in any form of anal stretching as this may result in anal incontinence.

Surgical manipulations through an endoscope have frequently been the source of injuries of the rectum and rectosigmoid. Thorbjarnarson reported on 10 iatrogenic perforations of the large bowel, five of which resulted from the use of biopsy forceps or a snare.[62] Two perforations were the result of taking too deep a bite during the biopsy of sessile colonic lesions, and another was the result of a biopsy of an ulceration which had

With collaboration of Frederic D. Nemer

resulted in extreme thinning of the bowel wall. Two perforations resulted from the use of a snare in the removal of polyps: the snare was brought too far down over the base of the polyp, thus bringing the full thickness of the bowel wall into its grip.

The risk of developing problems from biopsy and polypectomy are far greater above the peritoneal reflection. Usually full thickness biopsies, polypectomy or local excision of growths posteriorly, below 10 cm, in the adult rectum causes infrequent complications. This is contrasted to the often acute surgical emergency that will occur from a tiny pinpoint leak from an errant polypectomy or biopsy site above the peritoneal reflection. Colonoscopic complications such as hemorrhage and perforation present identical problems that require similarly swift attention. Jacobsohn and Levy, and Smith and Nivatvongs stress patience and gentleness to avoid complications in the performance of these procedures.[29,58]

Hemorrhage as a result of intraluminal manipulation is common. It is most likely to result after biopsy of a highly vascularized lesion such as polypoid adenoma or carcinoma, but also can occur from simple biopsy of the bowel wall. Proctosigmoidoscopic biopsy without the use of a functioning coagulation unit is not advised. Of course, blood dyscrasias or drug usage causing bleeding problems should be appropriately evaluated before the procedure. Excellent suction, a good coagulation unit, patience, and no panic in the face of profuse rectal bleeding will often allow one to arrest the hemorrhage, thus averting a trip to the operating room. Occasionally, constant pressure with a long cotton swab will allow hemostasis to be achieved.

## Diagnostic and Therapeutic Procedures

Few organ systems are as vulnerable to physicians' diagnostic and therapeutic procedures as are the colon, rectum, and anus. A vast array of diagnostic and therapeutic procedures exist for colon and rectal disease. Any of these procedures can cause injury if they are performed improperly or in tissues weakened by disease. Improper insertion of an enema tip for either therapeutic enemas or diagnostic barium enemas can result in laceration, perforation, or hemorrhage to the wall of the colon, rectum, or anal canal. Almost always, perforation results from insertion of the enema tip by unskilled or careless attendants, or by the patients themselves. Infrequently, excessive pressure in diseased bowel causes the perforation.

*Rectal Thermometers.* The taking of rectal temperatures has long been a clinical practice and is a "routine" procedure. However, in 1965 Fonkalsrud and Clatworthy reported on 10 accidental perforations of the intestine in infants.[17] They indicated that a major cause of the rectal perforation during the first few days of life was the use of rectal thermometers. These authors point out that the distance between the anus and the peritoneal reflection over the rectosigmoid in newborns is less than 3 cm, and that half the perforations of the bowel in these infants occur at this low level. In an article by Horwitz, an outbreak of peritonitis in a neonatal nursery was found to have been caused by a nurse using improper technique in taking of rectal temperatures, thus causing rectal perforation.[25]

*The "Simple Enema".* No procedure is so "simple" as never to have complications. Therapeutic misadventures occur as frequently as diagnostic ones, and frequently during supposedly "routine benign procedures". Errant instillation of improper liquid such as scalding water which can cause severe burns, or improper rectal solutions (such as formaldehyde instead of paraldehyde) can cause sloughing and severe rectal bleeding. A spectrum of anorectal injuries can occur during the "simple" enema.[15] Perforation from enemas can be classified into five types: (*1*) anal perforation, (*2*) submucosal perforation, (*3*) extraperitoneal perforation, (*4*) intraperitoneal perforation, and (*5*) perforation into adjacent organs. The vast majority of rectal injuries and perforations resulting from enema tips occurred in the anterior wall. This can be understood when one realizes that these injuries almost always occur with the patient in a sitting or lying position. Care in the insertion of any tube or tip rectally should prevent these injuries. Extraperitoneal perforation can cause abscess, fistula-in-ano, or severe hemorrhage.

*Proctosigmoidoscopic Perforation of the Bowel.* In 1967, Befeler reviewed the literature concerning more than 125 cases of iatrogenic perforations of the colon and rectum.[11] Most of them were at, or near, the peritoneal reflection of the rectosigmoid. Mortality rates in these cases were more than 25 per cent. In most of these instances, the bowel wall had been weakened by disease. Andresen reported a series of 94 proctosigmoidoscopic injuries, and concluded that mortality was directly related to the time between injury and operative intervention.[4] The mortality rate was 8 per cent if operation upon perforation was within six hours. If greater than 12 hours delay occurred between perforation and operation, death ensued in almost 20 per cent of patients.

In 1953 Klein and Scarborough reported 50 cases of perforations of the rectum and distal colon by proctosigmoidoscopy.[34] They listed a number of cases of these perforations in addition to those associated with biopsy examination and other forms of treatment. Some of the causes included blind introduction beyond the anal margin, re-insertion of the obturator to overcome spasm, injudicious use of a long cotton-tipped applicator, and the attempted forceful dilatation of rectal strictures with the proctosigmoidoscope. These authors recognized that the mortality in these cases was dependent upon the time lapse after perforation before definitive treatment was begun. Other instigating factors in perforation include full thickness biopsy and an uncooperative patient. While it is generally believed that injuries to the rectum are caused more commonly by those physicians who have less experience with these procedures, occasional perforations at the hands of experts occur, as well. Thus, it behooves all individuals doing these examinations to do them carefully, biopsy judiciously, and use a minimum of air insufflation during the procedures. A common error is made when the examiner attempts to overcome an area of spasm by forceful dilatation with vigorous compression of the insufflating bulb. This usually fails to dilate the spastic bowel, but does result in massive dilatation of the proximal bowel with subsequent pain. It is interesting to note that most perforations occur not during a routine screening examination but more often during an examination in an attempt to make a definitive diagnosis in an elderly patient with an acute disease, and frequently in the presence of an obstructive process.

*Barium Enema.* An extensive variety of complications has been reported associated with barium enema. Two of the most serious of these complications are the mechanical perforation of the bowel, either intraperitoneally or extraperitoneally by direct penetration of the enema tip, and over-inflation of the rectal (Bardex) balloon causing pneumatic rupture of the rectum during the performance of the study. Other complications include the formation of barium granulomas within the rectal wall, necrotizing proctitis, and barium embolism.

Kiser and associates reported one perforation of the colon in 1250 barium enemas performed at the Ellis-Fischell State Cancer Hospital in Missouri.[33] Most of the perforations reported were ruptures through ulcers, neoplasms, diverticula, or other areas of disease. It has not been the universal experience, however, that these perforations always occur through diseased areas. Rosenklint reported on six extraperitoneal perforations from barium extravasation during 20,000 barium enema examinations.[50] Four of the six patients died. The other two have permanent colostomies. None of the patients had disease in the colon or rectum. Prevention of this complication depended upon several factors: (*1*) keeping the "head of pressure" of the barium enema less than one meter; (*2*) not over-inflating the balloon; (*3*) keeping the balloon tip short, and making all those persons who perform these examinations aware of the possible complications; and, (*4*) deferring the barium enema in patients who had recently undergone biopsy or polypectomy of the colon or rectum for three to four weeks. Treatment of all the above perforations was by diverting colostomy, drainage of the peritoneal tissues, and antibiotics.

A spectrum of injury may result from injections of varying volumes of barium sulfate into the wall of the bowel. From small amounts injected submucosally, a simple barium granuloma may result. These may be asymptomatic or cause significant pain. More often they present several years later as isolated rectal nodules in a patient who has been otherwise asymptomatic. Larger amounts of barium injected in the same manner can result in a severe inflammatory reaction resulting in abscess formation or even necrotizing proctitis. Perforation above the peritoneal reflection results in intraperitoneal contamination by both barium and residual stool within the bowel. A number of reports indicate that even when perforation is into the free peritoneal cavity, the nature of the injury may not be suspected immediately because of the lack of significant symptoms suggesting that a free perforation has occurred. However, symptoms of peritoneal irritation occurring minutes or hours later should always be considered as possibly resulting from the preceding diagnostic barium enema study. Most of these cases, on repeat abdominal radiograph, show the presence of free air and/or evidence of barium outside the lumen of the bowel. The mere presence of air in the retroperitoneal tissues following endoscopy or enema is usually a benign process and is often asymptomatic.[52] This is compared to the drastic complications that usually ensue with combined barium and fecal contamination in the retroperitoneum.[14]

The mechanism of injury in the reported cases of rectal perforation during barium enema is not always obvious. It is clear that the balloon tip catheter is often responsible. In other cases, the inflation of the Bardex balloon forces the tip of the catheter into the mucosa causing deposition of barium into the submucosa where necrotizing proctitis may result. Rupture of the barium through a recent site of rectal biopsy or polypectomy is also another consideration. Excess hydrostatic or pneumatic pressure may be a significant factor. Most of the free perforations from barium have occurred at, or just above, the pelvic peritoneum at the rectosigmoid flexure. These are thought to be due to the relative fixation of the posterior rectal wall at the point where the rectosigmoid acutely flexes upon itself. Here, and at other areas above the dentate line where pain fibers are few, a forceful insertion may completely penetrate the bowel wall with little or no immediate patient reaction.

EFFECTS OF BARIUM ON TISSUE. There is general agreement that sterile barium by itself causes relatively little inflammatory reaction when injected into lungs, subcutaneous and retroperitoneal tissues, or the wall of the rectum and the peritoneal cavity. Kay and Sanders, as well as others, have shown that extraperitoneal or intraperitoneal contamination by sterile barium incites a rather benign reaction characterized by histiocytic granulomas that become progressively fibrous.[32,52] However, when combined with significant bacterial contamination from the bowel and stool, a massive, and often overwhelming, inflamma-

tory response occurs. Sisel experimented on rabbits producing colonic rupture following barium enema or enema with water soluble contrast material.[57] Without treatment, both types were uniformly fatal. However, surgical repair of the rupture with concomitant peritoneal lavage resulted in only 10 per cent survival in animals with feces and barium contamination. Fifty per cent of the animals with gastrografin and feces contamination were able to survive if surgery was performed promptly. Zheutlin reported a collected series of 53 patients with barium mixed with feces spilled into the peritoneal cavity.[72] The mortality rate in this group was 51 per cent. Thus, gastrografin is the preferred contrast in suspected perforations.

BARIUM EMBOLISM. A most uncommon, and usually fatal complication of barium enema is that of intravasation into the veins of the rectum resulting in massive pulmonary embolism and sudden death.[49] This is a rare occurrence, and can be decreased to nearly zero by not performing barium enema on patients with acute inflammatory disease of the bowel, or on patients who have had recent endoscopic procedures with biopsy or polypectomy.

## Parturition—Fourth Degree Vaginal Laceration

The process of childbirth is traumatic to the female genital tract. Cephalopelvic disproportion and the adjustments in local anatomy that take place during childbirth are extraordinary. Not infrequently, a deep laceration will occur in the perineum following parturition that will involve not only the vagina, but perineal body, the rectum, and anal canal. The anal sphincter mechanism is thus involved. The judicious use of an appropriately placed episiotomy during delivery has decreased the tendency for fourth degree lacerations involving the anal sphincter; however, if the episiotomy is performed in the posterior midline, a greater incidence of harm to the sphincter mechanism has occurred. Factors such as the size of the baby compared to the flexibility of the pelvic tissues, the parity of the patient, the obesity of the patient, the skill of the obstetrician, and the decision whether or not instrumentation is used are factors that dictate whether or not injury will occur.

The ability to accurately repair a fourth degree tear should be a well developed skill in all those who regularly attend deliveries; only occasionally should a colorectal surgeon be called upon to repair the acute laceration. Many of these repairs will heal uneventfully. However, others will require secondary repair in the form of a sphincteroplasty and repair of the perineal body.

Rectovaginal fistulae can also occur from difficult parturition. Pressure necrosis of the rectovaginal wall and instrumental injury are usually responsible. Repair, ideally, is deferred until the tissue edema has subsided and chance for spontaneous closure has been allowed. (See Chap. 25)

### Irradiation-induced Proctitis

Irradiation directed at neoplasms of the rectum or genitourinary tract may cause a number of immediate and delayed complications. Acute irradiation proctitis is an anticipated sequelae of irradiation for uterine, bladder, or ovarian malignancy. Quan reviewed 65 patients who underwent irradiation therapy for pelvic malignancies, 52 of which were for carcinoma of the cervix.[47] There was simultaneous injury to both bladder and intestine in many of the cases. The acute findings were an initial edema with inflammation of the rectal mucosa, and erythema with friability. This may actually progress to necrosis or ulceration. If healing does take place, ultimately, granulation tissue, fibrosis, and telangiectasia may ensue. If necrosis exceeds tissue repair, a rectovaginal fistula may develop. The result may be a stricture of the rectum, rectosigmoid, or the sigmoid colon. Microscopic examination of these tissues reveals irradiation-induced endarteritis causing deprivation of blood supply to the mucosa which leads to the above sequence of macroscopic events. Destruction of lymphatic channels also occurs. The onset of symptoms after radiotherapy varies from immediate, to weeks, months, or even years post-treatment. The most common symptom was rectal bleeding. In another series reviewing 80 patients with implantation of I$^{125}$ radioactive seeds versus external beam therapy, Quan noted that none of the patients treated by implantation developed rectal symptoms.[47] Proctitis developed in all the patients with external radiation therapy, and one-half of those patients developed chronic proctitis with constant mucus leakage and perianal pruritus. One of these patients who had been treated by 7000 rads of external radiation therapy developed rectal necrosis. This patient was diabetic and may have had pre-existing vascular disease. In reviewing patients who develop chronic proctitis, in a study from Memorial Hospital in New York, Quan reported on 50 patients with radiation-induced proctitis, 21 of whom required some sort of diverting colostomy to manage the condition.[47] Eleven patients subsequently maintained their colostomy as permanent; only 10 were temporary. The indications for colostomy were excessive bleeding; radiation necrosis of the rectum with or without fistulization to the vagina, bladder, or bowel; and bowel obstruction due to stenosis from radiation. The anterior rectal wall was the site for the worst radiation-induced changes. The extent of damage depends upon the size of the area treated, the total dose delivered, overall treatment time, and whether or not fractionation of the dosage was performed. Of course, individual techniques affected the outcome as well. Obliterative endarteritis occurs as a late effect following high-dose irradiation therapy. Mild proctitis usually requires no treatment. Sherman has reported good results using corticosteroid in the management of patients with acute and chronic irradiation proctitis.[55] Colonic obstruction due to irradiation colitis or proctitis is uncommon. If such complication occurs, colostomy is indicated.[43]

VanNagell, et al reported, in a series of patients with uterine carcinoma requiring irradiation, an increased incidence of rectal injury in patients who had pre-existing hypertensive vascular disease or diabetes mellitus. In addition, no rectal injuries occurred when the total dose to the rectum was less than 4000 rads. They also stressed the finding that severe proctitis often preceded bladder or bowel complications, and it is recommended that fractionation of the remaining irradiation dosage over longer periods of time prevents much of the later irradiation changes. They also recommended a two week "rest period" during the middle of the course with the utilization of topical steroid and cleansing enemas.

### Explosions

Explosions resulting from the use of cautery during proctosigmoidoscopy have occasionally been reported.[15] The injuries caused can vary from none to severe rectal or colonic lacerations and perforation. The danger of explosion when a spark is being used is an ever-present one. The gases that accumulate in the distal bowel may be hydrogen methane or hydrogen sulfide, or they may be gases produced by the electrocoagulation such as ethylene, acetylene, or hydrogen. It is of the utmost importance to evacuate these gases from the colon and rectum by suctioning the lumen clean before any kind of coagulation treatment is begun, and to repeat this process frequently during the coagulation process. Some endoscopists further attempt to prevent this accident by using a continuous flow of inert, non-flammable gas, such as nitrogen or carbon dioxide, through the course of the coagulation treatment. If the patient complains of abdominal or shoulder pain following an explosion, abdominal and chest radiographs are indicated to rule out free intra-abdominal air which would require emergency laparotomy.

### Ingested Foreign Bodies

Anal and rectal wounds resulting from ingested foreign bodies are decidedly uncommon.[15] Particles that are potentially injurious to the anus, rectum, or lower intestinal tract that occur in natural foods (such as pits, thorns, seeds, or soft bones) may undergo significant, if not near total, digestion by the time they reach the lower intestinal tract. However, other particulate matter, such as chicken or other animal bones, toothpicks, portions of glass, shells, or other sharp objects can pass through the intestinal tract into the colon and cause injury to the rectum and anus. Most frequently, foreign bodies that ultimately injure the intestinal tract are those ingested by infants, children, or mentally deranged adults. Of course, one can inadvertently swallow any object that enters the mouth, and parts of dentures have been known to break off and be swallowed by patients. Prevention of these injuries by keeping potentially dangerous objects out of the reach of infants, children, and incompetent adults is preferable to the treatment of the rare, but serious, injuries that occur. Perforation, hemorrhage, abscess formation, bowel obstruction, and death have all been reported in this regard.[48,54] It has been stated that 10 to 20 per cent of ingested foreign bodies fail to pass through the entire gastrointestinal tract, but fewer than 1 per cent cause perforation.[54] While ingestion of foreign bodies is not unusual, complications of ingestion are rare. "Intelligent neglect" or expeditious upper gastrointestinal endoscopy are the two best forms of initial therapy. One must decide if it is better to watch the foreign body pass, or to perform endoscopic removal within the first hour or two of ingestion. Surgical intervention is required for the 1 per cent of patients who perforate, and for the few patients who bleed or obstruct due to these objects. The most common sites for perforation in the gastrointestinal tract are the ileocecal valve and the appendix, where 75 per cent of gastrointestinal perforations occur.[54] Sequential flat plates of the abdomen show that most objects pass the gastrointestinal tract within a week, many within one to two days. Close observation for the development of complications is all that is usually necessary. Early endoscopic removal of selected objects may be a similarly acceptable approach.[54]

### Stercoral Perforation

Those individuals with chronic constipation and, in fact, impaction, have, in very rare circumstances, perforated either the rectum or the rectosigmoid colon by a process thought to be related to ischemic pressure on the previously jeopardized rectal and rectosigmoid blood supply. Impaired vascular supply in conjunction with bacteria of the stool is thought to cause necrosis of the wall itself, thus initiating the perforation.[8,69]

### Spontaneous Perforation

Rarely, spontaneous perforation will occur either in the rectosigmoid or cecum, either from distention, spasm, or pre-existing disease such as inflammatory bowel disease, diverticulitis and carcinoma.[39] Sometimes spontaneous perforation occurs in the absence of pathological disease.

### EVALUATION OF THE INJURED PATIENT

The symptoms and signs of anorectal trauma generally are not subtle. The multiple trauma patient evaluated in the emergency room setting or in combat after having suffered a penetrating wound to the abdomen will often disclose perineal or anorectal bleeding or bleeding from other orifices. The most dangerous situation occurs in multiple trauma when other life-threatening wounds such as cardio-respiratory and abdominal wounds and injuries take necessary priority in evaluation. This may cause the physician to overlook the more subtle perineal, anal, and rectal wounds until later. This delay in diagnosis and treatment can prove to be fatal.[7,13]

The examination and evaluation of the patient will go on only after resuscitation of the patient has been accomplished. The multiple injured patient, or the combat victim, requires hemodynamic stabilization, replenishment of body fluids and blood, antibiotic therapy to reduce the incidence of sepsis, and update of tetanus immunization. Many authors have shown the importance of initiating antibiotic therapy very early in the course of resuscitation no matter what kind of penetrating injury has occured. Altemeier showed that the results of surgical treatment were improved if antibiotics were delivered within the "golden period" of six hours of injury.[3] Contamination of the wound left untreated for longer than six hours met with an increased mortality and morbidity rate. Fullen and associates, and Polk and associates have similarly shown the benefit of prophylactic antibiotics in penetrating wounds of the abdomen, and the importance of an early administration of these medications if systemic and local sepsis are to be averted.[18,46] Simmons has shown the factors associated with the development of peritonitis, and states that not only is bacterial or fecal contamination important, but the presence of hemoglobin drastically inhibits the clearing of bacteria and contamination by the peritoneal surface.[56]

## History

Generally speaking, patients with isolated anorectal trauma complain of perineal, anorectal, and even abdominal pain. The pain has usually started abruptly, precisely at the time of injury. In less frequent cases, the onset of pain may be delayed as with delayed manifestations from subtle perforations of the rectum, or the pain that comes after foreign body placement which only later could not be removed. In a few instances a dull, lower abdominal pain may be the only manifestation of an upper rectal or rectosigmoid tear with perforation. Rectal bleeding suggests rectal trauma, and diagnosis depends on a complete history and a thorough examination.[6,16,70] The multiple trauma patient who is stabilized from a hemodynamic point of view may deteriorate one to two days later as infection from an overlooked rectal or colonic injury takes over. The first recognition of such an injury may come only when the patient becomes septic, hypotensive, or manifests other cutaneous or soft tissue changes of gas gangrene or septic shock. Unfortunately, once this late stage of sepsis has developed, the chances of saving the patient are remote.

## Physical Examination

In retrospect, it is always easy to say that evaluation of an acutely or multiple injured patient should be thorough and well performed. However, during the exigencies of resuscitation, the less acute injuries often take a secondary place to the life-threatening emergencies of an acutely bleeding patient or a patient with cranial or thoracic injuries. This is the common situation of patients injured on the battle ground or the patient suffering from multiple trauma from high speed vehicle injuries. Brief inspection followed by palpation of the perineum as well as rectal examination without finding blood is extremely helpful in ruling out any anorectal or colonic components of multiple trauma. Further, thorough examination includes an examination of the abdominal wall by palpation to rule out crepitus or hematoma formation. In addition, one should check for the proper position of the anal canal and rectum, and the presence of an attached levator sling. Obviously, a conscious patient can indicate whether or not abdominal pain is present. Anal examination can be performed most expeditiously with the patient in either the supine or left lateral position. With no observable evidence of perineal trauma, the digital examination is performed in the usual fashion. If rectal injury is suspected owing to the presence of bright red blood, anoscopy can be performed to attempt to visualize the lower part of the rectum and the anal canal. Should this fail to identify the bleeding point, proctosigmoidoscopy can be performed with the patient in the lateral or supine position.

One should be aware not to insufflate large volumes of air when the rectum is filled with blood secondary to trauma. The danger existing here is that one can create contamination of the peritoneal cavity or extraperitoneal soft tissues if a wound in the lower colon or upper rectum is present.

### Radiological

Radiologic studies can be very valuable in the diagnosis of gastrointestinal and rectal trauma. Flat and upright abdominal films as well as lateral films of the pelvis are most helpful. Visualization of free intraperitoneal air as well as extraperitoneal or extrarectal soft tissue densities, or gas shadows can be diagnostic of colonic or rectal injury. If one finds a separated symphysis pubis or other pelvic fracture, and if clinical findings concur, it is possible that there is an injury to the rectum.[13]

If the patient's condition permits, and one's clinical suspicion indicates such, diagnostic contrast studies can be performed. These would not be performed if the patient's abdomen was diagnosed as acute, and operative intervention was contemplated anyway. Use of water soluble substances such as gastrografin and hypaque, though not without some danger, are usually recommended in preference to barium. Well informed and gentle radiologists, aware of the possibilities of rectal or rectosigmoid injury, will be careful not to instill too much of the contrast material during the fluoroscopic examination, and will stop the flow immediately at the first sign of any bowel perforation.

Massive rectal bleeding after traumatic injury which is not responsive to supportive treatment by transfusion can be localized by performing arteriography of the inferior mesenteric vessels and the internal iliac vessels. When the bleeding point has been localized in the rectum, embolization of autogenous clots or gel foam may dramatically reduce or stop the bleeding. Otherwise, suture ligation or packing of the rectum with gauze will usually suffice to control diffuse bleeding. It has been reported by Getzen that rare situations exist of massive rectal bleeding secondary to trauma that is unresponsive to supportive or arteriographic measures. Abdominal perineal resection as an emergency may be required to save the patient and stop the bleeding. This, however, should be a rare occurrence.[20]

## MANAGEMENT
### Blunt and Penetrating Trauma: Mechanisms and Principles of Management

A vast array of mechanisms by which the perineum, anal canal, rectum, and colon may be injured result from our rapid means of transportation and hostile methods of dealing with interpersonal conflict both during war and in civilian life. Injury can occur by either sharp or dull penetration, or by blunt, nonpenetrating trauma. Vast clinical experience has developed through the history of mankind which has pointed to principles that we now hold to be important in the management of both blunt and penetrating trauma. Many disagreements concerning treatment still center around which specific operation to perform for a specific injury. Important, too, are the factors related to the degree of trauma, the length of time from injury to the initiation of definitive care, the amount of contamination to the peritoneal cavity and soft tissue by the injury, the overall health of the patient, the skill and experience of the medical and surgical team taking care of the patient, and, of course, associated injuries to other vital structures in the body.

For practical purposes, many types of dissimilar injuries will be grouped together, and discussion of therapy will center upon a continuum or a spectrum of injuries. The treatment of colorectal trauma will vary from close observation of the patient with absolutely no treatment being required, to life-saving operations consisting of multiple procedures and prolonged hospitalization. Colorectal trauma is seldom an isolated injury. More often colorectal trauma accompanies the more common injuries of pelvic fracture, intraabdominal emergency, pulmonary contusion, closed or open head injuries, and fractures of long bones.

*Impalement* injuries are usually caused by the patient attempting some sort of maneuver only to fall short of the mark, thus impaling himself on a sharp or blunt object. In this manner, rectal injury occurs, as does injury to soft tissues, urologic, and intra-abdominal organs. In far less injurious situations, the blunt trauma will result in hematoma and/or abscess formation alone in the perineal tissues. Kaufer reported an unusual case of impalement with an auto jack in a similar way.[31] The patient manifested signs of an acute abdomen, and was taken to the operating room with the impaled object in place. This is a key to the treatment of these injuries: the patient is evaluated more completely and resuscitated in the operating room. If the impaling object is not removed until the abdomen is opened, all the intra-abdominal organs can be examined and explored, and the impaling object can be removed under direct vision. In this way, as little damage to the organs as possible will ensue. Of course, the specific types of repair and treatment necessary depend upon the contamination, and the amount of injury to the rectum, sigmoid, and other organs.

*"Seat Belt Injury."* Another common mechanism of colon and rectosigmoid injury comes from auto and high speed vehicle accidents. The mechanisms of injury are numerous, but only a few will be mentioned. Pelvic fractures with subsequent rectal tear, blunt abdominal trauma with a sudden increase of intra-abdominal pressure and a "blow out" type injury to the rectum or sigmoid colon, perineal blunt trauma disrupting the rectosigmoid and anal canal from the levator muscular sling are some of the mechanisms mentioned in the recent literature on blunt injury.[7,26,60,64]

*Penetrating Trauma to the Colon, Rectum and Anus.* A vast spectrum of injuries and treatments exist for penetrating wounds that involve the colon, rectum, and anus. The last 50 years of medical and surgical therapy for these wounds has brought the care of these injuries to a high level. The most important factors in determining the type of treatment for penetrating injuries are: the general physical condition of the patient; the mechanism by which the injury occurred; the state of the bowel contents at the time of injury; the interval between injury and, if necessary, operative intervention; the presence or lack of shock or hemodynamic stability; the presence of peritoneal contamination; the injury or avulsion of the mesentery, colon, or rectum; as well as the application of mature surgical judgement to all these conditions. Multiple contributions to the literature have been made in the treatment of civilian and combat in-

juries, in intra- compared to extra-peritoneal injuries of the rectum, and high velocity and low velocity missile injuries to the colon and rectum. Care will be taken to separate specific therapy for each category.

Various mortality rates have been quoted for the treatment of intra-abdominal colonic injuries associated with multiple trauma and with battlefield injuries. A review of the literature shows that patients who experience multiple trauma as well as penetrating intraabdominal injury, namely the battlefield victim, experience mortality in the range of 10 to 30 per cent.[5,19,38,41,53] Mortality rates ranging from 6 to 15 per cent are the figures commonly given for penetrating colonic injuries in civilian practice.[9,67] The differences in mortality and survival seem to be based upon the velocity of the missiles used, the destruction that each causes upon the colon with subsequent contamination, the interval between injury and definitive care, the judgment and experience of the surgeon, and the early utilization of antibiotics.

ANTIBIOTIC PROPHYLAXIS. It has been shown by several workers in the field of antibiotics that preoperative utilization of a broad spectrum antibiotics that cover both the anaerobic and aerobic populations are definitely beneficial if given as close to the time of the inciting incident as possible. Thadepalli, in reviewing abdominal trauma, concluded that anaerobic bacteria are a significant cause of infection in the abdominal cavity, and that clindamycin was a significantly useful adjunct to therapy for such injuries.[61] The combination of clindamycin and kanamycin were much better than cephalothin and kanamycin in treating anaerobic infections. It is interesting to note that they had the same incidence of aerobic infections with each regimen. Fullen and colleagues reviewed 295 patients with penetrating abdominal wounds.[18] They found a 7 per cent infection rate in 116 patients who were given prophylactic antibiotics before operation. They found a 33 per cent infection rate in 98 patients who were given the antibiotic intraoperatively, and a similar infection rate in 81 patients when the antibiotics were started postoperatively. This work, following the earlier work of Polk and Altemeier, should reinforce the concept of early administration of prophylactic, high dose antibiotics covering both anaerobic and aerobic organisms.[3,46]

### Injuries to the Extraperitoneal Rectum

Unfortunately, our modern day treatment of extraperitoneal anorectal injuries results from extensive wartime experience. This has been accumulated particularly in the past 35 years. Numerous mechanisms of injury are recorded: knife, gunshot, and shotgun wounds; explosion; and the less frequent injuries incurred from diagnostic and endoscopic procedures. Surprisingly, injuries to the anorectum may be subtle, and at times difficult to diagnose. They may require no treatment if the injury is partial thickness or a hematoma is found without mucosal injury. When the injury creates full thickness tissue destruction with little tissue damage but in a relatively clean bowel as, for example, in bowel prepared for polypectomy, the defect can be closed primarily and the patient placed on antibiotics. Debridement of any devitalized tissue and foreign bodies should be performed as well. If the full thickness of the rectal wall is associated with significant soft tissue injury or pelvic fracture, there is very little controversy in the literature regarding the necessary treatment. Thorough debridement of the area, adequate retrorectal drainage combined with a closure of the rectal wound if possible, and mandatory, proximal, totally diverting colostomy has evolved as the therapy of choice. Copious irrigation with saline or antibiotic solutions into the contaminated tissues is recommended.

Several recent studies from wartime experience have shown that the treatment just mentioned is associated with the least mortality and morbidity. Armstrong showed from the Viet Nam war experience that in 32 missile injuries to the extra-peritoneal rectum, four patients died, giving a mortality of 12.5 per cent.[5] There was associated intraperitoneal injury in 18 of these patients. If colostomy alone was performed, the incidence of pelvic abscess was 36 per cent, but when colostomy, closure of the primary wound, and transperineal drainage were added to the regimen, there was 0 per cent incidence of pelvic abscess. Armstrong also used the distal wash-out technique to get the stool cleaned out of the distal segment of the injured rectum to prevent persistent contamination of the

perirectal tissues. He recommended a drainage technique pericoccygeally, and did not advocate the performance of coccygectomy. Excising the coccyx opens more tissue planes and creates the increased incidence of osteomyelitis. Allen reported 65 cases of high velocity, extrarectal injuries from the Viet Nam experience and further stressed the importance of adequate debridement and posterior dependent drainage, as well as evacuation from the distal segment of all retained fecal material.[2] A completely diverting, descending colostomy was also recommended. Several previous authors, writing from both civilian and military experience have shown the seriousness of these injuries, namely a death rate of over 20 per cent, and the importance of distal wash-out to decrease the incidence of further sepsis.[2,36,67,68] In addition, many more complications were experienced when a loop colostomy was created: 47 per cent complications with a 5.5 per cent mortality compared to a completely diverting colostomy at which time 29 per cent complications from sepsis occurred with a 0 per cent mortality. This form of therapy is quite advanced over the World War I therapy which recommended only careful debridement of the rectal wounds and colostomy for severe rectal injuries. At that time, diverting colostomy was not strongly recommended, and there was no idea that drainage of the presacral space was important.

Schrock and associates, and Gustavson have stressed the varying complications and high morbidity and mortality of rectal injuries to the extraperitoneal rectum.[23,53] The major complication from these wounds was sepsis. In Lavenson's series from Viet Nam, the complication rate due to sepsis was 60 per cent.[36] Schrock and Christenson mentioned that half of their patients with these rectal injuries were hospitalized for greater than 50 days, and four patients were hospitalized over 100 days.[53] Failure to clean out the distal segment by washing out the injured rectum will lead not only to generalized sepsis and local abscess formation, but also to the possibility of rectal fistulization and chronic osteomyelitis in the sacrum. For this reason, experts on the subject today recommend distal wash-out of the rectal segment. While creation of a mucous fistula is preferred, a Hartmann pouch is also acceptable. Suture materials, where necessary, should be absorbable rather than permanent, which may induce chronic sinus tract formation. Use of systemic antibiotics is a choice that is dictated by the operative findings, but most people recommend their use. When antibiotics are used, those covering both anaerobic and aerobic populations should be employed.[3,6,18,46]

In the special circumstance where the extraperitoneal rectum has been perforated during the performance of a barium enema, a situation where the bowel has been cleared of stool in preparation for a study, it is reasonable, in the absence of peritoneal signs, to feed the patient nothing by mouth, place him on intravenous fluids and broad spectrum antibiotics, and observe him very closely. Should peritoneal irritation occur, or should there be signs of sepsis, then the above outlined principles of a diverting colostomy and distal irrigation should be instituted together with better intrarectal drainage.

### Injuries to the Intraperitoneal Rectum

Once the peritoneal cavity has been soiled, an acute abdomen will almost always ensue. This will necessitate exploratory laparotomy, and repair of the injury to the intraperitoneal rectum or rectosigmoid. Relative contraindications to the use of primary closure without colostomy are: (*1*) delay in operation with spreading peritonitis; (*2*) high velocity rifle bullet wounds; (*3*) explosive and shot gun injuries with shattering wounds of the colon or rectosigmoid; and (*4*) severe tissue destruction with extensive intramural hematomas or mesenteric vascular damage.

The major discussion in most cases of intraperitoneal rectal or rectosigmoid injury revolves around the issues of whether or not a colostomy proximal to the repair of the bowel is necessary, whether primary repair of the injured bowel is good enough in itself, or whether exteriorization of the injured segment is required. The experience of war time injuries is worth reviewing in this regard. During World War I a mortality of 50 to 60 per cent was seen with simple primary closure of wounds. World War II brought the first real improvement when colostomy was recommended for all injuries to the rectum. In 1944 the Army issued a dictum that colostomy and retrorectal drainage be used in the management of all rectal wounds either intraperitone-

ally or extraperitoneally. This, together with improved management of shock, pre- and intraoperative antibiotics, as well as better anesthesia and earlier treatment lowered the mortality rate to 23 per cent.[30,37,53,63]

Since World War II numerous reports have advocated primary closure of wounds in selected cases of rectal or colonic trauma.[30,37,42] The proviso is a short interval from injury to operation, a low velocity injury (either a stab wound or a small caliber bullet), or some other object causing a clean, sharp wound to the colon or intraperitoneal rectum.

Since World War II numerous reports have also advocated primary closure of these wounds without fecal diversion.[2,9,28,30,71] However, the resultant mortality rates have all exceeded 20 per cent. Two reports from the Viet Nam experience gave mortality rates of 17 and 13.8 per cent which were achieved by using the principles of colostomy and drainage of the perirectal space which were adopted in World War II.[5,19,38] An experience with a large group of patients at the Parkland Hospital in Dallas, Texas was reported by Trunkey and associates.[63] They stated that for minor rectal trauma with injury to the mucosa or submucosa only, the extraperitoneal injury did not require colostmy. However, more extensive rectal injury which had a mortality of 11 per cent in 45 cases necessitated colostomy and presacral drainage. Loop colostomies were placed either in the sigmoid colon or the transverse colon. Thirteen of the colostomies were completely diverting, and these were performed in the most serious injuries. While primary repair without fecal diversion is acceptable when partial thickness or extraperitoneal rectal injury is present, the literature generally supports the view that any intraperitoneal rectal injury with any question about peritoneal soilage or size of wound is more safely managed with a proximal diverting colostomy. Most authors agree that a diverting colostomy is superior to a loop colostomy in preventing sepsis and further complications.[2]

In evaluating the patient with the colonic or intraperitoneal rectal injury from a high velocity missile or a civilian accident, Perry and co-workers, and Gumbert and co-workers have found that the use of diagnostic peritoneal lavage can be useful in helping to detect colorectal injuries. If properly performed, the incidence of false-positive and false-negative lavages is in the range of 4 per cent.[22,45]

### Injuries to the Anal Sphincter

The anal sphincter can be injured by any blunt or penetrating force. Wherever possible, a primary repair of the anal sphincter is recommended. If sphincter injury is isolated, primary repair without colostomy is generally acceptable. If perineal injury is extensive, repair of the sphincter with associated colostomy may be necessary. Other surgeons believe that a delayed repair is in order.[21,35] The newly developed polyglycolic acid or polyglactin sutures may be utilized in preference to permanent sutures so that suture sinuses do not remain a chronic problem. It should be kept in mind that sphincter injuries are rarely, if ever, life-threatening, and prior attention should be paid to the patient's more serious problems. If this means a proximal diverting colostomy with a delayed repair of the sphincter, the patient's best interests are protected for survival.

Lung, in studying wounds of the rectum in 24 patients from Viet Nam in 1970, stressed a primary repair of the anal sphincter musculature should it be injured, and noted the extended duration of these soldiers' hospitalization.[38] The mean hospitalization time for those patients was 207 days, and each had an average of 3.2 operations. For the technical details of sphincter repair refer to Chapter 22.

### FOREIGN BODIES AND SEXUAL TRAUMA

The variety of objects passed per rectum that become entrapped above the anal sphincter musculature and subsequently require removal is limited only by the imagination of the human mind. Practically any object that can be contemplated as fitting into the rectum has at one time been used either for sexual stimulation or for some sort of criminal assault. Aside from criminal assault, the entrapment of the object not only causes the patient social embarrassment, but also significant physical pain, and thus necessitates attention by the medical profession. Serious injuries to the rectum, the rectosigmoid, and other intraperitoneal structures can occur. Death from foreign bodies being placed per rectum has been reported numerous times.[1,6,12,16,59] Some of the more common foreign bodies that have been placed per rectum include rectal vibrators, plastic phalluses, baby powder cans, bottles of all shapes and sizes, flashlight batteries, flashlights, ball point pens, and thermometers. Eftaiha and associates have found it useful to classify the level of entrapment of the foreign body.[16] As will be seen, most objects in the rectum lying at a low or mid level of the rectum up to 10 cm can be removed transanally. Objects that become lodged in the upper rectum or lower rectosigmoid may very well require laparotomy to assist removal.

The circumstances under which foreign bodies are introduced into the rectum and colon have been summarized by Eftaiha and associates as: (1) diagnostic or therapeutic, for example, thermometers, barium, rectal tubes, disposable enema tips, or irrigation catheters; (2) self-administered treatment to alleviate symptoms of anorectal disease, for example, insertion of a broom stick to relieve itching or to reduce prolapsed hemorrhoids; (3) criminal assault with objects such as a glass bottle; (4) autoeroticism, for example, vibrators; and (5) accidental introduction.[16] Foreign bodies which become lodged in the rectum may, in fact, have been swallowed, causing symptoms only when they lodge in the rectum or cause rectal trauma such as laceration.

### Removal of Foreign Bodies

After the diagnosis and evaluation of a patient having a foreign body of the rectum, the task of removing the object must be undertaken. The creativity and skillfullness that is required to remove these objects almost always supasses the force or thought required to insert them. One of the greatest recommendations to physicians who care for these patients is to use one's ingenuity. While certain tried and true methods will be discussed, one should not become close-minded about new ideas that can be used to remove foreign bodies. If the principles as stated below are observed, modifications in extraction are certainly permissible.

There are several principles which should be followed in the removal of foreign bodies: (1) Abdominal and pelvic radiographs should be used to determine the type, number and location of foreign bodies. This often requires anteroposterior and lateral views. (2) Appropriate relaxation and sedation of the patient is necessary with removal of the object using anesthesia as necesary, and adequate lubrication of the anal canal. (*3*) An all-out attempt should be made to remove the object transanally keeping the anal sphincter intact. (*4*) Consideration must be given to the possibility of an internal anal sphincterotomy or opening of the external sphincter musculature to allow extraction of large foreign bodies with primary repair of the sphincter mechanism. (*5*) Laparotomy is used only as a last resort after failure of all transanal manipulations. (*6*) An attempt at removal by manipulation by intraabdominal and perineal operators without opening the colon should be made. use colotomy only when necessary. (*7*) Proctosigmoidoscopy should be performed following removal of foreign bodies. (*8* Proximal colostomy is the alternative if extraperitoneal rectal tear has resulted in considerable contamination with introduction or removal of the foreign body. (*9*) Inpatient observation must be followed to rule out bleeding or perforation with delayed symptoms in any patient upon whom transanal removal has taken place.

*Anesthesia Required.* Appropriate anesthesia, both to relax the patient and to totally relax the anal sphincter musculature, is usually necessary. This anesthesia can be applied in the outpatient area of the emergency room or in the operating room, if necessary. Extraction of foreign bodies can even take place in a physician's office.

LOCAL ANESTHESIA. Utilization of local anesthesia serves a two-fold purpose. First, it allows anesthesia to be applied to the perianal tissues so that an otherwise painful extraction will be made much more comfortable for the patient. Second, the anesthetic used, such as bupivacaine ¼ per cent with epinephrine 1 : 200,000, has the pronounced effect of relaxing the external sphincter. Injection of 20 to 30 cc of this solution takes effect within five minutes and causes complete relaxation of the external sphincter. Following this, the examiner can not only more easily insert instruments to examine the patient, but can also more easily, and without injuring the patient, insert instruments to remove the objects. Also, patients may voluntarily Valsalva, thus assisting the extraction.

INTRAVENOUS SEDATION. As an accompaniment to local anesthesia it is recommended that intravenous sedation be administered. The utilization of diazepam, for example, is very satisfactory. An intravenous line should be started so that the patient can be titrated to the exact level of sedation required. In addition, should the patient require any emergency medications, an intravenous line is already in place. Intravenous demerol or morphine can also be administered should more pain medication be necessary.

REGIONAL ANESTHESIA. Should the physician fail to remove the object utilizing local anesthesia, the next step is to use a caudal or spinal regional anesthesia. This should be performed in the operating room. The goal of this type of anesthesia is no different than that of the local anesthesia.

GENERAL ANESTHESIA. General anesthesia is usually not required unless abdominal laparotomy is anticipated. Objects that lodge in the low or mid-rectum almost always can be removed under local or regional anesthesia. Objects that lodge in the upper rectum or lower rectosigmoid may very well require abdominal laparotomy and, of course, general anesthesia.

*Procedures.* ABDOMINAL CELIOTOMY. The patient is prepared for laparotomy in the usual fashion with the preoperative blood work and preparation required as in any elective abdominal procedure. We prefer the lower abdominal transverse incision. Often no mobilization whatsoever of the rectum or sigmoid is necessary. The entrapped foreign body can be "milked down" into the mid- or lower rectum through the intact rectosigmoid so that the perineal operator may remove the object with his hand. If this procedure fails, a colotomy on the anterior wall of the rectum or rectosigmoid may be necessary to manually extract the object. Broad spectrum antibiotics, of course, are given to the patient.

SPECIAL TECHNIQUES. Several authors have suggested a variety of unique ways to remove foreign bodies transanally. Peet recommended the use of obstetrical forceps to remove impacted foreign bodies from the upper rectum.[44] Vadlamundi recommended the use of a Foley catheter inserted above the object and inflation of the catheter balloon, thus pulling the object down and hopefully out of the rectum.[65] This has the two-fold purpose of causing downward force on the object, and breaking the suction formed by the foreign body against the rectosigmoid wall. Hughes recommended that for hollow objects such as glasses with the open end distally, the use of a well-padded, special pliers might be beneficial.[27] Sachdev has reported the use of plaster of Paris inserted into glass-like objects and allowed to firm and harden, so that either a string or a clamp inserted in the center of the plaster would then be used to extract the object.[51] Occasionally the proctoscope, and less often, the colonoscope can be utilized to retrieve foreign bodies. The use of a Sengstaken-Blakemore tube passed through the proctoscope and into a glass has been reported for the removal of a foreign body from the rectum.

*Position.* For patients undergoing extraction of foreign bodies under regional or general anesthesia the lithotomy position is helpful because either a voluntary Valsalva maneuver or abdominal manipulation may prove useful. For those patients requiring laparotomy the legs should also be elevated as the procedure requires both an abdominal and perineal operator.

### Extended Injuries from Foreign Bodies

Beall, Barone, and Sohn have reported independently on rectosigmoid perforation caused by insertion of foreign bodies.[6,10,59] This may be incurred by the patient in an attempt at auto-eroticism, as an injury delivered by a sexual partner, or during a criminal assault. Actual splitting of the rectosigmoid has been identified with peritoneal contamination. The patient presents with an acute abdomen and often will not offer the information of the sexual or assaultive action that led to the patient's admission to the hospital. For this reason, radiographs are almost always taken to reveal the foreign body in the rectum. In patients with rectosigmoid perforation due to foreign body, the injury is handled as other intraperitoneal injuries to the colon and rectosigmoid. Rarely is primary closure alone, without a diverting colostomy, recommended

due to the contusion-type injury to the bowel and possible contamination of the peritoneal cavity. More often, the laceration or split is repaired with suture material, or if necessary, the involved segment is excised. A proximal diverting colostomy or colostomy and mucous fistula is suggested. The distal wash-out technique as discussed earlier is utilized as well.

### Sexual Assault

Either men or women may be the recipients of sexual assault. The assault may be intended to harm or it may be merely the result of a vigorous sexual act that was intended to be enjoyed by both partners. Whatever the motive, sexual assault can cause significant injury to the extraperitoneal or intraperitoneal rectum or rectosigmoid. These injuries have been discussed previously.

Sohn reports a previously undescribed act known as fist fornication in 11 patients over a four year interval.[59] The act of fist fornication is that of forcing a closed, clenched fist through the intact anal canal into the rectum for sexual gratification. The rectum or sigmoid colon were the recipients of the injury. Six of the patients had mucosal lacerations in the rectum that presented with rectal bleeding but no sphincter laceration. Simple suturing of the mucosal laceration was all that was necessary for those patients. Four patients developed an acute abdomen requiring laparotomy and resection as well as Hartmann's pouch. In addition, one complete anal sphincter incontinence resulted from severe sphincter laceration.

### REFERENCES

1. Abcarian, H., and Lowe, R.: Colon and rectal trauma. Surg. Clin. North. Am., *58:*519, 1978.

2. Allen, B. D.: Penetrating wounds of the rectum. Tex. Med., *69:*77, 1973.

3. Altemeier, W. A.: Bacteriology of traumatic wounds. JAMA., *124:*413, 1944.

4. Andresen, A. F. R.: Perforations from proctoscopy. Gastroenterology, *9:*32, 1947.

5. Armstrong, R. G., Schmitt, H. J. Jr., and Patterson, L. T.: Combat wounds of the extraperitoneal rectum. Surgery, *74:*570, 1973.

6. Barone, J. E., Sohn, N., and Nealon, T. F.: Perforations and foreign bodies of the rectum: Report of 28 cases. Ann. Surg., *184:*601, 1976.

7. Bartizal, J. F., et al: A critical review of management of 392 colonic and rectal injuries. Dis. Colon Rectum, *17:*313, 1974.

8. Bauer, J. J., Weiss, M., and Dreiling, D. A.: Stercoraceous perforation of the colon. Surg. Clin. North Am., *52:*1047, 1972.

9. Beall, A. C., Bricker, D. L., Alessi, F. J., Whisennand, H. H., and DeBakey, M. E.: Surgical considerations in the management of civilian colon injuries. Ann. Surg., *173:*971, 1971.

10. Beall, A. C., and DeBakey, M. E.: Injuries and foreign bodies of the colon and rectum. *In* Turell, R. (ed.): *Diseases of the Colon and Anorectum.* 2 ed. Philadelphia, W. B. Saunders, 1969.

11. Befeler, D.: Proctoscopic perforation of the large bowel. Dis. Colon Rectum, *10:*376, 1967.

12. Benjamin, H. B., Klamecki, B., and Haft, J. S.: Removal of exotic foreign objects from the abdominal orifices. Am. J. Proctology, *20:*413, 1969.

13. Berman, A. T., and Tom, L.: Traumatic separation of the pubic symphysis with associated fatal rectal tear: a case report and analysis of mechanism of injury. J. Trauma, *14:*1060, 1974.

14. Brunton, F. J.: Retroperitoneal emphysema as a complication of barium enema. Clin. Radiol., *11:*197, 1960.

15. Classen, J. N., Martin, R. E., and Sabagal, J.: Iatrogenic lesions of the colon and rectum. South Med. J., *68:*1417, 1975.

16. Eftaiha, M., Hambrick, E., and Abcarian, H.: Principles of management of colorectal foreign bodies. Arch. Surg., *112:*691, 1977.

17. Fonkalsrud, E. W., and Clatworthy, H. W. Jr.: Accidental perforation of the colon and rectum in newborn infants. N. Engl. J. Med., *272:*1097, 1965.

18. Fullen, W. D., Hunt, J., and Altemeier, W. A.: Prophylactic antibiotics in penetrating wounds of the abdomen. J. Trauma, *12:*282, 1972.

19. Ganchrow, M. I., Lavenson, G. S., and McNamara, J. J.: Surgical management of traumatic injuries of the colon and rectum. Arch. Surg., *100:*515, 1970.

20. Getzen, L. C., Pollak, E. W., and Wolfman, E. F.: Abdominoperineal resection in the treatment of devascularizing rectal injuries. Surgery, *82:*310, 1977.

21. Goligher, J. C.: Injuries of the rectum and colon. In *Surgery of the Anus, Rectum and Colon,* 3 ed. Springfield, Charles C Thomas, 1975.

22. Gumbert, J. L., Froderman, S. E., and Mer-

cho, J. P.: Diagnostic peritoneal lavage in blunt abdominal trauma. Ann. Surg., *165:*70, 1967.

23. Gustavson, R. G.: Rectal injuries. Am. Surg., *39:*456, 1973.

24. Haas, P. A., and Fox, T. A. Jr.: Civilian injuries of the rectum and anus. Dis. Colon Rectum, *22:*17, 1979.

25. Horwitz, M. A., and Bennett, J. V.: Nursery outbreak of peritonitis with pneumoperitoneum probably caused by thermometer-induced rectal perforation. Am. J. Epidemiol., *104:*632, 1976.

26. Howell, H. S., Bartizal, J. F., and Freeark, R. J.: Blunt trauma involving the colon and rectum. J. Trauma. *16:*624, 1976.

27. Hughes, J. P., Marice, H. P., and Gathright, J. B.: Method of removing a hollow object from the rectum. Dis. Colon Rectum, *19:*44, 1976.

28. Imes, P. R.: War surgery of abdomen. Surg. Gynecol. Obstet., *81:*608, 1945.

29. Jacobsohn, W. Z., and Levy, A.: Colonoscopic perforation: Its emergency treatment. Endoscopy, *8:*15, 1976.

30. Josen, A. S., Ferrer, J. M. Jr., Forde, K. A., and Zikria, B. A.: Primary closure of civilian colorectal wounds. Ann. Surg., *176:*782, 1972.

31. Kaufer, N., Shein, S., and Levowitz, B. S.: Impalement injury of the rectum: an unusual case. Dis. Colon Rectum, *10:*394, 1967.

32. Kay, S., and Choy, S. H.: Results of intraperitoneal injection of barium sulfate contrast medium: An experimental study. Arch. Pathol., *59:*388, 1955.

33. Kiser, J. L., Spratt, J. S. Jr., and Johnson, C. A.: Colon perforations occurring during sigmoidoscopic examinations and barium enemas. Missouri Med., *65:*969, 1968.

34. Klein, R. R., and Scarborough, R. A.: Traumatic perforations of rectum and distal colon. Am. J. Surg., *86:*515, 1953.

35. Large, P. G., and Murkheiber, W. J.: Injury to rectum and anal canal by enema syringes. Lancet, *2:*596, 1956.

36. Lavenson, G. S., and Cohen, A.: Management of rectal injuries. Am. J. Surg., *122:*226, 1971.

37. LoCicero, J. III., Tajima, T., and Drapanas, T.: A half-century of experience in the management of colonic injuries: Changing concepts. J. Trauma, *15:*575, 1975.

38. Lung, J. A., Turk, R. P., Miller, R. E., and Eiseman, B.: Wounds of the rectum. Ann. Surg., *172:*985, 1970.

39. Lyon, D. C., and Sheiner, H. J.: Idiopathic rec-

tosigmoid perforation. Surg. Gynecol. Obstet., *128:*991, 1969.

40. McLaughlin, A. P. III., and McCullough, D. L.: Successful urologic management of inadvertent rectal injuries. J. Urol., *106:*878, 1971.

41. Morton, J. H.: Perineal and rectal damage following nonpenetrating abdominal trauma. J. Trauma, *12:*347, 1972.

42. Mulherin, J. L., and Sawyers, J. L.: Evaluation of three methods for managing penetrating colon injuries. J. Trauma, *15:*580, 1975.

43. Novak, J. M., Collins, J. T., Donowitz, M., Farman, J., Sheahan, D. G., Spiro, H. M.: Effects of radiation on the human gastrointestinal tract. J. Clin. Gastroenterol., *1:*9, 1979.

44. Peet, T. N. D.: Removal of impacted rectal foreign body with obstetric forceps. Br. Med. J., *1:*500, 1976.

45. Perry, J. F. Jr., DeMeules, J. E., and Root, H. D.: Diagnostic peritoneal lavage in blunt abdominal trauma. Surg. Gynecol. Obstet., *131:*742, 1970.

46. Polk, H. C. Jr., and Miles, A. A.: The decisive period in the primary infection of muscle by Escherichia Coli. Br. J. Exp. Pathol., *54:*99, 1973.

47. Quan, S. H.: Factitial proctitis due to irradiation for cancer of the cervix uteri. Surg. Gynecol. Obstet., *126:*70, 1968.

48. Robbins, P. L., Sutherland, D. E. R., Najarian, J. S., and Bernstein, W. C.: Emphysema of the leg as a presenting sign of large-intestinal perforation: report of two cases. Dis. Colon Rectum, *20:*144, 1977.

49. Rosenberg, L. S., and Fine, A.: Fatal venous intravasation of barium during a barium enema. Radiology, *73:*771, 1959.

50. Rosenklint, A., Buemann, B., Hansen, P., and Baden, H.: Extraperitoneal perforations of the rectum during barium enema. Scand. J. Gastroenterol., *10:*87, 1975.

51. Sachdev, Y. V.: An unusual foreign body in the rectum. Dis. Colon Rectum, *10:*220, 1967.

52. Sanders, A. W., and Kobernick, S. D.: Fate of barium sulfate in the retroperitoneum. Am. J. Surg., *93:*907, 1957.

53. Schrock, T. R., and Christensen, N.: Management of perforating injuries of the colon. Surg. Gynecol. Obstet., *135:*65, 1972.

54. Schwartz, G. F., and Polsky, H. S.: Ingested foreign bodies of the gastrointestinal tract. Am. Surg., *42:*236, 1976.

55. Sherman, L. F., Prem, K. A., and Mensheha, N. M.: Factitial proctitis: a restudy at the University of Minnesota. Dis. Colon Rectum, *14:*281, 1971.

56. Simmons, R. L., Diggs, J. W., and Sleeman, H. K.: Pathogenesis of peritonitis. 3. Local adjuvant action of hemoglobin in experimental E. coli peritonitis. Surgery, *63:*810, 1968.

57. Sisel, R. J., Donovan, A. J., and Yellin, A. E.: Experimental fecal peritonitis: influence of barium sulfate or water-soluble radiographic contrast material on survival. Arch. Surg., *104:*765, 1972.

58. Smith, L. E., and Nivatvongs, S.: Complications in colonoscopy. Dis. Colon Rectum, *18:*214, 1975.

59. Sohn, N., Weinstein, M. A., and Gonchar, J.: Social injuries of the rectum. Am. J. Surg., *134:*611, 1977.

60. Stein, A.: Ano-rectal avulsion associated with crush injuries. South Africa J. Surg., *2:*43, 1964.

61. Thadepalli, H., Gorbach, S. L., Broido, P. W., Norsen, J., and Nyhus, L.: Abdominal trauma, anaerobes, and antibiotics. Surg. Gynecol. Obstet., *137:*270, 1973.

62. Thorbjarnarson, B.: Iatrogenic and related perforations of the large bowel. Arch. Surg., *84:*608, 1962.

63. Trunkey, D., Hays, R. J., and Shires, G. T.: Management of rectal trauma. J. Trauma, *13:*411, 1973.

64. Tumolo, M. A.: Complete loss of the anus and rectum due to crushing injury to the pelvis—treatment using a reversed ileal loop. Dis. Colon Rectum, *13:*34, 1970.

65. Vadlamundi, K., VanBockstaele, P., and McManus, J.: Foley catheter in removal of a foreign body from the rectum. JAMA., *221:*1412, 1972.

66. VanNagell, J. R. Jr., Parker, J. C. Jr., Maruyama, Y., Utley, J., and Luckett, P.: Bladder or rectal injury following radiation therapy for cervical cancer. Am. J. Obstet. Gynecol., *119:*727, 1974.

67. Vannix, R. S., Carter, R., Hinshaw, D. B., and Joergenson, E. J.: Surgical management of colon trauma in civilian practice. Am. J. Surg., *106:*364, 1963.

68. Wanebo, H. J., Hunt, T. K., and Matthewson, C. Jr.: Rectal injuries. J. Trauma, *9:*712, 1969.

69. Wang, S. Y., and Sutherland, J. C.: Colonic perforation secondary to fecal impaction: re-

port of a case. Dis. Colon Rectum, *20:*355, 1977.

70. Wolfe, W. G., and Silver, D.: Rectal perforation with profuse bleeding following an enema. Arch. Surg., *92:*715, 1966.

71. Woodhall, J. P., and Ochsner, A.: The management of perforating injuries of the colon and rectum in civilian practice. Surgery, *29:*305, 1951.

72. Zheutlin, N., Lasser, E. C., and Rigler, L. G.: Clinical studies on effect of barium in the peritoneal cavity following rupture of the colon. Surgery, *32:*967, 1952.

# 24

# Complications in Anorectal Surgery: Their Prevention and Treatment

Provided there has been careful attention to technical detail, perioperative or postoperative complications in elective anorectal procedures should be uncommon. Complications in wound healing almost always arise because operative techniques have not been executed to perfection, or because systemic disease causes a propensity to imperfect wound healing. The secondary situations might include chronic debilitation from malnutrition, chronic corticosteroid usage, deficiencies of vitamin C or zinc, diabetes mellitus, leukemia, inflammatory bowel disease, such as Crohn's disease or ulcerative colitis, immunoincompetence for any reason, and, of course, a combination of these factors.[11,15,23] Several complications will be discussed.

## SYSTEMIC COMPLICATIONS
### Cardiac Complications

Cardiac complications during anorectal procedures are uncommon. Preoperative screening by proper history, physical examination, and electrocardiogram suffices as proper evaluation in most cases. Patients with previously documented heart disease should be seen by an internist or cardiologist, and appropriate recommendations carried out. Care should be taken to see that appropriate medications are

With collaboration of Frederic D. Nemer

continued pre- and postoperatively, and that fluid and electrolyte balance is maintained.

### Pulmonary Complications

Special attention to pre- and postoperative pulmonary exercises should help to prevent major pulmonary complications in patients with preexisting pulmonary disease. Incentive spirometry, or the use of "blow bottles," will aid in preventing pulmonary atelectasis after general anesthesia.

Most physicians are aware of the catastrophic consequences of massive pulmonary embolism. Appropriate preventive precautions should be taken to decrease the likelihood of this occurrence. All ambulatory patients should be up and walking soon after the operative procedure. Elastic stockings may be used; however, if they are used improperly or are of poor quality these may actually embarrass circulation in the legs. Prophylactic, subcutaneous, low dose heparin should be considered for patients with a history of previous pulmonary embolism, for bedridden or obese patients, or for patients with a history of thrombophlebitis.[21] Proper positioning of the patient on the operating table and the expeditious performance of the operative procedure will further decrease the duration of venous stasis, and may decrease the chances for postoperative thromboembolic or phlebitic disease.

# SPECIFIC EARLY LOCAL COMPLICATIONS

## Hemorrhage

Massive postoperative hemorrhage which occurs within the first twenty-four hours after anorectal procedures, and requires a return to the operating room, should be very uncommon. In a review of over 2,000 hemorrhoidectomies performed at the Ferguson Clinic, Grand Rapids, Michigan, massive early postoperative hemorrhage occurred in less than 2 per cent of the patients, and only about half of these required suture ligation in the operating room.[10] Buls and Goldberg reported 0.8 per cent early postoperative hemorrhage in 500 patients undergoing hemorrhoidectomy.[5]

Causes of early postoperative bleeding include: (1) inadequate suturing of the hemorrhoidal pedicles or submucosal muscular bleeders; (2) previously undetermined coagulation defect; and (3) ingestion of medications known to prolong bleeding time such as aspirin and warfarin. Occasionally during the immediate postoperative period a patient may cough, or in some other way produce a Valsalva maneuver, thus increasing the intra-abdominal pressure and "popping a stitch". Epinephrine solutions have been implicated in early postoperative hemorrhage. Because they initially cause vasoconstriction they are used during the operative procedure, but, when the effect of the solution diminishes, small arteries and veins dilate and may bleed. However, Ganchrow and associates reported a 1.3 per cent incidence of subsequent suture ligation of early postoperative bleeders without the use of epinephrine solution, in patients receiving epinephrine locally, only 1.1 per cent of early postoperative bleeders needed suture ligation.[10] These statistics suggest there is actually no difference in the incidence of postoperative hemorrhage with or without epinephrine solutions if care is taken to achieve proper hemostasis at the time of operation. On the other hand, the advantage of an epinephrine solution is that there is a relatively dry field at the time of operation, therefore, significant arterioles may be more easily controlled. "Blind" clamping and mass ligation of the rectal wall should always be discouraged. Open dissection that includes exposure of the internal sphincter and subcutaneous external sphincter should be performed with meticulous cauterization of small muscular arteries and veins followed by continuous suture approximation of the mucosa anoderm to minimize postoperative bleeding.

There are a number of reasons why packing of the anal canal for hemostasis following any anorectal procedure should *not* be performed routinely. First, if postoperative bleeding should occur it may be masked. Second, the removal of a pack cannot be anything but painful. Finally, the presence of packing causes spasm which in turn causes pain, and may predispose to urinary retention. Because the colon and rectum offer a large reservoir for blood, significant bleeding may go undetected until the patient's vital signs are compromised. Without packing the rate and quantity of postoperative hemorrhage can be accurately assessed. If brisk, persistent bleeding should occur, an early reexamination under anesthesia is recommended. If there is no obvious bleeding site, all suture lines should be resutured, preferably, with a strong, synthetic, absorbable suture (polyglycolic acid or polyglactin). A light, oxidized, cellulose cotton may also be applied. The patient should then be evaluated for any coagulopathy that may have been missed on routine preoperative screening.

Delayed hemorrhage following anorectal, specifically hemorrhoidal surgery has a peak incidence between 7 and 10 days postoperatively.[5,10] This is generally secondary to wound separation following suture dissolution, or to trauma following the passage of a large, hard stool. The patient may state that straining at stool, vigorous physical activity, or the passage of a hard bowel movement precipitated the bleeding. However, the patient may also claim that no unusual or strenuous activity was being performed when the bleeding began. In fact, the patient may have been lying down in bed or sitting in a chair when the bleeding began. When massive bleeding begins, it is not unusual for one or two units of blood to be lost in a very short period of time; perhaps in 15 to 30 minutes. Replacement of blood should follow episodes of hypotension with continued bleeding. Most patients who lose two units of blood will already have their vital signs compromised.

Treatment for massive rectal bleeding consists, at least, of readmission to the hospital with bed rest, observation, stool softeners, and transfusions, if necessary. If hemorrhage continues, examination under anesthesia is required at which time bleeding points can be visualized, and appropriate suture ligations carried out. Should bleeding cease upon admission, at least 48 hours observation in the hospital is required. The passage of a normal, non-bloody bowel movement is required before discharge. Buls and Goldberg reported that in 500 patients undergoing closed hemorrhoidectomy 4 per cent had delayed hemorrhage, but only 0.4 per cent required reoperation.[5] The remaining patients responded to the conservative approach of observation as stated above.

When faced with an exsanguinating emergency of rectal or anal bleeding, the physician may place a temporary pack of rolled-up gauze covered by a plastic or rubber sheet over the wound to control hemorrhage until the operating room is made ready. The use of a Foley catheter placed in the rectum, inflated, and pulled down may also be helpful to stop bleeding but it is a painful technique and should only be used as a last resort on the way to the operating room.

## Urinary Retention

The occurrence of postoperative urinary retention following anorectal surgical procedures is a significant problem. Reported incidences of postoperative catheterization have ranged from a low of 1 per cent to high of 70 per cent.[6,19] A reasonable expectation would be within a range from 3.5 to 10 per cent.[1,5,7] Underlying the reason for this high incidence is the common innervation of the anal sphincter mechanism and the urethral sphincter. Any irritation to the anal sphincter may cause reflex spasm of the urethral sphincter and bladder trigone. This is the result of a reflex mechanism involving the pudendal nerve, sacral spinal cord, and pelvic parasympathetic nerves. The problem is precipitated and further aggravated by overdistention of the bladder caused by inappropriately administered, large volumes of fluid given intravenously during, or immediately following, operative procedures while the patient is still under anesthesia. Men are affected twice as frequently as women.[8]

Several factors, when controlled, will dramatically reduce the incidence of postoperative catheterization.[1,7] The preoperative physical examination should identify the patients who, because of their history or previous conditions, are at a higher risk to develop postoperative problems (e.g., borderline or overt benign prostatic hypertrophy). Patients should be encouraged to void immediately preoperatively. During anesthesia intravenous access is all that is really required; therefore, only a small amount of fluid ($<100$ cc) need be given. The intravenous fluid should be discontinued in the recovery room when the patient is stable. The patient is not allowed food or beverage until the anesthetic influence abates, and/or voiding ensues. The nursing staff should be aware that, because the patient was given minimal preoperative hydration, and a small amount of intraoperative fluid, postoperative voiding may be delayed as much as twelve or eighteen hours. However, if the patient becomes uncomfortable, or the bladder is palpably distended and the patient is unable to void, straight catheterization is recommended. Straight catheterization conveys less risk of urinary tract infection than an indwelling Foley catheter.[1,7,8,10]

The type of anesthetic agent used is thought to be a contributing factor in postoperative urinary retention. General anesthesia has very little effect on urinary retention. Spinal anesthesia, however, may often be associated with postoperative urinary retention secondary to the length of sensory motor block. Caudal anesthesia with local supplement probably has some effect on urinary retention but probably less than the spinal block (see Chap. 5). If one follows the above guidelines, it is reasonable to expect a 10 per cent or less incidence of postoperative urinary retention.

## Constipation/Fecal Impaction

Constipation with subsequent impaction should be infrequent following anorectal procedures. The first proviso is that the patient should not be discharged until the first good bowel movement occurs either spontaneously or following an enema. Almost all patients are apprehensive about the initial stool passage after anorectal procedures. Empathetic physician and nurse discussion will help alleviate some of the fears. Occasionally, patients may drastically alter their dietary habits or even refuse to eat because of fear of the first bowel movement. A psyllium seed bulk stool softener should be started during the patient's preoperative hospital stay. Postoperatively this is combined with lubricants (mineral oil) and mild laxatives (milk of magnesia) as well as adequate fluid intake (4–6 glasses per day). This tried and tested technique is generally responsible for spontaneous bowel movement on the third or fourth postoperative day. The physician should inquire daily as to the passage of flatus or stool. Each patient should be provided with adequate analgesia which will reduce postoperative discomfort, help alleviate anxiety, and aid in the first bowel movement. Prolonged use of strong narcotics, however, may be counterproductive. Rectal examination to rule out fecal impaction is generally not necessary prior to the third postoperative day. Anal examinations performed early postoperatively are always very painful, and should be reserved for the physician to perform only when absolutely necessary. A clue to the presence of impaction is the patient's complaint of increasing anorectal pain or pressure, or the presence of diarrhea on approximately the third or fourth postoperative day. At this time a rectal examination done gently may indicate a true impaction. An even less painful way to test for impaction is to use a moistened, cotton swab. If a large volume of firm stool is present, a single packaged phosphosoda, or tap water enema is recommended. This will almost always, totally relieve the patient's distress.

Prior to his return home the patient is encouraged to continue the bulk softener and adequate fluid intake. Mild cathartics such as milk of magnesia are used sparingly to stimulate a recalcitrant bowel. True fecal impaction necessitating readmission to the hospital for disimpaction is very uncommon. The delayed, acute onset of diarrhea and rectal pain should cause one to think of fecal impaction. True diarrhea can usually be managed at home by properly adjusting the patient's diet, providing a bulk-forming agent, and discontinuing any oil-type laxative after the first bowel movement. The development of severe pain after the patient is at home four to five days postoperatively is either due to an impaction or an abscess. If there are no signs of abscess, the impaction is generally relieved by a tap water or packaged phosphosoda enema. If a tap water enema is used, a rubber catheter should be gently inserted approximately 15 to 20 cm into the rectum prior to the instillation of fluid. In the case of a true fecal impaction, the treatment is actually quite simple, but the patient may require readmission to the hospital. Cleansing enemas utilizing a mixture of one four-ounce packaged phosphosoda enema, 100 cc of hydrogen peroxide, and water to a dilution of one liter have been found useful. This can be used as often as necessary to soften and flush the stool. In addition, mineral oil should be given by mouth until a soft, formed stool returns. If all of these measures fail, the patient can be taken to the operating room, where, under anesthesia (either general or caudal), with or without instruments, the fecal bolus can be manually removed. To help prevent this complication codeine should not be used as the postoperative analgesic.

### Infection

Despite a fertile milieu for potential infection, suppuration postoperatively in the anorectal surgery patient is very infrequent. Suppuration occurs more often in circumstances where the patient is diabetic, immunosuppressed as in the case of the transplant patient, or, occasionally, when the patient is suffering from malignant disease.[2,5,8,10,14,15] Only rarely do the usually healthy perirectal tissues become a site for suppuration. This generally occurs if these clean tissue planes are violated during the operation.

Early recognition and treatment is the key to a successful outcome. The physician or nurse may suspect early suppuration when the patient complains of inordinate or increasing perianal pain as the interval from operation increases. Simple, gentle inspection may reveal an early perianal or buttock swelling or cellulitis. An anal examination may be necessary to confirm the presence of an abscess. Adequate sedation or analgesia may be necessary for this. Abscesses, though uncommon, should be drained promptly and appropriately. They may occur in the perianal tissues, in the intersphincteric plane, or in the ischiorectal fossa. The source of most of these immediate postoperative perianal infections may either be an infected hematoma in an enclosed space, or violation of a previously uncontaminated tissue plane. Infection in the anorectal wound may be minimized by careful handling of the tissues, and elimination of dead space under the mucosal and anodermal suture lines. Patients with Crohn's disease, diabetes mellitus, or any type of immunosuppression are prone to develop persistent perineal infection and non-healing wounds.[14,22]

Overwhelming perineal infection (gas gangrene) that may crop up within 24 to 48 hours postoperatively must be diagnosed early because, if it goes unrecognized, death may ensue. These infections may occur spontaneously, or they may follow an operative procedure or trauma to the rectum. Pain which seems out of proportion to the problem at hand, anxiety and restlessness, progressive edema, cellulitis, and tissue crepitation should alert one to the severity of the infection.[15] Colostomy as well as the use of hyperalimentation may be necessary adjuncts in these patients.[12,22]

## SPECIFIC LATE LOCAL COMPLICATIONS

### Stricture

The true incidence of anal stricture following anorectal procedures is unknown. Two series report an incidence of approximately 1 per cent, but this is probably lower than the incidence experienced by most surgeons.[5,9,10] Bennett and co-workers, reported a 4 per cent incidence.[4] The problem, when it occurs, can be a serious one. Several factors contribute to its development. Excessive removal of normal anoderm or full thickness destruction of the skin elements is almost always the cause. When excessive anoderm is removed, the anal orifice becomes narrowed and markedly constricted when fibrosis and scar formation are complete. The preservation of normal anoderm should always be foremost in the surgeon's mind. The use of extensive cautery in the anoderm, as in electrocoagulation of anal condylomata, will also lead to scar formation and narrowing of the anal orifice. Rarely, the anorectal wound may become involved in a severe suppurative process that causes breakdown of the wounds, and slough of the normal skin. When the area subsequently heals by secondary intention, narrowing of the anal canal results.

Frequent digital or instrumental dilatation of the anal canal in the early postoperative period is not recommended because repeated trauma of anorectal tissues may cause fibrosis, inflammation, and scarring, and will certainly make the patient uncomfortable. For anorectal wounds, natural daily dilatation of the anal outlet is provided by the passage of a soft, formed stool. This event may be encouraged by providing the patient with a bulk stool softener of psyllium seed derivative. Because of the tendency to synechiae formation, it is important to see the patient soon after dismissal from the hospital. A gentle anal examination approximately two weeks after operation is often helpful in breaking up the superficial synechiae which may become dense scar tissue if left alone.

At the time of hemorrhoidectomy many surgeons perform partial internal sphincterotomy. They feel this helps reduce postoperative pain secondary to internal sphincter spasm, and prevent stenosis.[3,9] We agree with this theory. This additional measure should be used only for strict indications because permanent incontinence of flatus (at least) may result in the poorly selected patient. It is recommended for use in those patients in whom considerable sphincter spasm was demonstrated preoperatively. Treatment of established symptomatic anal strictures may require a formal anoplasty. (see Chap. 26).

### Painful and Unhealed Wounds

Painful scars or poor healing of anorectal wounds should be infrequent. They are generally caused by either excessive removal of anoderm, or traumatic factors such as digital or instrumental dilatations which are performed too early, too frequently, or in a rough manner.[2,5,8,11,13] Unhealed wounds may also result from early bridging of anoderm which may cause pocketing.

For reasons not understood at the present, Crohn's disease is a frequent cause of imperfect anorectal healing.[8,11,13,23,25] In addition, blood dyscrasias such as leukemia and polycythemia predispose to poor anorectal healing. In the absence of the above-mentioned etiologies a wound unhealed after three months should be searched for missed pathology. Rarely a retrorectal cyst or neoplasm may be responsible for persistent anorectal pain.[24] Sometimes reexamination will require anesthesia. Local anesthesia in the office may suffice, but one should not hesitate to return the patient to the operating room for a more thorough evaluation should this be necessary.

When a wound has failed to heal after three months it should be reexamined, and any excess granulation tissue should be curetted. The patient should be continued on bulk stool softeners. If these simple measures do not improve the wound healing process, examination and biopsy may be necessary. A small sinus tract or fistula-in-ano can be overlooked in an office examination; hence, the site of chronic infection may be missed. In difficult cases, a more thorough examination is best performed in the operating room under general anesthesia. The sinus tract can then be excised or unroofed. When the poorly healing wound is associated with anal sphincter spasm the patient may benefit from a lateral internal sphincterotomy regardless of the position of the unhealed wound. This is likely to alleviate the pain.[3] Another clinical observation is the propensity for poor wound healing in the posterior midline. For this reason an internal sphincterotomy, which inevitably causes a wound, should be performed in the lateral aspect of the anal canal.[3,13] Excessive granulation tissue occurs in poorly healing anorectal wounds or wounds healing by secondary intention. This granulation may be eliminated by careful curettage performed in the office with or without local anesthesia, followed by an application of silver nitrate. The use of a stick impregnated with silver nitrate or the liquid solution itself is often successful in suppressing the granulation tissue and allowing normal healing to take place. Electrocauterization is an alternative means of accomplishing this end. Hypertrophic granulation tissue may also indicate "pocketing"; an indication for further debridement or saucerization.

### Recurrence

Actually, when we speak of recurrence we usually mean residual disease. The problem could be residual hemorrhoids which have not been fully excised initially, or a residual fistulous tract that has not been completely unroofed. Anal fissures may actually recur.[3,9] This should suggest either inappropriate initial treatment (no internal sphincterotomy), a subtle presentation of inflammatory bowel disease, or persistent rectal trauma (homosexual acts).[3] Sometimes a return to the operating room is necessary to complete the job; however, much can be done in the office in situations such as residual internal hemorrhoids by using the Barron ligature or curettage of fistulous tracts under local anesthesia.

### Mucosal Prolapse

Mucosal prolapse is a common anorectal condition which is most often associated with mixed hemorrhoids. Development of mucosal prolapse may be averted at the time of hemorrhoidectomy by carrying the mucosal excision the full length of the anal canal, and even into the lower rectum when redundant mucosa is present, and fixing the suture line to the underlying internal sphincter. To avoid an ectropion it is important to maintain the mucocutaneous junction at the dentate line and not relocate the mucosal surface caudally.[5] This is an iatrogenic form of mucosal prolapse which may be seen following an incorrectly performed circumferential amputative hemorrhoidectomy (Whitehead deformity).[6] In the case of mucosal prolapse after hemorrhoidectomy, rubber band ligation (single or multiple) carried out high in the anal canal may obviate the need for re-operation. Sclerosing techniques with phenol-in-oil injection into the prolapsing hemorrhoidal cushion has proven satisfactory in selected cases. If the surgeon is confronted with the ectropion deformity where circumferential protrusion of the mucosa eventually replaces the anoderm, various plastic surgical procedures to create and mobilize full thickness skin flaps and fold them into the anal canal have been devised.[20] (See Chap. 26)

### Hypertrophied Anal Papillae

Hypertrophied anal papillae are frequently associated with anal fissures but may be an early or late manifestation following anorectal surgery. This is a benign process which when asymptomatic should be left alone. However, this tissue may protrude and cause patients to have some anxiety as to the nature of this mass. The patient should be reassured that it is benign with no malignant potential (a fibroepithelial histologically). Should it become symptomatic, excision can be performed as an office procedure.

### Skin Tags

A common postoperative sequalae is the development of unsightly and irregular tags of skin around the anal opening. They are usually mild, cosmetic imperfections that are, as a rule, totally asymptomatic. These tags, however, may be somewhat annoying to the patient: he may believe they represent a recurrence of the hemorrhoids or other disease. They may also be an annoyance to the fastidious surgeon who would like to see a "beautiful result". They should be excised only if they are a source of ulceration, induration, or when they cause chronic pruritus because of redundant folds and the inability to cleanse the anorectal region properly. Patients who have "cancer phobias", or who believe that their primary disease has recurred, should also have these tags excised under local anesthesia. Very often simply reassuring and explaining to the patient the etiology of the tags is adequate to allay his fears. Skin tags may be prevented by an adequate, but not excessive, excision of anoderm, and accurate apposition of the tissues. A closed technique of hemorrhoidectomy probably has a greater potential for development of skin tags, but the incidence decreases when the operator becomes more experienced.

### Fistula

Persistent or new anal fistulae may present postoperatively.[2,5,9,17,18] Either missed pathology or too rapid skin bridging over anal wounds may cause a fistula. In the latter circumstance, unroofing may be possible in the office under local anesthesia; the former usually requires operating room care.

### Temporary Incontinence

Temporary incontinence is a common phase after many anorectal procedures. This results from interference with the normal sensory and motor apparatus of the anal canal despite no mechanical injury to the sphincter mechanism. As a result, the patient cannot differentiate between flatus, solid, or liquid feces, and inadvertent soiling may occur. Discrete sensory perception is frequently lacking for approximately two to three weeks. The patient should be reassured that his sensory and motor functions will return to normal, and that he will once again develop proper discrimination. In the meantime, proper anal hygiene will tide the patient over during this period.

### Persistent Incontinence

This severe and dreaded complication most often follows fistula surgery in which excessive muscle mass has been divided. In a review of 800 cases of fistula surgery at St. Mark's Hospital, London, incontinence for liquid stool occurred in 17 per cent of the cases, incontinence for flatus in 25 per cent, and for soiling in 31 per cent.[17] These numbers are quite alarming, and, therefore, whenever one operates on the anorectum, care should be taken and thought should be given to the possibility of this complication.

Whenever the surgeon is concerned about the amount of muscle to be incised, a more conservative approach should be utilized. "Simple" core excision of the fistulous tract with preservation of the sphincter mechanism, or the use of the seton would be two alternative methods that offer greater safety and prevention as far as incontinence is concerned (see Chap. 8).[18] In addition to preserving the sphincter mechanism, care should be taken to preserve the anoderm and the mucocutaneous junction of the dentate line in its normal anatomical position. Also, careless traction and clamping procedures in hemorrhoidectomy

TABLE **24-1.** Complications in 500 Patients Undergoing
Closed Hemorrhoidectomy[5]

| COMPLICATION | INCIDENCE | TREATMENT |
|---|---|---|
| *Early hemorrhage* | 0.8% | Reoperation in all |
| *Delayed hemorrhage* | 4.0% | Reoperation in .04% |
| *Abscess formation* | 0 | |
| *Fistula-in-ano (superficial)* | 0.4% | Reoperation in all |
| *Anal fissure (painful wound)* | 0.2% | Reoperation |
| *Acute urinary retention* | 10.0% | Catheterization |
| *Incontinence (temporary)* | 0.4% | Complete resolution |
| *Anal stenosis (asymptomatic)* | 1.0% | Complete resolution |
| *Pruritus ani* | 2.2% | Complete resolution |
| *Fecal impaction* | 0.4% | Resolved with enemas |
| *Thrombosed external hemorrhoid* | 0.2% | Resolved |
| *Proctalgia* | 0.2% | Resolved |
| *Skin tags* | 6.0% | Excision under local anesthesia |

should be avoided because of the chance for inadvertent inclusion of the sphincter. When performing lateral internal sphincterotomy for fissure-in-ano the incidence of incontinence for liquid and flatus is insignificant in any critical appraisal of the operation. Division of the lower half of the internal sphincter only rarely results in any permanent disability. Care should be taken, therefore, to incise only the distal half of the internal sphincter (from the level of the dentate line distally).

As a point for consideration, a summary of complications seen in 500 patients undergoing closed hemorrhoidectomy is presented in Table 24-1.[5]

## REFERENCES

1. Bailey, H. R., and Ferguson, J. A.: Prevention of urinary retention by fluid restriction following anorectal operations. Dis. Colon Rectum, *19:*250, 1976.

2. Bautista, L. I.: Hemorrhoidectomy; How I do it: Complications of closed hemorrhoidectomy. Dis. Colon Rectum, *20:*183, 1977.

3. Bennett, R. C., and Duthie, H. L.: The functional importance of the internal anal sphincter. Br. J. Surg., *51:*355, 1964.

4. Bennett, R. C., Friedman, M. H. W., and Goligher, J. C.: Late results of hemorrhoidectomy by ligature and excision. Br. Med. J., *2:*216, 1963.

5. Buls, J. G., and Goldberg, S. M.: Modern management of hemorrhoids. Surg. Clin. North Am., *58:*469, 1978.

6. Burchell, M. C., Thow, G. B., and Manson, R. R.: A "modified Whitehead" hemorrhoidectomy. Dis. Colon Rectum, *19:*225, 1976.

7. Campbell, E. D.: Prevention of urinary retention after anorectal operations. Dis. Colon Rectum, *15:*69, 1972.

8. Crystal, R. F., and Hopping, R. A.: Early postoperative complications of anorectal surgery. Dis. Colon Rectum, *17:*336, 1974.

9. Ferguson, J. A.: Fissure-in-ano and anal stenosis. Clin. Gastroenterol., *4:*629, 1975.

10. Ganchrow, M. I., Mazier, W. P., Friend, W. G., and Ferguson, J. A.: Hemorrhoidectomy revisited—A computer analysis of 2038 cases. Dis. Colon Rectum, *14:*128, 1971.

11. Goligher, J. C.: Surgery of the Anus, Rectum and Colon. 3 ed. 1013-1039. Springfield, Charles C Thomas, 1975.

12. Gordon, P. H.: The chemically defined diet and anorectal procedures. Can. J. Surg., *19:*511, 1976.

13. Graham-Stewart, C. W., Greenwood, R. K., and Davies-Lloyd, R. W.: A review of 50 patients with fissure-in-ano. Surg. Gynecol. Obstet., *113:*445, 1961.

14. Granet, E.: Hemorrhoidectomy failures: Causes, prevention and management. Dis. Colon Rectum, *11:*45, 1968.

15. Hitchcock, C. R., and Bubrick, M. P.: Gas gangrene infections of the small intestine, colon and rectum. Dis. Colon Rectum, *19:*112, 1976.

16. Lee, P. W. R., Green, M. A., Long, W. B. III, and Gill, W.: Zinc and wound healing. Surg. Gynecol. Obstet., *143:*549, 1976.

17. Marks, C. G., and Ritchie, J. K.: Anal fistulas at St. Mark's Hospital. Br. J. Surg., *64:*84, 1977.

18. Parks, A. G.: Pathogenesis and treatment of fistula-in-ano. Br. Med. J., *1:*463, 1961.

19. Prasad, M. L., and Abcarian, H.: Urinary retention following operations for benign anorectal diseases. Dis. Colon Rectum, *21:*490, 1978.

20. Rand, A. A.: The sliding flap graft operation for hemorrhoids; a modification of the Whitehead operation. Dis. Colon Rectum, *12:*265, 1969.

21. Sagar, S., Koshi, M. M., and Kakkar, V. V.: Low dose heparin prophylaxis against pulmonary embolism. Br. J. Surg., *62:*163, 1975.

22. Sohn, N., and Weinstein, M. A.: Use of total parenteral nutrition as a "medical colostomy" in management of severe lacerations of a sphincter. Dis. Colon Rectum, *20:*695, 1977.

23. Turrell, R.: Diseases of the Colon and Anorectum. I. 2 ed. 723–760. Philadelphia, W. B. Saunders, 1969.

24. Uhlig, B. E., and Johnson, R. L.: Presacral tumors and cysts and adults. Dis. Colon Rectum, *18:*581, 1975.

25. Watts, J. M., Bennett, R. G., Duthie, H. L., and Goligher, J. C.: Healing and pain after hemorrhoidectomy. Br. J. Surg., *51:*808, 1964.

# 25

# Rectovaginal Fistula

A rectovaginal fistula is defined as a congenital or acquired communication between the two epithelial-lined surfaces of the rectum and vagina. A fistula between the anal canal distal to the dentate line and the vagina is not truly a rectovaginal fistula but is an anovaginal fistula. Rectovaginal fistulae account for fewer than 5 per cent of anorectal fistulae.[19]

## CLINICAL EVALUATION

Symptoms are dependent on the location, size, and etiology of the rectovaginal fistula, and on the woman's perceptiveness and tolerance of the condition. A few patients are asymptomatic, but for most women, the symptoms of rectovaginal fistula are distressing and totally unacceptable. Vaginal symptoms include a discharge with fecal odor, recurrent or chronic vaginitis, and passage of flatus or stool per vagina.[30] The last symptom may only be noted when the patient has diarrhea. Rectal symptoms of fecal incontinence because of associated sphincter damage, or of diarrhea, or blood or mucus discharge because of the underlying disease state may dominate the clinical picture.

Examination is essential to: (1) confirm the presence of a rectovaginal fistula; (2) accurately determine the size and location of the rectovaginal fistula; (3) assess the state of the anal sphincter; (4) exclude fistulae involving

With collaboration of David A. Rothenberger

other organs; and (5) search for signs of an underlying disease state such as an acute infection, Crohn's disease, irradiation injury, or a neoplastic process. Two recently reported cases emphasize that failure to recognize Crohn's disease as the etiology of a rectovaginal fistula can result in inappropriate surgical procedures which serve only to make the patient more symptomatic.[34] Most often, the fistula is palpable, and/or visualized easily by rectovaginal examination and proctosigmoidoscopy. Stool is often seen in the vagina, which may be the site of active infection. The dark red rectal mucosa contrasts with the lighter vaginal mucosa. If it is small, the opening of the fistula may appear only as a depression or pit-like defect. The gentle use of a probe may be necessary to define the fistula.

Ancillary studies may occasionally be necessary to outline the rectovaginal fistula, and to exclude underlying disease states, involvement of other parts of the bowel, or fistulae concomitant to other organs. An elusive rectovaginal fistula track can be identified by placing a vaginal tampon into the vagina and instilling methylene blue into the rectum. The anus is plugged for 15 to 20 minutes, and then the vaginal packing is removed. If it is unstained, the diagnosis of rectovaginal fistula is probably incorrect. A fistula involving other parts of the bowel such as an ileovaginal fistula should be excluded. Concomitant vesicovaginal, rectovesical, rectourethral, rectoperineal, and other fistulae should be sought since they may accompany rectovaginal fistulae.[19,25,31] Contrast media fistulograms, vaginograms, barium enemas, intravenous pyelograms, and endoscopic procedures may be of value.

## CLASSIFICATION

Rectovaginal fistulae may be classified on the basis of location, size, and etiology. Though somewhat arbitrary, such schemata are useful when comparing operative approaches and results of therapy, providing that the definition of terms is standardized.

### Location

The anterior rectal wall of the distal two-thirds of the rectum is subjacent to the posterior wall of the vagina. Depending on the underlying etiology, a rectovaginal fistula may occur at any site along this 9 cm rectovaginal septum. For convenience, many surgeons arbitrarily classify a rectovaginal fistula as "low" if it can be surgically corrected from a perineal approach, or as "high" if it can only be approached transabdominally. Bentley attempted to be more precise by defining a "low" rectovaginal fistula as one between the lower one-third of the rectum and the lower one-half of the vagina, while defining a "high" rectovaginal fistula as one between the middle one-third of the rectum and the posterior vaginal fornix.[4] Daniels, in his thesis on rectovaginal fistula, arbitrarily classified a rectovaginal fistula as "low" when it is located at, or just slightly above, the dentate line with the vaginal opening just inside the vaginal fourchette, as "high" when the vaginal opening is behind or near the cervix, and as "mid" when it is located between the "high" and "low" limitations (Fig. 25-1).[11]

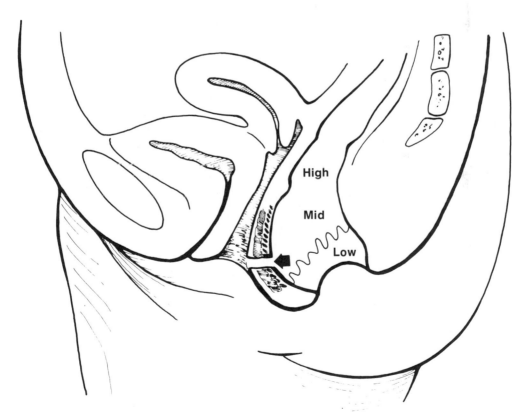

**FIGURE 25-1.** *Rectovaginal fistula, classification by location. Rectovaginal fistulae can be arbitrarily classified by location as "low" when at or just cephalad to the dentate line; as "high" when near the cervix, or as "mid" when located between the "high" and "low" types. A typical low rectovaginal fistula is illustrated.*

## Size

The size of rectovaginal fistulae varies greatly, though most are less than 1.0 to 2.0 cm in diameter. Daniels arbitrarily classified a fistula as "small" if it is less than 0.5 cm, "medium" if it is 0.5 to 2.5 cm, and "large" if it is over 2.5 cm in diameter.[11] Third degree defects involving the whole of the posterior vaginal wall up to the cervix can occur.[5,20]

## Etiology

A rectovaginal fistula may result from a congenital malformation, or from a variety of acquired disorders (see below). The precise incidence of a given etiology is difficult to determine since most series are small, and reflect the referral pattern of a particular author-surgeon or institution. In most series, obstetrical injuries account for the majority of rectovaginal fistulae.[16] Hibbard reported that 88 per cent of his 24 cases at the University of Southern California Medical Center were due to obstetrical trauma.[17] Given, in a review of 20 years' experience in a community hospital, reported that such injuries accounted for 32 per cent of his 38 cases, while irradiation and other operative trauma each accounted for 24 per cent.[13] Belt and Belt, however, reported that rectovaginal fistulae were most commonly caused by an infection originating in the anal tubular glands.[3] In the Mayo Clinic series of 252 patients with rectovaginal fistulae treated between 1947 and 1964, 24 per cent were secondary to inflammatory bowel disease, 12 per cent were secondary to congenital anomalies, and childbirth injuries accounted for only 11 per cent of the series.[21] Tuxen and Castro reported that almost half of the rectovaginal fistulae that they encountered during the past five years were related to inflammatory bowel disease.[34]

---

TRAUMA—Obstetrical, Gynecological, Colonic, Fulguration, Violence, Foreign Body
INFLAMMATORY BOWEL DISEASE
PELVIC IRRADIATION
NEOPLASTIC (Cervix, Rectum, Vagina)
    AND HEMATOLOGIC (Leukemia)
INFECTION—Anal Gland, Bartholin Abscess
CONGENITAL
MISCELLANEOUS

---

*Traumatic.* Childbirth injuries of perineal tears and obstetrical maneuvers such as episiotomies, especially when resulting in episioproctotomy, predispose to the development of rectovaginal fistula. Failure to recognize such an injury, inadequate repair, or development of a secondary infection in a repaired wound virtually assures development of a rectovaginal fistula. Prolonged labor with persistent pressure on the rectovaginal septum occasionally causes necrosis with resulting rectovaginal fistula.[20,22]

Operative trauma is often responsible for development of a rectovaginal fistula. Vaginal or rectal operative procedures can cause them, usually near the dentate line; while pelvic operations can be complicated by the development of high rectovaginal fistula.

Violence, either penetrating or blunt, can cause rectovaginal fistula. Impalement injuries and forceful coitus have also, reportedly, produced them.[16] Foreign bodies, such as pessaries or surgical sponges left after a previous procedure, have eroded through the rectovaginal septum, thus producing a fistula.[13]

*Inflammatory Bowel Disease.* Both ulcerative colitis and Crohn's disease can produce a rectovaginal fistula. Lescher and Pratt reported a 22 per cent incidence of ulcerative colitis compared to a 2 per cent incidence of Crohn's disease in 252 patients with rectovaginal fistula seen at the Mayo Clinic.[21] It must be pointed out that most of this large series was collected during a period when the pathologic distinction between Crohn's colitis and ulcerative colitis was unclear. A recent study by Faulconer and Muldoon of the Ferguson Clinic, Grand Rapids, Michigan, confirms our clinical impression that Crohn's disease, presumably because of its transmural involvement, is much more commonly responsible for rectovaginal fistula than is ulcerative colitis.[12] They reported that 15 of 77 patients (20%) with rectovaginal fistula had an associated colitis. One patient had chronic ulcerative colitis, while 12 patients had Crohn's colitis. Pathology reports for two patients were unavailable. DeDombal and associates reviewed 465 patients with ulcerative colitis at the General Infirmary, Leeds, England, and found that a rectovaginal fistula had developed in 10 of the 275 women (3.6%).[10] They noted that a rectovaginal fistula never developed during the 742 patient-years when the disease was in remission, and that the incidence of rectovaginal fistula increased with the severity of the attack from 0.2 per cent in mild attack years up to 2.1 per cent in severe attack years. They also noted an increased incidence in patients with involvement of the entire colon and rectum, and during the first twelve months of symptoms. Bagby and colleagues noted that Crohn's enterovaginal fistulae developed more commonly with severe disease.[1] Development of a rectovaginal fistula might imply the presence of colitis even in the absence of other signs of the disease.[12,34] A recurring rectovaginal fistula should make one think of the possibility of inflammatory bowel disease. Beecham, and Tuxen and Castro, each reported two such cases due to Crohn's disease.[2,34]

*Pelvic Irradiation.* Irradiation used in the treatment of pelvic cancers, especially carcinoma of the cervix or endometrium, can produce a rectovaginal fistula which is generally located high in the vagina. The incidence of rectovaginal fistula after irradiation for cervical cancer ranges from 1 to 10 per cent.[35] Graham noted that patients whose original tumors were small and superficial were six times more likely to suffer irradiation damage than those with large tumors.[15] Most irradiation-induced fistulae develop between six months and two years after therapy. Those that develop during therapy are probably due to dissolution of a tumor that had penetrated the wall of both the vagina and the rectum.

The development of irradiation-induced rectovaginal fistula is heralded by increasing looseness of the stool with passage of mucus and blood per rectum. next, irradiation proctitis, followed by ulceration of the anterior rectacl wall 4 to 5 cm above the dentate line, is noted. One-third to one-half of such ulcers progress to a rectovaginal fistula. When a patient complains of rectal pressure with the constant urge to defecate, fistula formation is imminent. These symptoms abate once the rectovaginal fistula is formed.[15]

It is critical that recurrent cancer be distinguished from irradiation change. A rectal ulcer with a gray, shaggy, friable base with an elevated perimeter is suggestive of carcinoma. Examination under anesthesia will often reveal firm masses or nodules adjacent to normal tissues in a patient with recurrent cancer, while those in patients with an irradiation-damaged pelvis will generally have a uniform tissue texture.[15] If any suspicion of neoplasm exists, appropriate biopsies must be taken, and a metastatic work-up instituted. Van Nagel and associates found, in a series of 271 patients, that five of eleven patients with rectovaginal or vesicovaginal fistulae arising after irradiation had recurrent cancer.[35]

*Neoplastic and Hematologic.* Primary, recurrent, or metastatic neoplasms can cause a rectovaginal fistula. Generally these processes are extensions of colorectal, cervical, vaginal, or uterine cancers. Occasionally leukemias, aplastic anemias, agranulocytosis, and endometriosis have been implicated in the etiology of a rectovaginal fistula.[16] Lock and coworkers recently reported a case of a giant condyloma of the rectum which produced a rectovaginal fistula.[24]

*Infections.* Any infectious process contiguous with the rectovaginal septum can produce a rectovaginal fistula. Diverticular disease, tuberculosis with a perirectal abscess, venereal disease such as lymphogranuloma venereum, perianal fistulae and abscess have all precipitated a rectovaginal fistula.[21,27] A pelvic abscess or Bartholin's abscesses in the pouch of Douglas can present by draining through the rectovaginal septum. Chemical burns can incite severe inflammatory reaction in local tissues with subsequent development of a rectovaginal fistula.

*Congenital.* In the 5 mm embryo, the urorectal septum divides the cloaca into a ventral urogenital portion and a dorsal rectal portion down to the pubococcygeal line. Lateral ingrowth of mesenchyma completes the division below this level. In the female, mullerian ducts are interposed between the dorsal and ventral portion, and give rise to the uterus and upper two-thirds of the vagina. The distal vagina develops from sinovaginal buds that originate from the epithelium of the dorsal wall of the urogenital sinus. Maldevelopment in this process can result in rectovaginal fistula which is almost always associated with an imperforate anus and rectum that ends as a blind pouch above the puborectalis sling.[32]

## OPERATIVE REPAIRS
### Timing of Operative Repair

The likelihood of spontaneous or nonoperative healing of a rectovaginal fistula is primarily dependent on its etiology and, to a lesser extent, its size, and will influence the timing of an operative repair. Mattingly states that one-half of small rectovaginal fistula secondary to obstetrical trauma will heal spontaneously.[26] He, therefore, recommends waiting at least six months prior to operative intervention. Removal of a foreign body is often followed by healing of the rectovaginal fistula.[13] Similarly, proper treatment of an infectious process may allow healing of fistulae without formal operative repair. On the other hand, fistulae due to inflammatory bowel disease fail to heal, even with aggressive medical therapy.[10,12] Once formed, irradiation of neoplastic-induced rectovaginal fistulae rarely heal spontaneously.[9]

Operative repair should not be attempted until the patient is in optimal condition. This can be achieved by aggressive treatment of underlying disease states. For some patients, this may involve the use of corticosteroids, azulfidine, antibiotics, antidiarrheal agents, or hyperalimentation to decrease the risk of operative repair and increase the chances of healing.

Finally, local tissues should be as close to normal as possible before operative repair. Resolution of pelvic sepsis may require drainage of abscesses, use of antibiotics, warm baths, and other local care. It may be necessary to wait several weeks or months to allow the rectovaginal septum to return to its normal soft, pliable state. Graham found it necessary to wait for over a year after colostomy in 12 of 21 patients with irradiation fistulae before local tissues regained their normal pliability.[15] Hibbard pointed out that for traumatic rectovaginal fistula, a shorter interval of several weeks to a few months is usually sufficient.[17]

## Preoperative Considerations

Bowel preparation including a mechanical cleansing regimen and the use of nonabsorbable oral antibiotics is recommended for all transabdominal repairs. It is less essential when other approaches are utilized for operative repair, though many authors recommend its use.[21,26,31] Vaginal preparation with a mechanical cleansing regimen is sometimes necessary.

Perioperative systemic antibiotics are probably justified when a trans-abdominal approach is utilized. Many surgeons also use such antibiotics when using a perineal approach to repair a rectovaginal fistula. Hibbard reported that four of 36 patients not given a bowel preparation or perioperative antibiotics developed a cellulitis, while none of the 15 patients so treated developed wound problems.[17]

A bladder catheter should be inserted just prior to the operative procedure. When one anticipates a difficult pelvic dissection, as with irradiation enteritis, ureteral catheters may be of value.

Because of the distressing symptoms, some form of operative therapy is indicated in all but extremely poor risk patients with rectovaginal fistula. Regardless of the specific repair utilized, adherence to the operative principles of gentle dissection, full mobilization, excision of the diseased bowel and in most cases the fistulous track, and accurate apposition of healthy tissues without tension is essential. No attempt will be made to discuss repairs of congenital rectovaginal fistulae because they are well presented in pediatric surgical literature.

## Approaches

Rectovaginal fistulae can be corrected by abdominal, rectal, vaginal, perineal, transsphincteric, and transsacral approaches, or by a combination of these methods. High rectovaginal fistulae can often only be approached transabdominally. Any of the other approaches may be suitable for low rectovaginal fistulae.

Most gynecologists prefer a vaginal approach. Russell and Gallagher advocate a rectal approach, emphasize that the primary opening is within the anorectal canal, not the vagina, and that correction of the rectovaginal fistula requires obliteration of the anorectal source of infection.[31] Greenwald and Hoexter agree, pointing out that a rectovaginal fistula joins the high pressure system of the rectum (25–85 cm $H_2O$) with the low pressure system of the vagina (atmospheric).[16] A rectal approach provides the best exposure of the high pressure side of the fistula. The literature is replete with various procedures for repair of rectovaginal fistulae. All are variations of several basic techniques.

---

*OPERATIVE REPAIR OF RECTOVAGINAL*
*FISTULA*
LOCAL REPAIRS
  Fistulotomy and drainage
  Conversion to complete perineal laceration
    with layer closure
  Inversion of fistula

Excision of fistula with layer closure ±
   muscle interposition
   vaginal approach
   rectal approach
   perineal approach
   transsphincteric approach (York-
      Mason[36])
SLIDING FLAP ADVANCEMENTS
   Mucosa and partial thickness internal
      sphincter (Laird[19])
   Anterior rectal wall (Noble[28])
   Segmental internal sphincter (Belt[3])
   Endorectal[30]
SPHINCTER-PRESERVING   TRANSAB-
   DOMINAL REPAIRS
   Mobilization, division and layer closure
      without bowel resection ± interposition
   Bowel resection ± interposition
   pull-through procedures
   low anterior resection—transsacral,
      EEA-stapler
   sleeve anastomosis (Parks[29])
Onlay Patch anastomosis (Bricker[6])
MISCELLANEOUS
   Sphincter-sacrificing bowel resections
   Colostomy
   Colpocleisis

---

*Local Repairs.* In the past, low rectovaginal fistulae have been treated by simple fistulotomy and drainage, laying open the entire track. This method works well for anovaginal fistula, but when used to treat rectovaginal fistula partial or total incontinence results. Belt and Belt reported partial incontinence requiring a second operation in all eight patients treated by fistulectomy and drainage.[3] In our early experience, two patients were treated by a fistulotomy followed by a second stage sphincter repair. One of the two fistulae recurred. Because of such dismal results, simple fistulotomy is not advocated for repair of rectovaginal fistulae.

A commonly used method of local repair is conversion of the fistula to a complete perineal laceration followed by a layer closure (Fig. 25-2). The entire rectovaginal fistula track including the adjacent sphincters and perineal body are excised. The vaginal wall is dissected from the remnants of the perineal body, and a two or three layer closure is performed. This technique is identical to the classical obstetric repair of a fourth degree perineal laceration, and is well described by many authors.[13,14,18,26] Given, and Hibbard have each used this tech-

nique successfully in ten patients with 100 per cent primary healing.[13,17] No long term follow-up was reported.

A transvaginal repair by inversion of the fistula into the anal canal is a third option for local repair (Fig. 25-3).[26] Such a repair is only suitable for small, low rectovaginal fistulae surrounded by normal tissues with a reasonably intact perineal body. A modification of this procedure, the Latzko technique, can be used to repair high, large rectovaginal fistulae. With this modification, both the anterior and posterior vaginal walls are used to invert the fistula into the rectum. This technique effectively closes off a small portion of the upper vagina (upper partial colpocleisis).[18,26]

A standard method of local repair consists of excision of the fistula with a layer closure. This can be accomplished through a vaginal, rectal, perineal, or transsphincteric approach, and can be accompanied by interposition of vascularized pedicles of muscle if necessary (see below).

Lescher and Pratt used a vaginal approach to treat 49 patients with rectovaginal fistula of traumatic or infectious origin.[21] Eighty-four per cent had recurrence in the postoperative period. Given treated 11 patients with rectovaginal fistula of traumatic origin and reported recurrence in three.[13] He treated two patients with post-irradiation rectovaginal fistula with this method of local repair and was unsuccessful in both. One patient had three recurrences, and the other two recurrences. Hibbard achieved primary healing of traumatic rectovaginal fistulae in 14 patients when he used this technique.[17] No follow-up was reported.

Most surgeons would not attempt a local vaginal repair of a high rectovaginal fistula. Lawson, however, has used a deep perineal (Schuchardt) incision which splits the vagina up to the lateral fornix, thus, providing access to fistulae located near the cervix.[20] If it is necessary for even greater exposure and mobilization, the pouch of Douglas can then be opened behind the cervix, and the rectum drawn down for layered repair. Lawson has had good success using this vaginal repair in 42 of 53 patients, opening the pouch of Douglas in 11 to facilitate closure of the fistula.[20]

Greenwald and Hoexter reported their experience with this method of local repair using the transanal approach (Fig. 25-4).[16] Twenty patients with rectovaginal fistula involving the

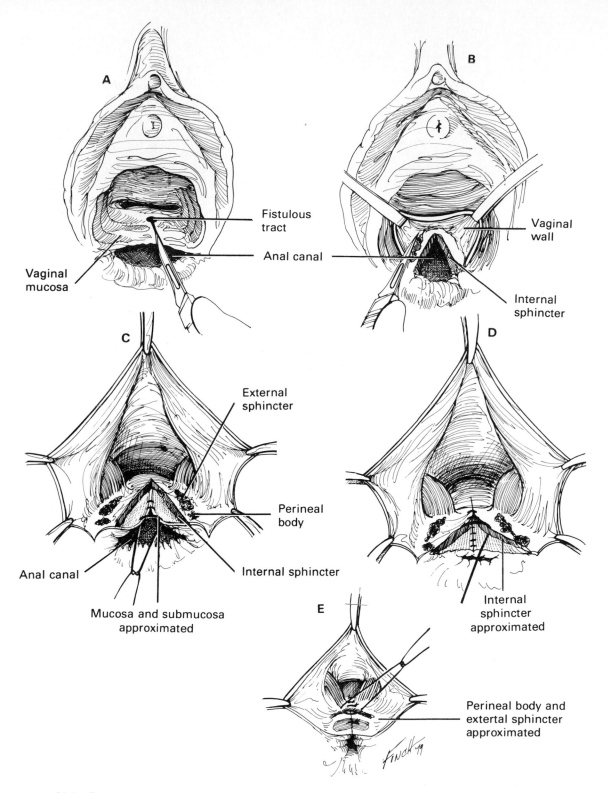

**FIGURE 25-2.** *Conversion to complete perianal laceration and layer closure. A transvaginal approach is illustrated. The entire rectovaginal fistula track including the sphincters and perineal body is incised (A). The vaginal wall is dissected off the remnants of the perineal body (B). A layered repair of the rectal mucosa and external and internal sphincter muscles is begun (C,D). The perineal body is reconstructed and the vaginal epithelium approximated (E). (After Hudson, C. N., in Operative Surgery. Rob, C., and Smith, R., (ed.): p. 385–386. Boston, Butterworths, 1977)*

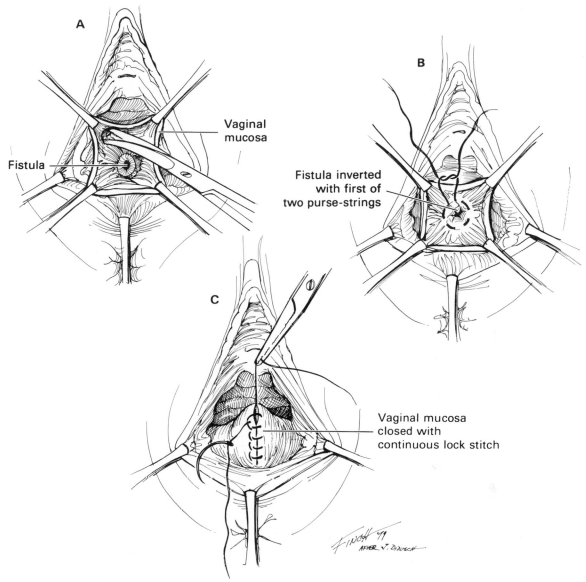

**FIGURE 25-3.** *Inversion of rectovaginal fistula. A transvaginal approach is illustrated. A circular incision is made through the vaginal mucosa about the fistulous opening and vaginal mucosal flaps are elevated from the margin of the fistula (A). Two or three concentric pursestring sutures are placed and tied to invert the fistula into the bowel lumen (B). The vaginal mucosa is reapproximated (C). (After Hudson, C. N., in Operative Surgery. Rob, C., and Smith, R. (ed.): p. 388. Boston, Butterworths 1977)*

middle portions of the rectovaginal septum were treated successfully without a recurrence during a three to twelve year follow-up period. They do not recommend this technique for treating rectovaginal fistulae arising from neoplasm, irradiation injury, or inflammatory bowel disease, or for fistulae located more than 6 cm cephalad to the dentate line.

Goligher points out two disadvantages of these methods of local repair: (*1*) excess tension on the suture line because of inadequate mobilization through the rectal or vaginal approaches, and, (*2*) direct apposition of the rectal and vaginal suture lines without much intervening tissue, which promotes a high recurrence rate.[14] He, therefore, proposed another

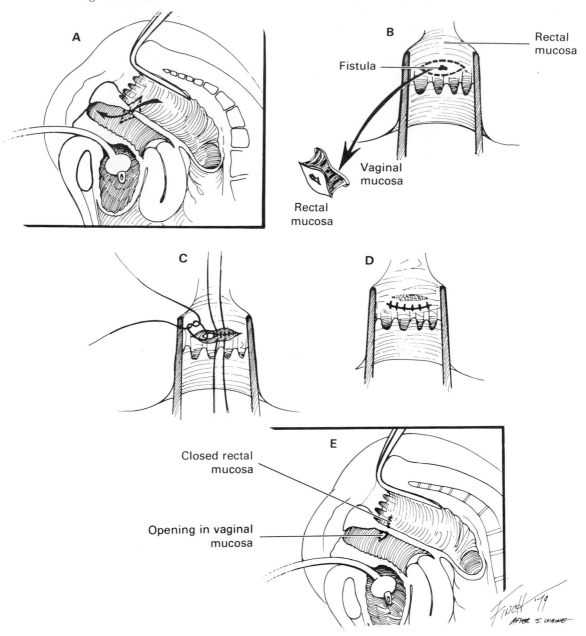

**FIGURE 25-4.** *Excision of rectovaginal fistula with layer closure. A transrectal approach is illustrated. A transverse elliptical incision is made around the fistula through the rectovaginal septum, thus excising the entire fistulous track (A and B). A two-layer closure of the defect in the rectovaginal septum is performed (C). The rectal mucosa is advanced distal to the deeper portion of the repair and reapproximated (D). The vaginal mucosa is left open for drainage (E). (After Greenwald, and Hoexter: Surg. Gynecol. Obstet., 146:443, 1978)*

approach involving the transperineal dissection of the rectovaginal septum. Through a slightly curved perineal incision, the anal canal and rectum are separated from the vagina. The rectovaginal fistula is divided, and the posterior vaginal wall and anterior rectal walls are widely mobilized. This approach allows layered closure of both the rectal and vaginal fistulous apertures without tension. In addition, by rotating the rectum and vagina slightly in opposite directions, direct apposition of the suture lines can be avoided.

The transsphincteric approach provides direct exposure of the anterior rectal wall and rectovaginal fistula which can then be repaired in layers. York-Mason, who developed this approach specifically to deal with a prostatorectal fistula, has used it to successfully repair rectovaginal fistulae in three patients.[36] This approach may obviate the need for transabdominal repairs of mid and high rectovaginal fistulae.

*Sliding Flap Advancements.* Various methods of advancing the internal fistulous opening to the anal margin have been described. Many authors feel this is the best means of correcting low rectovaginal fistulae.

Laird's mucosal flap advancement requires extreme care to avoid tearing, inadequate blood supply, or retraction of the flap composed of skin, rectal mucosa, submucosa, and some circular fibers from the rectal wall.[19] Though Laird reported good results utilizing this technique, others have been less successful.[3]

Mengert and Fish, and more recently, Russell and Gallagher, advocate advancement of the anterior rectal wall: a technique first described by Noble in 1902.[27,31] As Noble described it, the operation consists of "splitting the rectovaginal septum, dissecting the lower end of the rectum from the vagina, and drawing the anterior wall down through and external to the anus".[28] Mengert and Fish stress the importance of extensive mobilization up to the level of the cervix, and Russell and Gallagher similarly stress mobilization to a point 4 cm cephalad to the fistula in order to avoid retraction of the full thickness flap.[27,31]

Mengert and Fish used this technique to successfully treat nine patients with rectovaginal fistulae in the lower one-third of the vagina.[27] With a minimum of six months of follow-up per patient, there were no recurrences. Russell and Gallagher recently reported their results using this procedure on 22 patients with low rectovaginal fistula. These were caused by perianal infection involving the anterior midline anal crypt in 15 patients, childbirth injury in six, and inflammatory bowel disease in one. Three patients (14%) developed a recurrence and were reoperated.

With an average of over ten years of follow-up, good results were obtained in 15, fair results as denoted by occasional soiling and discomfort in six, and a failure in one patient despite four operative attempts. Belt and Belt have used this procedure with success in eight patients.[3]

To avoid the need for the wide mobilization required with the Noble operation Belt and Belt now advocate the use of a segmental advancement of the internal sphincter muscle with its attached overlying mucosa and the internal fistulous opening.[3] They claim that this approach lessens the need for wide mobilization, has a low incidence of flap retraction, and does not interfere with continence since the external sphincter is not disturbed. They also believe the technique cannot be used when the internal fistulous opening is at, or proximal to the anorectal ring. They have treated ten patients by this technique with good results, though length of follow-up is not specified.

Our own approach to the low rectovaginal fistula is an endorectal advancement of an anorectal flap consisting of mucosa, submucosa, and circular muscle (Fig. 25-5). Preoperatively, cleansing enemas are utilized, but a formal bowel preparation regimen is unnecessary. A colostomy is not used. After induction of general anesthesia, the patient is placed in the prone jackknife position over a hip roll with the buttocks spread by tape. In addition to the perianal field block, intermuscular injections of 0.5 per cent xylocaine, or 0.25 per cent bupivacaine with 1 : 200,000 epinephrine solution are made along the planned routes of dissection. Exposure is gained with the operating anoscope, and the rectovaginal fistula identified (Fig. 25-5A). The rectal flap is then outlined around the fistula extending approximately 7 cm proximally into the rectum, and at least 4 cm cephalad to the fistula. The base of the flap should be approximately two times the width of the apex of the flap to assure adequate blood supply (Fig. 25-5B). The flap is raised from the apex to the base (Fig. 25-5C). The cut edge of the circular muscle is mobilized laterally so that it may be approximated in the midline without tension (Fig. 25-5D). Hemostasis is achieved. The perineal body and rectovaginal septum are then reconstructed using 2—0 polyglycolic acid sutures which are first placed, and then tied serially (Fig. 25-5E). A final check for hemostasis is

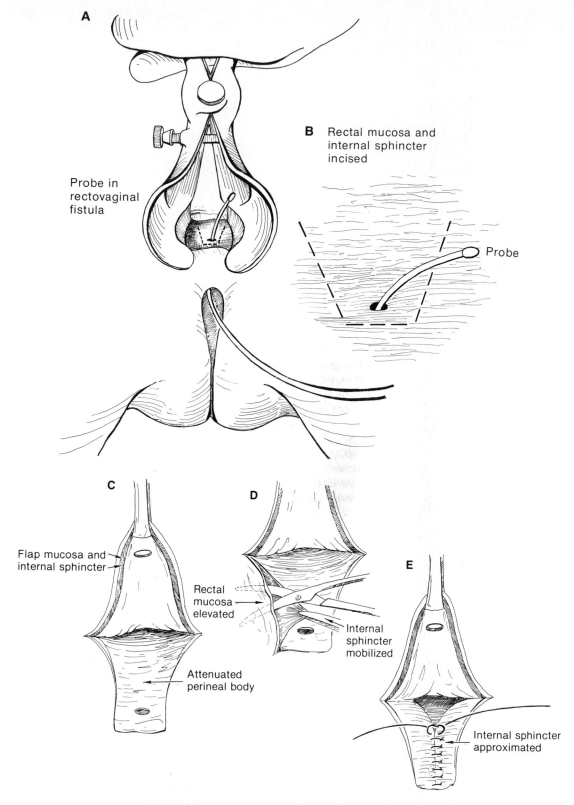

**A**

Probe in
rectovaginal
fistula

**B** Rectal mucosa and
internal sphincter
incised

Probe

**C**

Flap mucosa and
internal sphincter

Attenuated
perineal body

**D**

Rectal
mucosa
elevated

Internal
sphincter
mobilized

**E**

Internal sphincter
approximated

FIGURE **25-5.** *Endorectal advancement of rectal flap. See text for detailed description of technique. (Continued)*

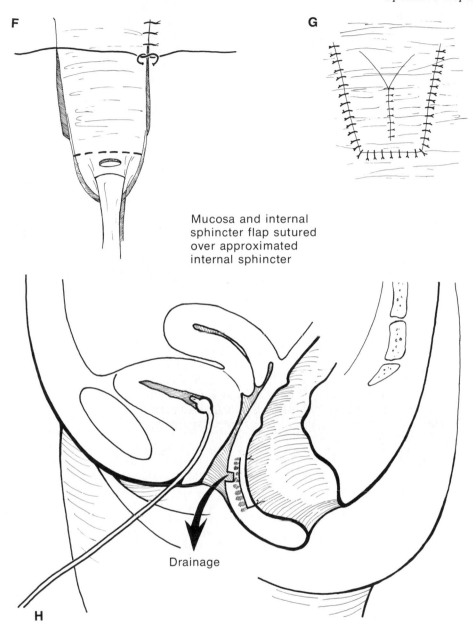

Mucosa and internal
sphincter flap sutured
over approximated
internal sphincter

Drainage

FIGURE 25-5 (*Conclusion*)

made before advancement of the flap. Excess flap including the rectovaginal fistula is excised (Fig. 25-5F). The flap is sutured in place restoring the normal anatomy using 3—0 polyglycolic acid sutures at the apex and along each side of the flap (Fig. 25-5G). Only small bites of the flap should be included in each suture. The vagina is left open for drainage (Fig. 25-5H). Postoperatively, the patient is given

analgesics and warm baths as needed to control the pain and spasm, as well as bulk stool softeners to avoid constipation. When she is comfortable, and after the first bowel movement, the patient is discharged.

We have utilized this procedure to treat 25 patients. The underlying etiology was an obstetrical or childbirth injury in 17, an operative injury in two, a childbirth injury and irradiation in one, and an unknown cause in five. In the cases of unknown origin, there was no evidence of neoplasm or inflammatory bowel disease, and no history of irradiation. All five women had multiple vaginal deliveries, therefore, the rectovaginal fistula most likely resulted from birth-related injury. In 22 patients, including the patient who had received irradiation, primary healing of the fistula was achieved with no recurrences during the follow-up period which averaged five months. In three patients, recurrence developed. One patient was cured after conversion of the fistula to a complete perineal laceration with layer closure. One patient refused further operative intervention. One patient remains a failure despite two additional repairs using the endorectal advancement technique.

*Sphincter-Preserving Transabdominal Repairs.* Local repairs and advancements generally cannot be used for high rectovaginal fistulae. In addition, they may be inappropriate if the fistula is due to irradiation change, neoplasm, or inflammatory bowel disease regardless of the location. Concomitant disease states may also warrant a transabdominal approach to a rectovaginal fistula. For such situations, a number of sphincter-preserving repairs have been advocated.

The simplest of these repairs involves mobilization of the recto-vaginal septum, division of the fistula, and a layer closure of the rectal and vaginal defects without bowel resection. Interposition of a live pedicle of tissue may be used to supplement this repair (see below). Bentley, Given, and Goligher have all had experience with this approach and find that it works well when normal tissues are available for the layered repair, and the fistula can be approached easily from above.[4,13,14]

When local tissues are abnormal, whether from irradiation change, inflammatory bowel disease, diverticulitis, or a neoplasm, bowel resection is most often an essential feature of the repair of a rectovaginal fistula. Whenever possible, the anal sphincter should be preserved. Several methods to accomplish this are available.

Pull-through procedures permit cure of the rectovaginal fistula, and elimination of diseased bowel by advancement of the entire colon, but are accompanied by many disadvantages related primarily to incontinence.

Cuthbertson and Buzzard, and Thomford and co-workers have all used such a technique to cure irradiation-induced rectovaginal fistulae.[8,33] Goligher has expressed dissatisfaction with his experience in using the Turnbull-Cutait pull-through procedure.[14]

Low anterior resection is another option. In the past, it was often difficult to perform an anastomosis deep in the pelvis at the site where high rectovaginal fistulae occur, though occasionally this was accomplished.[13] Goligher states he would no longer recommend an anterior resection in "cases in which a postoperative anorectal stump of less than 6 cm from the anal verge is the maximum that can be preserved."[14] Newer techniques make low anterior resection a more attractive choice. The abdominal transsacral approach has been utilized successfully by Marks to repair rectovaginal fistulae in four patients.[25] We would prefer, however, to utilize the end-to-end anastomosis (EEA) stapling device to perform a low anterior resection. This approach allows resection of the diseased bowel, including that portion involved in the rectovaginal fistula, and preserves continence.

Parks and associates have used a sleeve anastomosis technique to treat post-irradiation rectovaginal fistulae in five patients.[29] This involves complete mobilization of the colon so nonirradiated bowel can be brought down to the anal canal. The rectum is then mobilized down to the level of the rectovaginal fistula, and divided at that point. The irradiated colon is resected. Then, from a perineal approach, the mucosa is stripped off the underlying muscle until the entire remaining rectum is denuded of all mucosa. This leaves a rectal muscle tube which contains the fistula in its most cephalad portion. Next, the normal colon is threaded through the muscle sleeve, thus covering the fistula. Then, a per anal anastomosis of the colon to the anal canal is performed at the level of the dentate line.

Still another approach to irradiation-induced rectovaginal fistulae involves an onlay patch anastomosis as devised by Bricker and used successfully on four patients.[6,23] From a transabdominal approach, the rectosigmoid colon is mobilized, and the rectovaginal fistula exposed. The rectosigmoid colon is divided. An end-on sigmoid colostomy is established proximally. The distal rectosigmoid is turned down on itself so that the open end can be anastomosed to the freshly debrided edges of the fistulous opening in the rectum. This is accomplished with a combined abdominal and perineal approach (Fig. 25-6). At a second stage, after healing has been demonstrated radiologically, the proximal colostomy is sutured end-to-side to the intrapelvic loop of rectosigmoid colon. Bricker states that this technique has several advantages over other methods of repair of post-irradiation rectovaginal fistulae.[6] He feels this procedure is less difficult to perform than the alternative procedures. Because it is unnecessary to mobilize the rectum there is no risk of creating an iatrogenic defect in the posterior aspect of the rectum, there is no risk of hemorrhage from the presacral plexus, and the innervation of the ampulla and rectum is not disturbed, resulting in a better chance of continence. The technique can be used to reconstruct a strictured segment which often accompanies post-irradiation rectovaginal fistula. The theoretical disadvantages of the operation are: (*1*) the radiation-damaged rectum is returned to function which might result in exacerbation of proctitis or radionecrosis in the future; (*2*) the sigmoid loop used to patch the fistulous defect has been subjected to radiation, albeit a lesser dose; and, (*3*) there may be an increased risk of development of cancer in the radiated rectum.

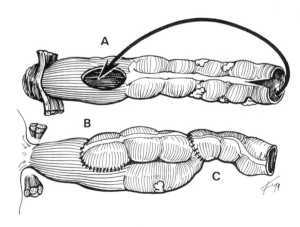

FIGURE **25-6.** *Onlay patch anastomosis. (A) The site of fistula is excised and the sigmoid colon prepared. (B) The end of the sigmoid colon is folded onto the site of fistula and an end-to-side anastomosis is carried out. The proximal end of the left colon is brought out as an end-colostomy. The continuity of the colon is established at a second stage (C). (After Bricker, et al.: Surg. Gynecol. Obstet., 148: 499, 1979)*

*Miscellaneous.* Sphincter-sacrificing bowel resections such as abdominoperineal resection or even a pelvic exenteration may be indicated for patients with neoplasm-induced rectovaginal fistulae. Similarly, patients with active, extensive inflammatory bowel disease may require proctectomy and/or colectomy to treat the rectovaginal fistula and the underlying disease. Faulconer and Muldoon reported that 11 of 15 patients with colitis and a rectovaginal fistula were treated by total proctocolectomy and ileostomy, and two of the 15 by subtotal colectomy with ileostomy and rectal mucous fistula.[12] Patients with irradiation-induced rectovaginal fistulae or rectovaginal fistulae associated with an unresectable malignancy, especially if they are poor operative risks, may be best treated by a permanent, totally diverting colostomy.[9] Still another choice for a poor risk patient is colpocleisis utilizing wire or some other permanent suture material to close the vagina at the introitus, thus forming a common chamber consisting of the vagina and rectum with the anus as the only exit.[13,15] This approach obviates the need for colostomy in elderly, incapacitated patients who would have difficulty with a stoma.

### Ancillary Procedures

A wide difference of opinion exists as to the need for a temporary colostomy when operative repair of a rectovaginal fistula is contemplated. Goligher, and Graham, routinely establish a preliminary temporary colostomy when repairing a rectovaginal fistula, while Russell and Gallagher emphatically state that a colostomy is unnecessary in most instances.[14,15,31] We would agree that for most rectovaginal fistulae which are low, and/or caused by trauma, infection, or inactive inflammatory bowel disease, a colostomy is unnecessary. However, when dealing with high, complicated rectovaginal fistulae caused by irradiation, neoplasm, active inflammatory bowel disease, and active infectious processes, a colostomy may be a useful adjunct to treatment. In such cases, a staged procedure may be beneficial. After establishing a diverting colostomy, direct repair of the rectovaginal fistula may be deferred as long as six to twelve months while waiting until local tissues are more normal. Another possible route is the creation of a comlementary colostomy at the time of the definitive repair.

Bricker emphasizes that when a patient with

a postradiation rectovaginal fistula requires a colostomy, it should be a left-sided, end colostomy, leaving a long distal segment with a mucous fistula.[6] This will facilitate later reconstruction; provide a means of study of the distal segment since contrast studies through the rectum are often unsatisfactory in the presence of a large rectovaginal fistula; and, leave the patient with a satisfactory colostomy if it is decided that reconstruction is not suitable.

Some surgeons utilize sphincterotomy either posteriorly or laterally, in the hope of preventing increased rectal pressure which might cause the rectovaginal fistula to recur.[36] This seems wise only when a stricture is present; but is otherwise unnecessary and meddlesome. Sphincter repair should be performed concomitant with operative correction of the rectovaginal fistula whenever fecal incontinence is associated.

Regardless of the approach used, many authors advocate interposition of vascularized pedicles of omentum or muscle between the rectum and vagina after dividing the fistula, especially when dealing with irradiation-induced rectovaginal fistulae. This avoids direct apposition of the suture lines in the two organs, and decreases chances of a recurrence. Bentley, and Goligher, have used omental pedicles based on the right gastroepiploic artery.[4,14] Given, Hibbard, and Mattingly have each used a Martius graft in which a flap of tissue consisting of the bulbocavernosus muscle and its adjacent labial fat is interposed between the rectum and vagina after a layer closure of the fistulous defects.[13,17,26] Graham describes the interposition of the gracilis muscle which, because of its proximal neurovascular supply, is highly suitable for transfer from its normal location in the thigh.[15] He, however, prefers the use of the rectus muscle based on the inferior epigastric vessels because of its width and proximity to the field, providing it has not been involved in an irradiation portal. Good results were achieved using this technique of muscle repair in 16 of 18 patients with rectovaginal fistulae following radiotherapy. Others have described use of the adductor longus, sartorius, or gluteus maximus muscles.[7,13] Hysterectomy with preservation of the ovaries may facilitate abdominal repair of a high rectovaginal fistula by improving access to its inferior margin. In rare situations, when there is dense pelvic fibrosis with obliteration of the pouch of Douglas and fixation of the uterus, cervix, and vaginal vault in solid scar, the only method of exposure may involve a subtotal hysterectomy and midline sagittal split of the cervical stump.[18] This exposes the fistula which can then be repaired in layers. Five of seven patients were treated successfully in this fashion by Lawson.[20] One developed a recurrence and one died of massive pelvic hemorrhage.

## Selection of Specific Procedures

The precise method of operative repair will vary with the location, size, and etiology of the rectovaginal fistula; with the number and type of previous repairs; with the associated abnormalities such as sphincter damage, rectal or vaginal stricture, or fistulae to other organs; with the patient's operative risk factors; and with the surgeon's training, experience, and interpretation of reported results of similar repairs. Of these many factors, etiology of the rectovaginal fistula is a primary determinant in selection of appropriate repair. Treatment of a rectovaginal fistula produced by a carcinoma, whether primary, metastatic or recurrent, should not interfere with the appropriate therapy of the underlying neoplasm. In many instances, bowel resection, often with sacrifice of the rectal sphincter, will be necessary.

Irradiation-induced rectovaginal fistulae challenge the judgment and skill of the surgeon because of the generalized nature of the irradiation effect. Diffuse tissue fibrosis makes dissection of the fistula difficult. Diffuse small vessel endarteritis results in vascular compromise with subsequent tissue loss from sloughing, and most often precludes use of local tissues for operative repair. There is often an associated stricture. For these reasons, a frequent method of treatment for irradiation-induced rectovaginal fistulae has been a permanent colostomy. Definitive repair must include the delivery of well vascularized tissue to the region.

In select, good-risk patients who are apparently cured of the condition for which they received irradiation but are plagued by a rectovaginal fistula, various procedures are available which will preserve normal anorectal function. In all such cases a temporary colostomy is established and maintained for six months to a year to allow necrosis to disappear and the inflammatory reaction to subside.

Then, a repair which utilizes non-irradiated tissue with a normal potential for healing can be undertaken. The fistula, because surrounded by abnormal tissue, cannot simply be closed, but must be occluded or patched by tissues unaffected by irradiation. Local or transabdominal repairs utilizing vascularized pedicles of omentum or muscle as described above accomplish this goal and are sometimes successful. A unique technique is the onlay patch anastomosis devised by Bricker.[6] Still another method of utilizing normal tissue for the repair involves resection of all irradiated bowel with a primary anastomosis of normal bowel. This can be done as a low anterior resection with the EEA stapler or with the sleeve anastomosis devised by Parks.[29]

Rectovaginal fistula in patients with active inflammatory bowel disease cannot be treated by local repairs or advancement flaps. We, and others, have successfully utilized such repairs for patients incapacitated by the rectovaginal fistula when the underlying inflammatory bowel disease is in remission and the rectum is apparently healthy.[2,12,34] Recurrence during a flare-up of the colitis is not uncommon, however. When a patient has persistently active disease not responding to medical therapy or has associated sphincter destruction and can no longer tolerate the incapacitating symptoms, proctectomy is indicated to treat the inflammatory bowel disease as well as the rectovaginal fistula.

For traumatic or infectious rectovaginal fistulae, the surgeon should select a procedure with minimal morbidity and a high likelihood of success. A transabdominal approach may be necessary to treat a high rectovaginal fistula near the cervix, though other means of exposure have been described. For low- or mid-rectovaginal fistulae, local repairs or advancement flaps work well. We prefer the endorectal flap advancement repair for all such fistulae. This procedure has a low morbidity because only minimal preoperative preparation is necessary, no colostomy or skin incision is required, operative time is short, the postoperative recovery is speedy, and continence is not disturbed. There have been only three minor complications in 25 patients. In addition, this procedure allows concomitant sphincter repair and rebuilding of the perineal body. Finally, it is highly successful at restoring the rectovaginal septum.

## REFERENCES

1. Bagby, R. J., Clements, J. L., Patrick, J. W., Rogers, J. V., and Weens, H. S.: Genitourinary complications of granulomatous bowel disease. Am. J. Roentgenol. Radium Ther. Nucl. Med., *117:*297, 1973.

2. Beecham, C. T.: Recurring rectovaginal fistula. Am. J. Obstet Gynecol., *40:*323, 1972.

3. Belt, R. L., and Belt, R. L. Jr.: Repair of anorectal vaginal fistula utilizing segmental advancement of the internal sphincter muscle. Dis. Colon Rectum, *12:*99, 1969.

4. Bentley, R. J.: Abdominal repair of high rectovaginal fistula. J. Obstet. Gynaecol. Br. Commonw., *80:*364, 1973.

5. Block, I. R., Rodriquez, S., and Olivares, A. L.: The Warren operation for anal incontinence caused by disruption of the anterior segment of the anal sphincter, perineal body and rectovaginal septum: Report of five cases. Dis. Colon Rectum, *18:*28, 1975.

6. Bricker, E. M., and Johnston, W. D.: Repair of postirradiation rectovaginal fistula and stricture. Surg. Gynecol. Obstet., *148:*499, 1979.

7. Byron, R. L., and Ostergard, D. R.: Sartorius muscle interposition for the treatment of the radiation-induced vaginal fistula. Am. J. Obstet. Gynecol., *104:*104, 1969.

8. Cuthbertson, A. M., and Buzzard, A. J.: Pullthrough resection of the rectum with vaginocystoplasty for repair of a rectovesicovaginal fistula. Aust. NZ J. Surg., *43:*72, 1973.

9. DeCosse, J. J.: Radiation injury to the intestine. In Sabistan (ed.): *Davis-Christopher Textbook of Surgery,* Philadelphia, W. B. Saunders, 1977.

10. deDombal, F. T., Watts, J. M., Watkinson, G., and Goligher, J. C.: Incidence and management of anorectal abscess, fistula and fissure in patients with ulcerative colitis. Dis. Colon Rectum, *9:*201, 1966.

11. Daniels, B. T.: Rectovaginal fistula; a clinical and pathological study. Thesis; University of Minnesota Graduate School, 1949.

12. Faulconer, H. T., and Muldoon, J. P.: Rectovaginal fistula in patient with colitis: Review and report of a case. Dis. Colon Rectum, *18:*413, 1975.

13. Given, F. T.: Rectovaginal fistula: A review of 20 years' experience in a community hospital. Am. J. Obstet. Gynecol., *108:*41, 1970.

14. Goligher, J. C.: Rectovaginal fistula; and Irradiation Proctitis and Enteritis. In *Surgery of*

*the Anus, Rectum and Colon.* Springfield, Charles C. Thomas, 1975.

15. Graham, J. B.: Vaginal fistulas following radiotherapy. Surg. Gynecol. Obstet., *120:*1019, 1965.

16. Greenwald, J. C., and Hoexter, B.: Repair of rectovaginal fistula. Surg. Gynecol. Obstet., *146:*443, 1978.

17. Hibbard, L. T.: Surgical management of rectovaginal fistulas and complete perineal tears. Am. J. Obstet. Gynecol., *130:*139, 1978.

18. Hudson, C. N.: Rectovaginal and other fistulae between the intestine and genital tract In Rob, and Smith (eds.): *Operative Surgery: Colon, Rectum and Anus,* 3 ed., London, Buttersworths and Co., 1977.

19. Laird, D. R.: Procedures used in treatment of complicated fistulas. Am. J. Surg., *76:*701, 1948.

20. Lawson, J.: Rectovaginal fistulae following difficult labour. Proc. R. Soc. Med., *65:*283, 1972.

21. Lescher, T. C., and Pratt, J. H.: Vaginal repair of the simple rectovaginal fistula. Surg. Gynecol. Obstet., *124:*1317, 1967.

22. Linke, C. A., Linke, C. L., and Worden, A. C.: Bladder and uretheral injuries following prolonged labor. J. Urol., *5:*679, 1971.

23. Lischer, C. E. in Discussion; Russell, T. R. and Gallagher, D. M.: Low rectovaginal fistulas: Approach and treatment. Am. J. Surg., *134:*13, 1977.

24. Lock, M. R., Katz, D. R., Samoorian, S., and Parks, A. G.: Giant condyloma of the rectum: Report of a case. Dis. Colon Rectum, *20:*154, 1977.

25. Marks, G.: Combined abdominotranssacral reconstruction of the radiation-injured rectum. Am. J. Surg., *131:*54, 1976.

26. Mattingly, R. F.: Anal incontinence and rectovaginal fistulas. In *TeLinde's Operative Gynecology,* 5 ed. Philadelphia, J. B. Lippincott, 1977.

27. Mengert, W. F., and Fish, S. A.: Anterior rectal wall advancement: Technic for repair of complete perineal laceration and rectovaginal fistula. Obstet. Gynecol., *5:*262, 1955.

28. Noble, G. H.: A new operation for complete laceration of the perineum designed for the purpose of eliminating danger of infection from the rectum. Trans. Am. Gynecol. Soc., *27:*357, 1902.

29. Parks, A. G., Allen, C. L. O., Frank, J. D., and McPartlin, J. F.: A method of treating post-irradiation rectovaginal fistulas. Br. J. Surg., *65:*417, 1978.

30. Patel, D. R., Rajendra, S., Nichols, J.: An unusual complication of rectovaginal fistula: Report of a case. Dis. Colon Rectum, *17:*246, 1974.

31. Russell, T. R., and Gallagher, D. M.: Low rectovaginal fistulas: Approach and treatment. Am. J. Surg., *134:*13, 1977.

32. Santulli, T. V.: Rectum and anus. In Benson, Mustard, Ravitch, Snyder, and Welch (eds.): Pediatric Surgery, Chicago, Law Book Medical Publishers, 1962.

33. Thomford, N. R., Smith, D. E., and Wilson, W. H.: Pull-through operation for radiation induced rectovaginal fistula: Report of a case. Dis. Colon Rectum, *13:*451, 1970.

34. Tuxen, P. A., and Castro, A. F.: Rectovaginal fistula in Crohn's disease. Dis. Colon Rectum, *22:*58, 1979.

35. VanNagell, J. R., Parker, J. C., Maruyama, Y., Utley, J., and Luckett, P.: Bladder or rectal injury following radiation therapy for cervical cancer. Am. J. Obstet. Gynecol., *119:*727, 1974.

36. York-Mason, A.: Transphincteric approach to rectal lesions. Surgery Annual, *9:*171, 1977.

# 26

# Strictures of the Anorectum

## CLASSIFICATION

A stricture is defined as an abnormal narrowing of a tubular structure. It may be the result of either an extrinsic process which impinges on its wall, or an intrinsic process arising from the wall itself. Strictures of the anorectum are classified on the basis of etiology, degree of severity, and structure. Etiologically, they are the result of benign or malignant processes. Benign strictures are most frequently caused by trauma, inflammatory disease, irradiation, and congenital malformations. Malignant strictures are usually caused by intrinsic bowel neoplasms, but may be secondary to neoplasms arising in proximity to the rectum, most commonly from urogenital organs (Fig. 26-1).

The severity and etiology of a stricture usually dictates its treatment. Strictures secondary to malignant disease clearly require the appropriate excision. Those benign strictures termed "mild" may be transient, and frequently respond to local measures such as removal of the offending agent, alterations of the diet, stool lubricants, and physiological dilatation with bulk agents. "Severe" strictures are usually recalcitrant to these measures and require surgical intervention.

Kark has described strictures in regard to structure as diaphragmatic, annular, or tubular.[19] "Diaphragmatic" strictures are characterized by a thin, constricting band of tissue which is also termed crescentic if it does not encompass the lumen. This type is frequently

With collaboration of Gregory W. Brabbee

seen in inflammatory disease of the anorectum such as ulcerative colitis, Crohn's colitis, or amebic proctitis. "Annular" strictures are defined as being less than 2 cm in length. They usually develop after trauma or surgical injury to the anorectum. Strictures which are greater then 2 cm in length are termed "tubular," and are occasionally caused by lymphogranuloma venereum and pelvic irradiation.

### Malignant Strictures

Malignant strictures may arise intrinsically from the rectum or from neighboring organs. Approximately 50 per cent of all colonic neoplasms develop in the rectum or rectosigmoid, and approximately one-third of these are within reach of the examining finger.[12] In these cases, the diagnosis is obvious. Strictures which are caused by extrinsic malignancies are usually distinguished by the sensation of normal mucosa on digital examination. Confusion exists, however, when an extrinsic malignancy invades the full thickness of the rectal wall, or a primary bowel neoplasm originates and remains in the submucosal plane. In most cases, a biopsy will help resolve this dilemma. In documented invasive cancers of the anorectum, a curative or palliative abdominoperineal resection is indicated, depending on the extent of the disease and the general condition of the patient. Electrocoagulation—with or without local resection—of cancers of the anorectum which have progressed enough to cause strictures are of limited value, but may afford some relief in the elderly, debilitated patient. These patients, or those in which extrinsic car-

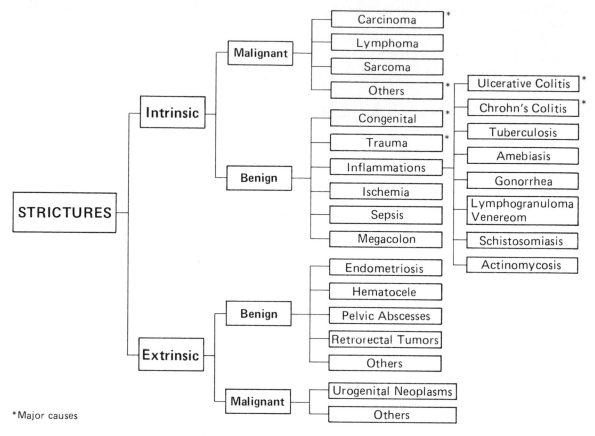

FIGURE **26-1.** *Classification of anorectal strictures.*

cinomas invade the rectum, may require a diverting colostomy.

**Benign Strictures**

Benign strictures may also be caused by processes which are intrinsic or extrinsic to the anorectum. Those which are extrinsic are uncommon and include retrorectal tumors, endometriosis, hematoceles, and pelvic abscesses.[29,33] The majority of benign strictures are caused by intrinsic processes, and except for congenital lesions, are primarily inflammatory in nature. The most important ones will be discussed individually.

*Trauma,* especially that caused by previous anorectal surgery, is probably the most common cause of benign stricture. It is estimated that between 5 and 10 per cent or more of all hemorrhoidectomies are complicated by some degree of stenosis, although most of these are asymptomatic and do not require any specific treatment.[9,25] Anal eroticism which lacerates or abrades the delicate mucosa may result in annular or radial scars which coalesce, and eventually lead to a stricture. Traumatic strictures also occur following low anterior resection, especially if it is complicated by an anastomotic leak or dehiscence; electrocautery or local excision of anorectal neoplasms; and as a complication associated with repair of rectal prolapse.[2,13]

*Inflammatory bowel disease* is a well known cause of rectal stricture. Although the exact incidence is unknown, 4 to 9 per cent of patients with ulcerative colitis, and an even greater percentage of patients with Crohn's colitis, develop `strictures of the anorectum.[7,14,15] Strictures seen in Crohn's colitis are characterized by a cicatrizing, transmural inflammatory process and are frequently associated with synchronous strictures occurring elsewhere in the colon, and extensive perianal disease. These important characteristics are often valuable in differentiating granulomatous from ulcerative colitis.

*"Disuse"* strictures are invariably located in the anal canal, and result in fibrosis of the internal sphincter. They sometimes occur in patients with a chronic anal fissure or in those who have abused saline or paraffin purgatives.[10] Because these agents produce liquid stools, there is no necessity for the anal canal to dilate; hence it strictures.

*Irradiation* injury to the rectum with subsequent stricture formation is an unfortunate, and not infrequent, complication of pelvic radiotherapy. In 1969 DeCosse reported a series of 100 patients with radiation injury to the gastrointestinal tract after pelvic radiotherapy.[5] The injuries, often multiple, included 44 patients with proctitis, 10 with rectal ulcers, 29 with rectovaginal fistulae, and 10 with rectal strictures. In 1976 Palmer reviewed patients treated with irradiation for carcinoma

of the cervix, and reported a 10 per cent serious complication rate.[26] Of those with gastrointestinal injuries, 17 per cent had low level rectal strictures. The incidence of complication is related to the dosage of irradiation (Fig. 26-2).

*Sepsis* has been recently identified as a cause of anal stricture. Greco reported the occurrence of a dense, circumferential anal stricture which required surgical intervention in an infant who had suffered from pseudomonas sepsis and enterocolitis.[16] Pseudomonas aeruginosa is known to produce characteristic infarcts of the mucosa which ulcerate.[16] In this case, ulcers clustered around the anus coalesced and caused a complete slough of the anoderm and perianal skin. Healing inevitably resulted in a stricture. Extensive chronic horseshoe fistula-in-ano may also result in stricture formation. The similarity of strictures caused by sepsis and ischemia suggests a similar pathogenesis, and has also been demonstrated in animals.[35]

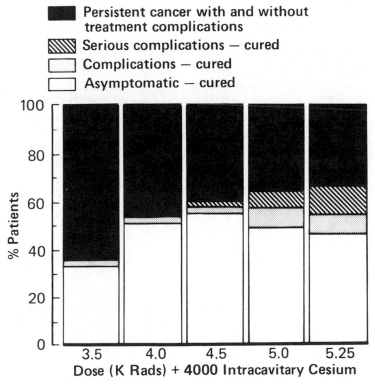

FIGURE 26-2. *Variations in survival and complication related to dosage of irradiation. (After Palmer, J. A., et al: Surg 80:458, 1976)*

*Ischemia,* well recognized as a cause of stricture elsewhere in the colon, has also been implicated in the pathogenesis of rectal strictures.[4,31] While the abundant collateral circulation to the rectum usually protects it from vascular insult, in rare instances, sudden occlusion of the superior rectal or interior mesenteric artery can result in significant ischemia to the rectum causing mucosal necrosis, fibrosis, and stricture. Recent experimental research conducted in animals lends support to this hypothesis.[35]

*Amebiasis* is a disease caused by the protozoa, Entamoeba histolytica, and transmitted by contaminated food stuffs and water. The cecum, ascending colon, and rectosigmoid are the areas of the gastrointestinal tract most commonly affected.[34] Rectal strictures are reported to occur in up to 5 per cent of patients with amebic dysentery. Although endemic in the United States, most carriers remain asymptomatic.[34] In patients with amebic dysentery, the invasive forms or Trophozoites penetrate the rectal mucosa causing necrosis and punctate ulcers. Secondary infection intervenes, resulting in acute proctitis manifested by bloody diarrhea mixed with mucus. Healing and repeated infection eventually cause fibrosis of the underlying muscle with thickening of the bowel wall and narrowing of the lumen. Grossly, amebic strictures may be difficult to distinguish from scirrhous carcinoma.[19] Patients with amebiasis sometimes develop amebomas or amebic granulomas of the bowel wall which may cause obstruction and are occasionally mistaken for submucosal neoplasms.

*Lymphogranuloma venereum* is a sexually transmitted disease caused by the organism Chlamydea trachomatis, and has a predilection for the anorectum. Following inoculation, the rectal and perirectal lymphatics are invaded causing lymphostasis. Secondary infection may occur, and this results in fibrosis and eventually the development of strictures. These are frequently long, and may extend up to the splenic flexure. Although in past years 25 to 35 per cent of patients with lymphogranuloma venereum reportedly developed strictures, the incidence of this disease has declined so sharply over the last 15 years that in the United States they are practically nonexistent. Levine, in 1964, reported a series of 472 patients with rectal stricture caused by lymphogranuloma venereum who were all seen at one institution, while ten years later between June of 1974 and July of 1975, only 374 cases of uncomplicated lymphogranuloma venereum were reported in the entire country.[22,34] Improved hygiene, patient education, and earlier treatment with effective antibiotics have played key roles in decreasing the morbidity of this disease.

*Gonorrhea,* a sexually transmitted disease caused by Neisseria gonorrhoeae, is endemic throughout the world but rarely a cause of rectal stricture. Following inoculation, the rectal mucosa becomes inflamed, edematous, and friable. In severe cases which have been neglected for long periods, fibrosis, and ultimately a stricture may develop.

*Tuberculosis, schistosomiasis (bilharziasis), and actinomycosis* involving the anorectum are uncommon in the United States, and are rarely the cause of strictures.

*Congenital lesions* of the anorectum account for a significant number of strictures. Embryologically these strictures are thought to be the result of excessive fusion of the anal tubules during the formation of the proctodeum.[28] In an analysis of 232 children with anorectal malformations, Partridge and Gough found 38 (11.8%) with strictures.[28] Men outnumbered women in a ratio of three to one, and most of the strictures were mild and confined to the anal canal. Several children had other associated abnormalities including sacral malformations, congenital heart disease, hypospadias, and absent or nonfunctioning kidneys.

## GENERAL SYMPTOMS

Although some patients are completely asymptomatic, most have a variety of complaints including constipation, tenesmus, rectal pain, and abdominal cramps.[33] Other symptoms include rectal bleeding and narrowing of the stools.

## DIAGNOSIS

While the diagnosis of anorectal stricture is straightforward, its etiology frequently requires further careful investigation. A thorough history should be elicited with special attention directed to genitourinary complaints, fever, weight loss, rectal discharge, previous irradiation or surgery, inflammatory bowel disease, anorectal trauma, and, where applicable, the patient's sexual proclivities.

Occasionally, perianal abscesses and fistulae are present. A bimanual exam may aid in detecting diseases outside the rectum. Severely stenotic lesions may require examination under anesthesia, and if necessary, a "stricture" sigmoidoscope should be used to view and biopsy the mucosa above and below the stricture. A barium enema should be obtained to evaluate the rest of the colon, especially if multiple strictures are suspected. Radiographically, benign strictures caused by inflammation are long and smooth with a central lumen. These are distinguished from those caused by malignancies which are usually characterized by overhanging edges, filling defects, and a lumen which is eccentric.[4,15] Further investigations may include stool for ova and parasites, smears and cultures of purulent exudate, a purified protein derivative of tuberculin (PPD), Frei Test, and lymphogranuloma venereum complement fixation test. A biopsy of the involved area is essential, but even if it is benign it does not necessarily exclude the presence of a malignancy. In some cases of stricture caused by pelvic tumor, a definitive diagnosis can only be made by exploratory laparotomy.

Congenital and acquired megacolon are sometimes manifested by spasticity of the rectosigmoid with proximal dilatation of the colon, and thus may simulate a stricture.[11] Histologically, both types are characterized by the complete lack of or degeneration of parasympathetic, myenteric nerve ganglia in the involved rectal segment. This results in a failure to relax this segment and, therefore, asynchronous peristalsis. The reader is referred to general and pediatric surgical texts for a more complete discussion of the physiology, diagnosis, and treatment of megacolon.

## TREATMENT

The approach to treatment of benign strictures of the anorectum is primarily based on the degree of stenosis and their location. Those which are low in the anal canal, short, and minimally symptomatic, may be managed by alteration of diet, bulk-forming agents, and periodic dilatation (see below). Most congenital strictures, and many of those caused by trauma, especially hemorrhoidectomy, can be treated in this manner.[21,28] Anal strictures which are more severe should be treated by some type of anoplasty (see below) as dilatation only tears the tissues, and does nothing to replace the loss of anoderm which is the basic problem. If the stricture is higher in the rectum, it may lend itself to resection. This may be the case in strictures caused by irradiation and inflammatory bowel disease and those seen in association with proctitis caused by lymphogranuloma venereum, amebiasis, or gonorrhea. Finally, extensive strictures which involve the sphincter mechanism are best treated by diverting colostomy, and/or abdominoperineal resection. This type of treatment is usually reserved for patients with long standing ulcerative colitis or severe strictures resulting from pelvic irradiation. Pull-through procedures such as those described by Swenson, Duhamel and Soave are usually reserved for patients with megacolon, and will not be discussed further. However, the colo-anal anastomosis described by Parks can be applied to rectal stricture caused by irradiation.[27]

### Non-Operative Measures

Non operative measures include the administration of laxatives of the lubricant or bulk-forming variety, and occasionally even enemas. Dilatation of anorectal strictures may be accomplished digitally, while a host of instruments including Hegar metal dilators, rubber bougies, sigmoidoscopes, and specially designed stricturescopes have been advocated for strictures occurring in the rectosigmoid. Denckler advocates the use of an ingeniously designed, expanding metal dilator which fits inside a 13 mm standard sigmoidoscope.[6] A technique for dealing with a low lying stricture was described by Mazier.[24] The principle utilized was the progressive dilatation of a stricture by pulling through an obturator of progressively increasing size (in this case a Foley catheter balloon) using the end of the sigmoidoscope as a fulcrum.[24]

### Anoplasty

The simplest treatment for the relief of an anal stricture is a lateral internal sphincterotomy. (For details of this procedure, see Chapter 7). Although primarily used in the treatment of chronic anal fissure, and by some as an adjunctive measure to hemorrhoidectomy, internal sphincterotomy is frequently used in conjunction with sliding or rotational skin flaps that have been constructed to reline or primarily close the anal canal due to the lack of sufficient anoderm.[3,17]

Flap procedures, if performed properly, probably afford the patient rapid healing and less discomfort than if the patient's wounds are allowed to heal by secondary intention. They are also invaluable in the treatment of mucosal ectropion, and as sources of donor skin necessitated by large defects resulting from radical excision of perianal or anal neoplasms.

The disadvantages of sliding skin flaps are significant. These procedures are more time consuming, require more technical expertise, and strict adherence to basic surgical principles, especially hemostasis and absence of tension along suture lines. The flaps must be elevated carefully and handled gently to assure the best possible result. Diligent postoperative care is required. Finally, the loss of a flap delays healing, increases the patient's discomfort, and may itself contribute to the formation of a stricture.

Y-V *Advancement Flap.* This procedure was first described by Penn in 1948 and has been modified by many surgeons since that time. The approach described is similar to that advocated by Nickell and Woodward.[25] A lateral sphincterotomy is performed from approximately the level of the mucocutaneous junc-

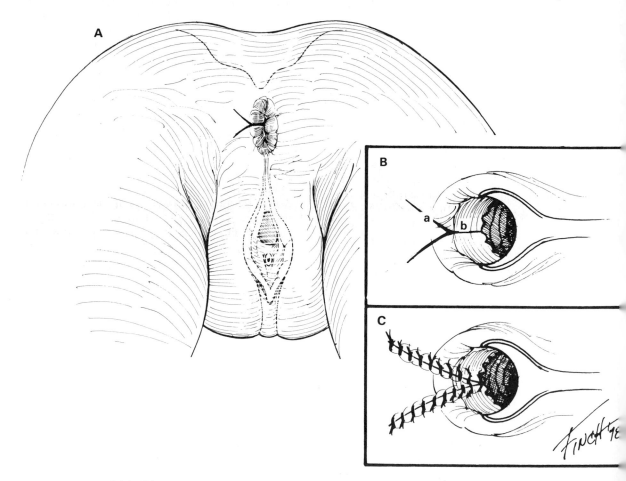

**FIGURE 26-3.** *Plastic repair of anal stricture using Y-V method. (After Nickell, W. B.: Arch Surg., 104:223, 1972)*

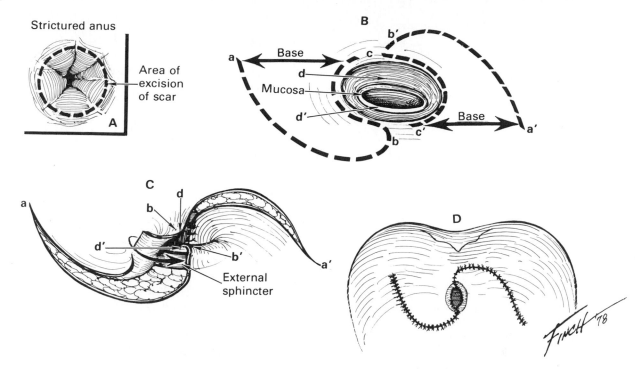

FIGURE **26-4.** S-Plasty for anal stricture. (*After Hudson, A. T.: Dis. Colon Rectum.,* 10:*57, 1967*)

tion and forms the base of the "Y" (Fig. 26-3A). This incision is then extended caudad into the gluteal skin in two directions, forming a "V" shaped flap and completing the "Y." The base of the flap should be broad, and the flap should be full thickness skin without subcutaneous tissue or muscle. It is undermined until it can be advanced (Point a to Point b) without tension (Fig. 26-3B). If it is possible, any remaining anal mucosa should be undermined to facilitate approximation to the flap. When hemostasis is ensured, the tip of the flap is sutured to the mucosa at the base of the sphincterotomy incision. The muscle and remaining anoderm are then sutured to each limb of the "Y" converting it to a "V" (Fig. 26-3C).

S-*Plasty.* This technique, first described by Ferguson, in 1959, for mucosal ectropion, utilizes two rotational flaps shaped in the form of an "S," and can be useful for the correction of circumferential anal strictures.[8,17] A circular incision is made and all scar tissue is excised cephalad to normal mucosa (Fig. 26-4A). A partial internal sphincterotomy is then performed. With the midpoint of the anal canal as the center, an "S"-shaped incision is then made (Fig. 26-4B), outlining two skin flaps (a,b,c—a',b',c'). These are elevated toward their bases, and then rotated until point b reaches point d, and point b' reaches point d' without tension. The grafts should be full thickness with their undersurfaces lined by a small amount of subcutaneous fat. After achievement of meticulous hemostasis, the flaps are swung into place and sutured in a manner such that a new 360° mucocutaneous junction is achieved (Fig. 26-4C). The resulting eliptical defects created on each side are closed only if this can be accomplished without tension (Fig. 26-4D). They are of little functional importance, and usually close rapidly by secondary intention.

*Two and Four Quadrant Sphincterotomy With or Without Sliding Skin Flap.* This technique, recently advocated by Sarner, is identical to that described for the sliding skin flap graft except that it is performed in two or four quadrants (Fig. 26-5).[30] It is useful in patients with tight anal strictures in whom a satisfactory diameter of the anal canal cannot be achieved

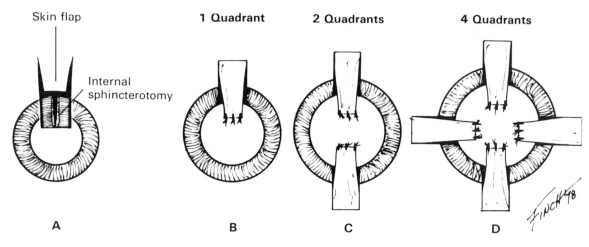

FIGURE **26-5.** *Sliding skin graft for repair of anal stricture.* (*After Sarner, J. B.: Dis. Colon Rectum., 12:277, 1969*)

with a single sphincterotomy and sliding graft.

The following suggestions are useful when dealing with sliding skin flaps:

1. Pre-, peri- and postoperative prophylactic antibiotics
2. Full thickness graft with a wide base
3. Meticulous hemostasis
4. Careful handling of the graft edges
5. Adjunctive internal sphincterotomy
6. Absorbable sutures
7. Diligent postoperative care with early detection and treatment of sloughed or infected grafts
8. Careful selection of patients—avoid patients with thin perianal skin

### Resection

Strictures of the rectum and rectosigmoid may be resected. Modern autosuture instruments such as the EEA stapler have not only facilitated, but also extended the limits of low anterior resection. Pull through procedures similar to those described for Hirschsprung's disease have also been advocated by some surgeons. The reader is referred to any standard pediatric surgical text for description of these techniques. As mentioned previously, severe strictures which involve the sphincter, and those accompanied by extensive perianal disease are best treated by diverting colostomy with proctectomy, if feasible.

Posterior extraperitoneal proctoplasty, originally described by Lloyd-Davies and Lockhart-Mummery in 1935, is another approach to treatment for strictures of the rectum.[23] The operation is performed as follows: using a posterior midline approach, the coccyx is excised exposing the strictured rectum; a vertical incision is then made in the strictured segment; and, the resulting defect is closed transversely, much like a Heineke Mikulicz pyloroplasty. This procedure has limited value, however, primarily because one is usually dealing with a thickened, fibrotic rectal wall which has a tendency to heal poorly, thus predisposing the patient to a suture line disruption and possible fecal fistula.

While many other surgical approaches for the treatment of rectal strictures have been advocated, most of them have been abandoned in favor of techniques already described. For historical purposes, the reader is referred to articles by, among others, Jelk and Keller.[18,20]

### REFERENCES

1. Colcock, B. P., and Hume, A.: Radiation injury to the sigmoid and rectum. Surg. Gynecol. Obstet., *108:*306, 1959.

2. Corman, M. L.: Rectal stricture secondary to Teflon sling repair of rectal prolapse. Dis. Colon Rectum, *17:*89, 1973.

3. Corman, M. L., Veidenheimer, M. C., and Collier, M. A.: Anoplasty for dual stricture. Surg. Clin. North Am., *56:*727, 1976.

4. Curr, J. F.: Rectal stricture due to ischemia following ruptured ectopic gestation. Gut, *8:*178, 1967.

5. DeCosse, J. J., Rhodes, R. S., Wentz, W. B., Reagan, J. W., Dworken, H. J., and Holden, W. D.: The natural history and management of radiation induced injury of the gastrointestinal tract. Ann. Surg., *170:*369, 1969.

6. Dencker, J., Johansson, J. I., Norryd, C., and Tromberg, K. G.: Dilator for treatment of strictures in the upper part of the rectum and sigmoid. Dis. Colon Rectum, *16:*550, 1973.

7. Edward, F. C., and Truelove, S. C.: The course and prognosis of ulcerative colitis. Part III: Complications. Gut, *5:*1, 1964.

8. Ferguson, J. A.: Repair of "Whitehead deformity" of the anus. Surg. Gynecol. Obstet., *108:*115, 1959.

9. Goligher, J. C.: *Surgery of the Anus, Rectum and Colon.* 3 ed., 148. Springfield, Charles C Thomas, 1975.

10. ———: p. 172.

11. ———: p. 366–405.

12. ———: p. 483–484.

13. Gordon, P. H., and Hoexter, B.: Complications of the Ripstein procedure. Dis. Colon Rectum, *21:*277, 1978.

14. Goulston, S. J. M., and McGovern, V. J.: The nature of benign strictures in ulcerative colitis. New. Engl. J. Med., *281:*290, 1969.

15. Greenstein, A. J., Sachar, D. B., and Kark, A. E.: Strictures of the anorectum in Crohn's disease involving the colon. Ann. Surg., *181.*207, 1975.

16. Greco, R.: Anal stricture following pseudomonas sepsis. J. Pediatr. Surg., *13:*91, 1978.

17. Hudson, A. T.: S-Plasty repair of Whitehead deformity of the anus. Dis. Colon Rectum, *10:*57, 1967.

18. Jelk, J. L.: A new operation for rectal stricture. Trans. Am. Proct. Soc., *32:*19, 1931.

19. Kark, A. E., Epstein, A. E., and Chapman, D. S.: Nonmalignant anorectal strictures. Surg. Gynecol. Obstet., *109:*333, 1959.

20. Keller, W. L.: Annular strictures of the rectum and anus. Treatment by tunnel skin graft. A preliminary report. Am. J. Surg., *20:*28, 1933.

21. Ladd, W. E., and Gross, R. E.: Congenital malformations of the anus and rectum. Am. J. Surg., *23:*167, 1934.

22. Levine, I., Romano, S., Steinberg, M., and Welsh, R. A.: Lymphogranuloma venereum: Rectal stricture and carcinoma. Dis. Colon Rectum, *7:*124, 1964.

23. Lockhart-Mummery, J. P., and Lloyd-Davies, O. V.: The operative treatment of fibrous stricture of the rectum. Br. J. Surg., *23:*19, 1935.

24. Mazier, W. P.: A technique for the management of low colonic anastomotic stricture. Dis. Colon Rectum, *16:*113, 1973.

25. Nickell, W. B., and Woodward, E. R.: Advancement flaps for treatment of anal stricture. Arch. Surg., *104:*223, 1972.

26. Palmer, J. A., and Bush, M. D.: Radiation injuries to the bowel associated with the treatment of carcinoma of the cervix. Surgery, *80:*458, 1976.

27. Parks, A. G., Allen, C. L. O., Frank, J. D., and McPartlin, J. F.: A method of treating post-irradiation rectovaginal fistulas. Br. J. Surg., *65:*417, 1978.

28. Partridge, J. P., and Gough, M. H.: Congenital malformations of the anus and rectum. Br. J. Surg., *49:*37, 1961.

29. Ponka, J. L., Brush, B. E., and Hodgkinson, C. P.: Colorectal endometriosis. Dis. Colon Rectum, *16:*490, 1973.

30. Sarner, J. B.: Plastic relief of anal stenosis. Dis. Colon Rectum, *12:*277, 1969.

31. Shanahan, M. K., and Steedman, R. K.: Inferior mesenteric artery occlusion. Br. J. Surg., *50:*533, 1963.

32. Sherman, L., Prem, K. A., and Mensheha, N. M.: Factitial Proctitis: A restudy at the University of Minnesota. Dis. Colon Rectum, *14:*281, 1971.

33. Sucre, A. J.: Inflammatory tumors as a cause of benign rectal stricture. Dis. Colon Rectum, *6:*356, 1963.

34. Top, F. H., Sr., and Wehrle, P. F.: *Communicable and Infections Diseases,* 8 ed. St. Louis, C. B. Mosby, 1976.

35. Wilcock, B. P., and Olander, H. J.: The pathogenesis of porcine rectal stricture, I & II. Vet. Pathol., *14*(1):36, 1977.

# 27

# Early Detection and Follow-Up of Rectal Neoplasia

## SCREENING OF GENERAL POPULATION

The high incidence of carcinoma of the large bowel is well recognized; 36 per cent of these carcinomas occur in the rectum.[25] Although the long term survival of patients with carcinoma of the colon and rectum has not improved much over the past 30 years it is well documented that those with Dukes' A lesions, when treated properly, have a five year survival of 90 per cent or better. However, the survival rate for patients with Dukes' B lesions is only 71 per cent, and 38 per cent for Dukes' C lesions.[33] There is no doubt that early diagnosis of carcinoma of the large bowel is urgently needed if we are going to achieve a higher cure rate. If one accepts the assumption that the majority of carcinomas arise from preexisting neoplastic polyps, one can conclude that if these are eradicated most carcinomas can be prevented. In order to screen a large population the tests have to be simple, economical, and accurate.

### Hemoccult Test

Recently the Hemoccult test has been used to screen the portion of the population "at risk". The person is on a meat-free, high roughage diet for 24 hours, after which a stool sample from each of several different areas is smeared on two Hemoccult slides. This is repeated on three consecutive days. The patient can send the specimens for the test by mail. Because of the low risk of carcinoma of the large bowel in the younger age group, such testing is recommended for patients between 50 and 80 years old. Preliminary results from a study conducted by Gilbertsen at the University of Minnesota have been most encouraging. During the first two years of the study approximately 500 of the 23,000 persons tested had stools positive for occult blood. Of these individuals, 475 were further studied by proctosigmoidoscopy, barium enema, and colonoscopy: 35 per cent were found to have polyps of the colon and rectum, and 10 per cent had carcinoma. Eighty per cent of the carcinomas detected by the hemoccult test were Dukes' A, compared to about 15 per cent of Dukes' A carcinoma in any large series of patients with carcinoma detected by other methods.[21,33] Although it is premature to draw any final conclusions at the present time, to date, Hemoccult testing is the most practical screening for the asymptomatic population.

### Proctosigmoidoscopy

There are only a few internal organs which lend themselves to direct visualization; the rectum is one. Proctosigmoidoscopy is a simple procedure which is well tolerated by patients if it is performed properly. However, it requires some preparation by the patient, and it must be done in an office or hospital where the facility is available. It is, therefore, not practical for screening the entire population. Nevertheless, it should be performed as part of a complete physical examination in people over 45 years of age. Between 5 and 10 per cent of asymptomatic patients are found to have rectal polyps. Gilbertsen found that the use of proctosigmoidoscopy to detect polyps, followed by their eradication, produced a significant decrease in the development of carcinoma of the rectum.[12] Of the more than 100,000 examinations of the 18,000 asymptomatic people 45 years and older undergoing an annual proctosigmoidoscopy 11 were found to have carcinoma, and 10 of these were at an early stage. This is compared to the estimated 75 to 80 people who were expected to develop carcinoma in the same age group and follow-up period. For asymptomatic people 45 years or older without a polyp, or a family history of a polyp or carcinoma, proctosigmoidoscopy every three years is probably adequate. One should always keep in mind that proctosigmoidoscopy is not a complete examination of the large bowel. If a polyp is found, further evaluation is indicated.

### Barium Enema and Colonoscopy

As screening examinations, these modes of investigation are neither practical nor necessary. They should be considered only if a patient's stool is Hemoccult positive, if a polyp is found at sigmoidoscopy, or if there are symptoms suggestive of colonic disease.

## POLYP REMOVAL FOLLOW-UP

The chance of developing a metachronous polyp is significantly higher in patients who have a neoplastic polyp in the colon or rectum than it is in the normal population; therefore, they require periodic surveillance.[2] A rectal polyp is a common incidental finding at routine proctosigmoidoscopy. A polyp smaller than 5 mm is of no immediate clinical significance, but biopsy to determine the histologic type of the polyp is desirable. A larger polyp should be totally snared and submitted for pathological examination. A neoplastic polyp found in the rectum may be a clue to more proximal polyps. These patients should have a barium enema and/or colonoscopy. Thereafter, an annual Hemoccult test and sigmoidoscopy, and a barium enema and/or colonoscopy should be performed every three years.

## CARCINOMA SURGERY FOLLOW-UP

The purposes of long term postoperative follow-up of patients who have undergone abdominoperineal resection or anterior resection for carcinoma of the rectum are: (*1*) to detect local recurrence; (*2*) to detect distant metastases; and, (*3*) to detect metachronous carcinomas or polyps.

### Detection of Local Recurrence

The incidence of local recurrence of carcinoma of the rectum varies from series to series depending upon the conduct and duration of follow-up. There is general agreement in the literature that the site of the malignancy, the grade, and the extent of the spread into the bowel wall greatly influence the tendency to local recurrence.[16] Hence, carcinoma of the lower part of the rectum, the Dukes' C lesion, and the poorly differentiated carcinoma have a greater tendency to recur. Most local recurrences are in the pelvic area: for women the most common sites are the posterior vaginal wall and the cul-de-sac; for men they are the posterior pelvic area, perineum, urinary bladder, periureteral area, and prostate gland.[11] It is obvious that many recurrences are difficult to detect by physical examination. In patients who have had low anterior resections, local recurrences which can be detected in the pelvis or by proctosigmoidoscopy are most commonly manifested at the suture line. Pelvic or perineal pain is a common symptom of pelvic recurrence. In Welch's series, half the patients with recurrence who presented with back pain had vertebral metastases demonstrated by radiograph.[32] Intravenous pyelogram (IVP) may detect pelvic recurrence earlier than the physical findings and, therefore, a base line IVP a few months after the operation is recommended for future comparison. The concept of the planned, second-look operation to detect local recurrence early and possibly convert it into a disease-free state is attractive and sound.[23] However, the high negative re-exploration rate, and the significant morbidity and mortality have limited its routine use.[14,15] Recently, serial postoperative carcinoembryonic antigen (CEA) determinations have been successful in detecting early recurrence. By obtaining CEA levels at four days, two weeks, one month, and every three months after an operation for cure, Herrera and co-workers found that three successive elevations of CEA gave a better than 90 per cent certainty of the presence of recurrent or metastatic disease.[18] Recurrence was detected five and one-half months earlier than by other clinical methods. These findings have also been confirmed by others.[19,29,30] Using CEA to aid in the selection of patients for the second-look in colon and rectal carcinoma has also been practiced.[19] Whether it will identify the patients early enough to permit curative operation remains to be seen. Preoperative determination of CEA levels have been shown to be of prognostic value with respect to mean time to recurrence in patients with Dukes' B and C lesions. Times ranged from 30 months for a level of 2 ng. to 9.8 months for a level of 70 ng./ml.[31] Computerized axial tomography has not been proved to be effective at the present time.[1]

## Detection of Distant Metastases

*Detection of Pulmonary Metastases.* Pulmonary metastases from colorectal carcinoma occur in 20 per cent of the patients who die of the disease.[27] Multiple, often bilateral, pulmonary metastases from colon and rectal carcinoma are frequently only one manifestation of generalized metastatic disease and, as such, are beyond any hope for cure. On the other hand, when there is no recurrence at the primary site, 30 per cent of patients who have a solitary pulmonary metastasis live five years after its resection.

In Schulten's series of 185 patients who underwent colorectal resection for cure, 14.5 per cent developed pulmonary metastases; of these, 15 per cent were solitary.[27] In this series the longer the interval between the removal of the primary carcinoma and the appearance of the metastatic pulmonary lesion the greater was the chance for long term survival. But in Cahan's series the interval between primary disease and metastasis did not influence the prognosis.[5] In general, the more extensive the carcinoma is, the greater the likelihood of the patient developing pulmonary metastases. Thus, a Dukes' C lesion has a greater chance of developing pulmonary metastasis than a Dukes' B or A one. Pulmonary metastases are best detected by routine chest radiograph.[5,9]

When a solitary lung shadow appears in patients who have had colorectal carcinoma, further work-up for documentation is necessary since not all of them are metastatic lesions. In Cahan's series of 54 patients in whom a solitary lung shadow subsequently developed, 25 proved to be metastatic and 29 were primary carcinomas of the lung.[5] He advocated that the following guidelines are useful in predicting the nature of a pulmonary lesion in a patient with a previously treated malignancy: (*1*) If a patient has a squamous cell carcinoma elsewhere, a solitary lung lesion usually indicates a separate primary. (*2*) If a patient has an adenocarcinoma elsewhere, a solitary lung lesion has an equal chance of being primary or metastatic. (*3*) If a patient has a soft tissue or skeletal sarcoma or malanoma, a solitary lung lesion usually indicates metastases. (*4*) If a patient has a lymphoma, a solitary lung lesion is usually a primary carcinoma.

Chest radiographs are accurate screening for metastatic colorectal carcinomas.[9] Bronchoscopy, biopsy, bronchial washings, and sputum cytology yield positive results in 76 per cent of the primary, and 12 per cent of the metastatic malignancies.[5] When a lung shadow is synchronous with a primary colorectal carcinoma it is not necessarily metastatic; in fact only one-fourth of Cahan's series were metastatic.[5] Definitive diagnosis frequently requires thoracotomy.

Since most pulmonary shadows are found by chance as part of a routine chest radiograph, and the probability of metastases or a new primary is highest within five years after detection of the primary carcinoma, this simple, non-invasive study should be done every 3 to 6 months.[5] It is also important to note that a significant number of patients who have had colorectal carcinoma and a second primary in the lung have a third or a fourth primary elsewhere.[5] This calls for a regular, thorough physical examination of all systems.

*Detection of Liver Metastases.* The incidence of liver metastases from carcinoma of the rectum in patients who undergo curative or palliative resection of the rectum is about 14 per cent.[33] The diagnosis of early liver metastasis is difficult, and at the present time there is no one reliable method to detect it. Alkaline phosphatase and lactic dehydrogenase (LDH) give an accuracy rate of 78 per cent with about 50 per cent false positives and 13 per cent false negatives.[24] Radionuclide imaging of the liver (liver scan) gives an accuracy rate between 75 and 84 per cent but false positives and false negatives are still unacceptably high.[7,10,24] Ultrasonography and computerized axial tomography may be useful to confirm the diagnosis.[15] Hepatic arteriography is the most accurate single study for identification of metastatic intrahepatic neoplasm (97% accuracy), but it is not practical for routine screening.[10] The present trend is toward the serial determinations of CEA postoperatively. A persistent rise in CEA from the postoperative baseline level indicates metastases.[18,19,29]

Experience with a highly select group of patients at the Mayo Clinic showed that multiple liver metastases are an ominous sign: there have been no five year survivals after hepatic resection.[35] In patients with a solitary liver metastasis, hepatic resection gives an amazingly high five year survival of 42 per cent, and 10 year survival of 28 per cent. The best results are those with a small solitary liver metastasis where wedge resection was undertaken.

### Detection of Metachronous Carcinomas or Polyps

The development of a second or a third carcinoma of the colon and rectum after the primary lesion has been removed is an infrequent occurrence. The incidence is about 3.5 to 4 per cent in patients who have been followed for 10 years; but, if the patient with a primary carcinoma had a synchronous polyp, the incidence of a metachronous carcinoma rises to about 8 per cent.[4,17] Any patient with carcinoma of the rectum should have a total colonoscopy at least once, if possible, before the operation. Thereafter, barium enema with air contrast alternating with colonoscopy should be done every two years. Stool should be tested for occult blood every six months. The patient can submit specimens and, if they are positive, repeat testing should be done with a three day, meat-free diet. If the stool is still positive for blood, a complete evaluation with proctosigmoidoscopy, barium enema with air contrast, and colonoscopy is in order.

Metastases to distant organs such as brain, bone, bone marrow, pancreas, thyroid, skin, aderenal glands, spleen, breast, ovary, penis, and nail beds are much less common. There are no specific or practical ways of detection, but an awareness of the possibility of their occurence is necessary.

It should be emphasized that the following suggestions for the postoperative follow-up of carcinoma of the rectum are entirely arbitrary. The interval of the follow-up should be adjusted to correspond to the extent to which risk factors such as stage of the disease by Dukes' classification, grade, location, and size are present. After five years, recurrence is a rather remote possibility; therefore, it is reasonable to double the length of the interval between follow-up procedures.

TABLE **27-1.** Postoperative Follow-Up For Carcinoma of the Rectum

MONTHS AFTER THE OPERATION

| | 3 | 6 | 9 | 12 | 15 | 18 | 21 | 24 | 30 | 36 | 42 | 48 | 54 | 60 |
|---|---|---|---|---|---|---|---|---|---|---|---|---|---|---|
| *Physical Exam* | X | X | X | X | X | X | X | X | X | X | X | X | X | X |
| *Chest X-Ray* | X | X | X | X | X | X | X | X | X | X | X | X | X | X |
| *Sigmoidoscopy* | X | X | X | X | X | X | X | X | X | X | X | X | X | X |
| *CEA* | X | X | X | X | X | X | X | X | X | X | X | X | X | X |
| *Hemoccult* | | X | | X | | X | | X | X | X | X | X | X | X |
| *IVP* | X | | X | | X | | X | | | X | | X | | X |
| *Barium enema* | | | | | | | | X | | | | | | |
| *Colonoscopy* | | | | | | | | | | | | X | | |

## TOTAL COLECTOMY FOLLOW-UP

Total colectomy with ileorectal anastomosis is the treatment of choice for the patient who has familial adenomatous polyposis coli, unless the entire colon is carpeted with polyps or the patient is unlikely to return for follow-up at regular intervals for the rest of his life. It should be emphasized that the anastomosis should be to the upper part of the rectum, and not rectosigmoid, or sigmoid colon. If this procedure is used the amount of tissue at risk is less, and a sigmoidoscope can be passed to the anastomotic area. A study by Bussey suggested strong circumstantial evidence that cancer arises in a preexisting benign neoplasm; therefore, destruction of polyps in the rectum should prevent the development of carcinoma.[4]

In the Mayo Clinic series of 178 patients who underwent colectomy and ileorectosigmoidostomy for familial multiple polyposis the incidence of carcinoma later developing in the rectum was 22 per cent.[20] When the patients were followed for 23 years, the figure rose to 59 per cent. By contrast, the experience at St. Mark's Hospital, London, in a series of 89 patients surviving total colectomy with ileorectal anastomosis was that there were only two who subsequently developed a carcinoma of the rectum, one at two years and the other at seven years after the first operation.[3] A third patient underwent excision of the rectum ten years after the colectomy because the rectum became carpeted with adenomas, but no carcinoma was found. The reason for this discrepancy of the risk of developing carcinoma from these two institutions is not entirely clear; it is possibly the result of different extents of resection or the method of follow-up. The experience at the Mayo Clinic suggests that the longer the rectum remains in situ, the higher is the risk of development of carcinoma.

It has been well documented that polyps in the rectum spontaneously regress after an ileorectal anastomosis, but this is usually temporary and one should not await or expect their regression.[28,34] Most of these polyps are 1 to 2 mm, therefore as many as possible should be destroyed by electrocoagulation. This should be done every month until all of them are gone. The patient should then be followed every three to six months for the rest of his life. Vitamin C (3 g daily), on the basis of its antioxidant property, has been suggested by DeCosse to cause regression of the rectal polyps in these patients.[8] Its efficacy has not been confirmed. Recently there have been several reports on the development of polyps or carcinoma of the stomach, duodenum, and small bowel in patients with familial polyposis.[22,26] These patients should therefore be followed with annual upper gastrointestinal and small bowel follow-through studies. Other carcinomas known to develop in patients with familial adenomatous polyposis are periampullary carcinoma, carcinoma of the thyroid, carcinoma of the adrenal gland, and carcinoma of the gallbladder. Finally, and most importantly, one must not forget to check the members of the patient's family. There is no rule of thumb to follow in deciding when to start examining the rectum. But since the polyps rarely develop before puberty, it is reasonable to start the follow-up at about this time.

## REFERENCES

1. Baker, C., and Way, L. W.: Clinical utility of CAT body scans. Am. J. Surg., *136:*37, 1978.

2. Brahme, F., Ekelund, G. R., Norden, J. G., and Wenckert, A.: Metachronous colorectal polyps and carcinomas in persons with and without histories of polyps. Dis. Colon Rectum, *17:*166, 1974.

3. Bussey, H. J. R.: Familial polyposis coli. Baltimore and London, The John Hopkins University Press, 1975.

4. Bussey, H. J. R., Wallace, M. H., and Morson, B. C.: Metachronous carcinoma of the large intestine and intestinal polyps. Proc. R. Soc. Med., *60:*2, 1967.

5. Cahan, W. G., Castro, E. B., and Hajdu, S. I.: The significance of a solitary lung shadow in patients with colon carcinoma. Cancer, *33:*414, 1974.

6. ———: Therapeutic pulmonary resection of colonic carcinoma metastatic to lung. Dis. Colon Rectum, *17:*302, 1974.

7. Cedermark, B. J., et al: The value of liver scan in the follow-up study of patients with adenocarcinoma of the colon and rectum. Surg. Gynecol. Obstet., *144:*745, 1977.

8. DeCosse, J. J., Adams, M. B., Kuzma, J. F., LoGerfo, P., and Condon, R. E.: Effect of as-

corbic acid on rectal polyps of patients with familial polyposis. Surgery, *78:*608, 1975.

9. Didolkar, M. S., Cedermark, B. J., Goel, I. P., Taketa, H., and Moore, R. H.: Accuracy of roentgenograms of the chest in metastasis to the lungs. Surg. Gynecol. Obstet., *144:*903, 1977.

10. DuPriest, R. W. Jr., Haines, J. E., Rosch, J., and Krippachne, W. W.: A comparison of scintiscans and arteriograms for identifying metastatic intrahepatic tumors. Surg. Gynecol. Obstet., *136:*705, 1973.

11. Gilbertsen, V. A.: Proctosigmoidoscopy and polypectomy in reducing the incidence of rectal cancer. Cancer, *34:*936, 1974 Suppl.

12. Gilbertsen, V. A.: Adenocarcinoma of the rectum: Incidence and locations of recurrent tumor following present-day operations performed for cure. Ann. Surg., *157:*340, 1960.

13. Gilbertsen, V. A., and Nelms, J. M.: The prevention of invasive cancer of the rectum. Cancer, *41:*1137, 1978.

14. Griffen, W. O. Jr., Humphrey, L., and Sosin, H.: The prognosis and management of recurrent abdominal malignancies. Curr. Probl. Surg., April:18, 1969.

15. Grossman, Z. D., et al: Radionuclide imaging, computed tomography, and gray-scale ultrasonography of the liver: A comparative study. J. Nucl. Med., *18:*327, 1977.

16. Gunderson, L. L., and Sosin, H.: Areas of failure found at reoperation (second or asymptomatic look) following "curative surgery" for adenocarcinoma of the rectum: Clinicopathologic correlation and implications for adjuvent therapy. Cancer, *34:*1278, 1974.

17. Heald, R. J., and Bussey, H. J. R.: Clinical experiences at St. Mark's Hospital with multiple synchronous cancers of the colon and rectum. Dis. Colon Rectum, *18:*6, 1975.

18. Herrera, M. A., Ming, C. T., and Holyoke, E. D.: Carcinoembryonic antigen (CEA) as a prognostic and monitoring test in clinically complete resection of colorectal carcinoma. Ann. Surg., *183:*5, 1976.

19. Minton, J. P., et al: The use of serial carcinoembryonic antigen determinations to predict recurrence of carcinoma of the colon and the time for a second-look operation. Surg. Gynecol. Obstet., *147:*208, 1978.

20. Moertel, C. G., Hill, J. R., and Adson, M. A.: Surgical management of multiple polyposis—the problem of cancer in the retained bowel segment. Arch. Surg., *100:*521, 1970.

21. Morgan, C. N.: Treatment of cancer of the rectum. Am. J. Surg., *115:*442, 1968.

22. Ohsato, K., Yao, T., Watonabe, H., Iida, M., and Itoh, H.: Small intestinal involvement in familial polyposis diagnosed by operative intestinal fiberscopy: Report of four cases. Dis. Colon Rectum, *20:*414, 1977.

23. Polk, H. C. Jr., Ahmad, W., and Knutson, C. O.: Carcinoma of the colon and rectum. Curr. Probl. Surg. *Jan:* 28, 1973.

24. Read, D. R., Hambrick, E., Abcarian, H., and Levine, H.: The preoperative diagnosis of hepatic metastasis in cases of colorectal carcinoma. Dis. Colon Rectum, *20:*101, 1977.

25. Rhodes, J. B., Holmes, F. F., and Clark, G. M.: Changing distribution of primary cancers in the large bowel. JAMA, *238:*1641, 1977.

26. Ross, J. E., and Mara, J. E.: Small bowel polyps and carcinoma in multiple intestinal polyposis. Arch. Surg., *108:*736, 1974.

27. Schulten, M. F., Heiskell, C. A., and Shields, T. W.: The incidence of solitary pulmonary metastasis from carcinoma of the large intestine. Surg. Gynecol. Obstet., *143:*727, 1976.

28. Sheppard, J. A.: Familial polyposis of the colon with special reference to regression of rectal polyposis after subtotal colectomy. Br. J. Surg., *58:*85, 1971.

29. Sorokin, J. J., et al: Serial carcinoembryonic antigen assays. Use in detection of cancer recurrence. JAMA, *228:*49, 1974.

30. Sugarbaker, P. H., Skarin, A. T., and Zamcheck, N.: Patterns of serial assays and their clinical use in management of colorectal cancer. J. Surg. Oncology, *8:*523, 1976.

31. Wanebo, H. J., et al: Preoperative carcinoembryonic antigen level as a prognostic indicator in colorectal cancer. N. Engl. J. Med., *299:*9:448, 1978.

32. Welch, J. P., and Donaldson, G. A.: Detection and treatment of recurrent cancer of the colon and rectum. Am. J. Surg., *135:*505, 1978.

33. Whittaker, M., and Goligher, J. C.: The prognosis after surgical treatment for carcinoma of the rectum. Br. J. Surg., *63:*384, 1976.

34. Williams, R. D., and Fish, J. C.: Multiple polyposis, polyp regression, and carcinoma of the colon. Am. J. Surg., *112:*846, 1966.

35. Wilson, S. M., and Adson, M. A.: Surgical treatment of hepatic metastases from colorectal cancers. Arch. Surg., *111:*330, 1976.

# 28

# Out-Patient Procedures

With a better understanding of the anatomy and pathophysiology of anorectal disease, along with acquired technical expertise, one can safely perform, under local anesthesia, a great variety of procedures in the office or out-patient department. A well-equipped office (which includes basic resuscitation equipment) permits the surgeon to perform the kind of procedures described below.

For the patient, the advantages of out-patient operations are numerous. There is no need for a formal hospital admission with its attendant psychological trauma. The necessity for a general anesthetic is obviated. In general, patients probably convalesce better, and are more comfortable in the familiar surroundings of their own homes.

At a time when costs for medical care are increasing steadily, great savings can be afforded the patient, third party carriers, and institutions, by performing many anorectal procedures in the office. In certain localities where hospital bed shortages occur, waiting periods are eliminated by out-patient operations.

In the minds of some surgeons, the threat of a malpractice suit for poor results or complications is restriction of the freedom of the use of their offices.[2] However, for selected procedures, in an adequately equipped office, this consideration should not be relevant. Proce-

dures which can be performed on a out-patient basis are discussed below.

## RECTAL BIOPSY

Various forceps or suction biopsy apparatus are available for obtaining specimens from the rectum for histological evaluation. The forceps technique is probably still the best for localized and proliferative lesions. In order for the pathologist to provide maximum information to the clinician, a correct anatomical orientation is necessary. Consequently, when the specimen is obtained, it should be submitted with the sub-mucosal surface downward against a flat, ground glass slide or paper to which it adheres by its own stickiness. After fixation, the biopsy is embedded. This facilitates detailed assessment of mucosal and sub-mucosal pathology. The advantages of a properly orientated biopsy specimen are apparent, and cannot be over emphasized. For biopsies of tumors and other localized or proliferative lesions, the tissue cannot be fixed and embedded in this way. It is suitable only for diffuse mucosal conditions, particularly inflammatory diseases.

Morson points out that rectal biopsies are becoming more and more useful for a wide range of local and systemic disorders.[1] It is essential for the diagnosis of neoplasms, particularly malignant ones. Indeed, no major operation should be carried out on the rectum without confirmatory biopsy. Its value is established in the diagnosis of inflammatory conditions including specific infections such as amoebic dysentery. Serial biopsies can be valuable in the diagnosis of ulcerative colitis and Crohn's disease as well as being useful in judging the response to treatment. Biopsy may detect changes which are not apparent to the endoscopist. The correlation between proctosigmoidoscopic observations and the histology of biopsies of the rectal mucosa is not always accurate. For this reason, biopsy can, in certain circumstances, add refinement to the clinical opinion. It also confirms the presence of normal rectal mucosa.

Unusual local conditions which can be identified by rectal biopsy include pneumatosis cystoides intestinalis, mucoviscidosis, melanosis coli, oleogranuloma, and parasitic infections such as schistosomiasis.[1] Rectal biopsy may be useful in the detection of certain systemic conditions such as neurolipidoses, metachromatic leukodystrophy, Hurler's syndrome, amyloidosis, the arteritis of rheumatoid arthritis, periarteritis nodosa, malignant hypertension, cystinosis, and Whipple's disease.[1]

## EXCISION OF THROMBOSED EXTERNAL HEMORRHOIDS

The treatment of a patient with a thrombosed hemorrhoid will depend upon the severity of pain that is being experienced. If the pain is subsiding there is no need for operative treatment. However, if the pain is excruciating, or an erosion has developed in the thrombosed hemorrhoid resulting in persistent bleeding, then an excision of the involved hemorrhoid is indicated. A complete ring of multiple confluent thrombosed external hemorrhoids is best treated in the operating room under proper anesthesia by a definitive hemorrhoidectomy.

### Technique of Local Anesthesia

The skin adjacent to the anus is richly innervated; therefore, the injection of a local anesthetic may be a painful procedure. An initial wheal is made with a small needle (gauge 25 or 26), and the anesthetic solution is *slowly* introduced into the tissue beneath and around the thrombosed hemorrhoid. Rapid injection will distend the tissues very quickly and cause increased pain. Lidocaine diffuses rapidly into the tissues, and hyaluronidase may be used to augment this diffusion. The addition of epinephrine aids hemostasis and prolongs the duration of anesthesia.

### Technique of Excision

The operative area is prepared with an aqueous antiseptic solution. Alcohol causes a burning sensation and may become ignited if cautery is used. An elliptical incision is made to encompass the thrombosed hemorrhoid, and dissection is carried down to the muscle but not into the anal canal. Incisions extended into the anal canal may result in a bleeding point that goes undetected. With the thrombosed hemorrhoid excised, the exposed edge of the external sphincter muscle is noted. Hemostasis may be obtained with a cautery, and the wound closed with a continuous absorbable suture such as 3—0 chromic catgut. The wound may be left open to granulate as the wound margins will fall together anyway. Mere incision and enucleation of the clot without removal of the hemorrhoid is not advisable because bleeding and clotting tend to recur within a few hours and the pain may be as intense as before.

## INTERNAL HEMORRHOIDS

The treatment of internal hemorrhoids is an office procedure in most situations. Because of the autonomic innervation of the tissues above the level of the dentate line, therapeutic procedures may be performed without anesthesia.

### Barron Rubber Band Ligature

The symptoms of bleeding and protrusion can usually be handled by the application of the Barron rubber band ligation technique. The method is simple and effective. Details of its application are described in Chapter Six.

### Sclerotherapy

Injection of sclerosing agents in the region of the offending hemorrhoidal tissue is effective for small internal hemorrhoids. The details of this technique are also included in Chapter Six.

## LATERAL INTERNAL SPHINCTEROTOMY

One of the most painful anorectal conditions is the acute fissure. When medical management proves unsatisfactory, a lateral internal sphincterotomy generally produces dramatic and immediate results in relief of pain. The operative technique and its numerous advantages are described in detail in Chapter Seven.

Associated with a fissure-in-ano may be a large prolapsing hypertrophied anal papilla. If it is symptomatic it can easily be removed by infiltrating a small amount of local anesthetic at the base of the pedicle, and transecting it flush with the wall of the anal canal. Hemostasis is easily controlled with cautery or suture.

## INCISION AND DRAINAGE OF ABSCESSES

Almost all perianal and pilonidal abscesses, as well as most ischiorectal abscesses, can be drained under local anesthesia in the outpatient setting. Such treatment affords immediate relief of the pain. Another advantage of draining abscesses around the anorectal region under local anesthesia is that the surgeon is not tempted to divide sphincter muscle at the initial sitting. Many patients will, therefore, be allowed to keep their sphincter muscle intact, rather than having portions divided at the initial procedure. Details of this technique are described in Chapter Eight. A simple incision is inadequate as the skin edges may coapt within 24 hours, and the abscess will recur.

The tiny abscesses and short subcutaneous fistulous tracks associated with hidradenitis suppurativa may also be opened and unroofed under local anesthesia as an out-patient. However, extensive disease requires more thorough treatment in the operating room. An intersphincteric abscess requires admission to the hospital because an adequate anesthetic will be required for sufficient drainage.

## POLYPS AND CARCINOMA

Most pedunculated polyps can be removed on an out-patient basis. A pedunculated lesion is easily snared and, when one is familiar with the electrosurgical equipment, there should seldom be any problem with bleeding. Details of this procedure are outlined in Chapter Nineteen.

An ulcerated or fungating neoplasm can easily be biopsied with a biopsy forceps. Electrocoagulation may be necessary to control bleeding.

Elevations of the mucosa less than 5 mm. in diameter are frequently seen, and there is a difference in opinion regarding their management. Some surgeons simply destroy such lesions by coagulation, while others insist upon biopsy and histologic examination. We strongly favor the latter approach because if the polyp proves to be neoplastic knowledge of its association to other synchronous and metachronous lesions becomes important, and patients require a life long follow-up with barium enema and/or colonoscopy. If the lesion proves to be hyperplastic, such close follow-up is not necessary.

Large sessile lesions are best removed in the operating room by lifting the lesion off of the underlying wall in the submucosal plane as described in Chapter Nineteen.

## CONDYLOMA ACUMINATUM

Although the application of podophyllin is easily carried out in the office, we do not recommend it as the treatment of choice because it is difficult to control, and can result in excessive destruction of normal anal canal mucosa.

Electrocoagulation has proven an effective means of destroying condyloma acuminatum. This can be performed on an out-patient basis. Care must be taken to rule out warts within the anal or vaginal canal. Cooperative patients with only a few scattered warts in the anal canal can have these coagulated under adequately administered local anesthesia. However, for patients with extensive warts located within the anal canal and perianal region a general or regional anesthetic is probably more satisfactory.

## PILONIDAL DISEASE

A considerably large percentage of patients with pilonidal disease can be adequately treated on an out-patient basis under local anesthesia. If the patient is cooperative, and the tracks are not too extensive, they can be unroofed, curetted of their granulation tissue, and marsupialized or left to heal secondarily. Details of this procedure are described in Chapter Nine.

## REFERENCES

1. Morson, B. C., and Dawson, I. M. P.: Gastrointestinal Pathology. 596. London, Blackwell Scientific Publications, 1972.
2. Rand, A. A.: Office and Outpatient Procedures. *In* Turell, R. (ed): Diseases of the Colon and Anorectum. 1273. Philadelphia, W. B. Saunders, 1969.

# 29

# The Pharmacology of Anorectal Preparations

In viewing the spectrum of human illness, one probably sees no area in which self treatment occurs more frequently than with the diseases of the anorectal region. Fear and embarrassment about this part of the anatomy often result in delay of the affected individual to seek medical attention. The ready availability of over-the-counter preparations makes such treatment easy. The troubled individual is undoubtedly influenced to a great extent by the unsupported advertising claims that some manufacturers make for the efficacy of their medications.[4] Undue reliance on these preparations, combined with the universal belief that almost all symptoms originate from hemorrhoidal disease, leads to the person's failure to seek medical advice, and this may have serious consequences.

Suggested indications for these preparations include the relief of pain and discomfort following anorectal surgery, hemorrhoids whether or not complicated by thromboses and prolapse, pruritus ani, proctitis, "cryptitis", fissures, fistulae, and other congestive, allergic, or inflammatory conditions. They are also suggested for use prior to rectal examination to anesthetize the area where it is too tender, or where there is too much spasm to admit the examining finger.

The pharmaceutical preparations available are of two types: the ointment and the suppository. The number of each type exceeds 100 products, and the total sales for 1971, according to Product Management, came to over $25 million.[7]

The available preparations contain combinations of traditional ingredients including topical anesthetics and analgesics, antiseptics, mild astringents, anti-inflammatory agents, emollients, and vasoconstrictors, in a host of bases and preservatives. Unfortunately, there is no documented evidence available regarding the efficacy of these drugs alone, or in combination in relieving the symptoms of anorectal disease.[4]

## CLASSIFICATION
### Topical Anesthetics and Analgesics

Topical anesthetics such as benzocaine, or topical analgesics such as diperodon or pramoxine hydrochloride are included in many ointments and suppositories. Reputedly, pramoxine hydrochloride provides surface analgesia within 2 to 3 minutes, lasts up to four hours, and is less toxic and sensitizing than benzocaine, cocaine, procaine, and dibucaine.

Frequently, dibucaine ointment is recommended as an independent therapeutic agent. Lidocaine hydrochloride ointment has been recommended by its manufacturer for the control of pain, itching, burning, and other unpleasant symptoms due to inoperable anorectal conditions, hemorrhoids, and fissures. Provided they are active on broken skin and mucous membranes, and are present in sufficient concentrations, topical anesthetics may be useful in relieving anal pain and pruritus. Surface or topical anesthesia blocks the sensory nerve endings in the skin or mucous membranes, but to reach these structures the drug must have good powers of penetration. Agents used primarily for surface anesthesia are amethocaine, benzocaine, cocaine, lignocaine, and prilocaine. However, the risk of contact sensitization and hypersensitivity common to nearly all the drugs must be considered. Of the topical anesthetics used, tetracaine, dibucaine and benzocaine have most often caused sensitization.

The main systemic toxic effect is excitation of the central nervous system, manifested by yawning, restlessness, excitement, nausea, and vomiting, and may be followed by depression, muscular twitching, convulsions, respiratory failure, and coma.[6] There is simultaneous depression of the cardiovascular system with pallor, sweating, and hypotension. Arrhythmias may occur. Repeated application to skin is more likely than systemic administration to give rise to allergic reactions.

In the treatment of fissures, anesthetic ointments, if applied only to the perianal region, are of absolutely no help. To have any effect they must be inserted into the anal canal. Since many patients find this rather distasteful as well as uncomfortable, success of this treatment is questionable.

## Antiseptics

Many preparations also include an agent such as phenol, boric acid, oxyquinoline, or phenylmercuric nitrate. Antiseptics are used to destroy or inhibit the growth of pathogenic micro-organisms. The inclusion of such agents in these preparations in such low concentrations could only have a marginal effect on the constantly renewed bacterial population of the anus and rectum. These agents, in all probability, are harmless but the risk of contact sensitization must be taken into consideration.[2]

Boric acid preparations should be applied only to intact skin. Absorption of boric acid from abraded skin areas and granulating wounds, or body cavities, may result in systemic toxicity.[1]

Phenylmercuric nitrate has antibacterial and antifungal properties but anorectal preparations were not listed among the uses suggested in Martindale's pharmacology textbook.[6]

## Astringents

Mild astringents, almost universally incorporated into all anorectal preparations, include substances like bismuth subgallate, zinc oxide, or balsam of Peru. These agents precipitate proteins, and when applied to mucous membranes or to damaged skin they form a protective layer and are not usually absorbed. They are designed to contract tissue and check exudative secretions. In the case of a thrombosed hemorrhoid, one cannot understand how they were intended to act, while in the case of fissures, frequently, they do not come in contact with the fissure itself.

## Emollients and/or Lubricants

Cocoa butter and liquid paraffin as well as other oils have been included in many of these products. As a soothing agent in the sense that these substances may better lubricate the anal canal during defecation, especially in the presence of painful conditions of the anus, some value might be perceived.

## Vasoconstrictors

Agents such as ephedrine and phenylephrine are intended to reduce bleeding from hemorrhoids, but clinical evidence to support this claim is not available. They produce capillary and arterial constrictions but their effect on veins is negligible.[4] In large doses, ephedrine may give rise to side effects such as giddiness, headache, nausea, vomiting, sweating, thirst, palpitations, difficulty in micturation, muscular weakness and tremors, anxiety, restlessness and insomnia. Some patients may exhibit these symptoms with the usual therapeutic dose.[6] Manufacturers caution against their use in patients sensitive to one of the ingredients, and in the presence of severe cardiac disease, diabetes mellitus, glaucoma, hypertension, or hyperthyroidism. It should not be given to patients being treated with a monoamine oxidase inhibitor.

## Corticosteroids

Numerous steroid preparations are currently available, sometimes to be used in combination with some of the already mentioned ingredients, while on other occasions they are prescribed independently. There is no clinical evidence that corticosteroids help hemorrhoids, anal fissures, or post-hemorrhoidectomy pain. These agents are available in three forms for the treatment of anorectal disease: ointments and creams, suppositories, and retention enemas.

*Steroid Ointments and Creams.* These preparations are frequently prescribed topically to provide symptomatic relief in the treatment of pruritus ani. However, the side effects of these agents must be recognized.[5]

ATROPHY AND TELANGIECTASIA. The long term use of potent topical corticosteroids in the perianal region may produce an itchy dermatosis. However, when the patient stops applying the drug, the rash and itching recur so that the medication is once again reinstituted. Atrophy and telangiectasia may take months or years to develop. The extent and degree will vary. In general, use of fluorinated steroid preparations on a long-term basis should be avoided in order to escape this complication.

MASKING OR CHANGING A PRE-EXISTING DERMATOSIS. The anti-inflammatory action of steroid removes or decreases the erythema and other findings in conditions such as scabes and tenia corporus. This can make identification of these conditions difficult unless one has a high index of suspicion.

SYSTEMIC ABSORPTION. Following lengthy use of steroids over large areas of the body, systemic absorption may occur, but if they are applied only to the perianal region it is probably of limited significance. As the safety of topical corticosteroids during pregnancy has not been confirmed, they should not be used in large amounts or for prolonged periods of time.

Jackson classified topical steroids into three groups: weak, medium, and strong.[5] He feels that almost all side effects can be avoided completely by restriction of the use of potent topical corticosteroids to small areas for short periods. In many conditions, maintenance therapy with 0.5 per cent hydrocortisone or another weak steroid preparation is adequate. Triamcinolone is more effective than hydrocortisone.[6] Jackson points out that potent steroids should not be used to treat undiagnosed conditions. The reader is referred to his extensive classification for detailed drug names.

*Steroid Suppositories.* Corticosteroid suppositories may prove to be of value for patients who suffer from a distal proctitis. This non-specific inflammatory condition of the rectum which involves the distal 8 to 10 cm of bowel frequently responds to the administration of hydrocortisone suppositories. Factitial proctitis (post-irradiation) may be another indication for the use of such suppositories, although no controlled studies have been done.[8]

*Steroid Enemas.* In patients who suffer from a distal proctitis who do not respond to hydrocortisone suppositories, the steroid enemas may be helpful. These proprietary enemas are aqueous suspensions of either hydrocortisone or prednisolone. They are administered as retention enemas once or twice daily. They may be effective in treating both distal proctitis as well as left-sided, non-specific ulcerative colitis. One must remember that some systemic absorption will occur with these agents.

**Miscellaneous**

A host of bases and preservatives are generally included and little is known about the effect of these agents. Adeps Solidus is a range of suppository bases consisting of mixtures of mono-, di- and triglycerides of saturated fatty acids. Theobroma oil, beeswax, and cetyl alcohol are also employed.

## PRECAUTIONS

General precautions usually mentioned in the pharmaceutical compendia for the use of these agent mixtures include avoidance by patients with a sensitivity to any of the components. Hydrocortisone preparations are not to be used in the presence of existing tuberculosis, or of fungal or viral lesions of the skin.

## GENERAL DISCUSSION

Suppositories are seldom helpful in treating the pain of thrombosed hemorrhoids or anal fissure.[3] Some commercially available suppositories contain opiates, but the mechanism of their analgesic effect is central and not local.[9] Steinberg also condemns the use of antibiotic suppositories in the treatment of inflammatory conditions in the anal canal both for their ineffectiveness and for the potential dangers of inducing local sensitivity.[9]

When suppositories are inserted they rest

well above the area of a fissure because they must rest above the puborectalis muscle, and therefore, are not in direct contact with the fissure. In addition, many patients complain that insertion is painful. The natural history of a fissure-in-ano is one of healing, and associated treatments such as warm baths to relieve sphincter spasm, and stool softeners to avoid straining, break the cycle of a hard stool, pain, and reflex spasm.

The continued use of the numerous available agents, and the credit given to them for their effectiveness, is almost certainly a function of the self-limiting nature of the diseases which they are treating. One must remember that the natural history of a thrombosed hemorrhoid is one of resolution with decreasing pain after two or three days. Patients will frequently relate that the suppository or ointment did not work for the first two or three days. By the same token, patients may use a given preparation for two or three days, and then switch to a second preparation which they then praise, but again this healing is almost certainly a function of the natural history of the disease. Had they used the preparations in reverse order, the praise and disdain for the two preparations would almost certainly have been reversed!

## REFERENCES

1. Compendendium of Pharmaceuticals and Specialties. 12 ed., Rotenberg, G. N., ed., Toronto, Canadian Pharmaceutical Association, 1977.

2. Drug and therapeutics Bulletin, 7:41, 1969.

3. Gordon, P. H.: Anal fissure—diagnosis and treatment. Consultant, *Feb.:*73, 1978.

4. Grosicki, T. S., and Knoll, K. R.: Hemorrhoidal preparations. *In* Griffenhagen, G. B., and Hawkins, L. L. (eds.): Handbook of Nonprescription Drugs. American Pharmaceutical Association, Washington D.C., 1973.

5. Jackson, R.: Side effects of potent topical corticosteroids, Can. Med. Asso. J., *118:*173, 1978.

6. Martindale: The Extra Pharmacopoeia. 27 ed. Wade, A. and Reynolds, J. E. F. (eds.) London, The Pharmaceutical Press, June 1977.

7. Product management. p. 37, Sept 1972.

8. Sherman, L. F., Prem, K. A., and Mensheha, M.: Factitial proctitis: A restudy at the University of Minnesota. Dis. Colon Rectum, *14:*4:281, 1971.

9. Steinberg, H.: Applied Pharmacology Related to the Colon in Diseases of the Colon and Anorectum. Turell, R. (ed.), Philadelphia, W. B. Saunders, 1969.

# 30

# Miscellany

## HIDRADENITIS SUPPURATIVA

Hidradenitis is an acute or chronic infection of the apocrine glands of the skin. In its chronic form it is an indolent inflammatory disease of the skin and subcutaneous tissue, characterized by abscesses and sinus formation. It may be located where apocrine sweat glands are found such as the axilla, mammary, inguinal, genital, perianal and scalp regions.[5]

### Clinical Features

This is essentially a disease of adult life as apocrine glands are structures activated at the time of puberty. Some authors state that hidradenitis is equally distributed between men and women, others state that it is more common in women, and still others that it is more common in men.[1,11,12,14] The disease is more prevalent in the black race than it is in the other races.[10] Affected individuals frequently have a seborrheic type of skin, are usually overweight, and perspire profusely.

### Etiology

Certain predisposing causes have been mentioned and include mechanical irritation, trauma, and the sequel to contact dermatitis.

### Bacteriology

The organisms usually found include Staphylococcus aureus, Streptococcus viridans, and coliforms.

### Clinical Course

The disease may start insidiously with burning, itching, local heat, and hyperhidrosis, and may eventually progress to produce pain. As the inflammatory process develops, sub-cutaneous nodules may be palpable with reddening or cyanotic discoloration of the skin. This may resolve slowly over a period of several weeks, or, more commonly, adjacent nodules may appear and coalesce to form a network of sinus tracks. Suppuration is usually slight, and only a few drops of pus may be evacuated from a nodule. Resolution and scarring may occur, or a series of recurrences and remissions may ensue with the formation of considerable induration, abscesses, and deep sinus tracks. Discharge may persist and, in later stages, ulceration may occur.[11] The average duration of the disease may be many years, and in long-standing cases squamous cell carcinoma has been found.[4,9]

### Pathology

This chronic inflammatory condition affects the skin and subcutaneous tissues. The affected area of skin has a red and white blotchy appearance, is thick and edematous with watery pus draining from multiple openings of sinus tracks. The persistent chronic nature of the disease leads to ulceration and scarring. Lesions may be localized, or involve large areas of perianal skin extending onto the buttocks. Microscopic examination of excised specimens shows an inflammatory exudate consisting of plasma cells, lymphocytes, and occasional giant cells of foreign body type with the formation of sinus tracks. These tracks become lined by squamous epithelium by downgrowth from the surface skin.[12] Squamous cell carcinoma has been reported.[8]

### Diagnosis

The pathological diagnosis may be difficult because the apocrine glands have been destroyed by abscess formation. The disease may be confused with pilonidal disease, anal fistulas, furunculosis, and Crohn's disease of the perianal skin.[7]

### Treatment

The surgical treatment of hidradenitis suppurativa in its acute phase is incision and drainage of a localized abscess.

Surgical treatment in the chronic stage may consist of: (*1*) excision, with the defect left open to granulate and epithelialize; (*2*) excision and primary closure; (*3*) excision and free skin grafting; and, (*4*) excision and closure with a pedicle flap.[2,11,13] Each of these procedures may have its place depending upon the location and extent of the pathology.[11] In mild chronic cases, unroofing of the area may be all that is necessary. For extensive lesions, wide excision may be necessary, and most surgeons combine this with split-thickness skin grafting.[2,11]

If there is extensive infection with abscess formation, incision and drainage may be necessary as a preliminary procedure. Following this, excision should include all sinus and epithelial skin bridges, along with all of the fibrous and inflamed portions of the subcutaneous fat. A primary skin graft may be applied if the area is relatively clean, but it may be necessary to delay skin grafting until healthy granulation tissue has formed.

Some authors believe that prior to any extensive grafting and radical surgical procedure, a diverting sigmoid colostomy should be performed.[1,3] At the same time, all sinus tracks and infected pockets are opened surgically. This usually results in a relatively clean area within a few weeks. Wide excision with skin grafting is then performed, and the colostomy is closed when healing is secured.

Although we entirely agree that for extensive disease, wide excision is necessary, establishment of a colostomy is, generally, unnecessary. A similar result should be obtained by adequate bowel preparation, and placement of the patient on an elemental diet and obstipating medications such as described by Gordon.[6]

## PROCTALGIA FUGAX

The term *proctalgia fugax* was first introduced by Thaysen in 1935.[5] Schuster has provided an excellent description of the clinical presentation.[4] There is abrupt onset of pain during day or night. Patients may be awakened with pain several hours after falling asleep. Pain varies in severity, but is often excruciating. Symptoms are of short duration lasting from a few minutes to less than a half an hour. Duration, although variable from patient to patient, is constant in a given patient. Pain is variously described as gnawing, grinding, cramp-like, sharp, or tightness. Pain is localized in the rectal region above the anus, varying in location from person to person, but constant in a given person. Symptoms disappear spontaneously without residue except for a weak, washed-out feeling after particularly severe attacks. There are no associated intestinal disturbances such as alteration in bowel habits, tenesmus, or paraesthesia.

The etiology of proctalgia is unknown. It has been suggested that it is due to spasm of the levator muscles.[1]

Between attacks, no consistent physical abnormality is evident. The lack of any objective abnormality suggests that at least a portion, if not all of these cases, are of psychogenic origin. A study by Pilling and associates of 48 patients with proctalgia fugax revealed that the majority of patients had professional or managerial occupations.[3] They were found to be perfectionistic, anxious, and tense; had a relatively high incidence of neurotic symptoms in childhood; and, were of above average intelligence. Pilling and co-workers felt that the tendency of this anxious, perfectionistic group to somatize emotional conflicts through the gastrointestinal tract, and by the use of pain is strong evidence that proctalgia fugax is of psychogenic origin.

Treatment of this condition is unsatisfactory. Firm upward pressure on the anus has been reported to provide relief. Other measures that have been employed include taking hot sitz baths, having a bowel movement, inserting a finger into the anus, or administering an enema.[2] Such maneuvers probably only pass time for a condition where the pain duration is self-limited. Inhalation of amyl nitrate or sublingual nitroglycerine have also been used. For patients who have frequent, repeated nocturnal attacks, nightly doses of quinine have been recommended.[5]

The importance of making the correct diagnosis is to avoid a mistaken diagnosis and subsequent misguided treatment, and to assure the perplexed and anxious victim that his condition is well recognized, and is neither a symptom nor a precursor of malignancy. Unfortunately, Douthwaite's sceptical but realistic appraisal holds true: proctalgia fugax "is harmless, unpleasant, and incurable".[1]

# PNEUMATOSIS COLI

The term *pneumatosis coli* is applied to the condition of pneumatosis cystoides intestinalis (PCI) when it is limited to the large intestine. This rare condition is characterized by cystic accumulations of gas in the submucosa or subserosa of the bowel. The peak incidence is between 30 and 50 years of age.[18] The condition may be seen in all sections of the gut, but is most common in the small intestine. Koss reviewed world literature and found 213 cases of which only 6 per cent had colonic involvement.[10] The entire colon and rectum can be affected, or only a part of the large intestine, more commonly the left than the right.[16]

## Etiology

The etiology of this condition is unknown, but the three most frequent hypotheses proposed are mechanical, pulmonary, and bacterial.[15]

Other hypotheses proposed have included biochemical, neoplastic, and nutritional theories but these have had little support in recent years.

*Mechanical Hypothesis.* It has been suggested that gastrointestinal gas, under abnormal pressure because of obstruction, is forced through mucosal defects, enters submucosal lymphatics, and is then distributed distally in the submucosa by peristalsis.[10] Marshak and colleagues reported pneumatosis of the descending colon after sigmoidoscopy without biopsy, and they suggested that instrumentation of the bowel may produce mucosal defects which then lead to localized pneumatosis.[12]

*Pulmonary Hypothesis.* Keyting and associates noted an association of pneumatosis intestinalis with chronic pulmonary disease.[9] They postulated that severe coughing produces alveolar rupture and pneumomediastinum. Gas then dissects downward to the retroperitoneum and along perivascular spaces to the bowel wall, and accumulates in a subserosal location. Elliott and Elliott implicated coughing, straining, and artificial inflation of the lungs as mechanisms capable of initiating dissection of air.[5]

*Bacterial Hypothesis.* This theory implicates gastrointestinal bacteria as the origin of gas found in the bowel wall. The typical location of gas in patients with pulmonary disease is subserosal, while pneumatosis secondary to gastrointestinal disease is linear in distribution, and is located in the submucosa. Pneumatosis intestinalis has been produced experimentally in the guinea pig by injecting a mixture of E. coli, Aerobacter aerogenes, and Clostridium welchii into the bowel wall.[17] Yale and Balish readily produced pneumatosis cystoides intestinalis in the germ-free rat by innoculating its peritoneal cavity with a pure culture of either Clostridium perfringens or Clostridium tertium.[21] Similar innoculation of the germ-free animal with any one of eight other clostridial species does not result in the formation of PCI. They felt, therefore, that the bacterial theory for the formation of at least some cases of PCI is now established, and treatment should be directed at controlling a possible clostridial infection.

## Associated Conditions

Yale listed a large number of conditions that have been found in association with PCI. Included among the pulmonary conditions were chronic lung disease, emphysema, and pneumomediastinum. It was, however, more frequently seen in association with gastrointestinal conditions, most commonly, peptic ulceration, carcinoma of the gastrointestinal tract, and pyloric stenosis.

## Clinical Findings

*Symptoms and Signs.* The symptomatology and prognosis of PCI are generally those of the associated condition. The presence of PCI is not associated with any characteristic clinical picture, and when symptoms occur they are non-specific. Manifestations range from the case which is found incidentally in an asymptomatic individual to the more severe form which may cause partial intestinal obstruction. Bouts of diarrhea, diarrhea alternating with constipation, constipation alone, melena, and flatulence are common.[3] Patients may complain of mucus, colicky lower abdominal pain, incontinence, and occasional flecks of bright red blood on the stools.

Physical findings occasionally include an abdominal mass. Rectal examination may reveal cysts in the rectum.

The length of history may vary from a few months to a few years.[10]

*Radiographically* the cysts may be suspected when a plain film of the abdomen reveals radiolucent clusters along the contours of the bowel. The presence of a pneumoperitoneum in an asymptomatic patient should suggest pneumatosis intestinalis, and a correct diagnosis will prevent an unnecessary operation. The diagnosis can be made from a chest film in which air cysts may be seen in the splenic or hepatic flexure of the colon. Retroperitoneal air may be present beneath the diaphragm bilaterally. It shows no shift regardless of the position in which the films are taken, and produces no specific symptoms. Barium enema studies demonstrate large polypoid defects on the wall of the intestine, or smooth filling defects which change in shape with distention or compression of the bowel.[12] Sometimes the barium practically obliterates the cysts, and they are not well visualized except on the postevacuation film where the mucosa appears swollen, thus suggesting ulcerative colitis.[3] The gas may also be evident as a linear radiolucent strip along the intestinal margin (Fig. 30-1).

*Pathology.* The cysts vary in size from a few millimeters to a few centimeters in diameter. They may occur either singly, or in clusters. Apparently, they do not communicate with the intestinal lumen, or with each other. In the colon they are located predominantly in the serosa, but they may be submucosal.

Morson described the macroscopic appearance of a surgical specimen of cystic pneumatosis as characteristic.[13] The mucosal surface has a coarse cobblestone appearance due to a large number of submucosal cysts, the apices of which may show intramucosal hemorrhage. Cysts also project from the serosal surface. The gas appears to be under pressure as rupture of cysts through the sigmoidoscope or in fresh surgical specimens causes a popping sound.

Rectal biopsy appearances are distinctive.[13] Cystic spaces lying in the submucosa immedi-

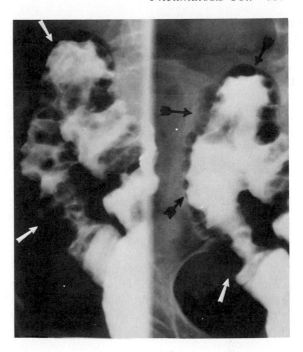

FIGURE **30-1.** *Pneumatosis coli. Barium enema showed a linear radiolucent strip of gas along the sigmoid colon (arrows).*

ately beneath the muscularis mucosae are lined by large macrophages, some of which may be multinucleate with much eosinophilic cytoplasm. The connective tissue between the cysts, which are often multilobular, shows little or no evidence of inflammation. The covering mucosa is attenuated, and sometimes contains small hemorrhages. The appearances are most likely to be confused with lymphangioma and oleogranuloma. In the former there are no macrophages, and the lymphatic spaces are lined by a flattened endothelium without any interstitial inflammation. In oleogranuloma, there is a macrophage response, but also much inflammation and fibrosis around fat filled spaces.

**Diagnosis.**

Very rarely, upon examination one may find a palpable colon to be present. Rectal examination may reveal the gas cysts. Sigmoidoscopic examination may disclose the clusters of cysts protruding into the bowel lumen. Simple radiograph of the abdomen may show the very striking appearance of pneumatosis coli. For more proximal involvement, colonoscopic examination will reveal the cysts. This might be useful when the diagnosis is in doubt, as when included in the differential diagnosis of multiple polyposis.[2] Barium enema will confirm the diagnosis.

The differential diagnosis includes familial multiple polyposis. Other causes of intestinal perforation in patients presenting with a pneumoperitoneum should be considered.

Careful sigmoidoscopic and radiological examinations, combined with biopsy should be performed to avoid errors in diagnosis, and hence, avoid unnecessary operations.

## Treatment

Asymptomatic intestinal pneumatosis does not call for any treatment. Historically, symptomatic patients were treated by operation. The problem of differential diagnosis of pneumatosis from polyposis and other neoplastic conditions lead Calne to favor operation.[2] He felt that the distinction was academic since the treatment of resection was common to both gas cysts and multiple polyposis.

However, in 1973 Forgacs and associates described a method of treatment that was both simple and effective.[6] It consisted of the administration of oxygen by face mask for a few days. The treatment is based on the theoretical consideration of gas exchange between the cysts and the surrounding tissues. They predicted that the cysts could be deflated if the total pressure of gases in venous blood was lowered by prolonged breathing of a gas mixture containing a high concentration of oxygen. Successful therapy has subsequently been reported by others.[1,4,7,8]

The paradoxical persistence of gas-filled cysts in the bowel wall implies that they are replenished at a rate that equals or exceeds the rate of absorption. Since a direct communication with the lumen of the bowel has never been demonstrated, gas presumably enters the cysts by diffusion. The rate of diffusion from bowel gas to cyst, and from cyst to capillaries is determined by the partial pressure of gases in each of these compartments, their solubility in tissue fluid, and the dimensions of the diffusing surface represented by the tissues separating them.

The object of treatment is to alter the balance between the diffusion of gases into, and out of the cysts in favor of absorption. This can be accomplished by lowering the total pressure of gases in venous blood by oxygen breathing, thereby increasing the pressure gradient between the cysts and the surrounding tissues. Investigators have described different quantities of intra-cystic gaseous constituents. Oxygen varied from 2.5 to 16 per cent, nitrogen 80 to 90 per cent, and carbon dioxide 0.3 to 7.5 per cent.[11,14] Breathing 100 per cent oxygen washes nitrogen out of the lungs and the tissues leaving only oxygen and carbon dioxide in arterial blood. Most of the oxygen is metabolized by the tissues so that the total pressure of gases at the venous end of the capillary is less than 100 mm Hg while the gas mixture in the cysts remains at, or above atmospheric pressure. The pressure gradient which determines the rate of removal of gases from the cyst is thus increased several fold. This approach has been used to hasten reabsorption of gases from a pneumothorax, to relieve postoperative abdominal distention, and prevent abdominal pain in airmen flying over high altitudes.

Down and Castleden suggested that the reason such therapy works is that the cysts are created and maintained by a fastidious anaerobic gas-forming organism that provides gas at a rate which exceeds the rate of absorption until an equilibrium is reached.[4] The high tissue/oxygen tension achieved with oxygen therapy kills the organisms, and the gas is then reabsorbed in the same way as gas contained within any natural or artificially created space in the body.

Pure oxygen cannot be safely administered over long periods because it damages the lungs. Concentration of oxygen in the gas mixture is, therefore, kept below 75 per cent with nitrogen making up the rest. To prevent the entry of atmospheric nitrogen into the lung the administration of oxygen must be continuous. Humidified oxygen at 8 liters per minute is delivered through a suitable mask, resulting in an inspired oxygen of 70 to 75 per cent, and $PaO_2$ levels in excess of 300 mm Hg.[19] Breaks in oxygen breathing of half an hour are allowed four times each day to permit meals to be taken, and other necessities attended to; however, at least four hours of unbroken administration are insisted upon, and the mask is worn all night.

Daily abdominal and chest radiographs are done. The plain radiograph will show gradual diminution in size of the cysts, while a chest radiograph will exclude atelectasis related to oxygen therapy.

The method of administration of oxygen, the amount given, and for what length of time are important practical issues that are, as yet, not fully defined. Aggressive oxygen therapy was initially recommended for six days, but it should be continued for at least 48 hours after complete radiological disappearance of all cysts has been obtained.[6] Long term follow-up is necessary to evaluate the continued benefit of this therapy.

## SOLITARY ULCER SYNDROME

The solitary ulcer syndrome of the rectum is a term coined by Madigan in 1964, and elaborated upon by Madigan and Morson in 1969, to describe unusual rectal ulcerations.[5,6] Its major importance is the fact that it may be confused with carcinoma, and lead to unnecessary radical operation. An extensive review of the subject was made by Rutter and Riddel, and the following information draws heavily from their comprehensive work.[8]

Solitary rectal ulcers occur most commonly between 4 and 10 cm from the anal verge. Sixty-eight per cent of lesions occur anteriorly or anterolaterally.[8]

The condition occurs equally in men and women, and most commonly between 20 and 29 years of age.

### Symptoms

The most common symptom is rectal bleeding, usually bright red and scant in amount. Mucus may be passed with resultant soiling. There may be an associated complete rectal prolapse. Pain, if present, is located in the perineum, sacral area, or left iliac fossa, and is usually trivial. Other symptoms include tenesmus and a feeling of anal obstruction which is manifested by straining. The necessity for straining is almost universal.

### Physical Examination

An area of induration may be felt, and ulcers visualized on the anterior rectal wall. Characteristically, the ulcer straddles or lies on the side of a rectal fold. The shallow, well-demarcated ulcers vary in size from 1 to 5 cm in diameter, and the base is covered with a greyish-white slough. Their shape is usually irregular with raised, rolled, or polypoid edges. The surrounding mucosa shows a mild inflammation, and may appear nodular due to the presence of misplaced mucous membrane in the submucosa at the edge of the ulcer. Occasionally, ulcers are seen on the apex of a complete rectal prolapse.

### Investigation

Routine blood tests, and radiographs, including barium enema, usually make no contribution to the diagnosis which is made on sigmoidoscopy, and confirmed by rectal biopsy. The diagnosis rests with the pathologist because the important differential diagnosis includes Crohn's disease, ulcerative colitis, villous adenoma, and rectal carcinoma.

Where facilities are available, cineradiography may be performed as such ulcers have been reported in association with internal procidentia, and the discovery of this condition may well influence the treatment.[3]

Electromyographic abnormalities have been found in patients with the solitary ulcer syndrome. The normal response to bearing down consists of relaxation of the external sphincter and puborectalis, but Rutter found that the puborectalis went into a state of marked activity with an increase in both the frequency and amplitude potentials.[8] This response persisted as long as the bearing down effort was maintained. This suggests that during bearing down efforts, the puborectalis behaves paradoxically. Instead of undergoing inhibitory lengthening to produce the necessary funnel shaped anorectum, it goes into a state of tight contraction, tending to maintain the integrity of the flap valve. Thus, defecation can only occur after forcible stretching of the puborectalis. The exact significance of this electromyographic abnormality has not yet been established.

### Histology

Biopsy reveals a characteristic appearance. There may be some superficial mucosal ulceration, the tubules show structural irregularity, and the epithelium is hyperplastic. The most significant change is a curious obliteration of the lamina propria by fibrosis and muscle fibers of the muscularis mucosae growing toward the lumen of the bowel.[7]

There is a tendency for the solitary ulcer syndrome to give rise to misplaced glands in the submucosa which are filled with mucus and lined by normal colonic epithelium. Rutter and Riddell feel that the most common association of this localized form of colitis cystica profunda is with the solitary ulcer syndrome. This situation may lead to the incorrect diagnosis of carcinoma. It is possible that the solitary ulcer is related to colitis cystica profunda, hamartomatous inverted polyp of the rectum, and enterogenous cyst.[1,2,11]

### Etiology and Pathogenesis

The appearances seen in the solitary ulcer syndrome are not specific, and are seen in a variety of other clinical situations, for example (*1*) at the apex of a complete rectal prolapse, (*2*) on the anterior mucosal prolapse in patients with the perineal descent syndrome, (*3*) at the apex of a prolapsing hemorrhoid, and (*4*) occasionally, at the tip of a colostomy or ileostomy.

The mechanism of the actual ulceration is postulated as the result of any one, or any combination of the following: (*1*) ischemia due to pressure necrosis when the tip of the prolapse becomes impacted in the upper end of the anal canal; (*2*) trauma, if the prolapse is replaced digitally (a proportion of solitary ulcer patients have a habit of passing a finger or intrument into the lower rectum as an aid to defecation and this may well be a contributory factor); (*3*) ischemia due to stretching and possible rupture of submucosal vessels at the time of maximum prolapse; and, (*4*) ischemia due to obliteration of the mucosal capillaries by the fibrous and muscular tissue filling the lamina propria. Other possible etiological factors include inflammatory bowel disease, hamartomatous malformations, and bacterial or viral infections.

The combination of prolonged straining efforts in the presence of a failure of inhibition of the puborectalis results in the adjacent anterior rectal mucosa being traumatized by the posterior bar of the puborectalis. The ulcers appear in these patients in the area of mucosa that bears the brunt of that straining effort, the "flap" of the physiological flap valve. Furthermore, the flap may also enter the upper end of the anal canal where it may be squeezed by an actively contracting sphincter which may render it relatively ischemic. The long term result of straining efforts is that eventual prolapse occurs either as a mucosal prolapse of the anterior rectal mucosa, or a full thickness prolapse beginning in the mid-rectum. In either case, rectal wall derived from higher up, enters the traumatizing mechanism. The relative importance of straining, prolapse, trauma, and ischemia in the pathogenesis of solitary ulcer syndrome of the rectum remains unknown.

### Treatment

Unfortunately, no local or systemic therapy has been shown to be reliably effective. Patients with few symptoms require no treatment. Tranquilizers may be of value since some of these patients have a marked preoccupation with their bowels and worry endlessly about defecation.

If the difficulty is due to faulty bowel training, re-education and attention to diet, in particular the taking of bran, may be helpful. If the concept of prolapse and eventual pressure necrosis is accepted, then it is clear that healing will not occur until the patient is able to cease straining. If EMG shows it to be due to a breakdown in the physiological behavior of the pelvic floor, then re-training will be useless. Straining may be reduced by liquifying the stool and using glycerine suppositories. Should the straining habit be broken the application of an agent known to heal ulcers elsewhere, such as carbenoxolone, might be helpful.[8] Should this fail, local excision of the ulcer transanally may be beneficial.

Should the ulceration be associated with a rectal prolapse, then a definitive repair as described in Chapter Twenty should be performed.[3] In very symptomatic patients, recalcitrant to other treatment, it has been recommended that a temporary diverting sigmoid colostomy be constructed.[10] Sulphasalazine and local steroids have been used without any obvious, or consistent improvement.[4] Based on the belief of the frequent association of the solitary ulcer with rectal prolapse, the use of a modified Ripstein procedure has met with considerable success.[9]

## COLITIS CYSTICA PROFUNDA

Colitis cystica profunda (CCP) is a benign disease characterized by varying sizes of mucin-filled cysts located deep to the muscularis mucosae. The chief importance of this entity lies in its differentiation from colonic mucinous adenocarcinoma. Failure to recognize this benign condition may lead to unnecessary radical operation.

## Etiology

The etiology of CCP remains unclear. A plausible explanation is that the condition is the result of invagination of the mucosa during the healing phase of an ulcer. Rutter and Ridell feel that the term colitis cystica profunda should be used as a purely descriptive term, and it should be recognized for what it is: an unusual complication of several different lesions.[5] The etiologies of the ulcer might include ulcerative colitis, bacterial colitides, resolution of lymphoid abscesses in the submucosa, radiation, instrumentation, biopsy of the colonic mucosa, and polypectomy.[6]

Others have considered the lesions to be inverted polyps, either acquired or congenital. If the condition were congenital, one would expect to find it in pediatric patients, but this has not been the case. Despite the suggestions of those who believe that CCP is of congenital origin representing hamartoma formation, chronic inflammation has been accepted by most of the investigators as the primary etiologic factor in the pathogenesis.[3]

## Clinical Findings

Tenesmus and mucous stools, hematochezia, diarrhea, and vague abdominal pain may occur alone, or in combination for many months or years prior to the diagnosis.[6] Other symptoms include rectal pain, weight loss, and previous rectal surgery.[3] Many cases involve only the anterior rectal wall between 5 and 12 cm from the anal verge.[4] Rectal examination may reveal single, or multiple nodules which frequently have a rubbery consistency. Polypoid masses have been described. Sigmoidoscopy may reveal the mucosa overlying the cysts to show irregularly distributed areas of edema, hyperemia, hypertrophy, and atrophy with occasional superficial ulceration or central umbilication. The mucosa is generally intact, but may be ulcerated in which case it may resemble carcinoma. Stenosis, as well as rectal prolapse, have been found, and ulcerative colitis may also be present.

## Pathology

CCP is a benign condition characterized by the presence of mucin-containing cysts in the submucosa of the colon and rectum. The disease may present as a localized process, a segmental process, or may be diffusely distributed. Grossly, there are nodular polypoid or plaque-like areas measuring 1 to 3 cm in diameter.

Microscopically, the cysts are deep to the muscularis mucosae. They are lined with normal appearing columnar epithelium, and may be filled with mucus which stains faintly basophilic. The overlying mucosa may be histologically unremarkable, or show focal ulceration. The surrounding submucosa is invariably fibrotic, and contains a mixed, inflammatory infiltrate of mild to moderate intensity.[6]

The distribution distinguishes it from colitis cystica superficialis in which multiple tiny mucous cysts are scattered throughout the colon but are confined to the mucosa. This latter condition is usually associated with pellagra.[6]

## Diagnosis

Barium enema may appear normal, or there may be single or multiple radiolucent filling defects. Included in the differential diagnosis are: adenomatous polyps, endometriosis, multiple polyposis, lipoma, leiomyoma, sarcoma, polypoid inflammatory granulomas such as those that occur with schistosomiasis, ulcerative colitis and Crohn's disease, ischemic proctitis or colitis with submucosal hemorrhage and edema and, most importantly, a mucus-producing adenocarcinoma.[3] Differentiation among these entities is possible with adequate biopsy.

Patients may have had numerous barium enemas, sigmoidoscopies, and removal of rectal polyps before CCP is diagnosed. The newest modality to help in making the diagnosis is colonoscopy.[2]

## Treatment

The treatment of choice is local excision.[4] This may consist of transanal excision for rectal lesions or local resection for higher lesions.[3] Incision or partial excision of cysts has corrected symptoms in some patients.[1] Management by diverting colostomy has also been effective.[4] The Kraske approach may also be used.

## COCCYGODYNIA

Coccygodynia (coccydynia, coccyalgia) is a term which denotes pain in the coccyx. It may be of functional origin, or it may be organic. The patient complains of aching, cramping, or sharp pain which is localized in the region of the coccyx, or may sometimes radiate to the buttocks, or down the backs of the thighs. At times, the attacks of pain can become sharp, shooting, or "breath-taking". These patients usually make the rounds of orthopedic surgeons, gynecologists, neurologists, and colon and rectal surgeons.

### Classification

*In functional coccygodynia,* more frequently seen in highly nervous people, no organic pathology causing this condition has been described. Spasm of the coccygeus and piriformis muscles has been mentioned as an accompaniment. The condition has been tagged as "T.V. watchers' disease," the implication being that sitting for long periods of time on sofas or soft chairs may be a causative factor. Sitting on hard chairs, frequent changes of position, supportive measures for reassurance, and occasionally tranquilizers are measures to be recommended. Surgery (coccygectomy) is never indicated because the pain often decreases without treatment, or is increased by any treatment.

*Organic coccygodynia* may arise either from rigidity of the sacrococcygeal joint or from traumatic arthritis. Fracture and dislocation of the coccyx with displacement is usually a result of direct violence, but may occur during a difficult delivery.

The symptoms of local pain on sitting as well as defecation are attributed to spasm of the surrounding muscles. Pain is exquisite and tenderness is sharply localized over the coccyx. In recent injury, swelling and ecchymosis may be found over the lower sacral region. The diagnosis is made if abnormal mobility at the coccygeal articulation, and accompanying sensitivity and tenderness are present.

Treatment consists of reduction by digital manipulation through the rectum, but that may fail because of the muscle forces continually in play.[2] Bedrest for approximately a week is usually sufficient to alleviate the majority of symptoms. Tight cross strapping of the buttocks lessens pain in some patients, but in others it aggravates it. The patient should sit on an inflated rubber ring. Sitting on one buttock at an angle may be sufficient to eliminate the discomfort of sitting squarely on both ischial tuberosities. Some patients prefer a hard surface which allows the ischia alone to bear the body weight.[4] Sitz baths help relieve muscle spasm, and stool softeners should be provided so that constipation does not aggravate symptoms.

These injuries should be treated conservatively for at least six months. The use of local hydrocortisone injection may be satisfying.[3] Watson-Jones stated strongly that coccygectomy should be considered for those patients who have severe disability following a coccygeal fracture.[5] To determine whether surgery is likely to be beneficial, Steindler advised infiltrating the region of the coccyx with a local anesthetic; if temporary relief is obtained, then coccygectomy will probably relieve the pain.

Surgery is contraindicated for acute sacrococcygeal injuries even when the coccyx is severely angulated anteriorly. Surgery is also contraindicated when the low back is painful because, occasionally, coccygodynia is an early symptom of pathologic change in the lumbosacral disc.[1]

## DESCENDING PERINEUM SYNDROME

As a result of study of the disordered physiology of patients with rectal prolapse, a distinct condition was recognized in which perineal descent is caused by excessive straining. The pelvic floor muscles are weakened by repeated straining and stretching, and perineal descent occurs. This was referred to as the descending perineum syndrome.[2]

### Symptomatology

Abdominal straining is such a potent inhibitor of pelvic muscle tone that, if the individual persists in straining at stool over many years, the effectiveness of the post-defecation reflex will be considerably reduced. During the straining effort of defecation, stool is passed followed by the anterior rectal wall mucosa. Further straining then follows in an effort to pass it. In advanced cases, prolapsing anterior rectal mucosa becomes so large that it occludes the upper end of the anal canal giving a feeling of anal blockage, and prevents further defecation by straining. The patient gives the typical story that after partial emptying of the rectum a sense of obstruction develops which he cannot overcome except by ceasing all straining. Indeed, some of these patients develop frank anal obstruction and may pass a finger into the anal canal to temporarily reduce this obstruction and allow defecation. If straining is repeated and prolonged, the anterior rectal wall mucosa will ultimately protrude. A vague, dull, aching pain in the perineum and sacral region may follow defecation. This is due to the anterior rectal wall mucosa in the upper anal canal, and the patient may continue straining in an endeavor to relieve it. Mucosa which prolapses becomes irritated and secretes mucus, causing perineal moisture, soreness, and irritation. The prolapsing mucosa may bleed, and anal leakage with soiling of the clothes and secondary pruritus may occur. Partial incontinence may also be present.

### Physical Signs

In the normal individual the anal margin lies just below a line drawn between the coccyx and the symphysis pubis. In patients with the syndrome, the anal canal is either situated several centimeters below this line, or it rapidly descends 3 or 4 cm when a straining effort is made. Digital examination reveals a lack of muscle tone, but the most characteristic change occurs when the patient is asked to strain: the puborectalis descends sharply and can no longer be felt as a separate bar, constituting the anorectal ring. On sigmoidoscopy during straining, the anterior wall bulges down into the instrument, and follows it as it is withdrawn. Solitary ulceration may be seen on the anterior rectal mucosa in these patients.[3]

### Electromyographic Studies

In the normal person, there is, at first, increased electrical activity in the sphincter muscles on straining followed, after several seconds, by inhibition which may be partial or complete. As soon as the straining ceases, there is a sharp return of exaggerated activity which is called the closing reflex. In patients with a descending perineum, the postural reflex (i.e., the continuous activity of the pelvic floor at rest) is usually normal, but upon straining inhibition occurs once the pelvic muscles are relaxed and allow rapid pelvic floor descent. Reflex recovery after straining may be delayed or grossly diminished.

### Treatment

The chief aim is to prevent further damage by eliminating all straining during defecation. Laxatives are of only limited value, as many of these patients have persistently liquid stool; a combination of liquid stool with lax sphincters causes soiling and sometimes partial incontinence. In those where the stool is hard, the patient is instructed to use liquid paraffin or a hydrophilic laxative, either of which is sufficient to soften it. Usually the most successful method of facilitating rectal emptying is by means of an irritant suppository such as glycerine or bisacodyl. Suppositories are inserted daily, and the patient is instructed to stop the straining efforts. The origin of these repeated calls to stool is explained to the patient, and he is told that once the bowel has emptied, all further calls should be ignored. Muscle weakness may be partially corrected by sphincter exercises, but it may be many weeks before any effect is noted. Submucosal injection of sclerosants such as phenol in oil may relieve symptoms. It will hopefully stop the bleeding and mucous discharge, and relieve the sensation of tenesmus.

In patients with large hemorrhoids, an extended hemorrhoidectomy removing the redundant lower rectal mucosa may be of considerable benefit.

When severe weakness of the perineal muscles results in anal incontinence, the post-anal repair described by Parks is recommended.[1] The effect of this operation is to raise the level of the pelvic floor and reduce the anorectal angle. Operation is not the end of the treatment, as it is essential that the patient avoid straining during defecation so as not to stretch the repair.

## PERIANAL ENDOMETRIOMA

Despite the fact that the presence of endometriosis is commonplace, the finding of a perianal endometrioma is no more than a surgical curiosity, even in the practice of a busy colorectal surgeon. Schickele, in 1923, was apparently the first to report a case of perineal endometriosis.[8] Cheleden, in 1968, reviewed the literature and found only 38 cases of endometriosis involving the perineum.[1] A few more had been mentioned by 1971 when Ramsey reported another case.[6] Paull and Tedeschi reported 15 cases of endometriosis occurring at the site of an episiotomy scar.[4] More recently, Gordon and co-workers described the varied manifestations of perianal endometrioma.[2]

### Histogenesis

The pathogenesis of endometriosis has been and continues to be controversial. The prevailing theories include: trans-tubal regurgitation of menstrual blood; the coelomic metaplasia doctrine; lymphatic dissemination; and, hematogenous spread. Although the histogenesis of perianal endometrioma is not clear, it is best explained by the implantation theory, a variation of the "retrograde menstruation" theme.[7]

### Pathology

Perianal endometriomas vary in size from microscopic to lesions 1 to 2 cm in diameter, and in color from reddish-blue to yellowish-brown. They may enlarge and coalesce. Because of the irritative effect of the blood, the nodules may provoke a marked fibroblastic proliferation, resulting in dense fibrous nodules. Because of periodic bleeding into the "cystic structures", the cysts have become known as "chocolate cysts". Paradoxically, the diagnosis can be most difficult in the advanced, florid, long-standing cases because, as the disease progresses, the fibroproliferative response progressively obliterates recognizable features. The definitive histologic diagnosis usually requires two of the three following features: stroma, glands, and hemosiderin pigment; the stroma being the most important element. Microscopically, the edematous endometrial stroma with an inflammatory infiltrate is often characteristic. Glands with their endometrial epithelial lining can be demonstrated together with hemosiderin-laden macrophages, which may be seen frequently. Collections of blood are also often present.

### Clinical Features

Endometriosis is characteristically a disease of the reproductive years of life, occurring most frequently between 30 and 40 years of age. The clinical manifestations of endometriosis are dependent upon the functional activity of the involved tissue. The lesion may present as an asymptomatic mass or, in the classic fashion, as a painful mass, this specifically being so during menstruation. The mass, in fact, may become noticeable only at the time of menstruation, when it becomes larger and more painful. It subsides several days after the termination of menses. On physical examination the lesions are usually found in old episiotomy scars. The onset of symptoms has become apparent as early as 45 days, and as late as 14 years from the time of delivery and perineal trauma.[4,5] The diagnosis is made on microscopic section.

Included in the differential diagnosis are anal fistula with abscess formation, thrombosed hemorrhoids, perianal melanoma, and other neoplastic and inflammatory conditions.[2]

### Treatment

Because this lesion is so readily accessible, and because the exact nature of it is frequently unknown preoperatively, the treatment of choice is undoubtedly local excision. In doing so, one should take great care not to injure the anal sphincter mechanism as these lesions are frequently intimately associated with the muscle. Plastic repairs and reinforcements of the sphincter may be necessary where the lesion is excised because the sphincter muscle may be considerably thinned in the area of the excision. Complementary hormonal therapy has been suggested, but the value of such treatment is not yet proven.[3] Ovarian ablative therapy may also be considered.

## MELANOSIS COLI

Melanosis coli is characterized by a deep pigmentation of the mucosa of the colon and rectum due to the presence of a melanin-like pigment. It may involve the large bowel from the rectum to the ileocecal valve with a sharp demarcation at this point. The color of the mucosa varies from shades of yellowish-brown to black. Adenomatous polyps and adenocarcinomas are free of pigment, and are therefore rendered more evident against the blackish background of the surrounding mucosa on sigmoidoscopy.

Melanosis may be obvious to the naked eye, but the vast majority of cases are apparent only on microscopic examination. Histologically, the melanin-like pigment is found in macrophages within the lamina propria. A few may be seen in the submucosa, and even in the regional lymph nodes.[3] There is a lack of inflammatory change in the colon.

The laxative family which consists of derivatives of anthraquinone (cascara, aloes, rhubarb, senna, and frangula) has been incriminated in causing this pigmentation.[1] In most instances, the laxative has been taken almost daily for a year or more. This distinct group of cathartics owe their activity to the presence of an irritating anthracene or emodin. The exact mechanism of pigment formation is uncertain. Perhaps the active principle of these laxatives contains a pigment, or elaborates a pigment within the colon which is phagocytized by the deep mucosal cells. Possibly there is some interaction that occurs between ferments and substances contained in the laxative which is responsible for the development of the pigment.[1]

Reports of the incidence of melanosis coli have varied from 0.04 to 11.2 per cent.[1] The frequency with which this entity is encountered has been decreasing, no doubt due to the decreasing use of the anthracene laxatives.

Earlier writers suggested that melanosis coli is found in the older age group. However, this is probably more related to the duration of the ingestion of these laxatives. There is a female preponderance ranging from 3 : 1 to 8 : 1, but this probably reflects the greater incidence of constipation and laxative habit among women patients. It occurs in all races.

Melanosis coli cannot be held responsible for any known symptom complex. A history of constipation is present almost universally, for it is in these patients that the laxatives are initially ingested. As a rule, following discontinuation of all anthracene laxatives, the pigmentation disappears within a period of 4 to 12 months.

# OLEOGRANULOMA

Oleogranuloma (lipoid granuloma, ileoma) is a foreign body reaction which usually results from the inflammatory reaction induced by unabsorbed, oil-based sclerosing agents employed in the injection treatment of hemorrhoids.[1,8] Mineral oil enemas may also be the cause of a rectal oleoma.[5] Retention of injected oil and consequent fibrosis have been held responsible for stricture in patients who have previously received such injection. Mineral oil was apparently the prime agent inducing chemical strictures in a series described by Rosser and associates.[6]

Experimental investigation in rabbits of the effects of different amounts of oils on animal tissue showed that only small quantities of oil are required to produce notable granulomatous lesions.[4] Lubricating oils appeared to be particularly dangerous since they permeated the tissues more readily than the solid greases, and produced greater pathological changes than liquid paraffin which had the same capacity for spreading.

Lipoid granulomas may give rise to symptoms of rectal pressure, or a sensation of incomplete evacuation, and occasionally to partial obstruction of the bowel.

Oleogranuloma generally occurs as a round, submucous mass in the anal canal just above the dentate line, but annular and even ulcerating lesions have been described.[2,7] They may extend as high as the recto-sigmoid junction, presumably, because the injected oil can track upward in the submucosal layer.

The histology of oleogranuloma is characteristic.[3] There is conspicuous fibrosis, and a variable degree of inflammatory cell infiltration according to the age of the lesion. Rounded spaces lined by large mononuclear or multinucleate histiocytes are scattered throughout. These spaces contain the oil which is removed from the tissues during the course of histological preparation, but can be demonstrated in frozen sections of formalin-fixed material. The histologic appearance can be confused with lymphangioma and with cystic pneumatosis, although the latter does not show any fibrous or inflammatory reaction.

Fewer granulomas are being seen at the present time because, during the past decade, the trend has been away from the injection treatment of internal hemorrhoids.

The principle interest in this tumor is from the standpoint of differential diagnosis. Clinically, the polypoid appearance can simulate adenomas or even carcinomas. The most important distinguishing feature is that the overlying mucosa is usually intact when an oleoma is present, in contradistinction to the usual ulceration of the mucosa when a neoplasm is present. Of course, a history of previous injections is of some help.

Because of the fixation and scarring of the tumor masses, surgical removal may be rather difficult.

# AMEBIASIS

## Etiology

Amebiasis is a water-borne disease caused by the protozoon Entameba histolytica (E. histolytica). Infection with E. histolytica is worldwide with the incidence as high as 50 per cent in an endemic area. Stool surveys indicate that the prevalence of infection in the United States is between 1 and 5 per cent.[5]

E. histolytica exists in two forms: the motile trophozoite and the cyst. The trophozoite is the parasitic form that dwells in the lumen or wall of the colon. When diarrhea occurs the trophozoites are passed, unchanged in the liquid stool. In the absence of diarrhea the trophozoites usually encyst before leaving the gut. The cysts are highly resistant to environmental change, and are responsible for transmission of the disease.[5]

## Pathogenesis

The infective stage of the disease is the cyst which gains entry to humans in food or drink contaminated by feces. Trophozoites release from the cyst in the small bowel, and are carried to the large bowel where they multiply and live commensally.

## Clinical Manifestations

The majority of patients infested with E. histolytica are asymptomatic (cyst-passers, carrier stage). Some patients have intermittent diarrhea, sometimes with blood and mucus. During acute or chronic attack there is frequently some degree of liver tenderness and hepatomegally. A fulminating attack of amebiasis is less common. The onset may be gradual or abrupt with diffuse and severe abdominal pain and tenderness associated with high fever which may simulate an acute surgical abdomen. The bloody diarrhea is usually profuse. Liver tenderness and enlargement are frequent.

## Complications

Liver abscess is the most common complication. Amebiasis may, in rare instances, involve the lung, brain, and skin. Perforation of the bowel occured in about 2 per cent of patients admitted to the hospital with amebiasis.[2] The distribution of bowel perforations in order of frequency are: cecum, ascending colon, transverse colon, terminal ileum, sigmoid colon, and rectum.[2] Penetration of trophozoites through the muscular wall of the large bowel may result in a large mass of granulation tissue called *ameboma*. This occurs most frequently in the cecum and sigmoid colon, where a palpable mass may lead to a mistaken diagnosis of carcinoma.

## Diagnosis

*Stool Examination*. When diarrhea is present, the trophozoites are usually identified in fresh stool. In the asymptomatic stage (formed stools) cysts may be found. There are certain drugs and substances which interfere with parasitologic diagnosis. These are: kaolin, barium sulfate, sulfonamides, oils, magnesium hydroxide, enema, and tetracycline.[3]

*Proctosigmoidoscopy* is the most useful examination in symptomatic patients.[1] During an invasive phase, the trophozoites penetrate the mucosa to produce characteristic flask-shaped ulcers. These may coalesce to form undermined ulcers with ragged edges. The exudate from the ulcers usually contain numerous trophozoites. Biopsy of the intervening normal mucosa may show trophozoites.

*Serologic Test*. The major advance in diagnosis has been the development of accurate serological techniques, especially the Indirect Hemagglutination test, Complement fixation, and Gel test. The positive test indicates past or present tissue invasion by E. histolytica, and may remain positive for months or even years. The accuracy of the test is approximately 90 to 95 per cent.[4] The more rapid serologic methods that have been developed recently are Cellulose Acetate Diffusion, and Latex Agglutination, but they are not as sensitive as the Indirect Hemagglutination.[7]

## Commonly Used Amebicides

*Emetine preparation* has remained universally successful whenever severe invasive amebiasis is encountered. However, the drug frequently fails to eradicate the amebas from the gut lumen, and hence, recurrence is common.[6]

*Tetracycline* acts on E. histolytica indirectly by modifying the bacterial flora of the bowel. Relapse may occur after an apparent cure.[6]

*Chloroquine* is used as a supplement medication for amebic liver abscess.

*Metronidazole* is a newer drug used for amebiasis. The precise mode of action against E. histolytica is not known, although it is definite that it is a direct-acting amebicide.[6]

## Treatment

*Asymptomatic or Mildly Symptomatic Patient.* Tetracycline, 1 to 2 gm per day for five days, is effective. Chloroquine can be added for its potentiating effect on tetracycline, as well as its ability to eradicate subclinical hepatic infection. Metronidazole is somewhat less effective in asymptomatic patients.[5]

*Mild and Moderate Dysentery.* Metronidazole, 750 mg three times a day for five days, is recommended. This regime will cure 90 per cent of the patients. The addition of tetracycline will raise the cure rate to close to 100 per cent.[5]

*Severe Dysentery.* Metronidazole, 750 mg three times a day for five days, plus tetracycline, 2 gm per day, are given. Emetine should also be added. It controls the acute attack, but because of its toxicity, administration of this drug should be discontinued as soon as the symptoms abate.[5]

## SCHISTOSOMIASIS (BILHARZIASIS)

Schistosomiasis is a major health problem in tropical and subtropical areas of the world. It is believed that 200 million people in 71 countries are affected by this condition. Because of the lack of appropriate snail hosts schistosomiasis is not transmitted in the United States.[3]

## Etiology

Schistosomiasis is a disease caused by trematodes or blood flukes. There are three species which are distributed in various parts of the world. *S. mansoni* has focal distribution in the Middle East, Africa, South America, and the Caribbean; *S. japonica* in China, Japan and South East Asia; and, *S. haematobium* in the Middle East and Africa.[2] The worm load among most patients in the endemic areas is low, and disease manifestations are absent. Because adult worms do not multiply within the body of the human host, heavy infections are the result of repeated reinfections occurring over a period of years. It is among this population that serious morbidity and mortality occur.[3]

## Life Cycle

The continuing presence of schistosomiasis depends on the disposal of infected human excrement into fresh water, the presence of suitable snail hosts, and the exposure of people to water contaminated with cercariae.[3]

Within the snail the miracidia (free-swimming larvae) are transformed by asexual reproduction into thousands of larvae called cercariae. The cercariae enter the human body by penetrating the skin and working their way into the venules, they are carried to the right heart, and then to the pulmonary capillaries. They finally enter the systemic circulation and live in different organs according to the different species: S. mansoni inhabits the left colon and rectum; S. japonicum inhabits the small intestine and right colon; and, S. haematobium inhabits the bladder and pelvic organs. Once the end-organs are reached the females deposit eggs which secrete an enzyme to destroy the surrounding tissue. The eggs then rupture into the lumen of the gut (or bladder in the case of S. haematobium), and are carried to the outside in the urine or feces. On reaching fresh water, the embryonated eggs quickly hatch, liberating more miracidia. These miracidia search out, and penetrate the specific snail host appropriate to the species.[3]

## Clinical Manifestations

The first sign of infection develops as an itchy rash (swimmer's itch) which lasts only a few days. The second stage of symptoms occurs during the maturation of the worms and the onset of eggs production. The symptoms at this time are primarily allergic causing fever, malaise, myalgia, cough, abdominal pain, urticaria, diarrhea, eosinophilia, lymphadenopathy, and hepatosplenomegaly. The final stage of symptoms usually begins several months after the infection, and is caused by the reaction of local tissue to the deposited eggs. Diarrhea and abdominal pain are common. Anorexia, weight loss, and signs of portal hypertension appear as the disease progresses. Urinary symptoms mays be present in S. haematobium. S. mansoni and S. japonica may cause multiple polyps in the colon and rectum which can be confused with adenomatous polyposis. Carcinoma of the bladder as a late complication of S. haematobium is well known in Egypt.[3] The relationship between carcinoma of large bowel and schistosomiasis has been reported.[5,6]

### Diagnosis

*Stool Examination.* The diagnosis of schistosomiasis depends upon detection of eggs in the stool (or urine in case of S. haematobium). Quantitative analysis of eggs per gram of stool has been developed.[1]

*Rectal biopsy (or bladder biopsy in S. haematobium)* is the single most reliable method of diagnosis. It is often positive when repeated stool examinations are negative. Eggs, often in hundreds, are clearly seen in the mucosa or submucosa.[3,4]

*Serological or intradermal test.* The test may be positive for years despite parasitologic cure. It is neither highly sensitive nor specific, and is of value chiefly as an epidemiologic tool.[3,4]

### Treatment

The treatment of schistosomiasis with drugs is not without risk; therefore, the aim is to reduce the worm load. It is not necessary to treat asymptomatic patients unless there are more than 50 ova per gram of stool.[2] Two drugs are available. Niridazole (Ambilhar) taken orally, 25 mg per Kg per day in divided doses for seven days. Stibocaptate (Astiban) given by intramuscular injection, 40 mg per Kg divided in four weekly doses.

## REFERENCES

### Hidradenitis Suppurativa

1. Adams, J. D., and Haisten, A. S.: Perianal hidradenitis suppurativa. Surg. Clin. North Am., *52*:2:467, 1972.

2. Chalfant, W. P. III, and Nance, F. C.: Hidradenitis suppurativa of the perineum: treatment by radical excision. Am. Surg., *36*:331, 1970.

3. Ching, C. C., and Stahlgren, L. H.: Clinical review of hidradenitis suppurative: management of cases with severe perianal involvement. Dis. Colon Rectum, *8*:349, 1965.

4. Donsky, H. J., and Mendelson, C. G.: Squamous cell carcinoma as a complication of hidradenitis suppurativa. Arch. Derm., *90*:488, 1964.

5. Goligher, J. C.: Surgery of the Anus, Rectum and Colon. 3 ed. 251. London, Bailliere Tindall, 1975.

6. Gordon, P. H.: The chemically defined diet and anorectal procedures. Can. J. Surg., *19*:511, 1976.

7. Hughes, E. S. R.: Inflammation and infections of the anus. *In* Turell, R. (ed.): Diseases of the Colon and Anorectum. 2 ed. Philadelphia, W. B. Saunders, 1969.

8. Humphrey, L. J., Playforth, H., and Leavell, U. W.: Squamous cell carcinoma arising in hidradenitis suppurativa. Arch. Derm. *100*:59, 1969.

9. Jackman, R. J., and McQuarrie, H. B.: Hidradenitis suppurativa: its confusion with pilonidal disease and anal fistula. Am. J. Surg., *77*:349, 1949.

10. Knaysi, G. A. Jr., Cosman, B., and Crikelair, G. F.: Hidradenitis suppurativa. JAMA, *203*:19, 1968.

11. Masson, J. K.: Surgical treatment for hidradenitis suppurativa. Surg. Clin. North Am., *49*:5:1043, 1969.

12. Morson, B. C., and Dawson, I. M. P.: Gastrointestinal Pathology. 614. London, Blackwell Scientific Publications, 1972.

13. Pigott, H., and Ellis, H.: Chronic hidradenitis suppurativa: a report of 9 cases. Br. J. Surg., *62*:394, 1975.

14. Tachau, P.: Abscesses of the sweat glands in adults. Arch. Derm., *40*:595, 1939.

### Proctalgia Fugax

1. Douthwaite, A.: Proctalgia fugax. Br. Med. J., *2*:164, 1962.

2. Goligher, J. C.: Surgery of the Anus, Rectum

and Colon. 3 ed. 1141. London, Bailliere Tindall, 1975.

3. Pilling, L. F., Swenson, W. M., and Hill, J. R.: The psychologic aspects of proctalgia fugax. Dis. Colon Rectum, 8:372, 1965.

4. Schuster, M. M.: Constipation and anorectal disorders. Clin. Gastroenterol., 6:643, 1977.

5. Thaysen, E. H.: Proctalgia fugax. Lancet, 2:243, 1935.

## Pneumatosis Coli

1. Britten-Jones, R.: A major advance in the management of pneumatosis coli. Aust. NZ J. Surg., 45:367, 1975.

2. Calne, R. Y.: Gas cysts of the large bowel simulating multiple polyposis. Br. J. Surg., 47:212, 1959.

3. Doub, H. P., and Shea, J. J.: Pneumatosis cystoides intestinalis. JAMA, 172:1238, 1960.

4. Down, R. H. L., and Castleden, W. M.: Oxygen therapy for pneumatosis coli. Br. Med. J., 1:493, 1975.

5. Elliott, G. B., and Elliott, M. B.: The roentgenologic pathology of so-called pneumatosis cystoides intestinalis. Am. J. Roentgen, 89:720, 1963.

6. Forgacs, P., Wright, P. H., and Wyatt, A. P.: Treatment of intestinal gas cysts by oxygen breathing. Lancet, 1:579, 1973.

7. Gruenberg, J. C., Batra, S. K., and Priest, R. J.: Treatment of pneumatosis cystoides intestinalis with oxygen. Arch. Surg., 112:62, 1977.

8. Hoflin, F., and Van Der Linden, W.: Pneumatosis cystoides intestinalis treated by oxygen breathing. Scand. J. Gastroenterol., 9:427, 1974.

9. Keyting, W. S., McCarver, R. R., Kovarik, J. L., and Daywitt, A. L.: Pneumatosis intestinalis: A new concept. Radiology, 76:733, 1961.

10. Koss, L. G.: Abdominal gas cysts (pneumatosis cystoides intestinalorum hominis). Arch. Path., 53:523,1952.

11. Lee, S. P., Coverdale, H. A., and Niccholson, G. I.: Oxygen therapy for pneumatosis coli: A report of 2 cases and a review. Aust. NZ J. Med., 7:44, 1977.

12. Marshak, R. H., Blum, S. D., and Eliasoph, J.: Pneumatosis involving the left side of the colon. JAMA, 161:1626, 1956.

13. Morson, B. C., and Dawson, I. M. P.: Gastrointestinal pathology. 590. London, Blackwell Scientific Publications, 1972.

14. Mujahed, Z., and Evans, J. A.: Gas cysts of the intestine (pneumatosis intestinalis). Surg. Gynecol. Obstet., 107:151, 1958.

15. Reyna, R., Soper, R. T. and Condon, R. E.: Pneumatosis intestinalis: Report of twelve cases. Am. J. Surg., 125:667, 1973.

16. Shapiro, B. J., Track, A. A., and Myers, E.: Pneumatosis cystoides intestinalis involving the left side of the colon. Can. Med. Assoc. J., 91:219, 1964.

17. Stone, H. H., Allen, W. B., Smith, R. B. III, and Haynes, D. C.: Infantile pneumatosis intestinalis. J. Surg. Res., 8:301, 1968.

18. Stone, H. H., Webb, H. W., and Kovalchik, M. T.: Pneumatosis intestinalis of infancy. Surg. Gynecol. Obstet., 130:806, 1970.

19. Wyatt, A. P.: Prolonged symptomatic and radiological remission of colonic gas cysts after oxygen therapy. Br. J. Surg., 62:837, 1975.

20. Yale, C. E.: Etiology of pneumatosis cystoides intestinalis. Surg. Clin. North Am., 55:1297, 1975.

21. Yale, C. E., and Balish, E.: Pneumatosis cystoides intestinalis. Dis. Colon Rectum, 19:107, 1976.

## Solitary Ulcer Syndrome

1. Allen, M. S. Jr.: Hamartomatous inverted polyps of the rectum. Cancer, 19:257, 1966.

2. Epstein, S. E., Ascari, W. Q., Ablow, R. C., Seaman, W. B., and Lattes, R.: Colitis cystica profunda. Am. J. Clin. Path., 45:186, 1966.

3. Ihre, T., Internal procidentia of the rectum—treatment and results. Scand. J. Gastroenterol., 7:643, 1972.

4. Kennedy, D. R., Hughes, E. S. R., and Masterton, J. P.: The natural history of benign ulcer of the rectum. Surg. Gynecol. Obstet., 144:718, 1977.

5. Madigan, M. R., and Morson, B. C.: Solitary ulcer of the rectum. Gut, 10:871, 1969.

6. Madigan, M. R.: Solitary ulcer of the rectum. Proc. R. Soc. Med., 57:403, 1964.

7. Morson, B. C., and Dawson, I. M. P.: Gastrointestinal pathology. 587. London, Blackwell Scientific Publications, 1972.

8. Rutter, K. R. P., and Riddell, B. H.: The solitary ulcer syndrome of the rectum. Clin. Gastroenterol., 4:505, 1975.

9. Schweiger, M., and Alexander-Williams, J.: Solitary ulcer syndrome of the rectum, its association with occult rectal prolapse. Lancet, 1:170, 1977.

10. Stavorovsky, M., Weintroub, S., Ratan, J., and

Rozen, P.: Successful treatment of a benign solitary rectal ulcer by temporary diverting sigmoidostomy: report of a case. Dis. Colon Rectum, *20:*347, 1977.

11. Talerman, A.: Enterogenous cysts of the rectum. Br. J. Surg., *58:*643, 1971.

## Colitis Cystica Profunda

1. Ballas, M., Nunel, L., and Miller, E. M.: Localized colitis cystica profunda. Arch. Surg., *103:*406, 1971.

2. Friedman, E., and Tueller, E. E.: Colitis cystica profunda: colonoscopic and pathological findings. Gastrointest. Endosc., *22:*40, 1975.

3. Green, G. I., Ramos, R., Bannayan, G. A., and McFee, A. S.: Colitis cystica profunda. Am. J. Surg., *127:*749, 1974.

4. Herman, A. H., and Nabbeth, D. C.: Colitis cystica profunda, localized, segmental and diffuse. Arch. Surg., *106:*337, 1973.

5. Rutter, K. R. P., and Riddell, R. H.: The solitary ulcer syndrome of the rectum. Clin. Gastroenterol., *4:*505, 1975.

6. Tedesco, F. J., Sumner, H. W., and Kassens, W. D.: Colitis cystica profunda. Am. J. Gastroenterol., *65:*339, 1976.

## Coccygodynia

1. Campbell's Operative Orthopedics, 5 ed. 955. Crenshaw, A. H. (ed.) St. Louis, Missouri, C. V. Mosby, 1971.

2. DePalma, A. F.: The Management of Fractures and Dislocations. 441. Philadelphia, W. B. Saunders, 1970.

3. Goldstein, L. A., and Dickerson, R. C.: Atlas of Orthopedic Surgery. 478. St. Louis, Missouri, C. V. Mosby, 1974.

4. Rockwood, C. A., and Green, D. P.: Fractures. 937. Philadelphia, J. B. Lippincott, 1975.

5. Watson-Jones, R.: Fractures and Joint Injuries. Baltimore, Williams and Wilkins, 1957.

## Descending Perineum Syndrome

1. Hardcastle, J. D.: The descending perineum syndrome. The Practitioner, *203:*612, 1969.

2. Praks, A. G., Porter, N. H., and Hardcastle, J. D.: The syndrome of the descending perineum. Proc. R. Soc. Med., *59:*6:477, 1966.

3. Rutter, K. R. P., and Riddell, R. H.: The solitary ulcer syndrome of the rectum. Clin. Gastroenterol., *4:*3:505, 1975.

## Perianal Endometrioma

1. Cheleden, J.: Endometriosis of the perineum: Report of two cases. South. Med. J., *61:*1313, 1968.

2. Gordon, P. H., Schottler, J. L., Balcos, E. G., and Goldberg, S. M.: Perianal endometrioma: Report of 5 cases. Dis. Colon Rectum, *19:*260, 1976.

3. Minvielle, L., and de la Cruz, J. V.: Endometriosis of the anal canal; presentation of a case. Dis. Colon Rectum, *11:*32, 1968.

4. Paull, T., and Tedeschi, L. G.: Perineal endometriosis at the site of episiotomy scar. Obstet. Gynecol., *40:*28, 1972.

5. Prince, L. N., and Abrams, J.: Endometriosis of the perineum: Review of the literature and case report. Am. J. Obstet. Gynecol., *73:*890, 1957.

6. Ramsey, W. H.: Endometrioma involving the perianal tissues: Report of a case. Dis. Colon Rectum, *14:*366, 1971.

7. Sampson, J. A.: Perforating hemorrhagic (chocolate) cysts of the ovary: their importance and especially their relation to pelvic adenomas of endometrial type ("adenomyoma" of the uterus, rectovaginal septum, sigmoid, etc.). Arch. Surg., *3:*245, 1921.

8. Shickele, M.: *Quoted by* Prince, I. N., and Abrams, J.: Endometriosis of perineum: Review of the literature and case report. Am. J. Obstet. Gynecol., *73:*890, 1957.

## Melanosis Coli

1. Bockus, H. L.: Melanosis coli in Gastroenterology. 3 ed., Vol. II, 1127. Philadelphia, W. B. Saunders, 1976.

2. Goligher, J. C.: Surgery of the Anus, Rectum and Colon. 3 ed. 1138. London, Balliere Tindall, 1975.

3. Morson, B. C., and Dawson, I. M. P.: Gastroenterology Pathology. 585. London, Blackwell Scientific Publications, 1972.

## Olegranuloma

1. Graham-Stewart, C. W.: Injection treatment of hemorrhoids. Br. Med. J., *1:*213, 1962.

2. Hernandez, V., Hernandez, I. A., and Berthrong, M.: Oleogranuloma simulating carcinoma of the rectum. Dis. Colon Rectum, *10:*205, 1967.

3. Morson, B. C., and Dawson, I. M. P.: Gastrointestinal Pathology. 618. London, Blackwell Scientific Publications, 1972.

4. Nairn, R. C., and Woodruff, M. F. A.: "Paraffinoma" of the rectum. Ann. Surg., *141:*536, 1955.

5. Neshat, A. A., Stone, D. H., and Price, H. P.: Self-induced lipoid granuloma of the rectum: Report of a case. Dis. Colon Rectum, *17:*5:696, 1974.

6. Rosser, C., and Wallace, S. A.: Tumor forma-

tion, pathologic changes consequent to injection of oils under rectal mucosa. JAMA, *99:*2167, 1932.

7. Webb, A. J.: Oleocysts presenting as rectal tumors. Br. J. Surg., *53:*410, 1966.

8. Wittoesch, J. H., Jackman, R. J., and McDonald, J. R.: Lipoid granulomas of rectum. Proc. Staff Meet. Mayo Clinic, *31:*265, 1956.

## Amebiasis

1. DeFord, J. W.: Amebiasis: Newer methods of diagnosis and treatment. South. Med. J., *66:*1149, 1973.

2. Eggleston, F. C., Verghese, M., and Handa, A. K.: Amebic perforation of the bowel: Experiences with 26 cases. Br. J. Surg., *65:*748, 1978.

3. Healey, G. R.: Laboratory diagnosis of amebiasis. Bull. NY Acad. Med., *47:*478, 1971.

4. Juniper, K. Jr., et al: Serologic diagnosis of amebiasis. Am. J. Trop. Med. Hyg., *21:*157, 1972.

5. Plorde, J. J.: Amebiasis in Harrison's Principles of Internal Medicine. 8 ed. 1066–1069. Ed. Thorn, G. W., Adams, R. D., Braunwald, E., Isselbacher, K. J., and Petersdorf R. G., (eds.) New York, McGraw-Hill, 1977.

6. Powell, S. J.: Latest development in the treatment of amebiasis. Adv. Pharm. Chemother., *10:*91, 1972.

7. Sodeman, W. A. Jr., and Dowda, M. C.: Rapid serological methods for the demonstration of Entameba histolytica activity. Gastroenterology, *65:*604, 1973.

## Schistosomiasis

1. Mahmoud, A. A.: Schistosomiasis (Letter). N. Engl. J. Med., *298:*850, 1978.

2. Mahmoud, A. A.: Schistosomiasis. N. Engl. J. Med., *297:*1329, 1977.

3. Plorde, J. J.: Schistosomiasis (Bilharziasis). *In* Thorn, G. W., Adams, R. D., Braunwald, E., Isselbacher, K. J., and Petersdorf, R. G., (eds.): Harrisons's Principles of Internal Medicine. New York, McGraw-Hill, 1977.

4. Schneider, J., and Fripp, P. J.: The diagnosis of Bilharziasis. S. Afr. Med. J., *51:*536, 1977.

5. Shindo, K.: Significance of Schistosomiasis Japonica in the development of cancer of the large intestine: Report of a case and review of the literature. Dis. Colon Rectum, *19:*460, 1976.

6. Wu, T. T., Ch'en, T. H., Ch'i, C.: The relationship of schistosomiasis to carcinoma of large intestine. Chin. Med. J., *80:*231, 1960.

## APPENDIX A: CRUDE FIBRE CONTENT
## OF VARIOUS FOODS

| FOOD | GRAMS OF FIBER* |
|---|---|
| HIGH FIBER FRUIT | |
| Apple (1 med. with skin 2½″ dia.) | 1.4 |
| Apple (1 med. without skin 2½″ dia.) | 0.8 |
| Apricots (½C. canned) | 0.5 |
| Banana (1 med.) | 0.6 |
| Cocoanut (½C. shredded) | 1.9 |
| Fig (1) | 0.5 |
| Fruit cocktail (1C. canned, drained) | 1 |
| Melon (honeydew, 1C. chunks) | 1 |
| Pear (1 raw, 3″ × 2½″) | 2.3 |
| Strawberries (1C. fresh) | 1.9 |
| Raspberries (½C. fresh) | 2.2 |
| HIGH FIBER VEGETABLES | |
| Baked beans (½C. canned) | 3.6 |
| Green beans (½C. fresh, cooked) | 0.7 |
| Green beans (½C. frozen, cooked) | 1.1 |
| Lima beans (½C. cooked) | 1.5 |
| Bean salad (½C. canned "3Bean") | 3 |
| Bean soup (½ can) | 1 |
| Broccoli (½C., ½″ pieces, fresh) | 1.2 |
| Broccoli (½C., ½″ pieces, frozen) | 1 |
| Brussels sprouts (1C. fresh, boiled) | 2.5 |
| Brussels sprouts (½C., frozen, boiled) | 1.4 |
| Cabbage (⅛C., shredded) | 0.6 |
| Carrots (½C., chunks, raw) | 0.7 |
| Carrots (½C., slices, boiled) | 0.8 |
| Celery (½C. chunks, raw) | 0.4 |
| Coleslaw (½C. shredded) | 0.8 |
| Corn (1C. niblets, fresh, boiled) | 1.2 |
| Corn (1 cob 5 oz., fresh, boiled) | 0.5 |
| Corn (½C., canned, boiled) | 0.7 |
| Corn (½C. frozen, boiled) | 0.8 |
| Eggplant (½C. boiled) | 1 |
| Lettuce (1C. chopped) | 0.4 |
| Green pepper (½C. fresh, chopped) | 1 |
| Peas (½C. fresh, boiled) | 1.4 |
| Peas (½C. canned, boiled) | 1.6 |
| Potato (2½″ dia. baked w/o skin) | 0.6 |
| Potato (2½″ dia. boiled w/o skin) | 0.6 |
| Squash (½C. boiled) | 1.7 |
| BREAKFAST CEREALS AND BREAD | |
| All bran (½C., 1 oz.) | 2.4 |
| Bran buds (⅓C., 1 oz.) | 2.1 |
| Kellogs bran flakes (¾C., 1 oz.) | 1.1 |
| 100% Bran, Quaker (½C., 1 oz.) | 3.6 |
| Kellogs Raisin Bran (½C., 1 oz.) | 1.2 |
| Bran muffin (1 med.) | 0.7 |
| Bread (1 slice 100% Whole wheat) | 0.4 |
| Peanuts (1 cup halves, roasted w/o skin) | 1.7 |

* Values for crude fiber are based on publications issued by the U.S. Department of Agriculture.

## APPENDIX B: SUGGESTED MENUS
## FOR 14 GRAMS FIBER

| MEAL | | GRAMS OF FIBER | |
|---|---|---|---|
| *BREAKFAST* | | | |
| | ½C. Kellogs' Raisin Bran | 1.2 | |
| | 2 slices whole wheat bread | 0.8 | |
| | 1 cup canned fruit cocktail | 1 | 3 |
| *SNACK* | | | |
| | 1 pear (raw 3″ × 2½″) | 2.3 | 2.3 |
| *LUNCH* | | | |
| | green salad (1C. chopped lettuce, ½C. chopped green pepper) | 1.4 | |
| | 1 bran muffin | 0.7 | |
| | ½C. canned apricots | 0.5 | |
| | | | 2.6 |
| *SUPPER* | | | |
| | 1 slice 100% whole wheat bread | 0.4 | |
| | ½C. cooked fresh broccoli | 1.2 | |
| | ½C. cooked fresh carrots | 0.8 | |
| | 1 fresh apple (2½″ dia., with skin) | 1.4 | |
| | | | 3.8 |
| *SNACK* | | | |
| | ½C. shredded cocoanut | 1.9 | 1.9 |
| *TOTAL* | | | 13.6 |

| MEAL | | GRAMS OF FIBER | |
|---|---|---|---|
| *BREAKFAST* | | | |
| | ½C. All Bran Cereal | 2.4 | |
| | 2 slices 100% whole wheat bread | 0.8 | |
| | | | 3.2 |
| *SNACK* | | | |
| | 1 Bran muffin | 0.7 | 0.7 |
| *LUNCH* | | | |
| | Salad (½C. chopped green pepper | 1 | |
| | 1C. chopped lettuce) | 0.4 | |
| | 2 slices whole wheat bread | 0.8 | |
| | 1 fresh pear (2½ × 3″ dia.) | 2.3 | |
| | | | 4.5 |
| *SUPPER* | | | |
| | 1C. coleslaw | 1.6 | |
| | ½C. canned peas | 1.6 | |
| | Baked potato (peeled) | 0.6 | |
| | 1 apple (with skin 2½″ dia.) | 1.4 | |
| | | | 5.2 |
| *SNACK* | | | |
| | 1 Bran muffin | 0.7 | 0.7 |
| *TOTAL* | | | 14.3 |

(*Continued on p. 376*)

| MEAL | | GRAMS OF FIBER | |
|---|---|---|---|
| *BREAKFAST* | | | |
| | 2 Bran muffins (med.) | 1.4 | |
| | 1 fresh pear (2½″ × 3″) | 2.3 | |
| | | | 3.7 |
| *SNACK* | | | |
| | ½C. shredded cocoanut | 1.9 | 1.9 |
| *LUNCH* | | | |
| | ½C. (4 oz.) ''3 Bean'' Salad | 3 | |
| | 2 slices 100% Whole wheat bread | 0.8 | |
| | | | 3.8 |
| *SUPPER* | | | |
| | ½C. cooked squash | 1.7 | |
| | ½C. cooked frozen corn | 0.8 | |
| | 1 slice 100% Whole wheat bread | 0.4 | |
| | | | 2.9 |
| *SNACK* | | | |
| | ½C. peanuts (roasted halves) | 1.7 | 1.7 |
| *TOTAL* | | | 14 |

*NOTE:* These are menu selections to be used to increase the fiber in your diet; they do not represent a complete, well-balanced daily diet, but will be included as a part of your usual daily eating plan. Use these items to replace similar items lower in fiber in your usual diet, or as additions to your usual diet, to achieve the required total of 14 grams of fiber every day.

The authors wish to thank Ms. Peggy Williams, B.A.Sc.P.Dt., who prepared the above menus.

# Index

Numerals in *italics* indicate a figure; "t" following a page number indicates a table.